ESSENTIALS OF LIFE & HEALTH

Fourth Edition

Reviewers of the Fourth Edition

Kenneth Ainley
Rhode Island College

William H. Anderman
Oregon State University

Lynda Anderson
University of North Carolina

Walter E. Ballou
Mount Wachusett Community College

Barbara Beier
University of New Mexico

Larry Bridges
Saint Francis Hospital Education Center, Tulsa, Oklahoma

Beverlee Ciccone

Charlotte C. Cook-Fuller
Towson State University

Jack Curtis
University of Wisconsin at LaCrosse

Darwin Dennison
State University of New York at Buffalo

Frank Egan
Queensboro Community College

Muzza Eaton
Brooklyn College

Mohammed Forouzesh
University of Illinois

Neil E. Gallagher
Towson State University

Frederick J. Goldstein
Philadelphia College of Pharmacy and Science

Ralph Grawunder
San Diego State University

Sue M. Gray

Richard Harrison
Augusta College

Harold Hauban
South Connecticut State College

Virginia R. Hogg
Bridgewater State College

Daniel Horn

Frederic R. Kahl
Wake Forest University

Gerald F. Lafferty
University of Florida at Gainesville

Lowell Levin
Yale University

J. N. MacCormick
North Carolina Division of Health Services

Richard L. Papenfuss
University of New Mexico

James Philp
Wake Forest University

Valerie Pinhas
Nassau Community College

Ann Carmen Pinna

David H. Reilly
University of North Carolina at Greensboro

Raymond Rosen
Rutgers Medical School

James Rothenberger
University of Minnesota

Becky Smith
Ohio University

Margaret M. Smith
Oregon State University

Robert Valois
Eastern Illinois University

Edward H. Wagner
University of North Carolina

Douglas R. White
Wake Forest University

Essentials of Life & Health

Fourth Edition

Marvin R. Levy
Temple University

Mark Dignan
University of North Carolina at Greensboro

Janet H. Shirreffs
Arizona State University

RANDOM HOUSE   NEW YORK

Fourth Edition
987654
Copyright © 1972, 1974, 1977, 1981, 1984 by Random House, Inc.

Library of Congress Cataloging in Publication Data

Levy, Marvin R.
  Essentials of life & health.

  Condensation of Life & health, 4th ed.
  Includes index
  1. Health I. Dignan, Mark B. II. Shirreffs, Janet H.
III. Title.
RA776.L655 1984b   613   83-24672
ISBN: 0-394-33262-8 (pbk.)

Text and cover design: Leon Bolognese

Cover photo: Sam Bass/SBA

Manufactured in the United States of America

PREFACE

We live in a time of change—scientific, technological, social, economic, and political—and the pace of change is accelerating now as never before. In recent years one notable response to the faster tempo of life has been a renewed emphasis on self-reliance. Individuals are increasingly expected to come to grips with their rapidly changing environment on their own and to decide for themselves what changes they must make if they are to meet the challenges of modern life. As in all aspects of American life, this holds true in the area of personal health: Each of us must make our own behavioral decisions in the light of advances in medicine and medical technology and research revelations about the causes and cures of health problems.

This new edition of *Essentials of Life and Health* reflects this trend. It is specifically designed to help readers assess their health status and make decisions about whether and how they should change their behavior to improve their health situation. We give readers all the information they need to understand important health issues—but then we go far beyond that: We also encourage readers to think about these issues, to explore their present attitudes toward health-related matters, and then to make informed decisions about choosing health-enhancing behaviors.

To get readers involved in thinking about their health behaviors, we present 32 pencil-and-paper activities, of three types:

- *Test Your Awareness.* These brief quizzes, which appear near the beginning of certain chapters, are designed to capture readers' interest. They ask students to indicate what they already know—or think they know—about the health topic covered in the chapter. For example: True or false?—Alcoholic beverages can be used to warm the body when a person is exposed to very cold temperatures (Chapter 5). True or false?—People with quick tempers usually have high blood pressure (Chapter 12). (Both of these statements reflect widely held beliefs—but both are false.)

■ *Exploring Health.* These activities, which appear within chapters, ask readers to assess some aspect of their current health status, including their attitudes and behaviors. For example, in Chapter 4 readers can work through an assessment questionnaire that explores the extent to which their use of drugs may be causing problems in their lives. In Chapter 9 readers can survey their views about which marriage partner—the wife or the husband—should have responsibility for various household tasks: cooking, taking out the garbage, doing the laundry, paying the bills.

■ *Making Health Decisions.* Each of these end-of-chapter activities invites students to set up an actual plan for change in some health behavior. For example, in Chapter 5 the decision activity helps students consider alternative ways they might behave at parties where alcohol is served. The decision activity in Chapter 8 asks students, "Which contraceptive method would be best for you?" and provides a series of questions to help them arrive at an answer. These activities are never prescriptive. They do not insist that readers make changes immediately; nor do they dictate the changes to be made. Rather, the decision activities guide readers through the steps they must take to think the situation through and find the way of dealing with it that is most appropriate and comfortable for them *if* they decide that they do want to change.

We have thoroughly revised the text in an effort to provide readers with the information that they need to make responsible health choices and decisions. This edition presents highly readable, up-to-date, thoroughly documented discussions of topics of great interest to today's college students, such as:

■ The effects of stress on physical and psychological health
■ Recreational drugs—marijuana, cocaine, alcohol, tobacco
■ Sexuality, reproduction, contraception, and sexually transmitted diseases (with the latest findings on herpes and AIDS)
■ Changes in family life—two-career families, marriage at later ages, smaller families, higher rates of divorce
■ Advances in cancer research and treatment and what individuals can do to detect the disease early

- Factors associated with cardiovascular disease and the steps individuals can take to reduce their risk of heart attack
- Issues and controversies concerning diet and nutrition —fad diets, fast foods, anorexia nervosa
- The role of physical fitness and weight management in promoting health
- The impact of individual, corporate, and governmental behavior on the environment (with discussions of the Times Beach dioxin incident and the Three Mile Island nuclear accident)
- Recent findings about the physiological basis of aging and about how health habits can affect the aging process

To go along with its new personal-health orientation, *Essentials of Life and Health* has a new look.

- The book has been redesigned and is now more open and accessible to student readers than ever.
- The text is profusely illustrated, with many new color and black-and-white photographs, charts, and drawings. Each illustration has been chosen for its effectiveness in making a pedagogical point. Thus, the diet and nutrition chapter contains a two-page "poster" summarizing the principles of a balanced diet; a graph in the alcohol chapter vividly illustrates the relationship between blood alcohol level and impairment of driving ability; the cancer chapter presents a pie chart reflecting the latest information on the extent to which various environmental factors have been linked to cancer.
- Throughout the text we present words of advice to students on facts they should know or preventive steps they can take. These pointers are set off from the text by distinctive ornamented rules—as, for example, in Chapter 5, "Alcohol":

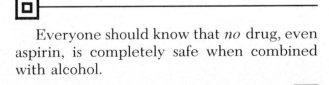

Everyone should know that *no* drug, even aspirin, is completely safe when combined with alcohol.

In Chapter 13, "Diet and Nutrition":

Those who frequently eat fast foods or processed foods should make sure that their other meals include whole grains and a variety of fresh fruits and vegetables.

In Chapter 6, "Health Care and the Consumer":

You should try to get into a group health-insurance plan if at all possible, because group plans offer the same basic coverage as individual plans, but are usually cheaper.

- We include a number of boxes on specific health issues and on practical ways the reader can deal with such matters as: how to use a prescription drug safely; how to host a party sensibly so that guests do not drive home drunk; how to avoid contracting herpes, and how to cope with it if it is contracted; how to recognize the signs of a heart attack; how to treat some common health problems at home.
- Full documentation is provided for all the findings discussed in the text. Footnotes appear at the end of each chapter.
- A glossary of the key terms used in each chapter (set in bold type where first used and defined in the text) appears at the end of the chapter, and a complete glossary of all key terms used in the entire text is presented at the back of the book, along with a complete index.

Essentials of Life and Health, Fourth Edition, is a paperback condensation of the fourth edition of *Life and Health.* It contains eighteen chapters, whereas *Life and Health* has twenty-two. As the title implies, we have condensed *Life and Health* to its essentials: Certain peripheral topics are discussed in somewhat less detail, and a number of boxes, illustrations, and activities have been dropped—but no major topic has been omitted. Our intention has been to make this material more accessible to students in the introductory health course by making it easier to cover the entire text in one term.

We could not have undertaken such a thorough revision of this important textbook without a great deal of help, and we are grateful for the uniformly high quality of the assistance we received. Our thanks go to the reviewers who did so much to guide us in orienting the text toward personal health and who gave us invaluable advice in revising the individual chapters; their names are listed opposite the title page. We would also like to acknowledge the contributions made by members of the Random House staff: Barry Fetterolf, editor-in-chief, special publications; June Smith, managing editor; Suzanne Thibodeau, manager, special projects; Cecilia Gardner, project editor; Pat Cahalan, copy editor; Leon Bolognese, designer; Laura Lamorte, production manager; R. Lynn Goldberg, photo editor; and Ilene Cherna, photo researcher. We thank Betty Gatewood for her judicious work in helping us distill *Life and Health* to its essentials. Above all, we owe a debt of gratitude to Susan Tucker, special projects editor, whose intelligence, dedication, skill, and unflagging enthusiasm were an inspiration to us.

We very much appreciate the contribution of our writer team: Betty Gatewood, Betty Holcomb, Gloria Jacobs, Roberta Meyer, Leila Mustachi, Dodi Schultz, and Gail Weiss.

MARVIN R. LEVY
MARK DIGNAN
JANET H. SHIRREFFS

CONTENTS

18
Aging and Death ▪ *429*

ESSENTIALS OF LIFE & HEALTH

Fourth Edition

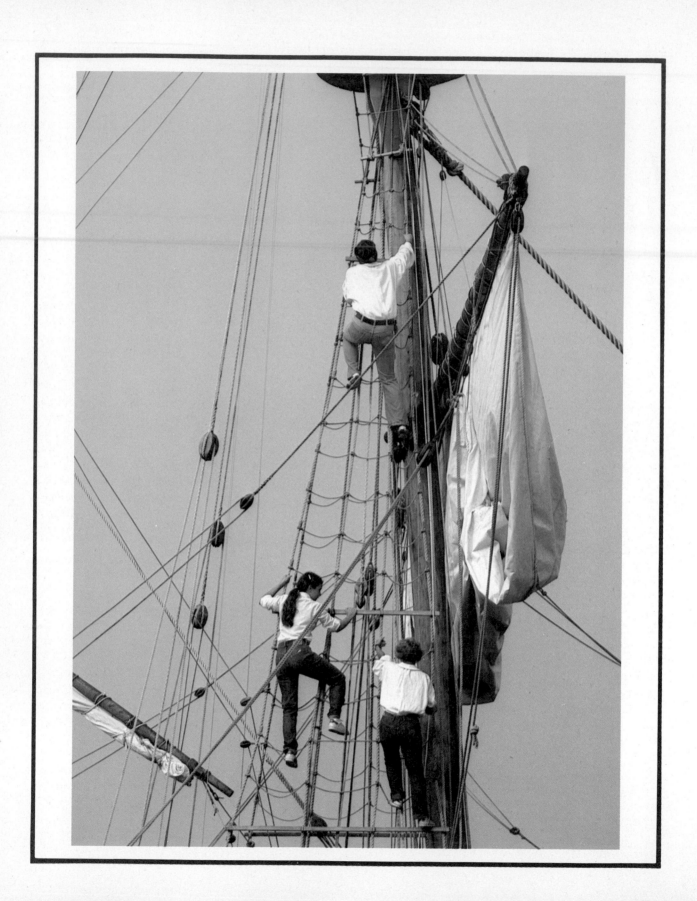

Introduction:
The Concept of Health

In the past ten years, the United States has experienced the beginning of a health revolution. Increasing numbers of Americans of all ages are turning to healthier lifestyles. Throngs of joggers head for the parks in the early morning. Business men and women walk or bicycle to work, rather than being transported passively by car or bus. Over 30 million people in the United States have successfully quit smoking; of those who haven't kicked the habit, two-thirds have tried, and 50 percent would like to quit.[1] In a two-year study of American health habits and desires, 80 percent of those studied were interested in learning about diet improvement; 75 percent wanted to learn techniques for reducing stress, and 88 percent wanted to make a commitment to an exercise program.[2] According to the National Center for Health Statistics, among adults aged seventeen years and over, almost two-thirds are trying to lose weight.[3] Public opinion polls report that close to half of the adult American population is actively concerned about the effects of lifestyle on health.[4]

Why is the American public so interested in healthy lifestyles, and why is health promotion coming to be recognized as a social movement of major proportions? Most diseases that affect Americans today are chronic diseases—such as cardiovascular disease, cancer, and emphysema—rather than infectious diseases such as smallpox and tuberculosis. We have begun to realize that our sophisticated drugs, hospitals, and surgical procedures are largely ineffective against chronic diseases: As one expert has put it, "As a society, we are becoming increasingly aware that our modern diseases and threats to health and life are heavily [associated with] problems of behavior."[5] It is true that our health status is in part a function of our heredity: The genetic makeup we inherit from our parents *may* predispose us to certain genetic diseases such as sickle-cell anemia and muscular dystrophy, and *may* predispose us to a higher risk of (or potential for developing) certain other diseases such as heart disease, diabetes, arthritis, or cancer. Health is also partly a function of our physical and social environment: Toxic wastes, noise, and air pollution can threaten our health, as can social conditions such as overcrowding, poverty, and unemployment. And our health is also partly a function of whether we have access to high-quality medical care.

But our lifestyles are even more important than these genetic and environmental influences. Years ago, the leading causes of death in the United States were infectious (communicable) diseases such as dysentery, tuberculosis, typhoid, and polio. Then, through improved public health measures, vaccination programs, and the discovery of antibiotic drugs, some of these acute infectious diseases were virtually eliminated and others brought under control. Today, the major causes of death and disability are diseases and problems such as heart disease, cancer, stroke, and accidents (see Figure 1). Today's killers are, to a certain extent, contributed to by human actions: They are strongly associated with such lifestyle behaviors as lack of exercise, reckless driving, abuse of alcohol, smoking, and improper diet.

It is because of these relationships that many Americans are modifying their behaviors—mini-

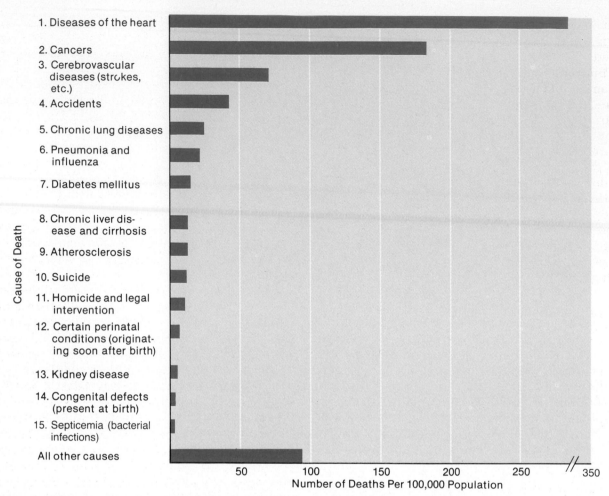

Figure 1   Chronic diseases have surpassed acute infectious diseases as causes of illness and death. This graph shows the death rates (number of deaths per 100,000 people) for the fifteen leading causes of death in the United States today. Of the twelve disease categories among these leading killers, ten are chronic conditions and only two—pneumonia and influenza, and septicemia—are acute infectious diseases.

Source: Adapted from National Center for Health Statistics, *Monthly Vital Statistics Report* 30, no. 13 (December 20, 1982): 22–23.

mizing those that could be injurious to their health and adopting health-generating ones instead. Hospitals and corporations are beginning to help by offering programs in alcohol and drug abuse, smoking cessation, weight control, nutritional awareness, physical fitness, stress management, and detection and treatment of high blood pressure.[6]

WHAT IS GOOD HEALTH?

Before we talk about "good health," let's look at someone who is *not* in good health—Bill, a forty-

five-year-old business-equipment salesman who is in the hospital recovering from his first heart attack. Bill is typical of many men in our culture who have spent much of their life pursuing the American dream. He married in his early twenties, had several children soon after, and has spent the last two decades striving for financial security and career advancement—external rewards that he has always thought would bring him inner satisfaction. Bill has been recognized many times for his fine salesmanship, his dedication to the company, and his achievements in a very competitive field; his family adores him and he has many friends. Now, at age forty-five, he is at the peak of his professional life. By all the outer standards of our society he is a successful man, and his future seems assured.

But Bill's future is *not* assured; in fact, his physician has told him that he has quite a considerable chance of suffering another, potentially fatal, heart attack. As she has noted, Bill's family history contains *genetic risk factors* (his father died of heart disease when he was fifty-five). *Environmental risk factors* have also increased Bill's chances of developing heart disease, since he lives and works in a city with high levels of air pollution. And his chance of heart disease has also been increased by a number of *lifestyle risk factors*—factors that she now recommends he try to minimize by making some big changes in his everyday living habits.

- Like most of us, Bill never considered the possibility of having a heart attack. Even though he has put on a good deal of extra weight over the years—much of it through business entertaining, which is an important part of his job—he thinks of himself as vigorous and "in good shape for a guy his age." Now, however, his physician has advised him to lose at least 10 pounds over the next two months and to begin exercising regularly.
- Smoking at least one pack of cigarettes a day has been part of Bill's lifestyle for the last twenty years. He thinks that smoking helps him relax, gets him going in the morning, and makes meals taste better—and, besides, all his friends smoke. Now his physician has advised him to stop smoking immediately.
- Drinking fairly heavily with friends and at meals with clients has been pleasurable for Bill, and it has helped him "fit in." Now, however, he has been advised to cut down his alcohol consumption drastically.
- Bill's life, with its long hours on the road and its high-pressure selling situations, has contained much of the stress that our society associates with the quest for success. This stress has not all been negative: Like other good salesmen, Bill thrives under pressure, and he has been energized by the push to make sales quotas and reach company goals. But now he has been advised to reduce the stress in his life.

What would you do if you were Bill? Put yourself in his position: Would you be able to make all the changes the physician has so persuasively recommended—and if you did, would you be healthy then? How will Bill feel if he changes the lifestyle from which he has derived so much satisfaction for the past twenty years? In the physical sense, it is clear that he will indeed be healthier. But what about his emotional health, and what about the social aspects of his life? If Bill can't function as well as he has in the past in his job or among his friends and colleagues, he will be upset; his family will feel the strain, too. Bill's problem is not an easy one to solve. Health for him includes many different aspects, and physical health is only one; he is also concerned with how he sees himself and how he thinks others see him. He is a complex creature, as all of us are, and limiting our attention to his physical problems greatly oversimplifies his heart attack.

As Bill's case shows, health is a quality that involves the psychological and social dimensions of our lives, as well as the greatest possible freedom from physical infirmities and disease. Hundreds of years ago, the word "health" meant "whole-th," or "wholeness," in our language; today, when health professionals speak of health, they mean the whole person. As the World Health Organization stated in its 1947 charter, health is "a state of complete physical, mental, and social well-being and not merely the absence of disease or infirmity." It's having all the parts of your life fit together in a way that is comfortable for you, so that you can function effectively from day to day.

Goals for Good Health

Health is a dynamic quality, changing from day to day. Even if you are in good health most of the time, you will have days when a cold, allergies, or other problems will make you feel not quite so well. But in general, good health would mean most of the following things for most people:

1. A HEALTH-PROMOTING LIFESTYLE

An extensive study has shown that people whose lifestyles include the following behaviors have a lower chance, statistically speaking, of developing diseases and a higher chance of living longer:[7]

- Not smoking cigarettes
- Drinking alcohol only in moderation (no more than two drinks a day), if at all

TABLE 1 · The Importance of Lifestyle in Good Health: Estimated Contribution of Four Factors to Ten Leading Causes of Death (Expressed in Percent)

	Factors			
Causes of Death	LIFESTYLE	ENVIRONMENT	GENETICS	HEALTH CARE SERVICES
Heart disease	54	9	25	12
Cancer	37	24	29	10
Stroke	50	22	21	7
Motor vehicle accidents	69	18	1	12
Other accidents	51	31	4	14
Influenza/pneumonia	23	20	39	18
Diabetes	34	0	60	6
Cirrhosis	70	9	18	3
Suicide	60	35	2	3
Homicide	63	35	2	0
All ten causes together	51	19	20	10

Source: U.S. Centers for Disease Control.

- Eating breakfast every day
- Not eating between meals
- Maintaining normal weight
- Sleeping seven to eight hours each night
- Exercising at least moderately

As Table 1 shows, lifestyle is the single most important contributing factor in eight of the ten leading causes of death.

2. ATTENTION TO THE BODY'S NEEDS

To stay in good health, you have to be able to deal with small problems before they become big ones. You have to be able to "read" the messages your body sends you about its needs—needs for more rest, for example; or different foods, or exercise, or a change in your environment—and respond accordingly. (Bill may have had some symptoms before his heart attack, but he may have ignored them thinking they would just go away.) You should have basic home health-care skills to cope with small medical problems at home. You should be able to deal with health-care professionals and institutions (such as hospitals) in the event of a larger medical problem; and you should take responsibility for obtaining regular checkups and tests, such as breast examinations and Pap smears for women.

3. SOCIAL HEALTH

Having good social health means being able to perform your roles in life—as a friend, neighbor, citizen, perhaps lover or spouse, perhaps parent—comfortably and with enjoyment, without doing harm to other people.

4. EMOTIONAL HEALTH

Essentially, emotional health includes:

- Being able to work, study, or pursue personal activities productively and with enjoyment.
- Understanding your emotions and knowing how to cope with everyday problems.
- Managing yourself in stressful situations, and not feeling compelled to turn to chemical sub-

Time spent with friends in enjoyable activities contributes to social health. (EPA-Documerica)

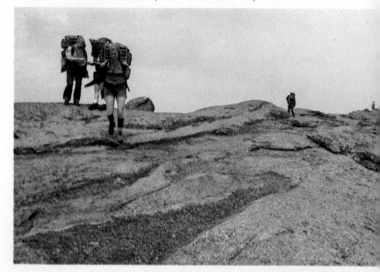

stances such as alcohol or psychoactive drugs to deal with or escape them.

For thousands of years, people have known that our emotional health can influence our physical health. For example, a person may be healed by a *placebo* (a medication that contains no active ingredients but is *believed* to be effective by the patient), or by faith or just by laughter. Physicians frequently see more commonplace demonstrations of the mind-body relationship. For example, people with good mental health have a lower rate of stress-related diseases such as ulcers, migraine headaches, and asthma, and people with intact families have lower rates of mortality (death) and morbidity (disease) than do people who have recently been widowed or divorced. We experience stress and emotional upheavals in the brain, which is part of the human nervous system and contains a network of specialized cells that send electrical impulses to every part of the body. The brain also contains areas that activate the endocrine glands releasing chemical substances called *hormones*, which help coordinate the various body systems. When stress or emotional turmoil continues for a long time, our nervous and endocrine systems may function improperly, wearing out our body defenses and putting us at greater risk of disease.

5. SPIRITUAL/PHILOSOPHICAL HEALTH

Some people believe that good health also includes a feeling that one's behavior is in rhythm with one's basic values. This feeling may also include a sense that life has meaning and is worthwhile, a sense of awe at the beauty and majesty of nature, or just a deep tranquility when you sit by yourself and ponder.

Of course, the challenge is—as we saw in Bill's case—to balance all these dimensions of good health so that they work for *you*. Health is partly a matter of personal values and preferences: Some people feel healthy only if they get at least an hour of strenuous exercise four or five times a week; others get depressed and fatigued unless they spend at least an hour a day with friends, no matter what other obligations are looming. The ingredients for health also vary with one's age and physical status: A twenty-year-old woman may want to be able to run four miles a day, an eighty-

year-old woman may feel satisfied with her physical health if she is able to walk a mile a day. The key is: Both these individuals have good health if they are able to do most of the things they want to do in their everyday lives, with a minimum of stress.

Wellness

Partly as a result of the trend toward disease-preventive lifestyles, some health experts have advocated that we strive for a level of health that is not just adequate, but much better than adequate. In their view, health may be thought of in terms of increasing levels of healthfulness—or increasing levels of *wellness,* a term that is currently popular —and the goal is "optimum health," or "high-level wellness" (see Figure 2).

Various viewpoints are represented in this approach. Some wellness advocates emphasize nutrition; some, the sense of well-being that can be derived from physical fitness activities; some, the rewards of stress-management techniques such as meditation and Yoga, which can calm people and help them get in touch with themselves. But most of the proponents of the "wellness movement" see health as not an end in itself, but as a means to a richer, fuller existence. As one writer has put it, the goal of the wellness approach is "optimal personal fitness for a fruitful and creative life."[8]

Whether or not you choose to make a conscious effort to gain "high-level wellness," it is worthwhile to think about the underlying message of the wellness movement. John Lennon once wrote, "Life is what happens to you while you're busy making other plans."[9] While your "other plans" are developing—education, career, marriage, adventure—it's a good idea to stop once in a while and think about your own daily well-being. Are you getting enjoyment out of your personal relationships? Are you finding time to explore your hobbies and interests—not just rushing to complete those tasks you're obliged to do? Are you taking steps to maintain and improve your physical health? All these are dimensions of your life that can help you derive more satisfaction from life every day. The key is to stay in touch with your own values and feelings; only you can decide exactly what combination of these elements will make your life more worthwhile.

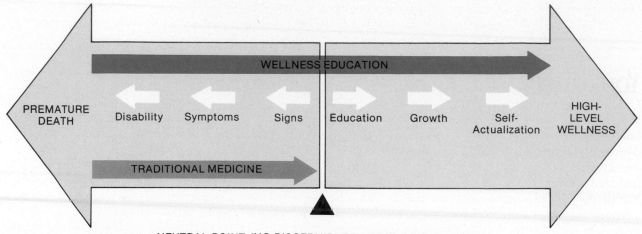

Figure 2   The illness-wellness continuum. Health may be thought of as a continuum, with high-level wellness at one extreme and premature death at the other. Traditional medicine can help us stave off premature death and can keep us at a neutral point where we are neither ill nor particularly well. Wellness education can take us even further, teaching us how to care for ourselves so that we can achieve the state of optimum physical, mental, and social health known as high-level wellness.

Source: Regina S. Ryan and John W. Travis, *The Wellness Workbook: A Guide to Obtaining High-Level Wellness* (Berkeley, Calif.: Ten Speed Press, n.d.), p. 122.

MAKING HEALTH DECISIONS

As you read this book, you *may* discover that you would like to change specific areas in your overall health behavior pattern. For example, you may decide that you want to modify the way you use drugs (if you use any drugs—and remember, coffee, alcohol, and tobacco are drugs). You may decide you want to lose some weight, or to change the way you relate to people. If cardiovascular disease runs in your family, you may want to try to avoid risk factors that make you more susceptible to heart attack. You may decide that you want to change the way you utilize health services or deal with physicians and other health care professionals.

We are all constantly in the process of evaluating ourselves in our surroundings and making decisions about our health. Some of these decisions are *unconscious:* Before his heart attack, for example, our salesman friend Bill might have unconsciously decided that keeping his weight down was not a high priority, since no one at home or in the office put much pressure on him to lose weight, and his job involved eating meals with clients on a regular basis. (He might have felt embarrassed ordering a salad—"Real men don't eat rabbit food," he might

have thought.) Some of our health decisions are *rationalizations* rather than rational decisions. For example, Bill thought smoking helped him get going in the morning and calm down later, and it was probably easy for him to justify his smoking habit. As you look at your own life, it may be helpful to try to see what unconscious decisions you may be making about your health. You might also consider which of your decisions may be rationalizations, rather than rational decisions. But don't deny your feelings and emotions. Bring them into your conscious, rational decision-making process. Otherwise, they're likely to trip you up on an unconscious level.

Steps to Behavior Change

Since your health affects your physical, emotional, social, and spiritual/philosophical well-being, whatever health-behavior changes you decide to make should include all these dimensions. You will have a better chance of making a lasting, psychologically acceptable change in behavior if you approach the change in steps rather than trying to do it all at once. Let's look at one common-sense approach to behavior change. It's a five-step process

ACTIVITY: EXPLORING HEALTH

Your Attitudes Toward Health and Illness

When you think about your own health attitudes, one of the most important points to explore is the degree to which you feel your own actions are effective in influencing your health. Some people feel that their actions have an influence on their health status. Others tend to believe that forces beyond their control (fate, luck, or health-care providers) largely determine their health status.

This activity is intended to assess your attitudes toward the control you believe you have over your health status—and about why you feel the way you do when you are sick. Responding to these questions may give you some insight into the conscious as well as unconscious decisions that you make regarding your health.

DIRECTIONS: Read each statement shown below and decide how well it describes you. Place a check (√) in the appropriate space.

	DEFINITELY TRUE	MOSTLY TRUE	DON'T KNOW	MOSTLY FALSE	DEFINITELY FALSE
If I become sick, I have something to do with getting well again.	_____	_____	_____	_____	_____
Often I feel that no matter what I do, if I'm going to get sick, I will get sick.	_____	_____	_____	_____	_____
I am directly responsible for my own health.	_____	_____	_____	_____	_____
When I stay healthy, I'm just plain lucky.	_____	_____	_____	_____	_____
I can generally stay healthy by taking good care of myself.	_____	_____	_____	_____	_____
I can maintain my health only by consulting health-care professionals.	_____	_____	_____	_____	_____

QUESTIONS

1. What pattern, if any, is evident in your responses? How would you describe your attitudes toward health? _____

_____

_____

2. How does your view of the role you play in influencing your health affect decisions you make about your lifestyle behaviors? For example, do you not wear a seat belt when traveling in a car because "when your time is up, it's up"? Are you putting off quitting smoking because

"everyone has to die sometime"? At the first sign of illness, do you rush to the doctor knowing that he or she will fix you up? _____

_____

_____

3. The following list includes five of the most common reasons why people are concerned about getting sick. Which are most important to you? Rank order the list, putting a *1* next to the reason that's most important for you and a *5* next to the least important reason.

RANK

Threat to my "health"   _____

Loss of income   _____

Loss of physical functioning   _____

Fear of death   _____

Loss of time   _____

a. Would you add other reasons to these five? If so, what are they? _____

_____

b. How does your ranking reflect the decisions you make in matters concerning your

health? (For example, many people seek out regular dental care to avoid more costly dental treatment.) _____

_____

c. Think back to the last time that you or a member of your family came down with an illness that required medical care. How did the factors listed above influence the decision to seek medical care? _____

_____

Sources: Adapted from B. Walston et al., "Development and Validation of the Health Locus of Control Scale," *Journal of Consulting and Clinical Psychology* 44 (1976): 580–585; R. H. Brook et al., *Conceptualization and Measurement of Health for Adults in the Health Insurance Study.* The Rand Corporation, R-1987/8-HEW, October 1979.

that is flexible enough to adapt to your own situation.

STEP 1: ESTABLISH YOUR TENTATIVE GOAL

When you decide to attempt to change your behavior (for example, by reducing the number of calories you take in daily), you are likely to do so on the basis of some idea of a tentative goal—let's say, to lose fifteen pounds in three months.

Why do we say this goal is "tentative"? At the beginning of your campaign you may not completely understand your own current behavior patterns. You may not know what social, psychological, and physical effects your proposed behavior change will have on you. The change may be ideal for you, and you may adapt readily to the new pattern. Or it may prove too challenging, and you may want to modify the goal: For example, you may finally decide to spread your fifteen-pound weight loss over five months, rather than three.

It's particularly difficult to predict what the emotional and social impact of your behavior change will be. For example, after attempting to cut out all desserts, you may discover that never having dessert makes you feel so deprived and frustrated that you are tempted to go back to your

former behavior. And turning down dessert might hurt someone's feelings—such as a mother or hostess who prides herself on her cooking.

STEP 2: ASSESS YOUR CURRENT BEHAVIORS AND ATTITUDES

Once you have established your tentative goal, you should assess your current behavior patterns. By taking stock of your current status and collecting information about yourself, you can develop a specific and realistic plan for the future.

If your tentative goal is to lose fifteen pounds in three months, you should collect information about your eating behavior that could reveal to you how you might best go about achieving the weight loss. One approach might be to keep a diary of your eating patterns for five days in a row. You would list everything you eat and determine how many calories you are getting. You would also note *when* you eat, in *what* situations, and specifically *what* you eat. This information would give you a picture of your eating patterns—the complex of personal habits you have developed that are associated with eating. Through self-monitoring, you would have a more specific idea of how your eating patterns contribute to your weight problem: You might, for example, discover that snacks—soft drinks, potato chips, candy bars—are

As health promotion becomes more widespread, we encounter more reminders of the need to take responsibility for changing our behavior to make our lifestyles healthier. (©Lincoln Russell 1980 /Stock, Boston)

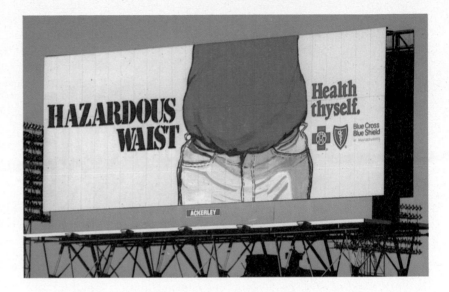

adding hundreds of extra calories a day, and it may be this extra calorie intake that is keeping you heavier than you want to be.

As you keep this diary, you need to realize that a subtle force is probably at work within you: the force of reactivity. That is, you may be changing your eating habits simply because you are keeping track: You may cut back on snacks during the assessment period because you are more conscious of snacking. Because of this tendency, you might get a biased picture of your eating habits, and you would have a difficult time getting a meaningful assessment. You can counteract the reactivity effect by keeping your diary for a longer time, or perhaps by getting someone else to keep track of your eating habits.

STEP 3: REDEFINE YOUR TENTATIVE GOAL

Once you have the results of your assessment, the next step is to redefine your tentative goal. Is it really going to be possible for you to lose fifteen pounds in three months, given your eating patterns, your psychological makeup, and your social environment? If not, then your goal should be modified. Don't forget, your goal should be measurable: You should try to choose a change that you can observe and document.

STEP 4: SELECT AND IMPLEMENT A CHANGE MECHANISM

The mechanism or procedure you choose for changing your behavior is the essential part of this whole process. In our weight-loss example, there are basically three procedures you could use to lose weight. You could eat less; you could exercise more; or you could choose to combine exercising more and eating less. Your assessment would have told you which approach might be most likely to produce the results you want. You may have discovered that you don't feel well when you greatly reduce your calorie intake, so you may decide to focus on exercise instead. Or you may have learned that you dislike exercise, but that you can reduce calories by giving up your 4 P.M. snack and selecting low-calorie foods at meals.

STEP 5: EVALUATE THE BEHAVIOR-CHANGE MECHANISM

This last step, evaluating your progress, is crucial to successful behavior change: Without it, you never know whether your program is working. Evaluation can also give you ideas about how you might modify your program to improve your results.

With a weight-loss program, the evaluation can be relatively simple—are you thinner? If not, why not? With a program designed, say, to increase your self-confidence, in contrast, evaluation may not be so simple. How can you measure an increase in self-confidence? Perhaps you could keep track of the number of times you have spoken out in class or carried out some other assertive behavior.

A Gradual Process

Changing your behavior involves changing the way you look at yourself. The more ingrained and habitual the behavior you are trying to change, the greater the challenge will be. It is important to remember that you don't behave as you do without good reason. Behaviors that you continue to use are valuable to you in some way. Even your dangerous behaviors are providing you with some benefit in your own mind.

To change your behavior, you must change the system that provides *reinforcement*—that *rewards* you for that behavior. You may have to substitute some other reinforcer that you value equally, or perhaps gain some additional insight about yourself that will allow you to overcome the power of your current reinforcement. In any case, you must be honest with yourself and expect only reasonable results. Many times a person fails to achieve a behavior change because he or she has tried to accomplish too much too soon.

This book contains a number of activities designed to help you assess your current health behaviors and make decisions about them. As you read the chapters, think about your current behavior and any changes you need to make; use the activities to focus on your behavior and begin the process of assessment. Keep in mind, however, that the assessment tools in this book are general ones. To understand your own behavior fully, you need to seek greater depth and expand the assessment into more dimensions (physical, emotional, social, spiritual/philosophical) of your health. Only you can determine which of these dimensions is most important to you in any health decision. Only you can fit the various aspects of health together into a unified, comfortable, effective way of living.

MAKING HEALTH DECISIONS

HOW HEALTHY IS YOUR LIFESTYLE?
A Personal Health Profile

There are many aspects of your personal lifestyle and forces in your environment that may help maintain your good health—or may contribute to illness. The following questions are intended to help you explore some of these areas.

THE PROFILE

DIRECTIONS: For each question, circle the number of the response that best describes your *typical* behavior.

I. Personal Health

A.	Do you experience periods of depression?	**1** never	**3** sometimes	**5** often
B.	Does anxiety interfere with your daily activities?	**1** never	**3** sometimes	**5** often
C.	Do you get enough restful sleep?	**1** often	**3** sometimes	**5** never

D. Are you aware of the causes and dangers of sexually transmitted diseases?

| 1 yes | 3 in part | 5 no |

E. Do you practice breast self-exam (if you are female) or testicular self-exam (if you are male)?

| 1 regularly | 3 sometimes | 5 never |

II. Exercise

A. What amount of physical effort do you expend during a typical work or school day?

| 1 heavy, physical work | 3 moderate work (walking, housework) | 5 light work (desk work) |

B. How often do you participate in *moderate* physical activities, such as skiing, golf, lawn mowing, gardening?

| 1 daily | 3 two or three times a week | 5 once a week or less |

C. How often do you participate in a *vigorous* exercise program—one that leaves you breathless and sweating?

| 1 daily | 3 two or three times a week | 5 once a week or less |

D. What is the average number of miles you jog or walk per day?

| 1 at least three | 3 one or two | 5 less than one |

E. How many flights of stairs do you climb per day?

| 1 at least ten | 3 five to ten | 5 fewer than five |

III. Nutrition

A. Are you overweight?

| 1 no | 3 5 to 19 pounds | 5 more than 20 pounds |

B. How often do you eat a wide variety of foods (items from all four food groups—meat, milk and other dairy products, grains, fruits and vegetables)?

| 1 each day | 3 three to five times a week | 5 once or twice a week |

IV. Alcohol

A. What is the average number of 12-oz. bottles of beer you drink per week?

| 1 0–7 | 3 8–15 | 5 16 or more |

B. What is the average number 1 1/2-oz. drinks of hard liquor you drink per week?

| 1 0–7 | 3 8–15 | 5 16 or more |

C. What is the average number of 5-oz. glasses of wine you drink per week?   1   0–7   3   8–15   5   16 or more

D. What is your average *total* number of drinks—beer, wine, or hard liquor—per week?   1   0–7   3   8–15   5   16 or more

V. Tobacco

A. How many cigarettes do you smoke per day?   1   none   3   fewer than 10   5   10 or more

B. How many cigars do you smoke per day?   1   none   3   fewer than 5   5   5 or more

C. How many plugs, pouches, or tins of tobacco do you chew per week?   1   none   3   fewer than 2   5   2 or more

VI. Automobile Safety

A. What is your mileage per year as driver or passenger?   1   less than 10,000   3   10,000 to 20,000   5   more than 20,000

B. How often do you exceed the speed limit?   1   never   3   sometimes   5   often

C. How often do you wear a seat belt?   1   always   3   sometimes   5   never

D. How often do you drive a motorcycle, moped, or snowmobile?   1   never   3   sometimes   5   often

E. If your answer to *D* is "sometimes" or "often," how often do you wear a regulation safety helmet?   1   always   3   often   5   sometimes or never

F. How often do you drive under the influence of alcohol?   1   never   3   sometimes   5   often

G. How often do you drive when your ability may be affected by drugs?   1   never   3   sometimes   5   often

SCORING AND INTERPRETATION

Now add the numbers you circled in each section and enter the totals in the spaces given.

Personal Health   _____

Exercise   _____

Nutrition   _____

Alcohol   _____

Tobacco   _____

Automobile Safety   _____

Total of all of above   _____

What is your total score, and which sections of the profile contributed most to the total? You can interpret your total score using the following criteria, but remember that the total can easily be distorted by an exceptionally high or low subtotal.

- If your total score was 52 or lower, then you scored very well indeed! Your health habits indicate a sensible lifestyle that will help to maintain your health.
- If your total score was 53 to 104, then there are some aspects of your lifestyle that could stand improvement. Look closely at your scores for the six sections of this profile and try to see where you can make positive changes.
- If your total score was 105 or higher, then it appears that you are taking unnecessary risks with your health. To get a total score this high, you must have several section scores that are also too high. What changes are needed in your life to get your score down? Which changes can be accomplished soonest? Now is the time to plan to alter your lifestyle to preserve your health.

You'll find information on most of the areas mentioned above in the following chapters in this book:

Personal Health: Chapters 14 and 16
Exercise: Chapter 15
Nutrition: Chapter 13
Alcohol: Chapter 5
Tobacco: Chapter 6

Source: Adapted from "Your Lifestyle Profile," Bureau of Health Education, Kansas Department of Health and Environment.

NOTES

1. K. Bauer, *Improving the Chances for Health: Lifestyle Change and Health Evaluation* (San Francisco: California National Center for Health Education, 1980), p. 8.

2. Mark Edwards, *American Health Habits and Desires, Employed People—All Levels in Organizations, 1978–79*, based on "Managerial Longevity: Maximizing Organizational Satisfaction, Performance, and Health," paper presented at the Gemini Conference, 1979.

3. U.S. Department of Health and Human Services, National Center for Health Statistics. *Health United States: 1980*, DHHS Pub. No. (PHS) 81-1232, October 1980, p. 414, Table and Source 4.

4. Bauer, *Improving the Chances for Health*, p. 8.

5. J. Rodin, "The Role of the Behavioral Sciences in Disease Prevention and Health Promotion," *Academic Psychology Bulletin* 2, no. 2 (1980): 237–242.

6. National Chamber Foundation, *A National Health Care Strategy: How Business Can Promote Good Health for Employees and Their Families*, 1978, p. 4.

7. N. Belloc and L. Breslow, "Relationship of Physical Health Status and Health Practices," *Preventive Medicine* 1 (1972), 409–421.

8. Howard S. Hoyman, "Re-thinking an Ecologic System of Man's Health, Disease, Aging, and Death," *Journal of School Health* 45, no. 9 (1975): 509–518.

9. John Lennon, "Beautiful Boy," © 1980 Lenono Music, Inc.

PART ONE

Feeling Well: Health and Mental States

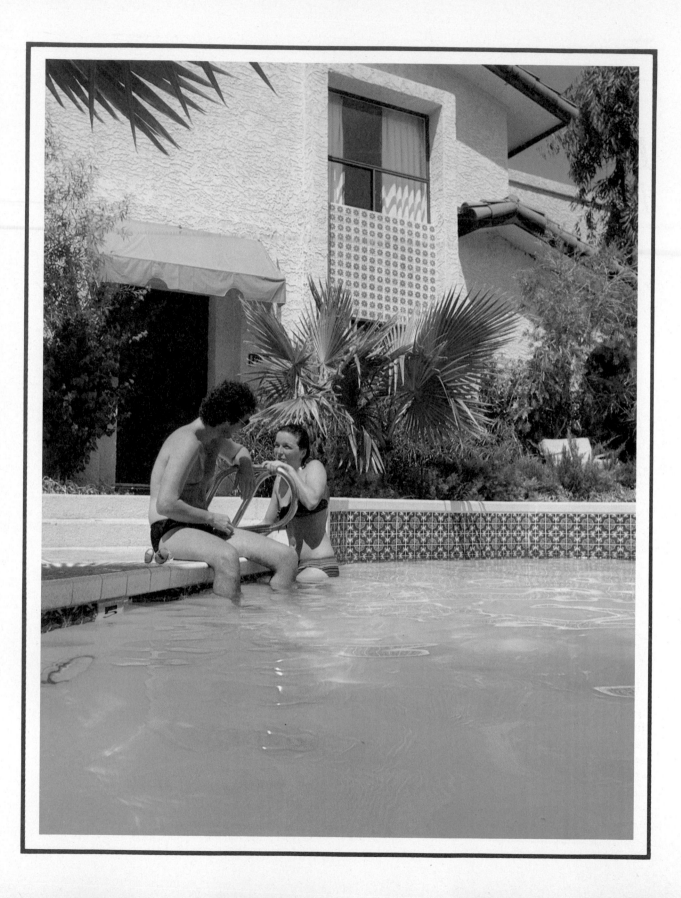

CHAPTER 1

Emotional Health and Mental Disorders

■ A student begins to feel more and more pressure on him as the term progresses and demands on his time increase. With exams, term papers, and laboratory assignments piling up, he finds he is constantly anxious and tense. Soon he begins to have occasional headaches and stomach upsets. As the weeks go by, he realizes that he has a problem dealing with tension in his life.

■ A mother has been furious all winter at her teenage daughter for repeatedly staying out past 11 P.M. without telephoning. She acts out her anger by screaming and yelling at her daughter. She loves her daughter, but, curiously, she shows her concern for her daughter's welfare through anger. The pattern seems to have been getting worse lately.

■ A thirty-four-year-old single man, who has always enjoyed his freedom as a bachelor, meets a new woman and slowly begins to change. He falls deeply in love with her, but he's terrified of making any sort of commitment, much less getting married.

What do these three people have in common? All three of them are experiencing conflict in their lives—conflict that results in emotional upheaval. We all have uncomfortable emotions at times—feelings such as anger, anxiety, and fear—but usually, under ordinary circumstances, these feelings just go away after a few hours, or perhaps a day or so. The people in our stories, however, are finding that they can't seem to shake their uncomfortable emotional patterns as the days and weeks go by. They are having problems with their emotional health.

WHAT IS EMOTIONAL HEALTH?

What do we really mean when we talk about **emotional health**? Like most of the other dimensions of health we will be discussing in this book, emotional health is a complicated quality. It doesn't mean total control over our emotions. Everyone feels some degree of emotion all the time. Sometimes we feel an intense emotion such as rage or passionate love, sometimes a much milder emotion such as boredom, a slight depression, or quiet cheerfulness and contentment. Emotional health means a balance among our emotions. When we are in good emotional health, we feel we can generally live with our emotional ups and downs. They do not get in our way to any great extent, or make it hard for us to lead our everyday existence.

To put this more clearly, emotional health means that we are not unduly troubled by ongoing conflicts among our emotions—feelings that pull the individual in many directions at once. We all get into emotional conflict from time to time—because of problems with our family, friends, teachers, or spouse; because of difficulties with our careers, our academic environments, or our communities; or because of other pressures that bear down on us. Some of this conflict comes from opposing forces within us: The bachelor in our story is torn between love and fear of commitment. Some conflict comes from forces in the environment: The student is being increasingly pressured by his school assignments. If we can resolve most of these conflicts within a reasonable time and go on living our lives more or less as we want to, then we are probably in good emotional health. If we can't resolve our conflicts, then we need to take steps to help ourselves.

The Emotionally Healthy Person

What are the basic qualities demonstrated by emotionally healthy people in our culture? (It's important to note that what we think of as emotional health depends to some extent on our culture. What we consider to be a normal way of dealing with a conflict might not be considered appropriate or healthy by a Brazilian or a Chinese, or by an ancient Roman, or by a person in the Middle Ages.) There are many exceptions to any rule about emotional health, of course, but most authorities agree that emotionally healthy people have at least the following characteristics:

- They are able to understand reality and deal with it constructively.
- They can adapt to reasonable demands for change.
- They have a reasonable degree of personal autonomy.
- They can cope with stresses.
- They have a concern for other people.
- They have an ability to love.
- They are able to work productively.

It is important to remember that our emotional health is not a static condition; it is a dynamic process. Our level of emotional health varies slightly day by day. All of us have days when we feel good about ourselves and the world around us seems friendly. We also have days when most things seem to go wrong for us and we feel bad about ourselves. But if our general emotional health is good, we can "roll with the punches." Emotional health is the quality that enables us to enjoy the good times and somehow make it through times when we are miserable—and keep both extremes in perspective.

Emotional and Physical Health

Our physical health is closely related to our emotional health. Have you ever had a stomach ache caused by the prospect of going to the dentist? Have you ever gotten a tension headache after dealing with a cranky two-year-old child all afternoon? If so, you know the close connection between feelings in the mind and feelings in the body. Feeling bad emotionally may make you feel bad physically. Conversely, if you feel well emotionally you may be able to help yourself feel better physically. Surgeons, for example, routinely evaluate their patients' emotional states before they operate on them, because they have learned that these emotional states can have an important impact on the patient's chances for recovery.

How does the connection between mind and body work? Scientists know about *some* of the links in the chain. First of all, it is widely accepted today that our emotions, which we may think we experience "in our minds," are actually physical states. Let's examine what happens to our bodies when we experience an emotion.

THE NATURE OF EMOTIONS

Two things happen when you have an emotion:

1. You experience certain physical sensations.
2. You label these sensations in terms of your environment. (This includes your internal environment, too, such as a memory or a thought. Often we blush and feel happy just remembering a time when we were with someone we love.)

In a fascinating 1962 study, psychologists Stanley Schachter and Jerome Singer set out to explore the way external events can influence a person's emotions. They decided to induce an emotionlike physical state in their subjects and then see if they could induce the mental part of the emotion too. The first step was to inject the subjects with a drug called epinephrine, which would cause their hearts to beat a little faster and their breathing rates to increase—the same physical changes that often occur when we have emotions in real life.

Next they put the subjects in a situation that might give them some cues to interpreting the emotional significance of their pounding hearts and fast breathing. The researchers sent a confederate into the room where the subjects were waiting. The subjects thought this person was another experimental subject, but he was actually assisting the researchers. The confederate was instructed

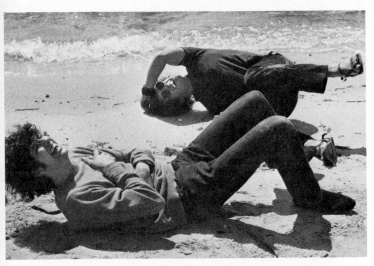

An emotion is a complex combination of mental perceptions and physical changes that can affect our behavior—though not often so strongly as this. (© Jeff Albertson/Stock, Boston)

to behave in a way that might lend an emotional flavor to the proceedings. He cracked jokes, made paper airplanes, clowned around with a Hula Hoop, and did everything else he could to make everyone in the room feel silly, happy, and euphoric. The subjects actually did feel an emotion: Not only did they feel their hearts pounding, they actually felt cheerful and euphoric. Schachter and Singer had proved their point: If you can induce an emotionlike physical sensation in a person and set up an environmental framework or series of cues, you can induce the person to have a specific emotion.[1]

The Body's Emotional Mechanism

How does the intricate relationship between emotions and bodily changes work? The answer lies in the way the brain and nervous system are set up. The human brain is somewhat like the central processing unit of a computer: It receives and processes information and controls body movements. Another part of the nervous system, the **autonomic nervous system (ANS)**, is like a video display terminal on which the emotional message from the computer is printed out. We read the message in the form of increased secretion of sweat glands,

tightening of the stomach muscles, or other physical reactions. When you stand in front of a classroom to give a report and your eyes survey the sea of faces waiting for your first word, a message goes from your eyes to your brain, which interprets what the eyes see and sends out its own message: panic. The ANS then "prints out" that message, and your hands turn clammy while your stomach churns.

KEY BODY RESPONSES IN EMOTIONS

There are six responses that scientists commonly look at to study emotions. These are heart rate, blood pressure, blood volume, electrodermal responses, muscle potential, and brain wave patterns, or electroencephalograms (EEGs). All are controlled by the nervous system.

HEART RATE This is the physiological response we think of first in connection with emotional situations, both because we recognize a thumping heart so clearly and because of the heart's mythic role as the center of emotions, where love, rage, and hatred supposedly hold sway.

BLOOD PRESSURE This term refers to the force exerted by the heart to push blood out of the arteries. There are great changes in blood pressure during highly charged emotional states.

BLOOD VOLUME Blood vessels can constrict and dilate (expand), which alters the rate of blood flow through them. When we grow pale with fear, the flow of blood to our faces has been restricted (vasoconstriction). In a person whose face is red with embarrassment, in contrast, the blood vessels are dilating, increasing the flow of blood to the face (vasodilation).

ELECTRODERMAL RESPONSES The skin, like all of the rest of our bodies, can conduct electricity. During strongly emotional states we sweat, and the added moisture makes the skin better able to conduct electricity than at other times. The degree of conduction can be measured by placing metal electrodes on the skin.

MUSCLE POTENTIAL Muscles often give us visible signs of emotion—the tightening of the jaw when angry, the activation of the facial muscles that form a smile. Each use of a muscle generates a burst of electricity, which scientists can measure to obtain an estimate of emotional activity.

EEG (ELECTROENCEPHALOGRAM) The brain also emits electrical waves that can be measured by placing electrodes on the skull. The resulting pattern of waves is called an electroencephalogram, or EEG for short. There are four types of brain waves, but only two are frequent in adults: alpha waves, which are the rhythm of the awake and relaxed adult, and beta waves, which indicate an alert or excited state.[2]

LEARNING AND EMOTIONS

As we've said, we interpret what's going on in our autonomic nervous system in terms of what's going on in our environment. The result is our emotional state as we intuitively sense it to be. Sometimes a series of events is involved in this process. First, there might be an environmental stimulus (perhaps we hear someone whisper "I love you"). Then our physical condition changes, and our autonomic nervous system "prints out" the change as, say, a tingling, excited feeling. Then we interpret this physical feeling as an emotion.

But what determines, in this instance, whether we will tell ourselves "What I'm feeling is joy" or "What I'm feeling is sheer panic"? It all depends on what we have learned in the past. We learn, over our lifetimes, how to interpret our environment and our own emotional sensations.

Learning Emotional Responses by Association

We learn some emotional responses by association. For example, a student whose palms sweat during history exams may discover, to her dismay, that they also begin to sweat as soon as the professor mentions that there will be an exam on Thursday. Psychologists call such learning by association **classical conditioning:** The person learns to associate an originally neutral stimulus (the word *exam*) with a meaningful one (the exam itself), and then responds to the neutral stimulus as if it were the meaningful one.

The student's nervousness at the thought of a history exam may not be very important in itself. But think what it may mean if the student comes to associate many different school-related situations with nervousness, anxiety, and panic. If enough of these small learnings take place, she may develop a painful emotional conflict—between her negative feelings about school and her wish to get good grades and feel satisfied with herself (and, maybe, please her parents). Her emotional health will suffer.

How Learned Emotional Reactions Can Affect Our Behavior

Suppose our nervous student gets an A on one particular history exam, which happens to be about a subject she's particularly interested in—the Vietnam war. Joy, excitement, relief! And she gets a bonus: Now she has positive emotions she will associate with the thought of exams. Will she study more willingly for the next test? Yes. The good grade gave her happy feelings. At the very thought of studying, she has some of these feelings again, and they take the edge off of that tense, clammy-palmed sensation she had before.

But note: Now an emotion is actually leading this student to *do* something—namely, study. And this new behavior on her part brings about a whole chain of events. The student acts on her environment—she studies hard and does well on the next test. The result is another A—the environment has responded back to her. Now she has more happy feelings. She has moved into a whole new emotional cycle.

Psychologists describe this process in terms of the **reinforcers** involved, such as the A and the happy feeling. These reinforcers, they say, strengthen the behavior in question, in this case, studying. In other words, the reinforcers make us more likely to repeat the behavior, because that behavior was reinforced in the past. Sometimes, therefore, our emotions can be the result of an interaction between our own behavior and our social environment. Our behavior can make our environment respond to us, with results that will then affect our emotions again.

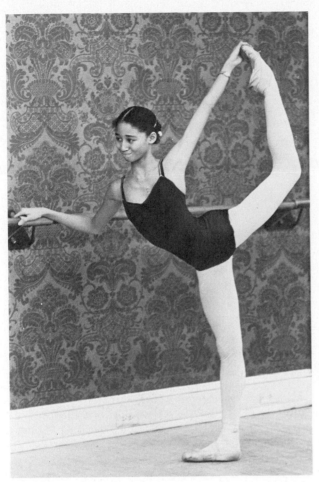

This girl is more likely to persevere with her dancing if it brings her personal satisfaction and the praise of others. Thus, her behavior and her social environment interact to affect her emotions about dancing. (© Joel Gordon)

We need not feel helpless or passive about our emotional lives. We can improve our own emotional experiences *if* we act on our environment so that it responds positively to us.

How We Learn Emotional Responses from Other People

We also learn emotional responses by observing the experience of others. (Psychologists call this process **social learning** or **modeling**.) Theorists suggest that the most powerful forms of social learning come when we see other people being rewarded for certain behaviors, and when we observe and imitate people we particularly admire and identify with. Our parents are important role models. Many of us voluntarily or involuntarily find ourselves acting just the way our mothers or fathers did in similar situations. This is not to say, of course, that behavior is fixed at an early age. Social learning continues throughout life, and as people grow older they can be more selective in choosing their models.

As an example of the way social learning can affect an emotional response, take the pattern often seen among American men with regard to crying and other displays of emotion. Do men in the movies cry? Not very often. Male characters in American movies who show emotion are of a special breed, and the emotions that they do show must be "packaged" very carefully. American men seldom cry in real life, either. Those who show emotion are sometimes viewed as weak. How then do small boys—who cry frequently in our society—grow into tough, noncrying men? Through social learning: They imitate real adults and those hard-jawed cowboys in the movies, and little by little they learn to hide their emotions.

HOW EMOTIONS DEVELOP THROUGHOUT OUR LIVES

We're all born with the capacity to experience emotions. This trait is something we've probably inherited from our animal ancestors. By the end of the first year, a child has identifiable, complex human emotions, including love, fear, and fascination. These occur in children all over the world at roughly the same age, a fact that shows that early emotions are maturational—that is, they are linked to physical development rather than learned.[3]

Yet despite this universality, specific events will trigger emotions of different intensity, depending on the child's environment. A child in a small, isolated village will tend to be more disturbed by seeing a stranger than a child of the same age who lives in a large city. Variations can even be found among children with the same ge-

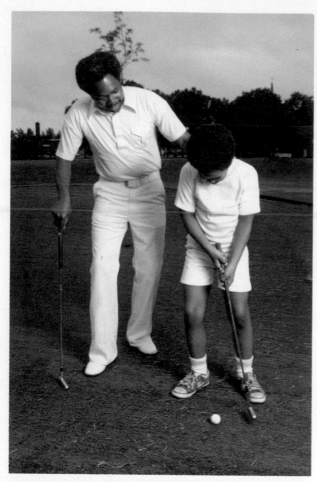

Social learning—especially imitation of parents—is a very important factor in emotional development. (© Menschenfreund/Taurus Photos)

netic background if they are raised differently. Zaslow found that at the age of eighteen months, Israeli children raised communally on a kibbutz were just as shy as children of similar genetic background raised at home. But by age two, the kibbutz children played with others more readily than those with a more traditional home life.[4]

The Role of Love in Early Emotional Development

It seems that there is a maturational sequence, programmed into the body, that leads to the development of what we would consider an emotionally "normal" human being —but only *if* the

early environment provides the right kinds of stimulation. What are these crucial environmental inputs? One of them is love. John Bowlby, René Spitz, and others have studied children who were deprived of their mothers at an early age. They concluded that severe personality problems can develop when an attachment is not formed or is forcibly broken (as by the death of the mother) before the age of seven. The child needs to have a constant source of tactile contact and comfort, whether provided by the mother or by other caregivers. Children need individual attention, warmth, comfort, security, and stimulation in order to develop properly. If they don't get these, not only will they fail to develop emotionally, but they will also have problems with sensorimotor skills (crawling, walking), language, and physical growth. Without a parent and family, they are less likely to receive this attention.[5]

Establishing Major Emotional Patterns

We've now set the stage for emotional development in the individual. All children have the basic capacity for emotion as part of their genetic heritage. If children get love and attention, their capacity to begin learning specific emotional responses will be unlocked and ready to function.

Now, what specific responses will each individual child learn? As we've noted above, some important learning tasks must be mastered for the child to become an emotionally healthy individual. The child must learn to love, to work, to be independent, to cope with reality, and to adapt to change when necessary. All these behavior patterns must be associated with at least some happy and pleasurable emotions if the child is to grow into an emotionally healthy adult.

A number of psychologists have outlined ways in which these emotional patterns are established in the healthy individual and ways in which they can be disrupted. Some of the earliest and most important contributions were made by Sigmund Freud.

THE INSIGHTS OF FREUD

According to Freud, emotional development involves a series of stages (see Figure 1.1). In the *oral*

Age	Stage	Aspects of Development
Birth to about one year	Oral stage	Pleasure centers around the mouth—eating, sucking, spitting, biting, chewing. Adults who fixate at this level may displace their oral impulses by being gullible, possessive, sarcastic, or argumentative, for example.
One year to three years	Anal stage	Pleasure centers around the retention and expulsion of feces; type of toilet training can affect the child's personality—depending on whether the training is too strict or too permissive, the child may become (as an adult) obstinate and stingy, or destructive and messy, or creative and productive, for example.
Three years to six years	Phallic stage	The child discovers and derives pleasure from his genitals; the Oedipal conflict and castration anxiety occur.
Six years to about eleven years	Latency stage	To relieve the anxiety stemming from the Oedipal conflict, the child represses a desire for the opposite-sexed parent and identifies with the like-sexed parent, repressing all erotic impulses toward the opposite sex.
Adolescence	Genital stage	Egocentric and incestuous love is replaced by heterosexual love and sexuality; the adolescent prepares for adulthood by channeling drives into group activities and preparation for work and marriage.

Figure 1.1 Freud's stages of emotional development. Freud noted that there is no sharp break or sudden transition between one of these stages and the next. The adult personality is the result of contributions from all the stages. (Freud's emphasis here was on males; he was less definite about stages of development in females.)

stage, infants derive pleasure from sucking at the breast or bottle. In the *anal* stage, young children experience pleasure from expelling feces. In the *phallic*—stage, which begins at three to six years of age, is interrupted by the *latency* stage at about age six to eleven, and continues through adulthood as the *genital*—stage, pleasure comes to be centered on the genital organs. Freud thought children needed to be able to interpret these pleasurable body experiences as acceptable, permissible, and good if they are to develop in a healthy way. If they connect these experiences with disapproval, anger, and fear, they will have emotional problems later in life.

Freud emphasized that these stages were connected: What we learn in one stage influences our experiences during other stages. He also emphasized the theme of conflict: The "self" wants one thing, and the "world" wants another.[6] Other psychologists have agreed with this perspective: As we progress from infancy to old age, our needs change and bring new conflicts with them.

THE VIEWS OF ERIK ERIKSON

Though Erik Erikson rejected Freud's emphasis on children's sexuality, he too saw emotional development in terms of a series of conflict situa-

Age	Stage	Result of Success	Result of Failure
Early Infancy (birth to about one year) (corollary to Freudian oral stage)	Basic Trust vs. Mistrust	Trust results from affection and gratification of needs, mutual recognition.	Mistrust results from consistent abuse, neglect, deprivation of love, too early or harsh weaning, autistic isolation.
Later Infancy (one to three years) (corollary to Freudian muscular anal stage)	Autonomy vs. Shame and Doubt	Child views self as person apart from parents but still dependent.	Child feels inadequate, doubts self, curtails learning basic skills like walking, talking, wants to "hide" inadequacies.
Early Childhood (about ages four to five years) (corollary to Freudian phallic locomotor stage)	Initiative vs. Guilt	Child has lively imagination, vigorously tests reality, imitates adults, anticipates roles.	Child lacks spontaneity, has infantile jealousy "castration complex," is suspicious, evasive, suffers from role inhibition.
Middle Childhood (about ages six to eleven years) (corollary to Freudian latency stage)	Industry vs. Inferiority	Child has sense of duty and accomplishment, develops scholastic and social competencies, undertakes real tasks, puts fantasy and play in better perspective, learns world of tools, task identification.	Child has poor work habits, avoids strong competition, feels doomed to mediocrity; is in lull before the storms of puberty, may conform as slavish behavior, has sense of futility.
Puberty and Adolescence (about ages twelve to twenty years)	Ego Identity vs. Role Confusion	Adolescent has temporal perspective, is self-certain, is a role experimenter, goes through apprenticeship, experiences sexual polarization and leader-followership, develops an ideological commitment.	Adolescent experiences time confusion, is self-conscious, has a role fixation, and experiences work paralysis, bisexual confusion, authority confusion, and value confusion.
Early Adulthood	Intimacy vs. Isolation	Person has capacity to commit self to others, "true genitability" is now possible, *Lieben und Arbeiten* — "to love and to work"; "mutuality of genital orgasm."	Person avoids intimacy, has "character problems," behaves promiscuously, and repudiates, isolates, destroys seemingly dangerous forces.
Middle Adulthood	Generativity vs. Stagnation	Person is productive and creative for self and others, has parental pride and pleasure, is mature, enriches life, establishes and guides next generation.	Person is egocentric, nonproductive, experiences early invalidism, excessive self-love, personal impoverishment, and self-indulgence.
Late Adulthood	Integrity vs. Despair	Person appreciates continuity of past, present, and future, accepts life cycle and life style, has learned to cooperate with inevitabilities of life, "death loses its sting."	Person feels time is too short; finds no meaning in human existence, has lost faith in self and others, wants second chance at life cycle with more advantages, has no feeling of world order or spiritual sense, fears death.

tions: The individual's needs and wants confront the demands of society, and the individual must resolve these confrontations, one after another, for optimal emotional development.

As the individual's life unfolds, Erikson felt, different needs and desires come to the fore. For example, infants need someone they can trust to provide consistent care; adolescents yearn for a sense of identity; and so on throughout life. Erikson, like Freud, saw these emerging needs in terms of a series of stages (see Figure 1.2).

Whether society will cooperate with the individual in satisfying every need and want, of course, is another matter. So, even though the individual may pass successfully through some of these stages of conflict, some anxieties and frustrations are bound to develop. The individual's success in resolving these conflicts helps to determine whether he or she will become emotionally mature or be troubled by recurring rage, nervousness, depression, or other distressing emotions throughout his or her life.[7]

DEALING WITH PAINFUL EMOTIONS

Emotions can be frightening. Our society places great stock in maintaining control over our emotions, and mature, healthy people are not expected to show their emotions often. From time to time, however, events are such that our control is challenged, and whether we like it or not, our emotions start to show more than we want.

The basic thing to keep in mind about emotions and control is that the control is not really a natural response; it is imposed on us by the particular culture in which we live. Emotions are a natural part of us and should be experienced freely, but

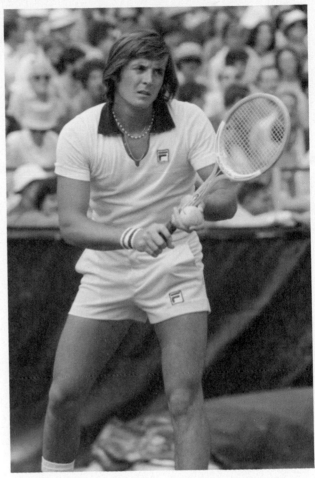

Anxiety is a very common emotion in competitive situations. (Peter Southwick/Stock, Boston)

at the same time we need to be able to cope with them. Let's examine some common painful emotions and consider some ways to deal with them.

Anxiety

Anxiety occurs when we have fear related to a loss or hurt. It doesn't matter whether the loss or hurt is real or imagined—the fear is very real. In most cases the fear is over some loss or hurt that might occur in the future. We often feel helpless at such times—we feel that things are out of our hands; and thus our anxiety is heightened.

Figure 1.2 Erikson's stages of emotional development. In Erikson's view, the success an individual has in resolving the conflict that characterizes each of these stages has a strong influence on whether the person becomes emotionally mature.

Source: Adapted from Ledford J. Bishof, *Interpreting Personality Theories*, 2nd ed. (New York: Harper & Row, 1970), pp. 578–580.

WHAT YOU CAN DO TO COPE WITH ANXIETY

The most effective way to deal with anxiety is to work toward regaining some feeling that you can control the events in your life—or at least your reactions to them.

Start by admitting to yourself that you are afraid of being hurt or of losing someone or something important to you. Once the sources of your anxiety are brought out into the open, you can examine them objectively. Imaginary fears can be seen for what they are; real threats to your well-being or self-esteem can be better understood.

Next, acknowledge your vulnerability. Sometimes simply admitting that you are vulnerable to a loss or hurt can help relieve the anxiety. Once you accept your vulnerability, you may be able to see that you can survive, even if your worst fears come to pass. True, a loss or hurt can be painful, unpleasant, or unfortunate, but you will survive it and continue to grow.

The key to coping with anxiety, then, is to accept your vulnerability and convince yourself that you can survive and grow despite your loss.

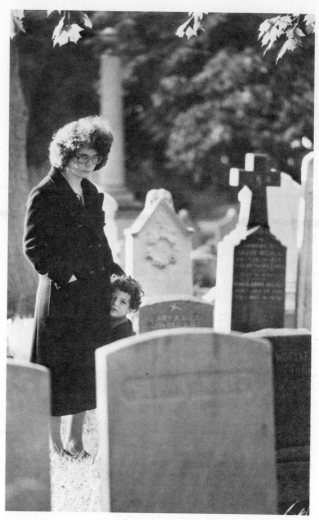

It is normal to experience depression for a considerable period after a loved one has died. (© Stephen Shames, 1982/Woodfin Camp & Assoc.)

Minor Depression

Minor depression is sometimes referred to as the "common cold" of emotional disorders. Most of us feel depressed at times. Depression is a "down" feeling that is usually associated with loss of self-esteem: Depressed people often feel worthless. Depression may also be due to anger that is directed inward: Depressed people often fight to hold anger back and, in some cases, have lost sight of the original reason for their anger.

WHAT YOU CAN DO TO COPE WITH MINOR DEPRESSION

To get over depression, start by directing energy away from yourself. Exercise, gardening, reading, or other distracting activities often help to break a depressed mood. Make a schedule for yourself for the day so that you can structure your activities toward some productive end.

Also, try to acknowledge the source of your anger, if possible, and allow trapped feelings to escape. Don't expect miracles in coming to grips with depression. Try to take one day at a time and remember that recovery will take time.

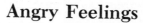

Angry Feelings

One writer, Walter S. Smitson, makes the intriguing comment that people who go through life making themselves and others miserable by being angry and frustrated much of the time may be too vulnerable to external stress and may need to desensitize themselves. They may need to learn to filter out more of the many hurts and hostilities the world aims in their direction. They may also need to "challenge" their own anger: to look under it to find out what other more subtle feelings—hurt, rejection, sadness, loneliness—it may be covering up, and try to face those feelings.[8]

WHAT YOU CAN DO TO COPE WITH ANGER

▶ Strengthen your "buffer zones" by developing your feelings of security and self-worth.
▶ You can drop some of your competitive feelings so that you're not constantly going forth to do battle with work, play, or other people. Then your "buffer zones" will help you ignore more of the painful stimuli from your environment.
▶ Figure out why you are reacting so strongly to this particular situation. Is it because you are particularly sensitive to criticism? Or are there certain types of people who annoy you? One tactic is to try to avoid situations or people who make you angry. Another is to see if you can change the way you perceive the situation.
▶ Some anger is caused by frustration. Take a look at the situation and see if you can figure out what is frustrating you—and then do something about *that*.
▶ Some anger can be constructive (if it's used carefully). It is speculated, for example, that tennis superstar John McEnroe *has* to get angry and behave as he does in order to go in for the kill on the court.
▶ Some anger gets even worse if you ventilate it, psychologist Carol Tavris claims. Yelling at your adversary just escalates the hostility and anxiety rather than clearing the air. It's better in some situations either to assert yourself and deal with the underlying difficulties or drop and simply walk away from the situation.[9]
▶ Use some good, healthy four-letter words (in private, if necessary). They'll help boost your self-esteem and keep you from feeling crushed by your circumstances. Psychologist Chaytor Mason says,

> The person using [four-letter words] is proving that at least he has a mastery over something, if only his own mouth. He is verbally hitting below the belt. It's a way of feeling powerful when one feels helpless. Show me a person who never swears, and I'll show you a person who is unduly afraid of people.[10]

Defense Mechanisms

Finding ways to cope with painful emotions is one of the most critical ongoing efforts of our lives. Whether we like it or not, stasis (standing still) is not part of the human condition. We find one way of living effectively and then everything changes —a family breaks up, a child leaves home, a mother or wife goes out to work for the first time, we find a new job, we go to a new school. The people we live with and rely on may change their values and habits. We are forced to adapt to all these changes—and, luckily, our minds and our bodies *are* adaptable. One of the ways we work through such adaptations is by using **defense mechanisms**—mental strategies for protecting ourselves from experiencing the anxiety associated with painful emotions.

COMMON DEFENSE MECHANISMS[11]

REPRESSION   **Repression** is considered the most basic of all defense mechanisms; with it we deny to ourselves any awareness of thoughts, feelings, memories, or wishes that are threatening. Repression is usually indicated by a person's refusal to acknowledge—through speech, emotion, or behavior—a response that would ordinarily be expected under specific circumstances. If, during the parents' divorce, a child displays no anger or distress, insisting "It doesn't matter," we may suspect that the child is repressing the fear, common to children, that he or she has done something to cause the divorce.

RATIONALIZATION   Those who rarely admit that their motives are anything but the highest may be using the defense mechanism of **rationalization**. The vice president of one tobacco company said, "A heck of a lot of people, if they didn't have cigarette smoking to relieve stress, would be one hell of a lot worse off."[12]

People often tend to use rationalization in situations where there is **cognitive dissonance**—an uncomfortable conflict between two realities that don't match. A person who smokes cigarettes while knowing that they cause lung cancer and heart disease experiences cognitive dissonance. She knows smoking is bad for her, and she would not normally choose to shorten her life by impairing her health; yet she continues to smoke. So she may employ a rationalization, insisting "There are plenty of valid studies that indicate that cigarette smoking and all those diseases are not related." She is reducing her emotional discomfort by altering her perception of reality.

PROJECTION Projection is an attempt to attribute our own undesirable feelings, wishes, and motives to other people or even inanimate objects. A man about to be married, for instance, may describe his roommate as interested in every good-looking woman who walks down the street, despite the fact that the roommate has never given him any cause to think that. The projecting person may be denying that he ever thought about other women and projecting onto his roommate the unacceptable feeling he has about his impending marriage.

DENIAL In repression we cover up truths about ourselves and our inner life. **Denial,** by contrast, is a defense mechanism in which we cover up truths about the outer world, ignoring those which threaten our self-esteem or create anxiety. Thus, we may not hear an insulting remark about us, even though it is spoken clearly and within hearing distance. A woman may insist that her son Johnny didn't hit Billy, even though the event occurred in plain sight.

PSYCHIC CONTACTLESSNESS Psychic contactlessness, first discussed by Wilhelm Reich, is a defense mechanism that involves an inability to communicate with or become intimate with others. A person who is deeply afraid of being hurt by intimacy, perhaps because he or she has been hurt in the past, is suffering from psychic contactlessness. Such persons never get to know others well, nor do others get to know them, but they keep their self-esteem intact: Nobody can hurt them because nobody is allowed to get close enough to do so.

DEPERSONALIZING OTHERS When we are unable to recognize that other people are fully human, with human feelings and emotions, we are engaging in **depersonalization.** Racial prejudice often contains strong elements of depersonalization: "That person doesn't experience the same needs or desires as I do, so it doesn't matter if he or she suffers socially or economically." On another level, depersonalization occurs when we view others only according to their social roles as, for example, workers, husbands, students. Depersonalization protects people from guilt they might feel at hurting others, or it may protect them from seeing that they cannot be intimate or loving with others.

SUBLIMATION Sublimation refers to the substitution of socially acceptable behavior for unacceptable impulses, such as hostility or aggression. Some people may become community leaders, constructively active outside the home all day, rather than face angry feelings they have about their home lives. A young person may go out for a sport, practicing all the time, sublimating uncomfortable feelings about the opposite sex. Such sublimation is often temporary; in fact, becoming proficient at a sport may help the individual feel more acceptable to the opposite sex.

IS IT UNHEALTHY TO USE DEFENSE MECHANISMS?

Defense mechanisms are normal; we all resort to them to one degree or another. Not all defense mechanisms are negative. They can serve as a moderating force in our lives when change is too stressful, giving us time to marshal our resources and gain the strength to go out and face a new challenge. Many defense mechanisms serve important positive purposes in our lives. In one study university students who used defense mechanisms were found to have significantly reduced their tension and anxiety.[13]

Basically, no defense mechanism is bad in itself; it depends on the degree to which you use it. A mentally healthy person needs to have a variety of defense mechanisms available, to be used when necessary in order to adjust successfully to stress and problems. The danger point occurs when defenses become our *only* way of dealing with reality.

HOW WE DEAL WITH MENTAL AND EMOTIONAL PROBLEMS

We all experience periods of extreme mental and emotional stress, times when we feel we just can't cope for another minute. We find ourselves acting in ways that make us uncomfortable, experiencing "strange" thoughts or feelings, unable to get through the day with energy or eagerness. When we feel this way, we may simply be having temporary emotional conflict. Or we may have an identifiable mental disorder. Mental disorders and emotional problems are extremely common: over 4 percent of all visits to health professionals are for treatment of mental disorders.[14] This means that a great many of us are likely to develop at least some mild mental or emotional problem at some point in our lives.

The key point here is that people shouldn't be frightened of the idea of having an emotional problem or a mental disorder. True, some mental disorders can be lifelong and require long periods of hospitalization. But some, like our second student's identity problem, are mild and short-lived. Many types of mental disorder *can* be controlled, and some can be completely cured. In most cases, seeing a therapist can help to ease the discomfort that often comes with an emotional problem.

When we are having difficulty coping and don't seem able to solve our own problems, it may be wise to see a guidance counselor or psychotherapist for some help and direction. In past years, many people were afraid to go to a psychiatrist or a psychologist—or almost any other sort of counselor, for that matter. They were embarrassed to admit they couldn't solve their problems on their own. Today, however, more and more people are realizing that there's no reason to be ashamed of seeking this kind of help. Having difficulties in your life doesn't mean you are officially "sick." You don't try to solve all your own medical problems; why should you expect to be able to solve all your own psychological problems?

People are often curious about what goes on behind the doors of the therapist's office. In reality, nothing mysterious happens. The therapist simply sees the client regularly, talks to him or her and listens very carefully, gives the client a sense of emotional support, analyzes the client's situation, and gradually helps the client figure out ways to approach daily life more comfortably and to function more effectively. Sometimes it's difficult, especially at first, for the client to face up to and discuss painful situations. But frequently the client comes away with a tremendous sense of relief. Therapists can often suggest new ways of looking at problems, and clients often come to realize that they have more options than they realized.

Today, the orientation of psychotherapy is shifting toward helping not only people with identifiable mental disorders, but also relatively "normal" people who are simply having difficulties with specific life problems such as divorce, the loss of a loved one, or worries about employment.

MENTAL DISORDERS

Health professionals view mental and emotional problems as a continuum, with many fine shadings between the "optimum health" end and the end representing serious mental illness. When an individual is having difficulty coping with life problems, there is no single moment at which he or she can be said to have developed an actual mental

Even severe mental problems need not always be crippling and need not permanently prevent the individual from functioning. One of history's great "madmen"—the artist Vincent Van Gogh—painted works of genius while in a mental institution. This is a self-portrait done in 1890. (The Louvre, Paris, EPA, Inc.)

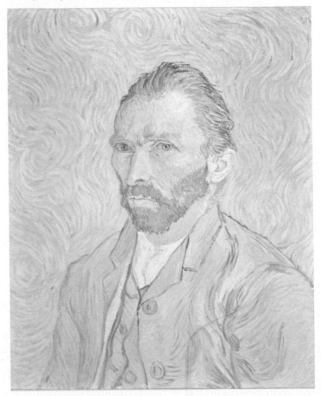

disease. Nevertheless, for the purpose of study and treatment, mental health professionals have identified a range of specific mental problems that they term "mental disorders." This term covers a wide variety of difficulties, ranging from disorders of behavior such as violent outbursts, to disorders of feeling such as depression, to disorders of thinking such as schizophrenia. Some are organically based, such as presenile dementia (Alzheimer's disease); others are associated with environmental factors, such as combat stress. The majority of mental disorders, however, probably fall somewhere in between: Physical problems, environmental stress, and problems of early psychosocial development may all play a role.

We should not be ashamed of mental disorders or think of them as "mysterious diseases," even though their causes are not always understood. People who suffer from these disorders are just as human as the rest of us—they may be the man or woman down the hall, your best friend, a family member, or yourself.

And let us make one more very important point: According to modern thinking, just being "different" does not necessarily mean that an individual has a mental disorder. When today's psychiatrists are considering whether an individual is suffering from a mental disorder, they look at the degree of distress or disability that is associated with the individual's condition. They try to see, for example, whether the abnormal behavior is disturbing to the individual or disrupts his or her life. A person may be socially deviant—he or she may be a thief or a transvestite, for example, or may do things that other people consider odd or unpleasant—but this does *not* necessarily mean the person is mentally disabled.

It is difficult to distinguish between mental health and mental disorder—and, not surprisingly, it is just as hard to classify the mental disorders themselves. Human behavior is far too complex to be easily categorized. Yet some definitions must exist so that mental health professionals can establish common ground for discussion and treatment. Over the years, most practitioners and researchers have come to accept—if with occasional misgivings—the categories suggested by the American Psychiatric Association in its *Diagnostic and Statistical Manual of Mental Disorders,* or *DSM,* as it is popularly known.[15]

The third edition of *DSM,* published in 1980,

raised a storm of controversy because it did away with many standard classifications—including neurosis, the familiar mental disorder everybody talked about at cocktail parties. Neurosis was gone; in its place the new *DSM* used such terms as "anxiety" or "personality disorder." Gone too was homosexuality as a classified disorder. Preferring not to label those who might simply be deviant, but not mentally disturbed, *DSM-III* stated that homosexuality is considered a mental disorder only if the individual is unhappy with his or her sexual orientation.

The categories we will discuss in this chapter all come from this new and controversial *DSM-III.* It is impossible for us to cover everything that is in the manual, but we will highlight the main disorders. It is important to remember that each mental disorder is not a separate, sharply defined condition. Sometimes an individual may suffer from more than one disorder.

PSYCHOTIC DISORDERS

The **psychotic disorders**—to oversimplify this complex topic greatly—are those in which the individual has significantly lost contact with reality. Two of the most common are schizophrenia and major depression; the category also includes paranoid disorders, organic disorders, and a number of other disorders, some of which we'll survey briefly.

Schizophrenia

Schizophrenia is considered the most serious of psychotic disorders. Because those suffering from it seem totally removed from reality, it is a frightening disorder for both patients and those around them. Patients may hear voices, believe that electronic devices are monitoring their activity, and laugh and talk for no reason at inappropriate times. Or they may sit motionless, in silence; although they seem to feel nothing, they are actually suffering a great deal.

What is going on in these patients' minds is just as disorienting as their behavior implies: Their thoughts are connected in random order, with little or no meaning. In speaking, patients may ramble, become increasingly vague, or repeat words or phrases without any awareness that they have lost the ability to connect ideas. The patient is very much separated from what we have come to describe as normality. And this is what makes it so difficult for the rest of us to respond to people suffering from schizophrenia with the sympathy and rationality they need. We have difficulty understanding them, we are afraid of them, and thus they become isolated.

Many people are surprised to learn that though schizophrenia is a grave disease, the outlook is by no means completely discouraging. Most patients do require hospitalization and drug treatment during the acute phase of the disorder, but the rest of the time they may live at home, interact socially, perhaps hold a job, and require only low maintenance doses of drugs for years at a time— although they may be subject to further acute phases. About 55 percent of all schizophrenics are chronically ill in this manner. In another 20 percent, the illness is more devastating: These patients have only rare remissions despite all treatment. But a surprisingly large 25 to 30 percent recover fully after a first attack.[16]

Despite their drawbacks, antipsychotic drugs have stabilized many patients to the extent that they can be released either permanently or for long periods. The relative calm that these drugs bring to the disordered life of many schizophrenics allows time for psychologically oriented therapeutic techniques. Once a patient is at home or stabilized in a hospital, he or she may be able to benefit from family, group, or individual therapy as well as social and vocational rehabilitation.

Affective Disorders

Schizophrenia is primarily (though not exclusively) a disorder in the patient's thinking processes. By contrast, the **affective disorders** are devastatingly painful disorders of mood or feeling. This category includes major depression and a disease known as bipolar disorder.

MAJOR DEPRESSION

We all experience *minor* depression at some time. As we noted earlier, it is often called the "common cold" of mental disorders because it affects so

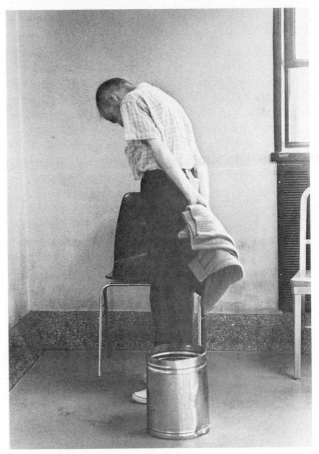

Some individuals suffering from major depression are so incapacitated that they must be hospitalized for intensive therapy. (© Chris Maynard/Stock, Boston)

many people: The National Center for Health Statistics recently reported over 6 million visits to therapists for treatment over a two-year period.[17] But some people develop much more serious **major depression**, which involves a range of incapacitating symptoms. There is a dysphoric mood —a profound unhappiness—and the individual loses interest in all aspects of life, even his or her favorite activities. This persistent unhappy mood may be accompanied by appetite disturbance, a change in weight, sleep disturbance, decreased energy, difficulty in concentrating, psychomotor agitation or retardation, feelings of worthlessness or guilt, and thoughts of death or suicide. Most of the pleasurable aspects of a person's life seem to disappear.

BIPOLAR DISORDER

In **bipolar disorder,** a less common affective disorder, the patient exhibits **mania** (a mood of extreme excitement), with or without depressive symptoms. The patient is hyperactive, convinced he or she can do everything—sometimes all at the same time. He or she may show inflated self-esteem and increased irritability. The mood may shift to anger or depression within minutes, the resulting depression lasting only a few moments, after which the patient becomes manic again. The two moods may alternate rapidly within a few days.

Other Psychotic Disorders

Space permits us to highlight only two of the other major psychotic disorders.

Paranoid disorders, which are quite rare, involve delusions of persecution. The patient may, for example, think he or she is being spied on, drugged, poisoned, or prevented from achieving goals. Although the paranoid disorders are similar to schizophrenia in that they involve some thought disorientation, the outlook for is somewhat more encouraging. Patients' personal lives are usually disrupted and full recovery is very unlikely, but they can often continue to function intellectually and in their work.

Organic mental disorders, which may involve symptoms such as delirium, dementia (mental deterioration), amnesia, and hallucinations, are caused by actual *physical* disorders of the brain. The dementia seen in some aging persons is an organic disorder many of us are familiar with. Organic disorders can develop at other times of life, sometimes as the result of disease or drug use. Often, friends and relatives of people with organic mental disorders don't realize how much emotional distress the disorder causes the patient. The patient may know perfectly well what is happening to him or her, but be unable to do anything about the psychotic symptoms.

NONPSYCHOTIC DISORDERS

The **nonpsychotic disorders** are the disorders once known as neuroses, such as panic attacks, hysteria, and unrealistic fears and anxieties that seriously inhibit a person's full functioning. In the nonpsychotic disorders the individual's thought processes are not as grossly distorted as they are in some of the psychotic disorders. Furthermore, the individual suffering from a nonpsychotic disorder recognizes and is disturbed by the symptoms. It is this very recognition that can make these disorders so painful: The patient's view of reality is distorted, but not completely—and not enough to make the patient unaware of how distressing and maladaptive his or her behavior is. In a sense, patients have double anxiety: They have the anxiety associated with the disorder itself, plus the anxiety of knowing "something is wrong." Their behavior —morbid fear of eating in public, for instance— does not actually violate social norms, but it does isolate these people. Even that isolation alone may be enough to cause the individual to feel chronically lonely, anxious, and sad.

Nonpsychotic disorders may occur with psychotic symptoms as well as independently. But —and this is a key point—they do respond to treatment. Getting help is essential: Without treatment a disorder may become chronic, enduring for the rest of the patient's life. It's important to recognize this fact, since so many of us experience nonpsychotic symptoms, if only very mild ones, at some point in our lives.

Anxiety Disorders

We all become anxious sometimes, from fear of exams, starting a new job, or wondering how a new friendship will turn out. Just living is an anxious business at times. But for some people, anxiety is not just a gnawing worry—it is incapacitating. A true **anxiety disorder** involves a severe and persistent level of fear or worry that can be almost as damaging to the individual's everyday functioning as psychosis. For example, the victim may be afraid to go out in public or to meet new people. These fears may prevent the person from functioning in a job or in other areas of normal life. According to *DSM-III,* "It has been estimated that from 2 to 4 percent of the general population has at some time had an anxiety disorder."[18]

Anxiety is not only an unpleasant emotion; it can also affect individuals physically, disturbing their breathing and increasing heart activity and sweating. These, of course, are the symptoms of fear; yet anxiety is different from fear. Fear is a correct response to a real danger, while anxiety is an irrational reaction to vague or imagined dangers. It may include panic attacks and a sense of impending doom or a consistently anxious feeling that lasts for months.

A typical anxiety disorder is *claustrophobia*—intense fear of enclosed spaces. When persons with this disorder enter a small area such as an elevator, they suffer a strong physical reaction. Other anxiety disorders include *agoraphobia,* a fear of crowded places; *social phobias,* such as the fear of having someone watch you while you write in public; recurrent *panic attacks,* some so bad they resemble heart attacks; and involuntary, irrational *obsessive thoughts* and *compulsive behaviors.* The obsessive thoughts are often about contamination or violence; the compulsive behavior is often ritualistic. Thus, a person with obsessive thoughts about germs may have a compulsion to wash his or her hands constantly, becoming extremely anxious if prevented from doing so.

TREATING ANXIETY DISORDERS

Many treatments have been tried for anxiety disorders, but so far none has proven to be consistently effective. Psychotherapy, in which the therapist helps the patient uncover underlying causes of anxiety, can be helpful in treating simple phobias and chronic, moderate anxiety. Behavior therapy has also been effective in relieving well-defined phobias. Patients with agoraphobia, for example, are trained to relax while role playing the experience of entering a big, bustling store. Sometimes they are actually taken into a store, but only after carefully monitored relaxation sessions. Other behaviorists believe the opposite approach works better: They favor "toughening" patients by bringing them right to the heart of their greatest fear. Patients with agoraphobia are taken directly to a large, busy store and allowed to experience the full force of their anxiety, in the expectation that they will see that nothing terrible

happens to them when they do so. According to some estimates, 50 percent or more of such patients can be cured by this method.[19]

Drug therapy remains the most common form of treatment for the greatest variety of anxiety disorders. Antidepressant drugs are generally considered more effective than tranquilizers, although both are still used. But drug therapy may be less helpful than psychotherapy or behavior therapy. Many researchers report a high relapse rate when drugs are discontinued; this may mean that the drugs "work" by suppressing the symptoms rather than by helping the patient deal with deep-rooted fears.[20]

Personality Disorders

Some people develop characteristic, deeply ingrained maladaptive reactions—**personality disorders**—that impair their social or occupational functioning. We see people with personality disorders often: They are the individuals we tend to perceive as odd or eccentric. Some seem overdramatic, theatrical, overemotional, or erratic; some seem dependent and passive-aggressive. One person may believe he can never succeed at anything and so refuses to work hard in school, at outside activities, or on the job. Another may experience persistent, intense symptoms, such as unwarranted suspicion of other people, or pathological jealousy.

What is the outlook for people with personality disorders? The disorders usually emerge during childhood or adolescence and continue throughout most of adult life. Treatment is difficult and time-consuming, and may have limited success. However, people who suffer from these disorders often tend to "mellow" as they get older. They seldom require hospitalization, either, unless the personality disorder is superimposed on another, more serious mental disorder.

OTHER CATEGORIES OF MENTAL DISORDERS

DSM-III describes other mental disorders that may be less familiar but are also of concern to us.

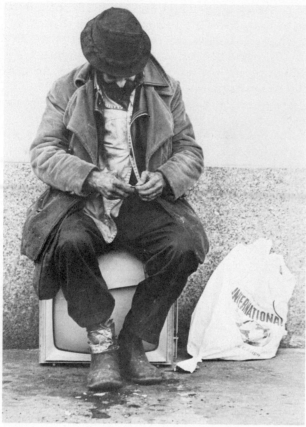

Substantial numbers of the homeless people who live in the streets of our nation's cities are former mental patients who have been discharged without adequate provision for follow-up treatment and assistance. (© Beatriz Schiller 1982/Int'l Stock)

may be broad, or it may be limited to specific areas: Some mentally retarded people, for example, can read but cannot understand arithmetic. In some cases, mental retardation is due to organic problems—chromosomal defects (as in Down's syndrome, once known as "mongolism"), genetic disorders (as in phenylketonuria), endocrine disorders (as in cretinism), and intrauterine factors (as in congenital syphilis). In other cases, the causes are unknown. One such condition is "cultural-familial retardation," the most common type of retardation. Here, the individual's IQ is low but borders on normal levels; why the deficiency develops is a mystery, but experts have noted that the disorder occasionally runs in families.

Today, it has been found that treatment can make a great difference in the extent to which mentally retarded individuals can function in society. If a retarded person is placed early in a carefully structured environment that provides training as well as shelter, he or she may progress to a point that was unheard of just a few years ago. Many mentally retarded people can be taught to carry out tasks accurately and reliably. Thus, the retarded are beginning to enter society on a much larger scale than before.

GETTING HELP WITH MENTAL PROBLEMS

How can you tell when you or someone you know needs treatment for a mental disorder or an everyday emotional problem? How can you better handle your psychological problems? How can you help someone else? Where can you turn to find professional help? And what types of treatment are available?

How You Can Help

One way to help is to listen. If someone has a problem, it often helps him or her to talk about it with another person who will listen empathically and uncritically. The most helpful approach is to acknowledge the person's feelings sympathetically with responses like "I can tell you are very worried," or "I've been down and unhappy, too. That can really be a terrible feeling." Usually it is

Not many people realize, for example, that children—even infants—are subject to mental disorders. These include schizophrenia, depression, anxiety, and others, plus developmental disorders such as infantile autism, which is defined as occurring prior to age 2½. Autistic babies are often silent, neither babbling nor speaking; they are unable to play with other children; and they often exhibit ritualistic, damaging behavior, such as banging their heads against a wall. Autism causes severe disturbances in emotional development, and the outlook for an autistic child is poor.

Mental retardation is also in the *DSM-III* classification system. **Mental retardation** can be defined as intellectual functioning at levels below those generally considered normal. The deficiency better to let the person work out a strategy for resolving the problem independently rather than rushing in with advice or a pep talk. It *is* appropriate, however, to encourage and reassure the disturbed person.

If it becomes apparent that the person is not feeling better and the problem is not being resolved, it is time to get outside help. It is better to get such help too early than too late. In many cases, tragic outcomes of mental illness might have been prevented if the people who knew about the problems had sought outside help sooner.

One step is to reinforce whatever inclination the troubled person has toward getting help. A good first contact might be a campus counseling service or a clergyman, a family physician, or someone else the person knows and trusts. Most communities also have mental health associations, clinics, and medical societies that can help with referral and advice. If the person has no interest in seeking help, a friend or family member can instead make this first contact and plan how the person can get help.

Crisis Intervention

In an emergency, if a disturbed person poses a danger to himself, herself, or others, those nearby must get professional help even against the person's overt wishes. One source of such ready help is a hospital emergency room. If the person is too violent to be taken there, one of the quickest sources of help is the police, who in most communities are trained to intervene humanely and effectively.

Many communities have a "crisis hotline," which is a quick and effective way to deal with emergency situations. People who are in trouble can telephone at any time and receive immediate counseling, sympathy, and comfort. Hotlines also provide information on the community services available to deal with various kinds of problems.

Which Therapist to Choose?

Does it matter which approach—psychoanalytic, behavioral, or whatever—the therapist takes? That depends, in part, on the nature of the client's

problem. But in most successful therapeutic relationships, regardless of the approach, the client and the therapist have a good personal relationship. Sometimes, this relationship is the only truly compassionate, honest, intimate relationship the disturbed person has—or has ever had. It can give the client a rock to stand on while learning to cope with the rest of the world.

Another question: Does it matter whether the therapist is a medical doctor? Again, this depends on the client's problem. Only M.D.s are permitted to prescribe drugs, and most psychoanalysts are M.D.s. But clinical psychologists, most of whom are Ph.D.s, are just as highly trained as M.D.s in many respects, and a clinical psychologist may be an excellent choice for many people. There are also other forms of technical training that can equip health care professionals to do therapy: Some social workers and psychiatric nurses, for example, have technical training in this field.

CHOOSING A THERAPIST: WHAT YOU CAN DO

Here are three more steps to take when you're considering a therapist.

1. Find out what counseling methods the therapist uses and what will happen during a session.
2. The therapist should be able to give you some idea ahead of time of how long the course of therapy may take—five weeks or five years? You should also ask how often you will be seeing the therapist.
3. Discuss fees openly before you begin therapy. Some therapists offer sliding payment scales, geared to the client's income. Or you may find that your health insurance policy will cover all or part of therapy.

Drug Therapy

Drug therapy is a useful aid in many different kinds of psychotherapy. *Minor tranquilizers* such as Librium and Valium are commonly used for treatment of anxiety. Two kinds of *antidepressants*, the tricyclics and the monoamine oxidase inhibitors, can be used to treat people with incapacitating depression. *Lithium* is used to treat

Suicide: America's Mental Health "Epidemic"

Every year some 35,000 people in the United States are officially recorded as having committed suicide. According to educated estimates, however, the true number of suicides may be as high as 100,000 a year, and there may be as many as eight to ten suicide attempts for every successful suicide. Over 5 million people now living in the United States have tried to kill themselves.

WHO IS AT HIGHEST RISK?

Over the last two decades, suicides among teenagers, young adults, and women have increased sharply. Since 1968, the number of suicides of people aged twenty to twenty-four has more than doubled. For the year 1982, the death rate from suicide was 11.7 per 100,000—as compared to a death rate of 7.4 per 100,000 for leukemia.

People who have attempted suicide are among the highest-risk groups for subsequent suicide: About 70 to 80 percent of suicides had previously attempted or threatened suicide. Among young adults, particularly, suicide attempts are often a cry for help that should be heeded. Those who attempt suicide are frequently trying to cope with a situation they find intolerable. Unfortunately, if their attempt succeeds, it is a permanent "solution" to what may actually have been only a temporary problem.

Suicide is 500 times more likely to occur among severely depressed people than among the general population. But people who are not depressed also commit suicide. If a person who is not depressed exhibits some of the warning signs, don't allow yourself a false sense of security.

Many American communities now have suicide prevention centers and hotlines, operated by volunteers trained to counsel callers who need help in coping with personal crises.

HOW TO RECOGNIZE A POTENTIAL SUICIDE

There's nothing subtle about a suicide attempt. It is a dramatic plea for help or proclamation of hopelessness. And often, suicide is not a spontaneous act, but one that a person plans consciously in order to escape an intolerable existence.

Yet far too often no one recognizes the potential suicide's despair, and a person dies who really wants to live. With life at stake, you should know how to identify the warning signs of suicide. Here are some things to be aware of:

1. Watch out for extremes in mood. Suicidal people may be hopelessly depressed and withdrawn from life or so agitated that they can't eat or sleep.
2. Be alert for extreme mood swings. A person who is severely depressed one day, elated the next, and depressed again the day after may be struggling with the desire to live and the even stronger desire to die.
3. Be concerned when people start giving away the things they love. They may be telling you that they no longer have any reason to live.
4. Be alert for a crisis that may precipitate a suicide attempt.

When suicidal individuals feel overwhelmed by external events—the loss of a job, the death of a parent, a pile of unpaid bills—they may feel that there is no way to cope with life as it is.

5. Listen for a suicide "plan." Suicidal people often talk about their death wish long before they try to kill themselves.
6. Take *every* suicide attempt seriously—no matter how ineffective it is. People who threaten to take their lives are crying for help. They want someone to save them from their intolerable situation.
7. Be aware that people who quickly bounce back from a suicide attempt and act as if nothing happened may try to kill themselves again within a short time unless they receive help.

Remember, most suicides really wanted to live. Suicide is preventable—if you know how to help.

Sources: Jan Fawcett, *Before It's Too Late: What to Do When Someone You Know Attempts Suicide* (American Association of Suicidology, prepared in cooperation with Merck, Sharp & Dohme Health Information Services, West Point, PA 19486); *Suicides: Do They Want to Die?* (New York: St. Vincent's Hospital and Medical Center of New York, n.d.); National Center for Health Statistics, "Births, Marriages, Divorces, and Deaths, United States, 1983," *Monthly Vital Statistics Report* 32, no. 1 (April 1983): 8–9.

people with manic-depressive psychosis. The *major tranquilizers* are widely used to relieve many symptoms of schizophrenia and some other serious mental disorders. Thorazine is perhaps the most widely used major tranquilizer; it is used commonly in mental hospitals for patients with symptoms of psychosis. These drugs cannot cure mental illness, and they do not work for all patients; but they have brought new control to many patients whose lives would otherwise have been much more seriously disrupted by mental illness.

Behavior Therapy

Behavior therapy attempts to alter a client's symptomatic behavior without worrying unduly about root causes. Behavior therapy is based on learning theory (discussed earlier in this chapter). We learn certain behavior under specific conditions and transfer the feelings, attitudes, and actual behavior associated with those conditions to other, once neutral, situations. The behavior therapist tries to help the client get rid of troublesome behavior by creating learning situations where it is possible, in a sense, to *unlearn* an unwanted response or to learn an alternate response. The therapist may also try to teach new and more adaptive behavior by changing the environment so that the person is systematically rewarded for developing desired responses.

Group and Family Therapy

It is sometimes useful for the psychotherapist to work with a couple or an entire family as a unit. In this way, the twisted web of relationships that have contributed to family members' suffering can be more easily untangled. Some people who are having problems with their lives can benefit from group therapy, which can give them the support and guidance of others who have similar problems. Group members learn to see themselves as others see them; they learn to understand other people's motivations and personality styles. Certain problems that are extremely resistant to individual therapy, such as drug dependence or alcoholism, seem to respond to the emotional support of the group.

MAKING HEALTH DECISIONS

How Do You Feel About Yourself?

Most mental health professionals agree that one of the basic foundations of mental health is self-esteem. If an individual has a low opinion of his or her self-worth, this *may* (though, of course, it does not always) contribute to the development of a period of poor emotional health. In a few instances it *may* be a contributing factor in the development of an actual mental disorder.

How well do you like yourself? How much do you approve of your own behavior? To find out more about this, try filling in the following questionnaire, which is a list of statements you might use to describe how you feel about yourself.

DIRECTIONS

Read each statement carefully, and place a check in the blank that best indicates how well the statement describes you. Note: There are no right or wrong answers.

	DESCRIBES ME EXACTLY	SOMEWHAT DESCRIBES ME	DOESN'T DESCRIBE ME AT ALL
1. I feel good about the way I look.	_____	_____	_____

	DESCRIBES ME EXACTLY		SOMEWHAT DESCRIBES ME		DOESN'T DESCRIBE ME AT ALL
2. I can get along with most people.	_____	_____	_____	_____	_____
3. I'm not much help to others.					
4. My friends seek my advice when they are in trouble.	_____	_____	_____	_____	_____
5. I enjoy being with members of the opposite sex.	_____	_____	_____	_____	_____
6. Sometimes I wonder if my family really cares about me.	_____	_____	_____	_____	_____
7. I have many good qualities.	_____	_____	_____	_____	_____
8. My future looks very bright.	_____	_____	_____	_____	_____
9. I take pride in my appearance.	_____	_____	_____	_____	_____
10. I often feel awkward.	_____	_____	_____	_____	_____
11. I avoid parties and other social functions.	_____	_____	_____	_____	_____
12. Sometimes I can't decide what I want to do.	_____	_____	_____	_____	_____
13. I enjoy making new friends.	_____	_____	_____	_____	_____
14. I can be an irritating person at times.	_____	_____	_____	_____	_____
15. I usually fail to achieve my goals.	_____	_____	_____	_____	_____
16. I would be happier if I were more attractive.	_____	_____	_____	_____	_____
17. I usually quit too soon.	_____	_____	_____	_____	_____
18. I don't learn as fast as most of my friends.	_____	_____	_____	_____	_____

	DESCRIBES ME EXACTLY		SOMEWHAT DESCRIBES ME		DOESN'T DESCRIBE ME AT ALL
19. I am happy with my sex life.	_____	_____	_____	_____	_____
20. My family relationships are a source of help and support for me.	_____	_____	_____	_____	_____
21. I sometimes behave badly toward other people.	_____	_____	_____	_____	_____
22. I am able to manage my life myself most of the time.	_____	_____	_____	_____	_____

EVALUATION

Now, let's analyze the way you responded to the questionnaire.

1. List the numbers of just those items where you indicated that the item "describes me exactly."

_____   _____   _____

_____   _____   _____

_____   _____   _____

2. List the numbers of just those items where you indicated that the item "doesn't describe me at all."

_____   _____   _____

_____   _____   _____

_____   _____   _____

3. Analyze the items that describe you exactly and compare them with those that don't describe you at all. What patterns emerge? Are there any aspects of your life that seem to have particular influence over your self-esteem?

    For example, if items having to do with your physical appearance—"I feel good about the way I look," "I take pride in my appearance," and so on—appear on one or both of the lists you have made, then you may conclude that physical appearance plays an important part in your self-esteem. If these items don't appear on your lists, this may mean that your physical appearance isn't important to you one way or the other.

    Or, take another example: If items having to do with the way you get along with other people—"I avoid parties and other social functions," "I enjoy making new friends," so on—appear on one or both of your lists, then you may conclude that interpersonal relationships are important in the way you feel about yourself. If these items don't appear on your lists, this may mean that interpersonal relationships simply don't affect your own feelings of self-worth, for either better or worse.

_____

_____

_____

_____

_____

Note that the purpose of this exercise is not to make you pass judgment on yourself. It's simply to help you get to know yourself a little better —to help you find out what personal qualities are important to *you*, and how you measure up in those particular areas in your own eyes.

4. Write a single sentence that summarizes the aspects of yourself that you like the most.

_____

_____

_____

_____

5. Think about what you've learned about yourself for a minute. If you find that doing this questionnaire has made you think about some

rather uncomfortable areas, and if you wish you felt a lot better about these areas, you *may* want to consider having a talk with a counselor or advisor of some sort—perhaps through your student counseling service. *You do not have to be ashamed of this,* or feel that it means you're inadequate. Sometimes just one conversation with a counselor is enough to help you think through your questions about yourself.

Remember: As with every other aspect of health, the smartest thing a healthy person can do is take steps to stay healthy.

SUMMARY

1. Emotional health means a balance among emotions and freedom from unduly troubling conflicts among emotions. Emotional health is defined within the context of one's culture.

2. Physical and emotional health are closely related. Emotions affect the functioning of the body, and physical states affect emotional states. When people feel an emotion, they feel certain physical sensations and then label these sensations in terms of their environment.

3. The key body responses involved in emotions are measured by: heart rate, blood pressure, blood volume, electrodermal responses, muscle potential, and brain wave patterns.

4. People learn some emotional responses by a process of association and reinforcement. People also learn emotional responses through social learning, or modeling, by watching others.

5. The capacity for emotion is a genetic trait. Love and attention in childhood are required for normal emotional development.

6. Sigmund Freud theorized that emotional development involves five major stages: the oral, anal, phallic, latency, and genital stages. Erik Erikson outlined eight stages of emotional development, each characterized by a conflict between the individual's needs and wants and society's demands.

7. One way to cope with painful emotions such as anxiety, depression, and anger is to employ de-

fense mechanisms. Repression, rationalization, projection, denial, psychic contactlessness, depersonalization, and sublimation are commonly used defense mechanisms.

8. Mental and emotional problems occur on a continuum between "optimum health" and serious mental illness. Psychotherapy can help when we are having difficulty coping with problems in our lives.

9. Some of the specific mental problems regarded as mental disorders are disturbances of behavior or of feeling, some are organically based, and some are caused by environmental factors. Most mental disorders, however, probably involve a combination of physical and environmental factors and problems of early psychosocial development.

10. The psychotic disorders are the most severe. The psychotic person has significantly lost contact with reality. Schizophrenia is the most serious psychotic disorder.

11. The affective disorders are severe disruptions of mood or feeling. Major depression involves profound, persistent unhappiness, a loss of interest in life, and a variety of other symptoms. Bipolar disorder is characterized by unpleasant feelings of depression alternating with mania.

12. Nonpsychotic disorders, once called "neuroses," include panic attacks, hysteria, and unrealistic fears or anxieties. They are less serious than psychotic disorders. They do impair a person's full functioning, however, and the individual usually recognizes and is disturbed by the symptoms.

13. Anxiety disorders, in which people suffer from incapacitating fear or worry, are a common type of nonpsychotic disorder. Current treatments for anxiety disorders include psychotherapy, behavior therapy, and drug therapy.

14. Personality disorders are nonpsychotic disorders in which the person develops characteristic reactions that impair social or job functioning. The cluster of traits involved may take different forms, but all personality disorders tend to persist into adult life and are difficult to treat.

15. Other mental disorders include problems in young children, such as depression, anxiety, schizophrenia, autism, and mental retardation.

16. To help a person with a mental disorder, listen sympathetically and reinforce any inclination to seek help. In an emergency, crisis intervention—by hospital personnel, police, or hotline counselors—can be valuable.

17. Other forms of therapy besides individual psychotherapy include drug therapy, behavior therapy, family therapy, and group therapy.

GLOSSARY

affective disorders   Devastatingly painful psychotic disorders of mood or feeling, such as major depression and bipolar disorder.

anxiety disorder   A nonpsychotic disorder, involving a severe and persistent fear or worry that interferes with the individual's everyday functioning and that may have physical effects as well.

autonomic nervous system   A part of the nervous system that works with the brain to produce emotions.

bipolar disorder   An affective disorder in which the individual exhibits mania, with or without depressive symptoms, alternating—sometimes rapidly—with anger or depression.

classical conditioning   A type of learning in which an individual comes to associate an originally neutral stimulus with a meaningful one, then responds to the neutral one as if it were the meaningful one.

cognitive dissonance   An uncomfortable conflict between two realities that don't match; often leads to use of the defense mechanism of rationalization.

defense mechanism   One of a number of mental strategies for protecting oneself from experiencing the anxiety associated with painful emotions.

denial   A defense mechanism in which an individual refuses to recognize truths about the outer world, ignoring those which threaten his or her self-esteem or create anxiety.

depersonalization   A defense mechanism in which an individual is unable to recognize that other people are fully human, with human feelings and emotions.

emotional health   A state in which we are not troubled by ongoing conflicts among our emotions, so that our emotions do not interfere with our everyday existence.

major depression   An affective disorder in which the individual experiences a dysphoric mood, loses interest in all aspects of life, and may suffer other incapacitating symptoms.

mania   A mood of extreme excitement; an aspect of bipolar disorder.

nonpsychotic disorders   Mental disorders in which the individual's functioning is seriously inhibited but in which thought processes are not as grossly distorted as in some of the psychotic disorders and the individual recognizes and is disturbed by the symptoms.

organic mental disorders   Psychotic disorders caused by actual physical disorders of the brain.

paranoid disorder   A psychotic disorder involving delusions of persecution.

personality disorders   Deeply ingrained maladaptive reactions that impair an individual's social or occupational functioning.

projection   A defense mechanism in which an individual attributes his or her own undesirable motives and feelings to other people or even inanimate objects.

psychic contactlessness   A defense mechanism in which an individual is unable to communicate with or become intimate with others.

psychotic disorders   Mental disorders in which the individual has significantly lost contact with reality.

rationalization   A defense mechanism in which an individual asserts acceptable motives for questionable behavior; often used in situations of cognitive dissonance.

reinforcers   Responses from the environment that strengthen a particular behavior, making an individual more likely to repeat it.

repression   A defense mechanism in which an individual rejects all awareness of threatening thoughts, feelings, memories, or wishes.

schizophrenia   A psychotic disorder in which the individual seems totally removed from reality.

social learning (modeling)   Behavior learned by observing the experience of others.

sublimation   A defense mechanism in which an individual substitutes socially acceptable behavior for unacceptable impulses, such as hostility or aggression.

NOTES

1. Stanley Schachter and Jerome Singer, "Cognitive, Social and Physiological Determinants of Emotional State," *Psychological Review* 69, no. 5 (September 1962): 379–399.

2. William W. Grings and Michael E. Dawson, *Emotions and Bodily Responses* (New York: Academic Press, 1978), pp. 6–19.

3. Kathleen Stassen Berger, *The Developing Person* (New York: Worth, 1980), pp. 238–248.

4. Ibid., p. 247.

5. René A. Spitz, "Hospitalism," *Psychoanalytic Study of the Child* (1945): 1.

6. Sigmund Freud, *The Basic Writings of Sigmund Freud*, ed. A. A. Brill (New York: Modern Library, 1938).

7. Erik H. Erikson, *Childhood and Society*, rev. ed. (New York: Norton, 1963).

8. Walter S. Smitson, "The Meaning of Emotional Maturity," *Mental Hygiene* 58, no. 1 (Winter 1974): 9–11.

9. Carol Tavris, *Anger: The Misunderstood Emotion* (New York: Simon & Schuster, 1983).

10. Quoted in John Leo and Hollis Evans, "A Good Word for Bad Words," *Time,* December 14, 1981, p. 77.

11. This discussion of defense mechanisms is based on Sidney M. Jourard and Ted Landsman, *Healthy Personality*, 4th ed. (New York: Macmillan, 1980), p. 214.

12. Washington Post News Service, November 1971, cited in Elliot Aronson, *The Social Animal,* 3rd ed. (San Francisco: Freeman, 1980), p. 106.

13. Jourard and Landsman, *Healthy Personality,* pp. 211–245.

14. National Center for Health Statistics, R. Gagnon, J. DeLozier, and T. McLemore, "The National Ambulatory Medical Care Survey, United States, 1979 Summary," *Vital and Health Statistics* Series 13, no. 66 (DHHS Pub. No. PHS82-1727) (Washington, D.C.: U.S. Government Printing Office, September 1982), p. 21.

15. American Psychiatric Association, *Diagnostic and Statistical Manual of Mental Disorders,* 3rd ed. (Washington, D.C.: American Psychiatric Association, 1980).

16. Dr. Robert Cancro, cited in Maya Pines, "Darkness of Schizophrenia Begins to Lift, a Little," *New York Times,* May 26, 1982.

17. National Center for Health Statistics, B. K. Cypress, "Patients' Reasons for Visiting Physicians," "The National Ambulatory Medical Care Survey, United States, 1977–78," *Vital and Health Statistics* Series 13, no. 56 (DHHS Pub. No. PHS82-1717) (Washington, D.C.: U.S. Government Printing Office, December 1981), p. 113.

18. American Psychiatric Association, *DSM-III,* p. 225.

19. Philip M. Boffey, "Anxiety: U.S. Seeks Improved Insight into Causes," *New York Times,* August 3, 1982.

20. Ibid.

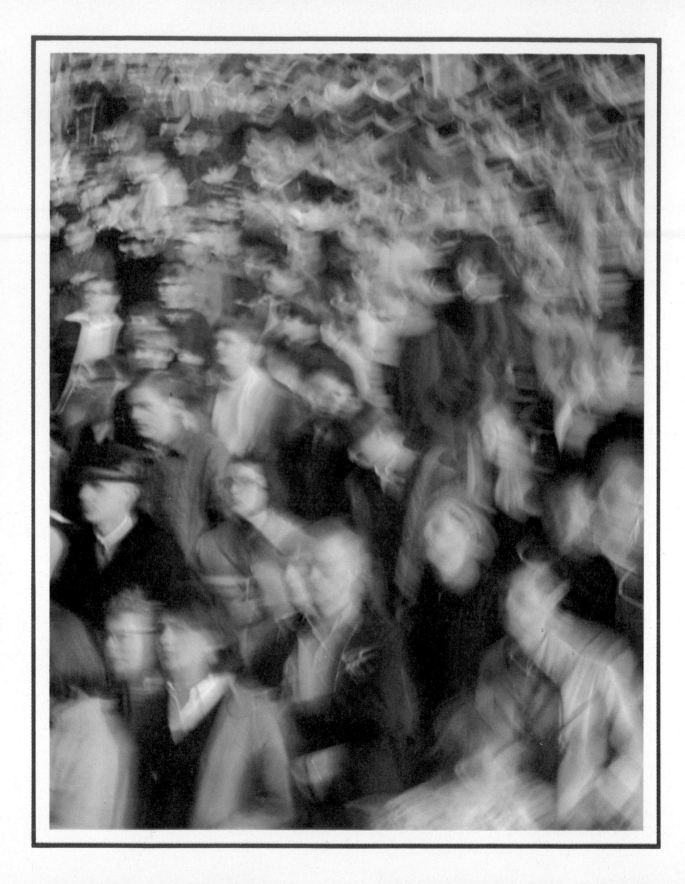

CHAPTER 2

Stress and Its Management

Through the ages, stress has been one of the most paradoxical of life's phenomena. We can't live without it, yet too much of it can threaten our well-being and even our life. Stress has been linked to the major diseases of the developed industrialized world. Stress spurs some people to new heights of achievement; it drives others to alcoholism, drug abuse, mental illness, or suicide. Some people who lose a loved one will die or become severely ill; others will rebuild their lives and thrive for many more years. A student who goes to bed knowing he has an oral presentation to make in the morning may sleep poorly and wake up feeling irritable and unable to eat; another in the same situation may wake up full of energy and jog five miles before breakfast.

THE NATURE OF STRESS

Stress is a term used to describe certain physical and psychological reactions that human beings (and other animals) exhibit in response to any **stimulus,** or marked change in their environment. For a long time, scientists have known that some of the ways we respond to a stimulus are *specific* to that stimulus: If we are exposed to extreme heat, we perspire; if we are exposed to extreme cold, we shiver. In the mid-1930s, however, the pioneering stress researcher Hans Selye observed certain similarities in our responses to any stressor—heat, cold, good news, bad news, winning money, losing money. These *nonspecific* physical reactions— pale skin, rapid breathing, quickened heart rate, elevated blood pressure, plus, often, extreme mental alertness, muscle tension, nausea, vomiting, and/or diarrhea—Selye called stress.[1]

With Selye's findings came the knowledge that euphoria (exaggerated feelings of well-being) can be as hard on the body as anger, fear, or frustration. A person who has graduated from college, found a job, and married within a relatively short period of time may be just as overloaded with stress as someone who has just lost a job and gotten a divorce. The body, Selye found, does not differentiate between different kinds of stress. It knows only that there has been an upheaval, adjustments must be made, and help may be needed.

Stress Can Be Beneficial—in Moderation

Essentially, stressful events—or one's perception of them—challenge the individual's ability to adapt. Changes in our environment encourage us to achieve and can make our lives more interesting—or they can produce despair. We are all familiar with the fact that most people study and learn better under the stress of an impending exam or other challenge. Similarly, athletes and other performers know that they need to "get up" for a game or a performance. Studies of young animals have shown that some stress in infancy is necessary for the processes of learning, sensing, and perception that equip the young animal with normal, adaptive behavior patterns. It is possible that humans need a moderate degree of stress for the same reason—both as children and as adults.[2]

The relationship between stress and efficiency follows what researchers call an inverted U-shaped curve. At very low levels of stress we are inefficient and tend to perform poorly; at moderate levels of stress, our efficiency and our performance improve; and at very high levels, they deteri-

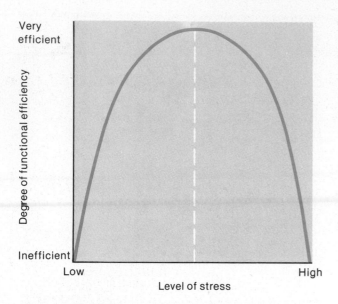

Figure 2.1   This inverted U-shaped curve diagrams the relationship between level of stress and degree of efficiency. We tend to perform inefficiently when we are experiencing very low or very high levels of stress. Under moderate stress, however, we are likely to function very efficiently.

orate again. The optimum level of stress (the top of the upside-down U) varies from person to person and from situation to situation for a given individual (see Figure 2.1).[3]

The Need to Manage Stress

Though moderate stress can be helpful, extreme or continual stress can harm our bodies—as well as our morale. Now that medical and public-health advances have brought many infectious diseases under control, most people can expect to develop some sort of chronic, stress-related disease at some point in their lives. It's not the stress itself that's at fault. It's the fact that many of us do not know how to handle it. We need to learn how to manage stress.

Much has been written and said about stress in the mass media, and we've been exposed to a lot of "information" about stress-related diseases. The marketplace is full of "stress management" programs that promise to help us ward off the ill effects of chronic tension. But the truth of the matter is that *some* programs work for *some* peo-ple. There are no simple solutions to stress-related problems. Most such problems are the result of long-established habits and require a lot of time and effort to overcome.

In short, our newly acquired awareness of how stress affects us will be helpful only if we use it appropriately. We compound our stress-related problems when we do not recognize the stressors in our lives and when we look for quick and easy answers. Our goal in this chapter will be to try to separate the facts about stress from the fallacies. Once you know the basic facts about stress, you will be prepared to plan a stress management program that works for *you.*

HOW AND WHEN DOES STRESS ARISE?

It's not possible to be alive without continually meeting stressors of all kinds, situational, biological, psychological, and behavioral—all the events and changes in our lives that require us to adapt, either physiologically or psychologically. Though many stressors affect us negatively, not all stressors are necessarily bad. Many of the good things of life —sudden wealth, a passionate love affair—are also stressors. How stressful a change will be depends, of course, on how the individual *perceives* it. What may be of little consequence to one individual may be severely stressful to another.

Situational Stress

CROWDING

Crowding is a familiar situational stressor. Most of us have had the experience of pushing our way into a packed subway or bus and feeling our heart rate go up—perhaps also feeling a slight sense of panic. Studies on animals show that crowding can lower their immunity to infection.[4] Urban crowding has been linked in some studies to liver disease, hypertension, and deterioration of the adrenal glands. An unfortunate by-product of crowding, which adds to the stress on our bodies, is environmental pollution—the fouling of air, water, and land with industrial and individual wastes.

Workers in some occupations—such as these commodities traders—are under continual severe stress, which may eventually have an adverse effect on their health. (© Eric Kroll 1979/Taurus Photos)

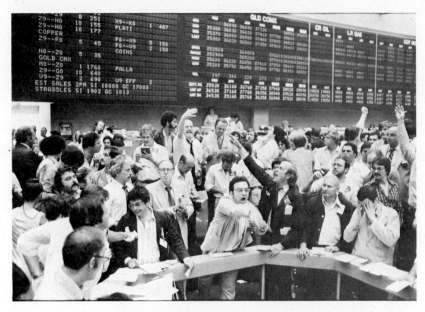

THE WORKPLACE

Many stressors are associated with the workplace. Some occupational pressures are mild—the continual nagging aggravations of getting to work on time, looking for typewriter ribbons, running to the photocopying machine—but some are severe. As one writer put it,

> Workers in manufacturing jobs are likely to suffer serious health problems as a result of the noise, the stress of working at piece rates, the strain of being paced by mechanical requirements of the assembly line or the sheer monotony of the tasks.[5]

Problems of minorities and women in the workplace can produce stress. So can anxiety about promotions and other job changes, boredom and the feeling that one is undervalued and excluded from important decisions. Job stress is so damaging and prevalent that in some states people suffering from work-related emotional disabilities—such as severe anxiety or depression—have qualified for workers' compensation payments.[6] Overstressed workers tend to be accident-prone and less productive, they are frequently absent due to illness, their judgment is impaired, and they make more mistakes.[7]

UNEMPLOYMENT

Unemployment is a significant source of stress. Ac-

The threat of unemployment, faced by these city workers in Boston, becomes a major source of stress in troubled economic times. (© Ellis Herwig/Stock, Boston)

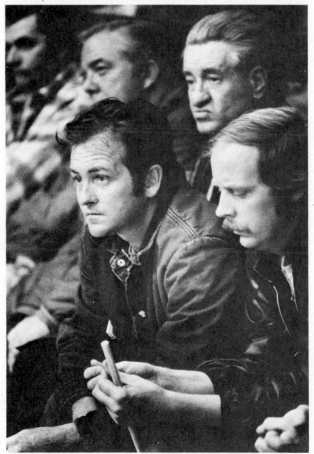

cording to one expert, when the nation's rate of unemployment rises 1 percentage point,

> 4.3 percent more men and 2.3 percent more women are admitted to state mental hospitals for the first time; 4.1 percent more people commit suicide, 5.7 percent more are murdered; 4 percent more people go to state prisons; and over a six-year period, 1.9 percent more people die from heart disease, cirrhosis of the liver, and other stress-related chronic ailments.[8]

STRESSORS IN THE PHYSICAL ENVIRONMENT

In the workplace and elsewhere, physical stressors make us uncomfortable and force our bodies to adapt. Fluorescent lights and extremes of temperature and humidity can put a constant strain on our body mechanisms, even if we are not aware of them. Also frustrating, much more so than we often realize, are situations where we cannot move about freely: Subway or bus breakdowns, traffic jams, and waiting in lines at the supermarket all take their toll.

SOCIAL STRESS

Work and school situations can generate social stress:

> Incompetent, domineering or insensitive supervisors and bosses or teachers create untold stress for the people who must work under them. Social stress can be returned, however, by recalcitrant subordinates or students unable to deal with authority. And as if this were not enough to make work and school unpleasant, co-workers and competitive students often victimize each other by playing politics, gossiping and ruthlessly competing.[9]

Social stress can also develop in the home or among friends. Children who demand expensive stereo equipment, parents who expect their children to get all A's on their report cards, sibling fights, conflicts the working mother faces as she tries to balance home and career—these are only a few of the stressful situations that crop up every day in family life. Dating and issues of sexual identity can be anxiety-provoking. Competition can

threaten friendships. Even casual acquaintances can make demands on our emotions and time. Moving to another town and trying to establish new roots and friendships can be more of a strain than people realize.

Perceived Stress

Just as we can encounter stress in dealing with the world around us, the way we *perceive* this world can also result in stress. We may experience **skill-related stress** when we are not sure whether we have the skills to do a task—drive a car, carry out an interview, solve a problem on a math test. We may have **cognitively mediated stress** when we label something negatively in our minds—for example, when we tell ourselves that we look terrible or that the interesting new person in our psychology class is sure to find us unattractive. Or we may have **conditioned anxiety** if we have learned to fear specific situations, such as riding in elevators or crossing streets.[10]

Stress Associated with Life Stages

Some stresses develop as a result of transitions from one stage of life to another. Childhood and the college years may be particularly stressful.

STRESS IN CHILDHOOD

Children, most of whom are impressionable, insecure, and vulnerable, are especially prone to stress-related disorders. It has long been known that extreme neglect and lack of touching and handling can permanently harm a baby, but so can living in an atmosphere of tension and disharmony—as might be the case if parents are having marital or financial difficulties.[11]

Harsh, excessive discipline and its counterpart, over-permissiveness, are also distressing to children, who thrive best in a relaxed setting where limits are firmly set and gently enforced.[12] Pressure to perform can backfire, too. With today's emphasis on sports and fitness, for example, doctors are seeing more and more children whose stomach pains and other ills can be traced to their parents' anxiety about their athletic performance.[13]

STRESS AND THE COLLEGE STUDENT

Not all adults realize that college students are under a variety of stresses that can make their college experience quite difficult. Some of these are discussed below.

POOR TIME MANAGEMENT   The college experience places large demands on students' time. Students often feel rushed and overextended. Many do not budget their time effectively, do not set priorities for tasks, or put things off until the last minute—and some do all three. Usually, students' problems are due not to the work load, but to poor time management. (We discuss ways you can manage your time better later in this chapter.)

LACK OF BALANCE BETWEEN WORK AND PLAY
Fearing failure and under pressure to meet deadlines for assignments, some students turn to a pattern of "all work and no play." Yet without some form of recreation, rest, and relaxation, we set ourselves up for chronic stress problems.

NOISY AND CROWDED LIVING CONDITIONS   A physical environment that is noisy and cramped (as dormitory rooms typically are) can be a significant source of stress.

FEAR OF REJECTION AND FAILURE   Certain learning and testing situations are a source of stress, especially if undue emphasis has been placed on grades or the attainment of specific skills. Competitive students often victimize one another with merciless competition, and social organizations such as fraternities and sororities can put students under physical, emotional, and social pressures.

PRESSURE TO CONFORM   Many college students, especially freshmen, are living away from home for the first time, and this alone can be stressful. The situation is often made worse when wanting to be accepted by the peer group makes students accept and participate in behaviors that conflict with their established values and standards.

CAREER ANXIETY   A common concern for today's college student is finding employment after graduation. The high costs of college education mean that many young people are deeply in debt by the time they graduate. Even if the student has a marketable skill, his or her future is less assured in uncertain economic times.

Personality and Stress

Some people seem to *invite* disproportionate amounts of stress into their lives. Hurried, aggressive, impatient, and easily angered, these people have been labeled "Type A" by Meyer Friedman and Ray H. Rosenman. These researchers define Type A people as those engaged in "a relatively *chronic* and *excessive* struggle to obtain an unusually excessive number of things from the environment in too short a period of time." In contrast, the typical Type B person is low-keyed, contemplative, and relaxed. (Contrary to what one might

The "Type A" person is impatient, aggressive, and seemingly always under stress. (© Hank Morgan/Rainbow)

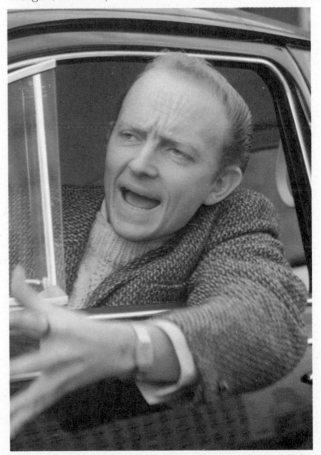

expect, Type A people are not necessarily more successful than Type Bs, because Type A behavior is often disruptive and counterproductive, and Type B behavior may be more organized and efficient.)[14]

Not all stress experts agree that people can be so neatly classified as Type A or Type B. But the Type A/Type B distinction is an interesting one to bear in mind when we look at our own behavior.

Stressful Life Events: The Holmes-Rahe Scale

Certain stressful life events have been shown statistically to play an important role in illness. In the early 1970s Thomas H. Holmes of the University of Washington, Seattle, and Richard H. Rahe of the San Diego Naval Health Research Center developed their Social Readjustment Rating Scale. This scale, now widely used and frequently modified or adapted, gives a numerical value to events in a person's life that have occurred within a given period of time, such as the preceding year. According to Holmes and Rahe, a high stress score —the result of several life changes within a relatively short time—indicates increased susceptibility to illness. The highest rating, 100 Life Change Units (LCUs), is given to the death of one's spouse. Being fired from a job rates 47 units; having sexual difficulties rates 39 units; and changing schools rates 20 units. Note that a degree of stress is associated even with joyful, pleasant life events such as getting married (50 LCUs) or going on vacation (13 LCUs).[15]

The most significant stressors for children are loss of a parent (through death, divorce, or desertion), physical mutilation (such as the loss of a cancerous limb), hospitalization, and the birth of a sibling. As an individual grows older, new stressors take on importance: marriage, out-of-wedlock pregnancy, drug addiction, or alcohol abuse.

HOW DOES STRESS AFFECT THE BODY?

Whenever we react to a stressor, whether it is a physical or a psychological one, an intricate physiological stress mechanism that affects our entire body is set in motion. This mechanism may gear us up to either fight or flee the stressor. Or it may cause us to "freeze"—and find ourselves unable to move in any direction. (These responses are rooted in the early days of the human race, when a typical stressor might have been the sight of an enemy or a menacing animal.)

How the Stress Mechanism Works

Whenever we are confronted by a stressor, we must decide how to cope with it. In effect, a stressor represents a problem that has to be solved. Some scientists believe that stress generates an increased blood flow to the parts of the brain that are crucial to problem-solving or "coping" activity. The brain's arousal level increases; it's as if more of its millions of electrical circuits were "turned on." Meanwhile, the hypothalamus, a key control center in the brain, puts the rest of the body on "red alert." It activates two interrelated physiological systems: the autonomic nervous system and the endocrine system.

THE ROLE OF THE AUTONOMIC NERVOUS SYSTEM

The autonomic nervous system helps control the involuntary muscles of the blood vessels and internal organs. It has two divisions, the sympathetic and the parasympathetic. In a highly emotional or stressful situation, the sympathetic division takes over. The blood pressure rises and the pulse quickens; blood leaves the skin and races toward the brain and the skeletal muscles for fast action. Digestion slows so that more of the body's energy can be devoted to combating the stressor. The pupils of the eyes enlarge to take in more visual information.

These are reactions that can help us cope in short-term stress situations—when we are running to catch a plane, for example. Once the crisis has passed, the reactions activated by the sympathetic division normally subside and the parasympathetic division—the division responsible for "nonemergency housekeeping chores" such as digestion and normal respiration—will take over.

THE ROLE OF HORMONES

A second mechanism, involving the **endocrine system,** is also activated by stress, especially long-

ACTIVITY: EXPLORING HEALTH

The College Readjustment Rating Scale

How would *you* score on a Holmes-Rahe scale? Try testing yourself on the following scale, which is a Holmes-Rahe scale adapted for college-age people, and see.

To determine your level of stress during the past year, add up the number of Life Change Units corresponding to the events listed below that you have experienced.

Life Event	Life Change Units
Death of spouse	100
Female unwed pregnancy	92
Death of a parent	80
Male partner in unwed pregnancy	77
Divorce	73
Death of a close family member (other than parent)	70
Death of a close friend	65
Divorce between parents	63
Jail term	61
Major personal injury or illness	60
Flunk out of college	58
Marriage	55
Fired from job	50
Loss of financial support for college (scholarship)	48
Failed important or required course	47
Sexual difficulties	45
Serious argument with significant other person	40
Academic probation	39
Change in major	37
New love interest	36
Increased workload at college	31
Outstanding personal achievement	29
First quarter/semester in college	28
Serious conflict with instructor	27
Lower grades than expected	25
Change in colleges (transfer)	24
Change in social activities	22
Change in sleeping habits	21
Change in eating habits	19
Minor violations of the law (e.g., traffic ticket)	15
TOTAL	_____

Source: Adapted from T. H. Holmes and R. H. Rahe, "The Social Readjustment Rating Scale," *Journal of Psychosomatic Research* 2 (1967): 213–218.

INTERPRETING YOUR SCORE

If your score is 150 or more, you have about a 50–50 chance of experiencing an adverse health change. If your score is below 150, you have 30 percent chance of becoming more vulnerable to illness.

Note that your subjective reaction to stressful life events can be modified into a positive one by rational thinking, and your coping skills can minimize the negative side effects. This chapter can help you develop these behaviors.

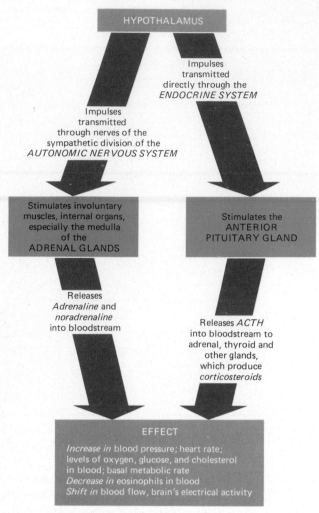

Figure 2.2   Stress activates the endocrine system to increase its output of both adrenal hormones and pituitary hormones.

term stress. This system releases **hormones,** chemical substances that act as messengers within the body and help regulate the body's responses. Hormones play an important role in many bodily functions, not just in the stress alert. Some hormones guide our reproductive cycles, some help our digestive systems function properly, some help children grow, and many others regulate equally vital processes. Hormones are produced by a variety of cells and tissues, known collectively as **endocrine glands.**

The hormones that are more heavily secreted under stress tend to decrease urine output and to raise the levels of certain chemical substances in the blood, such as glucose, which the cells need for energy. They fall into two main categories, adrenal hormones and pituitary hormones (see Figure 2.2).

ADRENAL HORMONES: EPINEPHRINE AND NOREPINEPHRINE   One of the key glands in the stress alert reaction is the inner portion *(medulla)* of the paired **adrenal glands,** which are located just above the kidneys. In response to a stress signal from the **hypothalamus** in the brain, the adrenal medulla pours two hormones into the bloodstream: **epinephrine (adrenaline)** and **norepinephrine (noradrenaline).**

PITUITARY HORMONES AND CORTICOSTEROIDS   At the same time, the hypothalamus signals the **pituitary,** a tiny "master gland" located at the base of the brain, to secrete hormones that travel via the bloodstream to the adrenal, thyroid, and other glands. One of the most important of these pituitary hormones is **ACTH (adrenocorticotrophic hormone),** which stimulates the outer portion (the *cortex*) of the adrenal glands to produce hormones called **corticosteroids.** Studies have found high corticosteroid levels, for example, in men who were starting underwater demolition training and jumping out of helicopters into the ocean—and also in people who were going through periods of anguish and anger over personal disappointments and changes in their work.[16]

The Stress Mechanism's Effects on the Body

Today, the "fight or flight" response is still useful if a physical reaction (such as dodging a speeding car) is called for, or if we have to meet some short-term psychological challenge (such as giving a speech or taking an exam). Our bodies are equipped to handle stress without damage—*if* we are able to relax after we have mobilized our physical resources and taken the short-term action that was called for. After the stressful situation has passed, we need a chance to regain our original balanced state—what is known as our bodily **homeostasis.** Just as our bodies need to maintain a normal temperature of about 37°C (98.6°F) most of the time, so do they need to keep other aspects of functioning in balance most of the time. These aspects include blood pressure, the volume of fluids, and the level of hormones in the blood.

Trouble arises when one arousal reaction is piled on top of another and the body does not get a chance to return to normal. Many of our modern stressors are psychological. We can neither fight them nor flee them. Stress tends to build up and disrupt our body's functioning, particularly through the action of hormones released by the endocrine glands under stress. Epinephrine, for example, may keep muscles tense and the blood pressure and heart rate high for several days, or even longer. It may also interfere with the immune system, lowering our resistance to disease. As a result, we may develop one or more of many different, subtle symptoms without even being aware of the degree of stress we are under.

HOW TO SPOT STRESS

For a quick way to spot hidden stress, take a look at the following list. You *may* find you have one or more of these stress warning signals.

- ▶ Feeling unable to slow down and relax
- ▶ Explosive anger in response to minor irritation
- ▶ Anxiety or tension lasting more than a few days
- ▶ Feeling that things frequently go wrong
- ▶ Inability to focus attention
- ▶ Frequent or prolonged feelings of boredom
- ▶ Fatigue
- ▶ Sexual problems
- ▶ Sleep disturbances
- ▶ Tension headaches
- ▶ Migraine headaches
- ▶ Cold hands or feet
- ▶ Aching neck and shoulder muscles
- ▶ Indigestion
- ▶ Menstrual distress
- ▶ Nausea or vomiting
- ▶ Loss of appetite
- ▶ Diarrhea
- ▶ Ulcers
- ▶ Heart palpitations
- ▶ Constipation
- ▶ Lower back pain
- ▶ Allergy or asthma attacks
- ▶ Shortness of breath
- ▶ Frequent colds
- ▶ Frequent low-grade infections

- ▶ Frequent minor accidents
- ▶ Overeating
- ▶ Increased consumption of alcohol
- ▶ Increased dependence on drugs

Can People Adapt to Stress?

We may *think* we are adapting successfully to continuing stressors, but in resisting or becoming acclimated to a stressor, we are often unaware of the compromises and adjustments that we are actually making. We may not consciously recognize the stress generated by such situations as being late for an important meeting, performing hard labor in extreme heat, or carrying on a frustrating romantic relationship. Or we may think we have become accustomed to poor eyesight, insufficient light, glare, or continuing family conflict. Yet chronic exposure to such stressors is likely to set in motion our physiological stress mechanism, with potentially damaging effects.

STAGES OF ADAPTATION

Researchers have suggested that our bodies go through stages in adapting to continual stress. Selye and others distinguish three stages in a process known as the **general adaptation syndrome (GAS)**—the sequence of events that takes place in the body's efforts to adapt to stress (see Figure 2.3). The first stage is the *alarm stage,* in which physiological adjustments take place as the body reacts to the stressor. Next is the *resistance stage,* in which the mind and body struggle to combat the stressor—or to learn to live with it. Finally, if the stressor is not removed or if the individual is unable to overcome it, the body reaches the *stage of exhaustion:* the body's adaptation energy is used up and the person or animal may actually die.[17]

Marita Frain and Teresa Valiga have suggested that stress situations can be broken down into four levels of severity, with correspondingly severe physical responses. Least serious are Level I situations, in which the individual copes with everyday stress, such as driving in heavy traffic or receiving poor service in a restaurant. Level II situations involve new or unexpected events, such as a job interview or a blind date. Level III situations involve more sustained stress, such as a parent's or

Figure 2.3 Stages in the general adaptation syndrome. The individual's level of functioning increases during the resistance stage, as the body tries to battle or cope with the stressor. If the stress persists and the individual advances into the stage of exhaustion, the level of functioning plummets.

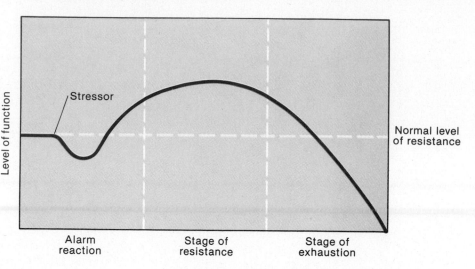

spouse's life-threatening illness; this level is especially likely to be reached if the individual under stress is unable to take command of the situation. At this level, physical responses may intensify and may include palpitations, digestive upsets, and other symptoms. Level IV is a crisis stage—it is usually incapacitating and may lead to psychosis or serious physical illness.[18]

Regardless of how the theorists view stress, the main point is clear. The body's ability to deal with stress is limited, and if the body does not get a chance to return to its original balanced state, the damaging effects of stress may pile up, leading to uncomfortable symptoms or to actual disease.

STRESS AND DISEASE

If an individual already has a disease such as heart disease or diabetes, the increased muscle tension and elevated blood sugar caused by stress can be particularly dangerous. But stress may also cause, or help cause, disease.

Some researchers have identified a cluster of problems they link with "failure to cope"—that is, with failure of the electrical circuits in the brain to come down from a state of high arousal over a period of time. If a person is faced with too much stress, the problem-solving areas in the brain may stay "turned on," resulting in insomnia, changes in sexual processes, infertility, weight changes, and compulsive behavior such as overeating, drinking, or gambling. Sometimes—paradoxically—the

high level of arousal will cause depression, which the individual will not recognize as long as his or her brain stays in the hyperaroused state. Hyperaroused people, it has been suggested, sometimes drive themselves to delinquent behavior (if they are children) or overwork (if they are adults) in order to stay "up" and avoid feeling the depression.[19]

Somehow—researchers do not yet know how—persistent stress can also alter the body's hormonal and nervous systems, creating a fertile climate for disease. Stress can directly affect the immune system—the group of mechanisms in our bodies that work together to fight infection: It can lower the effectiveness of these mechanisms (for example, phagocytes, T-cells, and B-cells) that play a role in our immune response.[20] (We discuss the immune system in greater detail in Chapter 10.) And stress can act indirectly on our resistance to infection if we respond to tension and anxiety by not eating properly, not exercising enough, not getting enough sleep, or smoking and drinking too much.

Diseases That May Be Linked to Stress

Researchers have been able to show that there is a strongly positive correlation, or connection, between stress and certain physical and psychological responses. However, they have *not* demonstrated *direct cause-and-effect relationships*. What this means is that we cannot yet conclude that stress—in itself—actually causes any specific disease. We do know, of course, that stress may affect the way people *deal with* disease (their "illness behavior"). It may make them slower (or faster) to recognize that something is bothering them, and it may alter the way they react to the resulting discomfort. With these cautions in mind, we will briefly review some of the connections between stress and specific diseases that have been suggested—but not yet proven.

CAN STRESS CAUSE HEART DISEASE?

Coronary heart disease is the leading cause of death and disability among adults in industrialized societies, and stress *may* be a factor in this group of disorders. Friedman and Rosenman believe that stressful Type A personality traits are a major cause of heart and blood vessel ailments. In a ten-year study of more than 3,500 men, Friedman and Rosenman found that those with Type A traits were twice as likely as those with Type B behavior to develop coronary disease. In addition, Type A people were five times more likely to suffer a *second* heart attack than were their Type B counterparts.[21]

Other researchers are not convinced, however, that personality differences and ability to handle stress are major or direct factors in heart disease. A more recent study suggests that Type A behavior affects the processes involved in heart attacks only in societies that already have a high rate of coronary heart disease.[22] So the direct connection between the Type A behavior, in itself, and heart disease may not be as definite as Friedman and Rosenman originally thought. It is possible that Type A behavior leads to other physical problems, which *in turn* may have something to do with heart disease. At this point, the consensus seems to be that although stress may be a secondary factor in the incidence of coronary heart disease, it should not be considered a primary factor.

CAN STRESS LEAD TO HYPERTENSION?

Since an individual's blood pressure rises temporarily in reaction to a stressor, researchers have come to suspect a possible connection between stress and hypertension. Chronic hypertension, the sustained abnormally high blood pressure that can be a forerunner of cardiovascular disease, is believed to be stress-related. A number of studies reveal that people who work under great psychological pressures (such as air traffic controllers) and those who are subjected to sustained environmental stress (such as people who work in places with high levels of noise) are more likely to develop high blood pressure than people who live and work in less tension-filled atmospheres.

ARE THERE CONNECTIONS BETWEEN STRESS AND CANCER?

The role of stress in the development of cancer is still much debated. Nevertheless, there are indications that tensions may play a part in the onset of cancer in certain individuals who, due to genetic, constitutional, and environmental factors, may be predisposed to cancer.

One theorist has noted that a disproportionately high number of cancer patients have suffered a devastating personal loss—of a child, parent, sibling, or spouse—before the onset of the disease.[23] Other researchers have found a link between cancer and depression, feelings of hopelessness, and inability to express hostile feelings. It is important to remember, however, that these connections are not firmly established. Many members of the medical community question their validity. They note that the onset of cancer—and especially the patients' discovery that they have the disease—may be the cause of the patients' negative emotions, and not the other way around.[24]

Somewhat more widely accepted is the theory that once an individual is diagnosed as having cancer, his or her emotional state will be one of the factors in the success of treatment. The medical annals are full of reports of patients who believe they will get well again or who discover something to live for, and go into remission (a state in which the disease's symptoms disappear) or recover completely. Conversely, severe emotional traumas have been associated with the reappearance of cancer in certain patients who had been in remission.[25]

WHAT OTHER CONDITIONS MAY BE LINKED TO STRESS?

HEADACHES Tension headache, a condition common among people who suppress their emotions (and thus build up tension in their bodies), is

Stress and Sudden Death

Sudden death from emotional shock or a broken heart has always seemed to be more the stuff of opera and Shakespearean drama than real life. Yet for centuries it was assumed that there was a relationship between intense emotion and sudden death. How else to explain this mysterious phenomenon—the unexpected arrival of death while the victim was in the throes of fear, rage, grief, humiliation, or joy?

The notion fell into disrepute during the late nineteenth and early twentieth centuries as modern scientific theories of germs and disease began to take hold. But it surfaced again during the last half of the twentieth century. In 1957 psychologist Curt Richter tried an experiment: He confined rats in such a way that escape would seem impossible to them, tying them in a bag and dropping them into a tank of water. The rats died of cardiac arrest rather than trying to free themselves: Confronted with what they believed to be overwhelming odds, they simply gave up and expired. Was it possible that human beings could react the same way? The speculation was a tempting one.

Later researchers, studying the sudden-death phenomenon and the phenomenon of hexes and voodoo death in certain cultures, suggested that the individual might get into a psychological "bind." These researchers called it a "giving up–given up complex," and thought it might be related to the overstimulation of the nervous and endocrine systems observed in stress:

▶ Such people feel their world is falling apart and they are powerless to do anything about it.
▶ They lose faith in themselves and those around them.
▶ Finally, unable to obtain help from either the environment or their own inner resources, they adopt a "what's the use" attitude and conclude that their situation is hopeless.
▶ Disease—or sudden death—may follow.

Researcher George Engel found sudden and unexplained death among some people who had lost a loved one in an auto accident or other traumatic circumstances; some who had been in situations of danger or struggle; some who had suffered defeat or lost self-esteem; and, ironically, some who had just experienced moments of triumph or great happiness.

Nevertheless, these connections between stress and sudden death—like the connections between stress and cancer—have not been firmly established. Many scientists are not convinced that a connection exists, and additional studies are needed before any conclusions can be drawn.

Sources: David Lester, "Voodoo Death: Some New Thoughts on an Old Phenomenon," *American Anthropologist* 74, no. 3 (1972): 386–390; George Engel, "Emotional Stress and Sudden Death," *Psychology Today,* November 1977, pp. 117, 118, 153.

usually caused by a tightening of the muscles of the head and neck. The muscles use up oxygen more rapidly than usual, and this causes the blood vessels to expand, which the body senses as painful.

IRRITABLE BOWEL SYNDROME The diarrhea some people get in anticipation of a visit to the dentist, the constipation some people develop when they are away from home, the nausea an actor experiences on opening night, and indigestion, vomiting, flatulence, abdominal pain—all these are symptoms of irritable bowel syndrome (IBS). Researchers have found strong, though not conclusive, evidence of a relationship between psychological stress factors and IBS.[26]

ECZEMA Stress is believed to aggravate several skin conditions, the most severe of which is eczema, a maddeningly itchy rash that tends to recur and persist for months or even years.[27]

MENTAL DISORDERS Mental health practitioners have developed a number of theories about a possible relationship between stress and mental dysfunction, and studies have noted a high incidence of major life events shortly before the onset of schizophrenia, depression, and nonpsychotic disorders. According to one theory, some individuals are born with a predisposition to mental disorders, which surface under unusual stress.[28] (We discussed mental disorders in detail in Chapter 1.)

DIABETES AND PEPTIC ULCER Diabetes mellitus is a metabolic disorder in which the body's utilization of carbohydrates is reduced. It is believed to be caused by a deficiency of insulin. If untreated, it can produce serious consequences, including degeneration of blood vessels, loss of electrolytes, coma, and death. Peptic ulcer is a sore in the lining of the stomach; it is thought to be caused by an excessive secretion of gastric acid. It produces pain and, in advanced cases, can perforate the stomach wall, producing internal bleeding. Both diabetes and peptic ulcers have been shown to be associated with exposure to prolonged stress.[29]

ALLERGIES AND ASTHMA   Asthma is a disease in which the air passages to the lungs become constricted due to swelling and edema of the bronchial mucous membrane. It is considered to be an allergic response to a foreign substance in the body called an antigen (discussed in detail in Chapter 10). The antigen causes the body to produce chemicals that constrict the air passages. As with other allergies, there is some evidence that stress is associated with the onset of asthma.

COPING WITH STRESS

In setting up your personal stress management program, you should begin by deciding which of the stressors in your life are unavoidable, or at least beyond your control. There is, for example, little you can do about the troubled economy or long, cold winters. Then make a mental list of the stressors you can avoid *totally*. There may not be very many of these, unfortunately. Dropping out of school to avoid the stresses of college life is not a very effective coping strategy.

All the other stressors in your life are ones you can do something about. Some stressors you can modify: If you can't stand the noise in your dormitory, for example, you can at least get on a dorm committee and work to have rules imposed to limit the noise to certain hours. Other stressors may be subject to even more control: those you contribute to, or even create for yourself, through poor planning, putting things off, expecting the worst (though it seldom happens), and so on.

Make some notes about concrete ways you can reduce some of the stresses you are under—from "Start studying in the library, where it's quiet" to "Do lab assignments earlier in the week" to "Stop worrying about what my parents will say about my future."

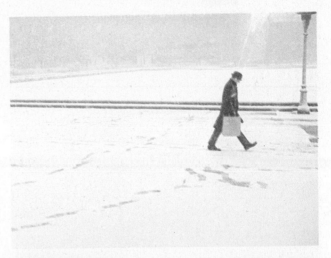

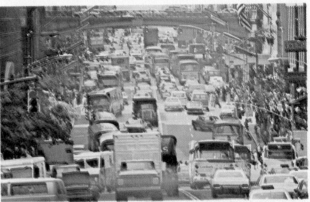

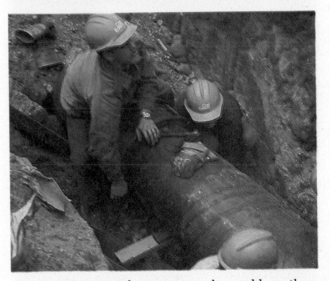

Many environmental stressors—such as cold weather, urban pollution and overcrowding, and strenuous physical labor—cannot be avoided; but we can devise strategies for coping with them successfully.
(© Leonard Speier; © Allen Green/Nancy Palmer Photo Agency; © Leonard Speier)

Some Techniques for Relaxing

DIAPHRAGMATIC BREATHING

Normally, when you take a breath, you probably expand your upper chest and raise your shoulders a little. In diaphragmatic breathing, you breathe air deep into your lungs, allowing your abdomen to expand while your chest and shoulders stay still.

> Lie on your back with your knees bent slightly. Place your hands over your navel. Completely relax, especially your shoulders and chest, so that they are not moving as you breathe through your nose naturally. Let your stomach relax. Feel your hands rise as you breathe in, and fall as you breathe out. Concentrate on your breathing, noticing some of its characteristics.
>
> As you breathe in, you might feel slightly refreshed and alert. As you breathe out, tension is released as your diaphragm and rib muscles relax. You will feel a calming, relaxing feeling as your body seems to sink down into the floor or bed. After a few breaths, your breathing becomes slower and more regular. Now try this for a few breaths: At the very end of each exhalation phase, pull your upper abdomen back and up slightly to push "stale" air out of the lungs (actually, you're just trying to move your diaphragm). Then completely relax your stomach area. Without any effort, air will flow in naturally. . . . Practice until diaphragmatic breathing becomes smooth, natural, and effortless.*

PROGRESSIVE RELAXATION

To practice Edmond Jacobson's progressive relaxation, you should first lie down in a comfortable place and then alternately tense and relax each major muscle group in turn—from the hands and arms to the head, eyes, mouth, neck, shoulders, back, chest, abdomen, buttocks, thighs, calves, and feet.

MEDITATION: THE BASICS

Here are some general directions for meditation:

▶ Set aside a block of time (about twenty minutes) twice a day, preferably before breakfast and before dinner (an active digestive system interferes with meditation).
▶ Take a comfortable sitting position in a quiet place where there are few distractions.
▶ Remove glasses or contact lenses and loosen any restrictive clothing.
▶ Assume a passive frame of mind, close your eyes, and concentrate on a calming mental image, word, or phrase, slowly repeating it to yourself over and over again.
▶ Attend to physical discomforts (the need to blow your nose, scratch an itch, or go to the bathroom), or you will end up meditating on them.
▶ If your mind wanders, gently return your attention to the meditation technique.
▶ Open your eyes to check the time. Don't use an alarm clock—it can tense up muscles when it goes off.

Next, consider some specific coping strategies for dealing with those stresses you can't avoid. The trick to handling potentially stressful situations is:

■ Prepare yourself in advance by setting up coping strategies.
■ Give yourself pep talks instead of giving in to discouraging thoughts.
■ Try to relax as much as possible.

Learning Stress Management Techniques

What specific coping strategies are available to us? In recent years, many people have tended to turn to drugs to get relief from stress. But drugs do not give an individual internal control over the stress.

They just give him or her an escape—and only a temporary one, at that.

The better route is to use one or more of a variety of stress management techniques developed by specialists in this area, which we'll describe below. In each of these techniques, individuals learn to *monitor* their own stress reactions and to *control* them through self-regulated relaxation techniques. Some stress management techniques are briefly described below; for the specific skills you'll need to use some of these techniques, see the box above.

RELAXATION

Some theorists herald the "relaxation break" as a potentially major tool in preventive health care. Relaxation methods are based on "the principle of

▶ Emerge from a meditative state slowly and smoothly. If you are interrupted shortly before you are finished (by a ringing telephone, for instance), sit down again and meditate for five minutes longer.†

THE RELAXATION RESPONSE

Here is a well-known meditation method developed by Herbert Benson of Harvard University.

1. Sit quietly in a comfortable position.
2. Close your eyes.
3. Deeply relax all your muscles, beginning at your feet and progressing up to your face. Keep them relaxed.
4. Breathe easily and naturally through your nose. Become aware of your breathing. As you breathe out, say the word "one" silently to yourself.
5. Continue for 10 to 20 minutes. You may open your eyes to check the time, but do not use an alarm. When you finish, sit quietly for several minutes, at first with your eyes closed, and later with your eyes opened. Do not stand up for a few minutes.
6. Do not worry about whether you are successful in achieving a deep level of relaxation. Maintain a passive attitude and permit relaxation to occur at its own pace. When distracting thoughts occur, try to ignore them by not dwelling upon them and return to repeating "one." With practice the response should come with little effort.

7. It is recommended that this be done twice a day for 10 to 20 minutes, but not within 2 hours after any meal.**

AUTOANALYSIS

Autoanalysis is similar to meditation in that it reduces tension by lifting your mind away from the troublesome thoughts buzzing around in it.

Sit or lie down comfortably, close the eyes, and pay attention passively to anything which goes on in the body. Put into audible words whatever happens. Do not analyze, do not intellectualize, but just pay attention and report what is sensed. Scan the body and feel more clearly what is happening in different places. For example, "Pressure in the stomach; eyes fluttering; right ear rings; throat tight; left foot itches." Omit all unnecessary words and all references to yourself such as "I" or "my." Just observe and verbalize the location and the sensations felt. Such attending brings gradually a quieting of spontaneous restlessness and a clearing of the mind. After a few minutes, sensations become fewer and a calm state, possibly sleep, follows.‡

Sources: *Glenn R. Schiraldi, *Facts to Relax By* (Provo, Utah: Utah Valley Hospital, 1982), p. 11; †Gay G. Luce and Eric Peper, "Learning How to Relax"; **Herbert Benson, *The Relaxation Response* (New York: Morrow, 1975), pp. 114–115, as cited in Schiraldi, *Facts to Relax By*, p. 21; ‡Beata Jencks, *Respiration for Relaxation, Invigoration, and Special Accomplishments* (Salt Lake City, Utah: Private Printing, 1974).

inhibition of anxiety: it is impossible to be relaxed and anxious at the same time."[30] They range from simple exercises to complex systems that require extensive—and expensive—training.

PROGRESSIVE RELAXATION More than fifty years ago, long before the scientific study of stress, Edmond Jacobson, a Chicago physiologist, developed a technique he called *progressive relaxation* for relieving muscle tension. Jacobson believed that in order to relax, the individual must first deliberately "do" (contract a group of muscles) and then "not do" (relax that muscle group). In this way, the individual can contrast the sensation of tension with that of letting go.[31]

DEEP BREATHING Another way to reduce anxiety is through deep, controlled, *diaphragmatic breathing*. Tension headache sufferers who learn deep-breathing techniques often report a marked decrease in the frequency and severity of headaches.[32]

AUTOGENIC IMAGERY TRAINING

Autogenic imagery training adds to the relaxation techniques described above: While the individual relaxes the major muscle groups of the body, he or she also tries to imagine sensations of heaviness and warmth.

MEDITATION

Effective **meditation** produces a state of deep physiological and mental repose by reducing blood pressure, muscle tension, pulse rate, and

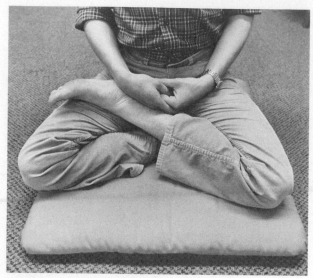

Meditation can be an effective method of reducing stress by inducing relaxation.

level of stress hormones in the blood. The **relaxation response,** a method for stress management similar to meditation, developed by Herbert Benson of Harvard University, has been shown to increase the "alpha" brain waves that are associated with feelings of relaxation and well-being. Done daily, Benson's studies show, this technique can help lower blood pressure in patients with hypertension, and it tends to discourage body tissues from responding to stress hormones as strongly as they otherwise do.[33]

BIOFEEDBACK

Biofeedback is a technique for developing conscious control over involuntary body processes such as blood pressure and heartbeat. Biofeedback has helped some people cope with problems such as hypertension, headaches, menstrual cramps, and gastrointestinal disorders. Here's how one author describes it:

> Biofeedback is not a treatment at all but rather a learning process based on the same principle of deep relaxation which underlies the practice of yoga, TM [Transcendental Meditation] and their Western parallels, Jacobson's Progressive Relaxation and Luthe's Autogenic Training. . . . In most biofeedback training sessions, the subject listens to tape-recorded relaxation in-

structions derived from, for example, autogenic training, at the same time that he is being given auditory or visual feedback about what is happening to one or more functions such as heart rate, skin temperature, muscle tension. Gradually, he becomes aware of state of mind, attitudes or thoughts associated with these functions, and can summon them forth at will without the machine.[34]

Some biofeedback devices are available to the public, but many of the skills are difficult to master on one's own; if you are interested in learning the technique, it will be better for you to do it with professional help. Certified biofeedback therapists or clinics are sometimes affiliated with a university medical center. If there is none in your area, check the medical school or psychology departments of local universities, or write to the Biofeedback Society of America, Department of Psychiatry, University of Colorado Medical Center, 4200 East Ninth Avenue, Denver, Colorado 80220. The society has lists of doctors and psychologists throughout the country who can help.

PSYCHOLOGICAL APPROACHES TO STRESS MANAGEMENT

COGNITIVE REAPPRAISAL Many effective coping responses are not instinctive—they have to be learned. One such technique, called *cognitive reappraisal,* teaches individuals to consciously alter their perception of a situation so that it becomes less stressful. For instance, when a professor, boss, or friend is suddenly brusque, we might react by worrying. "What did I do wrong?" we ask ourselves, or "Perhaps he (or she) doesn't like me any more." But we can, through the use of cognitive reappraisal, teach ourselves to give equal consideration to less threatening explanations. Maybe the other person is not feeling well; maybe anxiety about a personal problem is causing the person to be short-tempered and irritable. The cognitive reappraisal approach is consistent with the time-honored advice, "Don't take it personally."

PSYCHOTHERAPY Traditional psychotherapy can sometimes help control chronic stress by enabling us to develop other ways of perceiving anxiety-provoking situations (as described above) and to gain insights into our stress responses.

Changing Your Behavior to Avoid or Reduce Stress

Another effective approach involves examining your own attitude and behavior for ways of making changes to keep stress—and your physical response to it—at a healthy minimum. In one study, it was found that executives who worked under stress, but had low levels of illness, tended to have a relatively vigorous attitude toward their environments (what might be called a "can do" attitude). They had a sense of meaningfulness; an **internal locus of control** (they believed that *they,* not outside forces or other people, were largely responsible for what happened to them in life); and a strong commitment to themselves. In other words, they took a positive, active stance in their everyday dealings with the world.[35]

Such a positive attitude can work for you. Let's consider two areas in which you can readily make changes that will help you avoid or reduce stress: managing your time better and improving your program of nutrition and exercise.

MANAGING YOUR TIME BETTER

You will greatly reduce your stress level if you adopt some of the "time management" techniques that stress experts have been discussing recently. Time management requires you to plan everything you do carefully, and really get tough with yourself about putting aside nonessential tasks and doing essential things *now.* Interestingly, time management also requires you to set aside some of your ego-involvement in your activities. You have to give up the feeling that you can do *everything,* and all at the same time. You have to stop feeling that you must be at the center of all activities and that no one can replace you.

WHAT YOU CAN DO TO MANAGE YOUR TIME MORE EFFECTIVELY

For really constructive time management, some experts recommend that you take a long look at your values and goals and try to determine which of them *really* matter. Decide which ones represent what *you* believe in and want, not what other people think you should want. Then divide these goals into three categories: self, work, and family. Most of us have to balance goals from all three of these categories. No single category can be sacrificed in favor of the others without producing inner psychological conflict or rebellion. As one writer put it:

> Without an organized and systematic way of ranking what is important for yourself, work, and family, it is easy to get caught spending your time (that means life) on someone else's priorities or wasting time. When this happens, you worry about how to cram more and more things to do in less and less time. Anxiety develops, frustration sets in, and you move a lot faster but still don't accomplish what you set out to do.[36]

As this quote indicates, the most important step is to establish priorities among all your goals in each of the three categories. You might label the most urgent goals A and the least important ones C; all others would be rated B. If you can't decide whether an item is a B or a C, make it a C for the time being; you can upgrade it later, if necessary. You should always have your list of priorities clearly in mind, so that trivial tasks don't distract you from pursuing important goals.

You should also bear in mind that these priorities are flexible, subject to revision as emergencies, conflicts, and compromises arise. It would be self-defeating to use time-management techniques to lock yourself into a pattern that imposes *more* stress on you. There is no point in clinging rigidly to a set of time priorities that no longer apply to your situation. The idea is for you to learn to manage time, not to let time manage you.

IMPROVING EXERCISE AND NUTRITION

New insights into the relationship between mind and body have shown that exercise can be an important means of reducing stress. Exercise helps us "come down" from the stress alert state by lowering the level of adrenal hormones in the bloodstream. This in turn cuts down the effects of these hormones on the rest of the body.[37] Exercise may stimulate the brain to release **endorphins,** natural chemicals that are similar to morphine and that help the individual feel relaxed and elated after a good workout. People who are in good physical shape, moreover, look and feel better, and thus have more natural resources to draw on when battling a stressor. In one study, researchers found that having moderately depressed people get out and run relieved their depression as much as psychotherapy did.[38] (For more about the effects of exercise, see Chapter 15.)

The specific role of nutrition in stress management is more controversial. Some researchers believe that during times of stress, the body needs high levels of vitamin C and certain B-complex vitamins to keep the nervous and endocrine systems functioning properly—but as yet there is no consensus on this question. It *is* well established that vitamin C helps maintain resistance to infection; when the body is under any major stress such as injury or illness, its supply of vitamin C is depleted more rapidly than usual, and it is particularly important to keep the intake of vitamin C high at these times.[39] (Nutrition is discussed in detail in Chapter 13.)

MAKING HEALTH DECISIONS

Your Responses to Stress

Below are listed a wide range of physiological and psychological responses that can occur from undue pressure or stress. Check the appropriate boxes to indicate which of these signs and symptoms you have actually experienced when exposed to a stressor.

Legend: NE: I never experience this reaction.
OE: I occasionally experience this reaction.
FE: I frequently experience this reaction.
CE: I constantly or almost constantly experience this reaction.

SYMPTOM/SIGN	NE	OE	FE	CE
Excessive fatigue				
Urge to sleep				
Insomnia				
Nightmares				
Lower back pain				
Tension headache				
Migraine headache				
Shortness of breath				
Feeling faint				
Dizziness				
Pounding heart				
Indigestion				
Nausea or vomiting				
Constipation				
Diarrhea				
Dry mouth				
Excessive sweating				
Clammy hands				
Lowered sex drive				
Preoccupation with sex				
Menstrual distress				

SYMPTOM/SIGN	NE	OE	FE	CE
Erectile problem				
Orgasmic problem				
Respiratory problems				
Skin problems				
Indecisiveness				
Disorganized habits				
Forgetfulness				
Confusion				
Tendency to blame others				
Depression				
Fearfulness				
Anger				
Panic				
Feelings of helplessness				
Feelings of hopelessness				
Lethargy				
Apathy				
Accident-proneness				
Increased food intake				
Decreased food intake				
Increased smoking (tobacco)				
Increased drinking (alcohol)				
Increased use of other drugs				

SCORING: You can score this checklist if you like. Give yourself 4 points for every CE, 3 points for every FE, 2 points for every OE, and 1 point for every NE. Scores can range from 44 to 176 points. A rough estimate of the consequences follows.

Score	Stress Level	Probability of Negative Side Effect	Example
44–54	Very slight	10%	Rare cold
55–67	Mild	30%	Low resistance to infection
68–80	Moderate	50%	Psychosomatic distress
81–103	Serious	70%	Depression
104 +	Major	90%	Major illness

INTERPRETING YOUR RESPONSE

Considering your family health history and environmental factors and in light of your stress response as shown above, what is the most probable negative side effect that is a logical consequence of your situation? _____

What adaptive coping responses could you use to neutralize or minimize the chance of experiencing this negative side effect? _____

_____

_____

What specific coping response(s) could provide a specific benefit to you? (Note: try to list the coping responses that *you* would choose when under stress.) _____

_____

_____

SUMMARY

1. Stress is the physical and psychological reactions that human beings exhibit in response to marked changes in their environment. Hans Selye noted that nonspecific physical responses to stressful stimuli include paleness, rapid breathing and heart rate, elevated blood pressure, mental alertness, muscle tension, and gastrointestinal symptoms.

2. Great happiness can generate stress just as anger, fear, or frustration can. Moderate stress can improve a person's coping abilities. Very low or very high levels of stress, in contrast, diminish a person's efficiency and performance.

3. Stress may arise from our situation in the workplace, in the physical environment, in the social situation, or in our own perceptions, as a result of our stage of life, as an aspect of our personality, or as a result of stressful life events (as measured by the Holmes-Rahe scale).

4. Stress affects the body by inducing a "fight, flight, or freeze" response: blood flow increases to the "problem-solving" parts of the brain, and the hypothalamus activates the autonomic nervous system and the endocrine system. The sympathetic division of the autonomic nervous system reacts during short-term stress. The endocrine system reacts to long-term stress. The body needs to return to its original balanced state once stress has passed; if it cannot achieve this homeostasis, illness may result.

5. The body goes through several stages in the general adaptation syndrome, its response to stress. In Hans Selye's model, first comes the alarm stage, then the resistance stage, and finally the stage of exhaustion. Another model describes responses to stress at four levels: everyday stress, unexpected situations, sustained stresses, and crises. Both models posit that the body's reserves are eventually exhausted by stress, at which point illness may set in.

6. Unrelieved stress may produce a "failure to cope," in which the brain's electrical circuits do not recover from arousal and the person suffers from hyperarousal or, paradoxically, from depression. Unrelieved stress may also lower resistance to disease.

7. Theories of how stress actually hurts the body are still unproved, but some of these theories suggest possible connections between stress and heart disease, hypertension, cancer, headaches, irritable bowel syndrome, eczema, certain mental disorders, diabetes, peptic ulcer, allergies, and asthma.

8. Stress management means first monitoring one's own reactions to stress and then controlling them by means of such techniques as relaxation,

autogenic imagery training, meditation, the relaxation response, biofeedback, or psychological approaches, including cognitive reappraisal and psychotherapy.

9. Another effective approach to managing stress involves changing one's behavior to avoid or reduce stress. Such changes can be readily achieved in two areas: learning to manage one's time better and improving one's program of nutrition and exercise.

GLOSSARY

ACTH (adrenocorticotrophic hormone) A pituitary hormone that stimulates the cortex of the adrenal glands to produce hormones called corticosteroids.

adrenal glands Two glands located just above the kidneys; the inner portion (medulla) secretes the hormones epinephrine and norepinephrine in response to stress; the outer portion (cortex) secretes corticosteroids.

biofeedback A technique for developing conscious control over involuntary body processes such as blood pressure and heartbeat.

cognitively mediated stress Perceived stress that occurs when we label something negatively in our minds.

conditioned anxiety Perceived stress that comes from having learned to fear specific situations.

corticosteroids Hormones produced by the cortex of the adrenal glands.

endocrine glands Body cells and tissues that produce hormones.

endocrine system The body's mechanism for producing and secreting (releasing) hormones.

endorphins Brain chemicals that are similar to morphine.

epinephrine (adrenaline) One of the hormones secreted by the medulla of the adrenal glands in response to stress.

general adaptation syndrome (GAS) Hans Selye's term for the series of stages that occur in the body's efforts to adapt to stress; it consists of the alarm stage, the resistance stage, and the stage of exhaustion.

homeostasis A state in which bodily functions are in normal balance.

hormones Chemical substances that are produced by glands and that act as messengers within the body and help regulate the body's functioning.

hypothalamus A structure in the brain that produces certain hormones that, in turn, stimulate the pituitary gland to secrete hormones.

internal locus of control A person's belief that he or she, not outside forces or other people, is largely responsible for what happens to him or her in life.

meditation A technique by which a person can induce in himself or herself a state of deep physiological and mental repose.

norepinephrine (noradrenaline) One of the hormones secreted by the medulla of the adrenal glands in response to stress.

pituitary gland The tiny "master gland," located at the base of the brain, that is stimulated by the hypothalamus to secrete hormones that, in turn, stimulate other glands to secrete other hormones.

relaxation response A method of stress management similar to meditation, developed by Herbert Benson of Harvard University.

skill-related stress Perceived stress that occurs when we are uncertain whether we have the skills to do a task.

stimulus Any marked change in an organism's environment.

stress Certain physical reactions that human beings (and other animals) exhibit in response to any stimulus.

NOTES

1. Hans Selye, *The Stress of Life* (New York: McGraw-Hill, 1976), p. 74.

2. Seymour Levine, "Stress and Behavior," *Scientific American* 224, no. 1 (January 1971): 26–31.

3. Clinton G. Weiman, "A Study of Occupational Stressors and the Incidence of Disease/Risk," *Journal of Occupational Medicine* 19 (1977): 119–122; Jerrold S.

Greenberg, *Comprehensive Stress Management* (Dubuque, Iowa: Brown, 1983), p. 16.

4. George W. Carey, "Density, Crowding, Stress, and the Ghetto," *American Behavioral Scientist* 15, no.4 (March–April 1972): 495–509.

5. Lyle H. Miller, Robert Ross, and Sanford I. Cohen, "Stress: What Can Be Done?" *Bostonia* 56 (December 1982): 17.

6. Joann S. Lublin, "On-the-Job Stress Leads Many

Workers to File—and Win—Compensation Awards," *Wall Street Journal*, September 17, 1980, p. 33.

7. Gary L. Calhoun, "Hospitals Are High-Stress Employers," *Hospitals,* June 16, 1970, pp. 171–172.

8. M. Harvey Brenner, cited in Maya Pines, "Recession Is Linked to Far-Reaching Psychological Harm," *New York Times,* April 6, 1982.

9. Miller, Ross, and Cohen, "Stress: What Can Be Done?"

10. Ibid., p. 19.

11. R. E. Steen, "Stress Disorders in Childhood," *Journal of the Irish Medical Association* 65 (December 23, 1972): 609–611.

12. Ibid.

13. Glenn Collins, "Forcing Children into Sports," *New York Times,* January 31, 1983.

14. Ray H. Rosenman and Meyer Friedman, "Neurogenic Factors in Pathogenesis of Coronary Heart Disease," *Medical Clinics of North America* 58 (March 1974): 269–276.

15. Thomas H. Holmes and Richard H. Rahe, "The Social Readjustment Rating Scale," *Journal of Psychosomatic Research* 2 (1967): 213–218.

16. Richard H. Rahe, Robert T. Rubin, and Ransom J. Arthur, "The Three Investigators Study: Serum Uric Acid, Cholesterol, and Cortisol Variability During Stresses of Everyday Life," *Psychosomatic Medicine* 36, no. 3 (May–June 1974): 258–268.

17. Selye, *The Stress of Life,* pp. 36–38.

18. Marita Frain and Theresa M. Valiga, "The Multiple Dimensions of Stress," *TCN/Stress Management* 1, no. 1 (April 1979): 43–52.

19. Ivor H. Mills, "The Disease of Failure of Coping," *The Practitioner* 217 (October 1976): 529–538.

20. George F. Solomon, Alfred A. Amkraut, and Phyllis Kasper, "Immunity, Emotions and Stress," *Psychotherapy and Psychosomatics* 23 (1974): 209–217.

21. Rosenman and Friedman, "Neurogenic Factors."

22. A. Keys, *Seven Countries: Death and Coronary Heart Disease in Ten Years* (Cambridge, Mass.: Harvard University Press, 1979).

23. Mary G. Marcus, "The Shaky Link Between Cancer and Character," *Psychology Today*, June 1976, pp. 57–59, 85.

24. Nora Scott Kinzer, *Stress and the American Woman* (Garden City, N.Y.: Doubleday/Anchor, 1979), pp. 86–90.

25. Gotthard Booth, "Psychobiological Aspects of 'Spontaneous' Regressions of Cancer," *Journal of the American Academy of Psychoanalysis* 1 (1973): 303–307; Theodore R. Miller, "Psychophysiologic Aspects of Cancer," *Cancer* 39 (1977): 413–418.

26. Douglas Drossman, "The Irritable Bowel Syndrome," *Gastroenterology* 73 (1977): 811–822.

27. Dennis G. Brown, "Stress as a Precipitant Factor of Eczema," *Journal of Psychosomatic Research* 16 (1972): 321–327.

28. G. W. Brown et al., "Life Events and Psychiatric Disorders," Parts 1 and 2, *Psychological Medicine* 3 (1973): 74–87, 159–176; B. Cooper and J. Sylph, "Life Events and the Onset of Neurotic Illness: An Investigation in General Practice," *Psychological Medicine* 3 (1973): 421–435; Arthur Schless et al., "The Role of Stress as a Precipitating Factor of Psychiatric Illness," *British Journal of Psychiatry* 130 (1977): 19–22.

29. S. Cobb and R. M. Rose, "Hypertension, Peptic Ulcer, and Diabetes in Air Traffic Controllers," *Journal of the American Medical Association* 224 (1973): 489–492.

30. Norman L. Corah et al., "The Use of Relaxation and Distraction to Reduce Psychological Stress During Dental Procedures," *Journal of the American Dental Association* 98 (March 1979): 390.

31. Edmond Jacobson, *Progressive Relaxation,* 2nd ed. (Chicago: Chicago Press, 1938).

32. Daniel Goleman, "Migraine and Tension Headaches: Why Your Temples Pound," *Psychology Today,* August 1976, pp. 41, 78.

33. Herbert Benson, with Miriam Z. Klipper, *The Relaxation Response* (New York: Morrow, 1975).

34. Ruth Rosenbaum, "The Body's Inner Voices," *New Times,* June 26, 1978, p. 48.

35. Suzanne Kobasa, "Stressful Life Events, Personality, and Health: An Inquiry into Hardiness," *Journal of Personality and Social Psychology* 37, no. 1 (January 1979): 1–10.

36. D. G. Danskin and M. A. Crow, *Biofeedback: An Introduction and Guide* (Palo Alto, Calif.: Mayfield, 1981), p. 196.

37. John D. Curtis and Richard A. Detert, *How to Relax: a Holistic Approach to Stress Management* (Palo Alto, Calif.: Mayfield, 1981), pp. 214–215.

38. John H. Greist et al., "Running as Treatment for Depression," *Comprehensive Psychiatry* 20, no. 1 (January–February 1979): 41–54.

39. Curtis and Detert, *How to Relax*, pp. 211–213.

PART TWO

Deciding About Drugs: Health and Chemical Substances

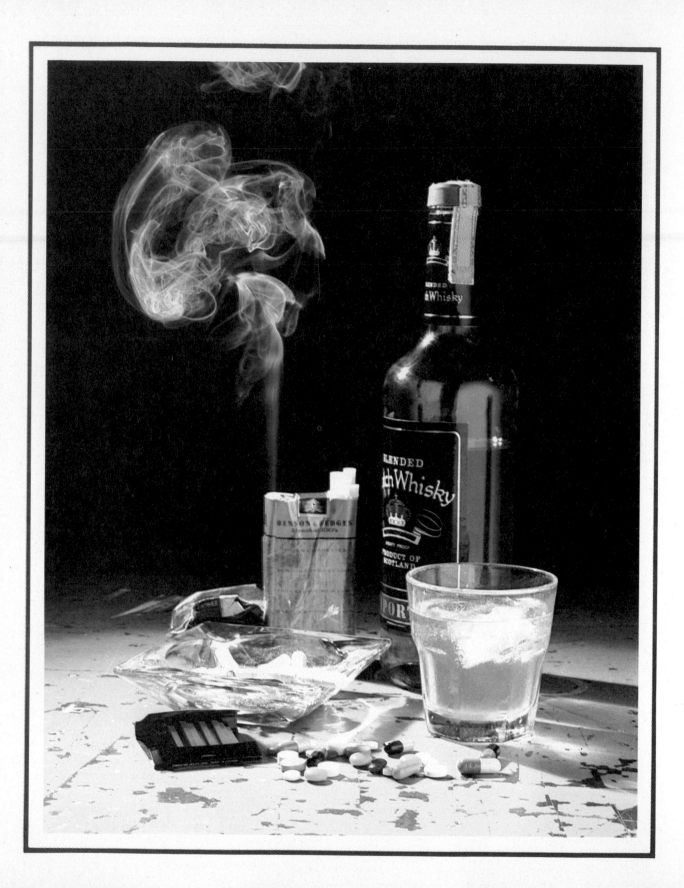

CHAPTER 3

Patterns of Drug Use

Many Americans begin their day with a drug, though most probably do not think of it as such: a cup of coffee, tea, or cocoa. As the day goes on, other drugs may be added: a cigarette, a vitamin pill, a cola drink, or a martini; perhaps—if the individual is not feeling well—an over-the-counter remedy for a headache or upset stomach or a prescription drug for a more serious condition.

The United States has been called the most drug-oriented society in history, with an enormous variety of chemical substances available both legally and illegally. Drugs are a part of almost every medical treatment, and they are widely used to ease social occasions. People use drugs freely out of habit, or to give themselves a lift, or to help themselves relax, or to feel better or not so bad, or just because it is the thing to do. Americans are continuously barraged by advertisements touting different brands of alcohol or tobacco, aspirin, cold remedies, or other drugs. Not only do these ads sell products, they also sell the idea that drugs can provide immediate solutions to human problems.

Not all advertising claims are exaggerated, of course. Many drugs do effectively provide what people need or feel they need. Some drugs do save lives and improve human health—by curing diseases, for example, or by helping to limit the size of families, or by controlling mental illness. Drugs are easy to take, and their effects are often immediate. It is no mystery, then, why so many people believe that "relief is just a swallow away" or why chemical means of escaping and coping are—and will continue to be—so popular.

The question is not whether people will use drugs; the evidence is that virtually everyone does and will (see Table 3.1). The real issues are who

TABLE 3.1 ▪ Reported Use of Drugs Among Young Adults Aged 18 to 25

Drug	Percent Who Say They Have Used Drug at Least Once	Percent Who Say They Continue to Use Drug
Alcohol	95.3	75.9
Cigarettes	82.8	42.6
Marijuana	68.2	35.4
Cocaine	27.5	9.3
Hallucinogens	25.1	4.4
Stimulants	18.2	3.5
Sedatives	17.0	2.8
Tranquilizers	15.8	2.1
Inhalants	16.5	1.2
Heroin	3.5	−0.5

Source: National Institute on Drug Abuse, *National Survey on Drug Abuse: Main Findings, 1979* (Washington, D.C.: U.S. Department of Health and Human Services, 1980).

will use what drugs, for what purposes, with what benefits and risks, and with what short- and long-term consequences. The challenge is to maximize the benefits of these substances while reducing the risks.

DRUGS AND THEIR EFFECTS

What is a drug? Broadly, one could define a drug as any chemical substance that is not one of the basic nutrients (proteins, fats, carbohydrates, and vitamins and minerals) and that, when taken into the body, alters the body's structure or function. By that definition, though, ordinary table salt could be labeled a drug. And so could a host of other substances—pesticides, or the venom injected by a rattlesnake, for example—which might find their way into the body accidentally, with devastating impact.

But most people would not think of either table salt or pesticides as drugs, so we can narrow our definition a bit and establish a specific one for our purposes. The term **drug,** as used in this text, will mean a nonfood substance that is *deliberately* introduced into the body in order to produce some physiological or psychological effect.

Drug Effects: "Targeting" Body Problems

"Take two aspirins and call me in the morning," says the physician in the old joke. But in real life a physician cannot be so casual. He or she must prescribe the *right* medicine for your particular problem, choosing from a huge assortment of drugs, each with its own specific effects in the body.

A vast range of medical conditions can be aided with specific drugs. Prescription drugs are available to

- *relieve symptoms* (examples: nasal decongestants; headache relievers; lotions applied to itchy insect bites)
- *prevent illness* (example: vaccines used against diseases such as polio)
- *control chronic conditions* (examples: drugs used to control high blood pressure; anti-inflammatory drugs used for arthritic problems)
- *treat certain diseases* (example: antibiotics used to treat tuberculosis)

There is also a wide range of medical problems for which people can purchase "over-the-counter" (OTC) drugs—you can buy drugs off the shelf for many minor ailments, from reddened eyes to sniffles to corns on your toes.

How Drugs Interact with Body Cells

How is it that each of these drugs can act on a specific problem? Why, for example, does one drug act on the blood vessels and another on the spinal cord? The answer to this question has to do with the concept of **receptor sites**—the idea that a drug has its effect only at specific spots within cells where the drug molecule "fits." (A **molecule** is the smallest unit of a chemical substance such as a drug.) The drug molecules don't act on the whole cell—only on the receptor sites. Furthermore, the drug will act only on those cells that have receptor sites that are compatible with the drug molecule.

This compatibility (or "fit") between the drug molecule and the receptor site in a cell is similar to the mechanism of a key in a lock. If the teeth of the key match the tumblers in the lock, the interaction produces the desired effect (the lock responds by opening). So if we want to know whether a drug will act on a given type of cell in the body, we have to find out *how much* compatibility there is between the drug molecule and the receptor sites in the cell. In other words, we have to find out the "degree of fit." (See Figure 3.1.)

SIDE EFFECTS OF DRUGS

If a drug acted on only one site in the body—the place where you had a problem (such as, let's say, an aching knee joint)—the physician's task would be simple. Unfortunately, however, drugs can't be counted on to act this way in all circumstances. All drugs have **side effects**—effects that are unwanted and are not related to the essential purpose of the drug. Some drug side effects may occur immediately, some only over a period of time; some are transient, some permanent; some mildly annoying, some much worse—perhaps even life-threatening. Even aspirin, whose purpose is to relieve pain, can have the side effect of upsetting your stomach if you don't take it with plenty of water. An over-the-counter antihistamine (intended to relieve sniffles or allergic symptoms) can make you drowsy.

What causes the side effects of drugs? Basically, the problem is this: Some drugs are much less selective than others about the receptor sites they will interact with. Certain drugs used to treat cancer, for example, interlock with the receptor sites on the rapidly dividing cancer cells and cause them to reduce their activity or to die. Unfortunately, these drugs also interlock with receptor sites on normal cells. Particularly when such "unselective" drugs are taken in highly concentrated doses—as they often must be in cancer therapy—the drug *may* produce more harm to the

TEST YOUR AWARENESS

Do You Know How to Use a Drug Safely?

Have you ever taken a drug on the advice of a physician? dentist? pharmacist? friend? If you answer yes to any of these questions, answer the following:

1. Did you know the name of the drug?   YES   NO
2. Were you certain that the substance you were taking was actually the drug it was supposed to be?
   YES   NO
3. Did you know the specific effect you were supposed to experience?   YES   NO
4. Did you know how much to take in order for the drug to produce the specific effect?   YES   NO
5. Did you know when to take it in order to make it most effective?   YES   NO
6. Were you aware of the side effects produced by the drug *before* you took it?   YES   NO
7. Did you ever borrow the drug, or lend it to someone else?   YES   NO
8. Did you ever mix it with any other substance with which it could interact to produce side effects?
   YES   NO

SCORING

Answering no to any of the first six questions or yes to either of the last two questions indicates that you *might* have been taking a dangerous chance. You'll find out why as you read this chapter.

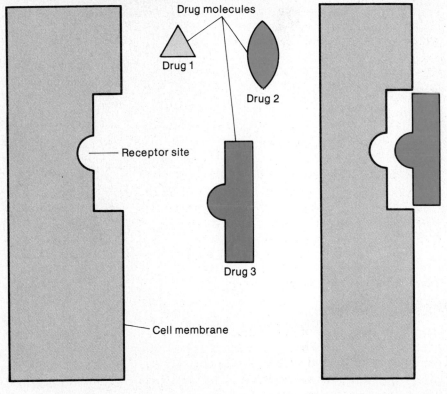

Figure 3.1   A schematic illustration of the idea that a drug has an effect only on the specific cell receptor sites into which the drug's molecules fit. (A) Drugs 1 and 2 are not compatible with the receptor site shown, so they will have no effect on it. (B) Drug 3 does fit the receptor site; *how well* it fits determines its pharmacological effect.

Drug molecules

Drug 1

Drug 2

Receptor site

Drug 3

Cell membrane

A

B

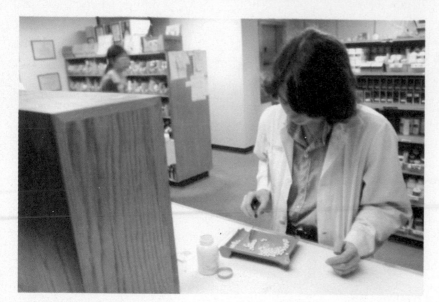

The modern pharmacy can provide relief for almost all our medical problems. But no drug is a completely safe cure-all. Before taking any drug, you should consider such factors as potential allergic reactions and side effects.
(© Bill Gallery 1979/Stock, Boston)

body than benefit.[1] To cite another example: Some *antibiotics* (drugs that fight bacterial infections) can cause blood-cell defects or have a major impact on vital organs of the body.[2] In medical descriptions of a drug, the specific hazard is sometimes designated by a word denoting the organ that may be injured—for example, ototoxicity (harm to the ears), nephrotoxicity (the kidneys), or hepatotoxicity (the liver).

Sometimes, the risk is there but not for everyone. Certain over-the-counter antacids, for instance, contain relatively large amounts of sodium, because the active ingredient is a sodium salt, such as sodium bicarbonate. For some people, these antacids may be helpful and safe, but for those who have hypertension (high blood pressure), the antacids may pose a serious risk of complicating the condition. Similarly, many drugs are relatively riskless *except* if they are taken by a pregnant woman. Although they are unlikely to injure the mother, they can interfere with crucial stages of the baby's prenatal development. Such drugs associated with birth defects are said to be potentially **teratogenic.**

When a physician gives or prescribes *any* drug (especially if there is a possibility of critical or permanent injury), he or she always takes into account the risk-versus-benefit ratio. That is, the physician weighs the good the drug may accomplish (such as curing or controlling a life-threaten-

ing or disabling illness) against any threat it poses to the patient.

DRUG ALLERGIES

An **allergy**—also called **hypersensitivity**—is an acquired overreaction to a specific substance by the body's immune system (see Chapter 10). Allergies to drugs may produce many reactions, ranging from mild rashes to the life-threatening **anaphylactic shock,** where blood pressure can drop so low that the person dies. Allergy to drugs is not so widespread a problem as is popularly believed. With some drugs, however, it can represent a major difficulty. This is especially true when a patient has, say, an infection and is allergic to the antibiotic that is known to fight that infection most effectively. Fortunately, alternative medications are often available, particularly in the area of antibiotics: A person who is allergic to the antibiotic drug penicillin, for example, can be given another antibiotic known as erythromycin, which is effective against many of the same infectious organisms and is far less likely to cause allergic reactions.

In some instances, allergy to one drug will warn of possible similar reactions to other, chemically related ones, a situation known as **cross-sensitivity.** Cross-sensitivities are known to exist among some of the antibiotics, as well as among some other groups of drugs.

HOW YOU TAKE A DRUG

We've now pinpointed two fundamental principles of safe, responsible drug use: Be sure you are taking the *right* drug for the specific effect you need or want, and be aware of other effects the drug could have. This isn't all you need to know, however. *How* you take the drug can make a big difference in whether the drug will have the desired effect.

Which Route of Administration Is to Be Used?

First, let's look at how the drug actually enters your body—what's known as the **route of administration** of the drug. Drugs may be taken by mouth, injected, inhaled, implanted, applied to the skin, or administered through body orifices (as with rectal suppositories). Which route is used can be crucial: The same drug can have a very different effect if injected, for example, than if swallowed.

The three most common routes of administration are by mouth, by injection, and by inhalation. Let's look at them in more detail.

ORAL ADMINISTRATION

Most drugs used for medical purposes are administered **orally** (taken by mouth), and this route is often the safest and most convenient. (Imagine having to inject yourself with every prescription medicine, and you see the advantage of pills and capsules that can simply be swallowed.)

HOW IT WORKS Drugs designed to be taken orally are dissolved and liquefied in the stomach, and they mix with the contents of the stomach and small intestine. This way, they can pass through the walls of the gastrointestinal (GI) tract into the bloodstream, where they are circulated, first to the liver, and then to other tissues and organs of the body.

WHICH DRUGS ARE SUITABLE Fat-soluble drugs (drugs that can dissolve in fat) and water-soluble drugs with small molecules are readily absorbed by the GI tract.

FACTORS TO CONSIDER IF YOU ARE TAKING A DRUG BY MOUTH

An important factor with oral administration is whether there is food in the stomach. The drug will be absorbed more rapidly if the stomach is empty. (The ethyl alcohol found in alcoholic beverages, for instance, has a much more pronounced effect when the stomach is empty than when it contains food.)

- ▶ If rapid absorption is desired, a doctor may specify in the prescription that the drug be taken *before meals.*
- ▶ Some drugs tend to irritate the stomach, and these are best taken when the stomach is "cushioned" with food. In this case, the prescription will specify that the drug is to be taken *after meals.*
- ▶ Fat-soluble drugs should not be taken with a fatty meal. The reason is that the drug will be taken up by fat in the meal, and since fat is digested slowly, the drug may not be absorbed into the bloodstream as rapidly as is desirable.

WHEN MIGHT ORAL ADMINISTRATION NOT BE APPROPRIATE? Some drugs simply can't be taken by mouth: Once in the stomach, they are destroyed by digestive juices. (An example is insulin, the hormone many diabetics must take regularly.) Sometimes a person may be so nauseated that he or she can't "keep down" anything taken by mouth. And some people have difficulty swallowing a pill—a small child or an unconscious person, for example, may not be able to take a pill.

PARENTERAL ADMINISTRATION

When a drug is administered **parenterally,** usually by injection, it does *not* go through the digestive tract to reach the bloodstream. This approach avoids the problems of oral administration: Anyone can be given a drug by injection—even a person who is nauseated, unconscious, or uncooperative.

HOW IT WORKS In this route, drugs are introduced directly (or nearly so) into the bloodstream. The drug does not have to be dissolved, liquefied, or mixed in order to be swallowed, and it cannot be destroyed by digestive juices or by interaction with food.

ADVANTAGES AND DISADVANTAGES One great advantage of injection is that it is the quickest way of getting a drug into the bloodstream—and in life-threatening situations this time advantage can be crucial. Another advantage is that the walls of the blood vessels are relatively insensitive; they can tolerate certain irritating substances better than the stomach can.

A word of caution: A disadvantage of parenteral administration is that injecting a drug requires special equipment and skill. It should not be attempted by anyone who does not have medical training.

INHALATION

Inhalation involves breathing a drug into the lungs. This route of administration allows the drug to be rapidly absorbed into the bloodstream without the paraphernalia required for injections. It eliminates problems with stomach irritation or with drug disactivation by digestive juices. Inhalation does have certain disadvantages, however. Dosage levels are more difficult to regulate when a drug is inhaled, and inhalation simply does not work with some drugs—certain drugs will not diffuse effectively through the lung tissues to reach the bloodstream.

HOW IT WORKS A drug that is inhaled comes into direct contact with the rich supply of capillaries (tiny blood vessels) in the nose, throat, and lungs. The drug is absorbed into the bloodstream through the walls of the capillaries.

WHAT KINDS OF DRUGS CAN BE TAKEN VIA INHALATION? Most drugs must be in a gaseous state in order to be inhaled. Gases such as nitrous oxide, ether, and chloroform; fumes from cleaning fluids, gasoline, and airplane glue; vapors from paints, solvents, and thinners—all these are fairly quickly absorbed via inhalation. The smoke from tobacco, marijuana, or any plant material can also carry

some drugs into the bloodstream via the lungs. Certain fine-particled dusts or sprays can also be inhaled.

A word of caution: Not everyone realizes that inhalation of some drugs can injure the body. Some drugs in these forms (gases, smoke, fumes, and so on) can irritate the delicate tissues that line the respiratory system. It is wise to bear this in mind.

In What Form Is the Drug to Be Taken?

If the route of administration used is important to the drug's final effect, so is the form in which you take the drug.

SHOULD THE DRUG BE TAKEN IN DISSOLVED FORM?

Drugs are absorbed better into the bloodstream when they are *in solution* (dissolved) than when they are in a solid state. For example, aspirin is most quickly absorbed when it is dissolved in water. If you swallow aspirin tablets without water, the tablets will still dissolve in your stomach acid—but more slowly than they would with the help of a glass of water.

THE CONCENTRATION LEVEL OF THE DRUG

Drugs in highly concentrated solutions are absorbed more quickly than those in weaker solutions. (A *highly concentrated* solution is one where there is a relatively high proportion of drug molecules to molecules of water.) Generally, the larger the absorbing surface in the part of the body where the drug is to be absorbed, the faster the drug will be absorbed. The lining of the intestinal tract, for example, with its thousands of tiny folds (called *villi*) has a large surface area—as do the lungs, with their many tiny sacs (called *alveolae*).

THE TIME–RESPONSE RELATIONSHIP

The third important factor, when we are asking about the effect of any drug, is time. We want to know how long it will take for the drug to produce the desired effect and how long the effect will last. If there is the possibility of dangerous side effects, we are particularly interested in how long it will be before the body can "fend off" the drug—by transforming it chemically, by *excreting* it (expelling it from the body), or both.

First, what actually happens to drugs inside the body? Have you ever wondered what happens to those tiny grains of aspirin after you swallow the tablets and they arrive in your stomach? Where do they go once they're in your body, and what happens to them when they get there? These concerns are part of the study of **pharmacokinetics** (a word that literally means "the movement of drugs"). We'll look at some aspects of pharmacokinetics below.

Distribution

Different drugs have different ways of spreading themselves throughout the body. Most drugs begin to affect the parts of the body that are most richly supplied with blood vessels (the brain, the heart, the liver, and the kidneys) before the rest of the body. They then move on to the other internal organs and to the muscles, fat tissue, and skin. But some drugs tend to end up in specific spots. Iodine, for example, usually winds up in the thyroid gland by way of the bloodstream; heavy metals, such as lead, accumulate in bone tissues.

In addition, the parts of the body where a drug will go may be determined by the drug's specific chemical characteristics. Drugs that have fatlike characteristics tend to affect the brain and central nervous system particularly: The barbiturates, LSD, heroin and morphine, cocaine, marijuana, and the antianxiety drugs such as Librium and Valium work this way. Hardly any penicillin, by contrast, ever reaches the brain.

Figure 3.2   A schematic illustration of the time-response relationship. The time it takes the body to begin responding to a drug, and the time the drug's effect lasts, vary with the size of the dose and with the route by which the drug is administered. For example, a drug administered intravenously (by injection into a vein) reaches a high level in the bloodstream quite rapidly, and its effects wear off relatively soon; the same drug administered orally takes longer to reach the bloodstream and to begin having an effect, and its action on the body lasts longer.

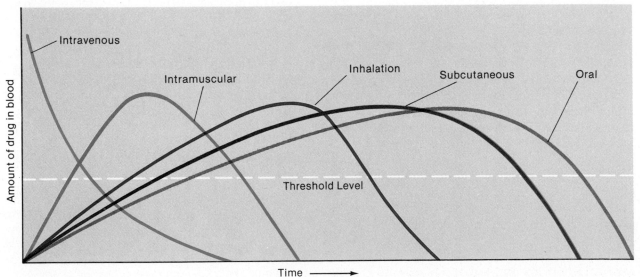

HOW DISTRIBUTION AFFECTS SPEED OF EFFECT

How fast does the drug take effect? This can vary, depending in part on the drug's distribution pattern. Some drugs react with the body almost immediately: Ethyl alcohol, for example, moves quickly via the bloodstream right to the brain because it is fat-soluble.

How long will the drug's effect last? The effects of most drugs that act quickly are not as long-lasting as those of drugs that act more slowly. The duration of effect can also depend in part on the drug's distribution pattern. Drugs stored in fat tissues, for example, remain in the body for longer periods of time than drugs stored elsewhere.

Biotransformation (Metabolism)

Certain reactions inside the body may chemically alter the drug, or **biotransform** (**metabolize**) it, so that it is a quite different compound by the time it leaves the bloodstream. Some drugs, for example, combine with body proteins as they move through the bloodstream, which prevents these drugs from entering the cells where they were intended to act. Others are broken down into smaller chemical components by the liver, the kidneys, and the gastrointestinal tract.

BIOTRANSFORMATION AND DURATION OF EFFECT

A drug that becomes biotransformed in one of these ways is less likely to linger in the body in active form long after it is needed or wanted. Research has shown that heroin and morphine, ethyl alcohol, amphetamines, nicotine, and even insecticides are metabolized by liver enzymes into other compounds. Thus, they have only a relatively short time to work their effects, good and bad, on the body.

LSD, in contrast, does not appear to be transformed by the body. Therefore, it is more slowly excreted and can continue to be active in the body over a period of days. Small amounts of diazepam (Valium) may also remain in the body as long as eight days after a single dose. Certain chemicals such as lead, DDT, and marijuana are known to be actually stored by the body tissues; these chemi-

cals are difficult to remove and are retained long after absorption.

Some drugs are digested in the gastrointestinal tract before they have a chance to take effect. We have noted, for example, that insulin can be deactivated by stomach acids before it can act on the body; hence, it must be injected rather than swallowed if it is to have the desired effect.

Excretion: How the Body Gets Rid of Drugs

Drugs may be eliminated from the body either unchanged or as **metabolites**—the new substances they have become through biotransformation, or metabolism. The kidneys do most of the work in eliminating drugs and metabolites, by excreting them in the urine. But there are other exit routes as well. Some drugs are excreted in the feces. Some are exhaled—anesthetic gases are exhaled after an operation, for example. Other substances (for example, mercury, lead, ethyl alcohol) leave the body in tiny amounts dissolved in tears, sweat, or saliva.

An often overlooked route of excretion is mother's milk. If drugs such as barbiturates, laxatives, nicotine, salicylates (aspirin products) and THC (the psychoactive ingredient in marijuana) are taken by a nursing mother, they are often excreted into breast milk, sometimes in concentrated form. Since this can pose a danger to the nursing infant, lactating mothers should take drugs only under medical supervision. One drug dangerous to infants that is excreted in breast milk is metroindazol (Flagyl), a drug used to treat a sexually transmitted disease known as trichomoniasis. Women should not breastfeed their infants while taking Flagyl, or vice versa.

KNOWING THE TIME FACTORS: A KEY TO SAFE DRUG USE

Clearly, the time factor is one of the crucial points you need to consider when taking *any* drug.

► If you are taking a prescription medication, follow your physician's directions exactly. If the directions tell you to take the drug three times a day, for example, be sure to do so—otherwise the drug's effects in your body may taper off to the point where the drug isn't doing you much good at all.

▶ If you are using a drug such as alcohol recreationally, be sure you know the time factors involved. Know how long it will take for the effects of the drug to die down, and wait before you do anything that requires coordination and judgment—from driving a car to making a business deal.

THE DOSE–RESPONSE RELATIONSHIP

How much of a drug does a person have to take in order to produce a particular effect? For example, how much aspirin does he or she have to take to relieve a headache? If this amount—sometimes called the "threshold dose"—were the same for everyone, responsible drug use would be simpler. In reality, however, the threshold dose varies from person to person. Some tranquilizers, for example, are used in dosages from 2 milligrams to 50 milligrams or more. In this case, the large dose needed

to exert a calming effect on a seriously disturbed person would probably make a person who was only mildly anxious feel dazed and extremely drowsy.

The Effective Dose

To have a reference point, doctors refer to the dose that causes the desired effect in 50 percent of the population. This is called "Effective Dose 50" (ED 50). (Also available are statistics concerning the effective dose for other percentages of the population—for example, 30 percent of the population, for which the effective dose would be called ED 30.) To repeat: the effective dose for *you* is not necessarily the same as that for 50 percent of the population. Depending on your weight, your gender, your health, your overall metabolism, and other factors (such as other drugs you may currently be using), you may need to take much less (or perhaps much more) of a particular drug than someone else does for the same therapeutic effect.

Figure 3.3   A schematic illustration of the dose-response relationship. The drug in question—let's say it's an analgesic, or pain reliever—has an effective dose 50 of 100 mg (that is, a 100-mg dose effectively reduces pain in 50 percent of the population). Its lethal dose 50 is 700 mg. Thus, its therapeutic index, or the margin of safety between the effective dose and the lethal dose, is 700 ÷ 100, or 7.

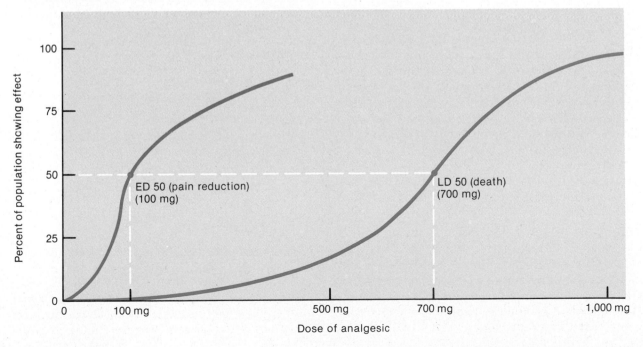

The variation in effective dosages is one reason why people are warned against borrowing prescribed medications from friends or relatives. Your friend's 50-milligram dose of a medication may be right for him, but it may be far too much for you—enough to make you ill or produce unpleasant side effects. (And, of course, you may be allergic to the medicine, or there may be medical reasons why it would be dangerous for you.)

The Lethal Dose and the Therapeutic Index

There is also a Lethal Dose (LD) level for every drug. It is determined in much the same way as the effective dose: Statistical studies on animals have enabled researchers to establish the dose that could cause death in 50 percent of the human population (LD 50). This is crucial, of course, because doctors want to be sure there's a reasonable margin of safety between the effective dose and the lethal dose levels. They refer to this safety margin as the **therapeutic index.** Obviously, a drug with a high therapeutic index (a wide separation between the effective dose and the fatal dose) is safer than one with a low index!

The picture is further complicated by the fact that a drug will usually have not one but a number of different effects, depending on how much of it the individual takes. Aspirin, for example, relieves headache at relatively low doses, but it can reduce inflammation of the joints in arthritis in a much higher dose. In the context of a headache problem, aspirin has a high therapeutic index, or safety margin. When it's taken for arthritis, however, its safety margin is not as high.

WHICH DRUGS CAN A PERSON OVERDOSE ON MOST EASILY?

With many drugs, the potential to cause harm is specifically related to the amount of the drug taken. Overdose is *least* likely to occur with such drugs as anti-infectives—no one has ever been known to take a lethal overdose of an antibiotic, although some people can experience a severe allergic reaction to antibiotics.

Fatalities are *most* likely with drugs that affect the vital functions (such as respiration and circulation) and the central nervous system. For example, many deaths have occurred, accidentally and otherwise, by overdoses of hypnotics (sleeping pills) and other depressants such as alcohol, as well as powerful stimulants such as amphetamines. Some drugs may not be very dangerous by themselves, but if taken with other drugs they can have lethal consequences (for example, anxiolytics taken together with alcohol; we'll discuss these later).

The main problem with most psychoactive drugs—heroin, LSD, amphetamines, and the like—is that they may have numerous and severe side effects. Thus, if an individual is wondering whether or not to take a particular psychoactive drug, he or she should find out not only about the safety margin but also about the prevalence and severity of side effects.

WHAT YOU CAN DO TO AVOID DRUG OVERDOSE OF ANY KIND

▶ Know how *you* respond to common prescription and over-the-counter drugs, and be sure to tell your physician about your individual response pattern.
▶ Know how much alcohol it takes to make *you* high . . . drunk . . . really sick. This amount may be very different for you than it is for your best friend. (We'll say more about this in Chapter 5.)
▶ Know how much coffee or tea makes *you* nervous or makes it difficult for you to sleep.
▶ If you have taken other recreational drugs, be aware of your own past experiences with specific doses. But remember: Reactions can vary from one time to the next; we'll give more detail on this in Chapter 4.
▶ Know the lethal dose of *any* drug you are thinking of taking, and be sure the amount you take is nowhere near the lethal dose.

Drug Interactions: One + One = Two—Or Maybe More

A serious and often unpredictable risk is that of interaction between two or more drugs. Such interactions occur in three main ways.

BLOCKING OF DRUG EFFECTS

One drug interaction problem is that drug *A* may counteract the beneficial effects of drug *B*. An over-the-counter antacid, for example, may prevent an antibiotic from effectively battling an infection, by decreasing its absorbability.[3]

INCREASING SIDE EFFECTS

A second interaction problem is that drug *A* may, by its own side effects, provide a setting that heightens the side effects of drug *B*. One effect of ordinary aspirin, for example, is that it interferes with the clotting of the blood; aspirin has in fact been experimentally used in patients to prevent the formation of circulatory clots. The result is an increased tendency to bleed—especially in people who suffer from peptic ulcers.[4] If alcohol is taken at the same time as aspirin, the effect may be additive—that is, the possibility of the aspirin's having a blood-thinning action may be increased.

SYNERGISM

The third major type of drug interaction is the phenomenon called **synergism**. When drug *A* and drug *B*, both with similar effects, are taken together or in rapid sequence, the end result may be not simply additive, but much more extreme: The first drug may be *potentiated*—made more powerful—by the addition of the second. One plus one may equal not two (as in additive effects), but three, four, or more.

A classic, and potentially lethal, synergistic combination is that of alcohol with any of a number of sedatives—ranging from mild anxiety-reducing drugs such as Valium to barbiturates. All of these drugs are, in a broad sense, depressants—meaning not that they necessarily create emotional depression, but that they relax, soothe, slow things down, decrease excitability and anxiety. When they are combined, these effects can be increased to the point that the effect is not merely to calm the individual but to kill him or her. Many people, including a number of famous personalities, have died as a result of drinking several cocktails combined with several doses of sedatives.

Do *not* take alcohol in combination with a sedative of any sort, regardless of the dose of either.

Even OTC preparations can interact with other drugs to cause undesirable effects, as Table 3.2 indicates.

TABLE 3.2 · Possible Interactions with OTC Drugs

Use of OTC	Ingredient That Causes Interaction	Interacts With	Result
Decongestants	Antihistamines	MAO inhibitors	Hypertensive crisis
		Phenothiazines	Increased drowsiness
		Alcohol	Increased drowsiness
Pain	Aspirin	Anticoagulants	Increased effect
Fever	Aspirin	Oral antidiabetics	Increased effect
Indigestion	Magnesium hydroxide	Irontetracycline	Reduced effect
Constipation	Gut irritants	Oral anticoagulant, by reducing vitamin K absorption	Increased effect
Cough (mixture); sore throat (lozenges)	Iodine	Diagnostic test for thyroid function	Falsely high PBI
Many preparations	Sugar	Diabetic therapy	Decreased effect
Multicontent products	Paracetamol, aspirin, codeine, caffeine, antihistamines	Paracetamol, aspirin, codeine, caffeine, antihistamines	Increased danger of toxic effect

Source: Jill David, "Do-It-Yourself Medicine, Part 2," *Nursing Times,* February 19, 1981, p. 329.

How to Use a Prescription Drug Safely

A seventy-year-old woman who was on vacation in Atlantic City went to a pharmacist to refill a prescription for Synthroid, a thyroid medication. The label on her prescription specified that she was to take one tablet of Synthroid per day, but it did not indicate the strength of the dose. As a result, the pharmacist would not refill the prescription at first. However, after the woman insisted she was taking the "pink pill," he gave her a one-month supply of the drug.

Less than a month later, the woman was in the hospital. She was suffering from weight loss, loss of appetite, tremors, and rapid heartbeat. The tablet she was supposed to be taking was *orange;* the "pink pills" the Atlantic City pharmacist gave her were *ten times* the dosage her doctor had prescribed. "I guess I'm just not good with colors," was the woman's explanation.

This is a dramatic example of how a prescription drug may be misused. To avoid such consequences, you should know as much as possible about any prescription drug you are taking.

BASIC FACTS YOU SHOULD KNOW

Whenever your doctor prescribes a medication, you need to know:

1. *The name(s) of the drug.* The same drug may go by different names. For instance, the antibiotic known by the generic name tetracycline is also sold under the brand names Achromycin (made by Lederle) and Sumycin (made by Squibb).
2. *The reason you are taking the drug.* This is especially important with a "silent" disease such as high blood pressure, which people often do not realize they have. At first, the medication for this problem may make patients feel *worse,* and unless they know why they are taking the drug, they may stop using it.
3. *How you should take the drug.* Drugs can come in pills, liquids, or other forms. They can be swallowed, injected, inhaled, or taken via some other route of administration. Should you take the drug before or after meals? If you are to take it orally, should you take it with or without water or other liquids? Many drugs need to be taken with water to dissolve them or dilute their strength. Aspirin may be taken with milk to avoid stomach upset. On the other hand, tetracycline, a commonly prescribed antibiotic, should not be taken with milk or milk products.
4. *The strength of the dose* the physician has prescribed. The story of the woman on vacation highlights the importance of this information. Overdosing with a prescription drug can lead to serious side effects; underdosing may lead to the continuation of whatever ailment you are being treated for.
5. *The frequency of administration* that the physician recommends. If you take the correct dosage —but take it too often or not often enough—you may suffer an unpleasant reaction or a prolongation of your disease. Be sure the directions are clear. Instructions to "take three times a day," for instance, do not tell you whether you should take the drug every eight hours around the clock, or at evenly spaced intervals over your time awake.
6. *The length of time you should continue to take the drug.* Generally, you should keep taking it until your supply is used up. Your doctor will then tell you whether or not to get the prescription refilled. It is a mistake to stop taking your medication as soon as you start feeling better. This is often true of antibiotics: If you stop taking them too soon, the infection is likely to recur.
7. *Does taking the drug require any change in your diet or activities?* A number of drugs are dangerous if you drink alcohol while you are taking them. Certain other drugs may cause drowsiness or interfere with your coordination: if you are taking any of these you should avoid driving, working with dangerous machinery, or other hazardous activities.
8. *What if you accidentally miss a dose?* With some drugs that have a cumulative effect, missing a dose may lower the level of the drug in your body to a point where it does little good—yet it might be dangerous to double up the next dose.
9. *What side effects can you expect?* All drugs can cause side effects, ranging from trivial to serious. You should know whether to expect serious adverse effects—and how these effects can be treated.

To make sure that you know these essentials, you should review them with your doctor when he or she gives you the prescription. Then you should be sure the pharmacist includes the relevant information on the label he or she prepares for you.

THE PRESCRIPTION FORM

A prescription is an authorization that a physician prepares so that a patient may buy a certain drug from a licensed pharmacist. To be legal, a prescription must be written on a special prescription form in ink or indelible pencil.

The typical prescription form contains the following elements:

1. The *heading.* This consists of the doctor's name, office address, and telephone number, preprinted, and the blanks where the doctor will write in your name, your address, and the date. The doctor should write in your *full* name so that other members of your family will be less likely to use your drug by accident.
2. The *superscription.* This is the well-known *Rx* symbol, which stands for "Take thou" in Latin. It is an abbreviated form of a prayer that the ancient Romans offered to bless the remedy.
3. The *inscription.* This is the name of the drug and its dosage. The doctor will list the drug by either its brand name or its generic name. Ask your doctor if he or she can prescribe the drug by its generic name; it will cost less than a specific brand. Of course, there are cases in which the doctor will have a good reason for prescribing the brand name.
4. The *subscription.* This contains, often in the form of Latin abbreviations, the information the phar-

macist needs to prepare the prescription—what ingredients, how much to include, and whether the prescription can be refilled, for example. Some of this information may be translated into English when the pharmacist types up your prescription label. Some common Latin abbreviations and their translations are:

- ▸ *a.c.*   before meals
- ▸ *b.i.d.*   twice daily
- ▸ *caps.*   capsule
- ▸ *h.s.*   at bedtime
- ▸ *ung.*   ointment

5. The *signature.* This is the part of the prescription that the pharmacist will type on the label that will be attached to your medication. Be sure that these instructions are clear and complete. For example, if the pharmacist has typed "Take as directed," give it back and ask to have the doctor's complete instructions typed in. It is extremely important to have all the instructions for taking the drug *in writing* so you can refer to them. Pay attention to any special instructions that may appear on the label; the common antibiotic tetracycline, for instance, should not be taken with milk.
6. The *doctor's signature.* If your doctor has not signed the prescription, it is not legal.

Finally, remember what the label of every prescription drug must say: "Caution: Federal law prohibits dispensing without prescription." It is illegal to obtain a prescription drug without a valid prescription from a doctor. It is also illegal—and potentially dangerous—to share a prescription with another person, unless the prescription specifically applies to more than one person.

---

① **JOHN H. JONES, M.D.**
1501 Wisconsin Blvd.
Atlanta, Ga. 30340

BNDD No. AH 8741906
Office hours by appointment   Phone: 403-2222

Name .*Ms. Ticia Edwards*........ Date *11-16-84*
Address *1911 Belfield Road*..........

② ℞

③ *Tetracycline mgms. 250*

④ *Capsules No. 16*

⑤ *Sig: one capsule y 6 h*

REP. ⓪ · 1 · 2 · 3 · PRN   ⑥ *John H. Jones* .... M.D.

Source: A. Hecht, "On Reading Prescriptions," *FDA Consumer,* January 1977, p. 18.

Sources: Michael R. Cohen, "Reducing Errors in Health Care," *Alumni Review* (Spring 1982), pp. 11–13; Brent Q. Hafen, *The Self-Health Handbook* (Englewood Cliffs, N.J.: Prentice-Hall, 1980), pp. 119–124.

WHEN THE USER BECOMES ACCUSTOMED TO THE DRUG

Not least among the risks that we all need to be aware of, in order to make informed decisions about drugs, is the risk of becoming too accustomed to the drug. This subject has received a great deal of attention, much of it sensational; but here we'll try to define some terms objectively.

Tolerance

First of all, there is the possibility of developing a dangerous tolerance to a drug. *Tolerance*, in the sense of patience and understanding for others, is a virtue. Tolerance to drugs, however, may mean serious trouble. Here, **tolerance** means that the body becomes adapted to the drug, so that increasingly larger dosages are needed to produce the original desired effect—and this increases the hazard of any *un*desired effects the drug might have.

Tolerance has been known to develop to non-psychoactive drugs—drugs that do not affect mental functioning. Mainly, though, when we talk about tolerance, we are speaking of the psychoactive drugs, which include potent drugs prescribed for insomnia, anxiety, or pain (such as the barbiturates, anxiolytics, and analgesics) and the various drugs that some people use nonmedically to change their mental status—such as alcohol, narcotics, and similar drugs.

Dependence

Often, particularly with drugs such as heroin or alcohol, there is a very fine line between tolerance and **dependence**—a situation in which individuals become so accustomed to the drug that they cannot, or feel they cannot, function without it.

Dependence may refer either to psychic dependence or to physical dependence. Both conditions can, of course, exist at the same time, but we should recognize the distinction between the two.

PSYCHIC DEPENDENCE

In psychic dependence the user who is deprived of the drug may feel restless, irritable, or anxious but will usually not become physically ill.

PHYSICAL DEPENDENCE

In physical dependence the body's very systems have been altered. The body is in a condition in which an abnormal situation—the continuous presence of the drug—has become the norm. If a physically dependent individual is deprived of the drug, he or she will always experience a **with-**

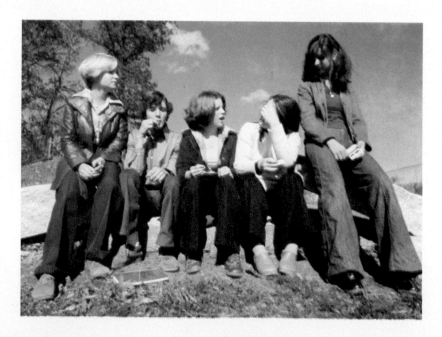

Peer pressure is a strong influence on many young people to begin experimenting with drugs. (©Arthur Grace/Stock, Boston)

drawal syndrome (sometimes known as "abstinence syndrome")—invariably an unpleasant and possibly painful experience, and sometimes even a life-threatening one.

The well-known DTs *(delirium tremens)* of the alcoholic is an example of a withdrawal syndrome. Contrary to popular belief, the condition occurs not while the alcoholic is "under the influence" but after the effects of the alcohol have worn off. The unfortunate victim may suffer nausea and vomiting, tremors, hallucinations, and convulsions.

In withdrawal from heroin there may also be nausea and vomiting, as well as a runny nose, sweating, fever, racing pulse, heightened blood pressure, tremors, joint and muscle pains, and other signs and symptoms. Many of these same symptoms may occur in withdrawal from barbiturates. In fact, barbiturate withdrawal is one of the most dangerous forms of withdrawal.

DO ALL THREE FORMS OF DEPENDENCE DEVELOP TOGETHER?

It should be noted that these three phenomena—tolerance, psychic dependence, and physical dependence—can operate quite separately.

- With caffeine or tobacco, for example, tolerance is not likely to develop. Psychic dependence is quite common with these drugs, though, and some people seem to develop physical dependence as well.
- With cocaine or marijuana, tolerance and physical dependence may develop, and psychic dependence occurs frequently.
- With barbiturates, there is comparatively small tolerance—and essentially *no* tolerance to lethal doses—but there is still a high risk of physical dependence.
- With heroin, many users have a pattern of tolerance–psychic dependence–physical dependence. Nevertheless, some users have been known to restrict their use for long periods to small doses—essentially developing both psychic and physical dependence, but never developing the tolerance that requires increased dosages.

ADDICTION AND HABITUATION

What, you may have been wondering, is a "drug addict"? Does this term refer to a person who has

developed a physical dependence, or at least psychic dependence, as described above? *Addiction* is a term that has received mixed usage by professionals, in part because it has come to imply criminality and other socially value-laden ideas. Some experts use the term **addiction** when they want to emphasize a compulsive quality in an individual's use of a drug or drugs. This pattern is marked both by tolerance (a tendency to increase the dose) and by psychic and physical dependence.[5]

Habituation, another term that's less commonly used today (many professionals prefer to use *psychic dependence*), also involves the idea of compulsive drug use. It usually refers to the compulsive use of a drug for the sense of well-being it gives the individual. A person who is habituated to a drug usually has little or no tendency to increase the dose.

How Do People Become Dependent on Drugs?

Dependence can develop both with drugs used medically and with those, such as alcohol and marijuana, that are taken from the start for purely recreational or social purposes. With either, the individual gets trapped in the pattern in essentially the same way.

RELIEF OF DISCOMFORT: ONE ROUTE TO DEPENDENCE

Whether physician-prescribed or self-"prescribed," drugs are sometimes taken to relieve an uncomfortable condition such as physical pain or anxiety (which may be general, or may relate to a specific situation). Let's take as an example a runner who has torn a leg muscle and is waiting for it to heal. She may have a drug that has been prescribed by her physician, to be used at her discretion for pain. (Let's say it is a compound that contains an opiate among other ingredients.) She has almost undoubtedly been warned that the medication is potentially addictive—and that she should use a minimum amount of it, and only when the pain becomes intolerable.

If the patient follows those instructions, fine. But she may deviate from them in either of two ways, and either one may lead to dependence:

- If the drug acts very quickly to banish the pain, she may unconsciously begin to lower her level of "intolerable" pain. Remembering what the welcome rush of relief feels like, she may begin to take the medication for lower and lower pain levels—in other words, more and more often. (This pattern is less likely to develop with a drug that acts more slowly.)
- Or, the patient may reason as follows: Since the drug creates a pain-free state, why not *anticipate* the recurrence of pain and take the drug ahead of time, thus avoiding the discomfort entirely? This pattern may be mentally reinforced as the patient recalls the experience of pain, which itself may create additional anxiety. Now she is on an "avoidance schedule," which can lead rather quickly to regular but unnecessary use of the drug, vastly increasing her chance of developing both psychic and physical dependence.

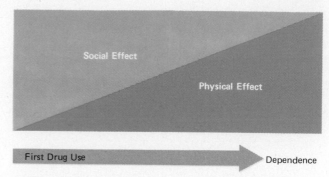

Figure 3.4 The first use of a drug is usually experimental—the result of peer pressure or other social forces. As use continues and dependence increases, the person becomes more and more involved with the physical effect of the drug and less and less concerned with its social aspect.

Replace the word *pain* with *anxiety* or *depression* or just plain *nervousness* in the preceding paragraph, and it is clear how this pattern can develop with an antianxiety drug, alcohol, heroin, or any other substance that promises relief from unpleasant feelings.

LEVELS OF DRUG USE

Not everyone who uses a drug a few times, of course, is doomed to a destructive dependency. There are actually several levels of nonmedical drug use. Whether a person is likely to develop a drug dependency depends in part on which of these patterns he or she tends to follow.

Here are the levels, in more or less chronological order:

1. *Experimental use:* The individual "samples" a drug, typically in social situations, but uses it only very occasionally or infrequently. At this level, the risk of dependence is usually low.
2. *Recreational use:* The individual uses modest amounts of a drug in a social setting where such use is accepted or even expected. The widespread use of alcohol and marijuana in this country, as well as the use of cocaine in some circles, typifies recreational use. Such use occurs when the drug is commonly provided and its use commonly accepted as part of the social events or gatherings in which the individual generally participates. The individual's level of use, in these circumstances, reflects that of his or her social stratum or milieu. Again, the risk of dependence is relatively low.
3. *Situational use:* The individual deliberately uses a drug in order to experience effects that he or she sees as beneficial in a particular situation or under certain circumstances. There need be no one else present—in contrast to recreational use, which involves social settings. At this level, the risk of dependence may be considerable, depending on the situation, frequency, and particular drug used.
4. *Intensified use:* The individual uses a drug regularly, over a period of time, to reduce perceived physical, psychological, or social discomfort, with a distinct deviation from the pattern of use prevailing in the individual's social milieu. The frequency of use generally increases and becomes self-reinforcing, and—depending on whether tolerance occurs—the amount of the drug the individual uses may also increase. The risk that dependence may develop is usually high.
5. *Compulsive use:* In this dependence pattern, tolerance has often developed. The drug has become *less* able to produce the anticipated pleasure or relief from discomfort, and the individual has become preoccupied with obtaining and using the drug. At this stage, normal functioning is

markedly impaired. The individual's social relationships are superficial, he or she usually develops some degree of physical debilitation, and vocational or academic pursuits are markedly imperiled or totally abandoned. There is, at this point, a critical risk to the individual's physical and emotional health.[6]

SOCIETY'S CONCERNS AND THE LAW

It may be that—at least among adults—the use of certain drugs is accepted and indeed viewed as "normal" and unlikely to impair the functioning of most individuals. Nevertheless, some areas of legitimate concern are clearly within society's realm of jurisdiction. Even the most outspoken libertarian would not object to some degree of regulation in these areas pertaining to drug use.

The Role of the FDA

As we've seen, drugs can be dangerous. That's why some are available only by prescription. And even over-the-counter drugs—familiar sights in every drugstore—are closely monitored and regulated by governmental agencies. Control of drugs marketed in this country is the legal responsibility of the Food and Drug Administration (FDA).

DRUG CATEGORIES: PRESCRIPTION VERSUS OTC

The FDA decides whether a drug will be sold by prescription or OTC. By and large, those drugs the FDA designates as OTCs are most likely to be symptom relievers: the drugs that act on such problems as headaches, itches, coughs, and stuffy noses. There is an exception: The more potent or potentially dependence-producing painkillers and sedatives are *not* available OTC.

Those drugs the FDA allows to be sold only by prescription are likely to be more powerful drugs with major impact on body systems and organs. For these drugs, dosage must be carefully established and monitored by the doctor for each patient.

OTHER FDA FUNCTIONS

The FDA has the right to decide whether a new drug is to be available at all. The FDA also checks the accuracy of drug advertising in medical journals and other professional media. It may confiscate or recall a drug that is found to be unduly hazardous, misleadingly labeled, or manufactured or handled improperly. It also reviews all drugs to determine their safety and effectiveness. In 1972 the agency began reviewing more than two dozen categories of OTC drugs—a massive task that involves hundreds of thousands of products and is expected to be completed in the mid-1980s.

Attempts to Control Use of Psychoactive Drugs

Most people in our society agree that psychoactive drugs, including alcohol, pose *some* dangers that should be dealt with by government. For example, there is substantial evidence that some drugs used even in moderate amounts may impair the physical and psychological development of children and adolescents. The government has regulated the use of alcohol for this reason; alcohol may legally be sold only to adults. Some people have suggested similar regulations for marijuana.

Another widely recognized problem is the control of illegal drug distribution by organized crime. That control, particularly of heroin, has driven many drug-dependent individuals to commit robberies, burglaries, and other crimes to obtain cash for the drugs they need. Many solutions to this extremely serious problem have been suggested, ranging from enforced drug withdrawal for those apprehended to free heroin for dependent individuals.

Aside from these two relatively clear-cut issues, however, there is much disagreement about the regulation of many drugs—notably widely used ones such as marijuana and cocaine. Even those who are knowledgeable about the legal and moral questions involved frequently express conflicting views. At present, it is difficult for even the most well-informed individual to reach a conclusion on the benefits versus the risks of such drugs. In the next chapter, we'll summarize the known facts about these and other specific drugs.

MAKING HEALTH DECISIONS

Does Your Lifestyle Invite Drug Dependence?

Are your the type of person who is likely to become dependent on a drug? The answer depends, in part, on your lifestyle. To get some indication of the extent to which your health behaviors contribute to a drug-free lifestyle, try completing the following scale.

DIRECTIONS: Next to each of the following statements, place a check mark in the blank that most closely applies to you.

	MOST LIKE ME		UNDECIDED		MOST UNLIKE ME
1. I prefer to socialize with friends who do not use drugs.	_____	_____	_____	_____	_____
2. I engage in regular exercise for relaxation.	_____	_____	_____	_____	_____
3. I maintain good habits of diet and nutrition.	_____	_____	_____	_____	_____
4. I enjoy responsible sexuality.	_____	_____	_____	_____	_____
5. I feel competent in college work.	_____	_____	_____	_____	_____
6. I make friends easily and enjoy lasting friendships.	_____	_____	_____	_____	_____
7. I prefer natural highs to chemical highs.	_____	_____	_____	_____	_____
8. I am able to manage the stress in my life.	_____	_____	_____	_____	_____
9. I am happy most of the time.	_____	_____	_____	_____	_____
10. I belong to a goal-directed social group.	_____	_____	_____	_____	_____
11. I engage in creative hobbies and games.	_____	_____	_____	_____	_____
12. I enjoy intellectual conversation and reading.	_____	_____	_____	_____	_____
13. I practice responsible citizenship.	_____	_____	_____	_____	_____
14. I am concerned about environmental conservation.	_____	_____	_____	_____	_____
15. I act as a responsible consumer of health products and services.	_____	_____	_____	_____	_____
16. I attend workshops and seminars on social issues.	_____	_____	_____	_____	_____
17. I am looking forward to a challenging career.	_____	_____	_____	_____	_____

	MOST LIKE ME		UNDECIDED		MOST UNLIKE ME
18. I am proud of my race, nationality, or religion.	_____	_____	_____	_____	_____
19. I have a set of goals for my life.	_____	_____	_____	_____	_____
20. I am happy with my lifestyle.	_____	_____	_____	_____	_____

SCORING

Give yourself a 5 for every check mark you made under "Most Like Me," a 4 for every check mark in the next row of blanks, and so on down to 1 for every check mark under "Most Unlike Me." Add up your score. A score above 75 indicates a lifestyle that is more likely to be drug-free. A score below 50 may indicate a lifestyle that is less likely to remain drug-free.

The next step is: If you have scored below 50, you may decide that you want to change the way you live to some extent—in order to be less susceptible to drug problems or for other reasons.

Do any items in the above list suggest areas that you would like to explore more fully?

List them here. _____
_____
_____

What major changes would have to take place in your life in order for you to explore these areas? Check the ones that apply, and indicate whether the change would be relatively easy, moderately easy, or relatively difficult to accomplish.

	EASY	MODERATELY EASY	RELATIVELY DIFFICULT
_____ I might have to drop most of my friends and make a whole set of new friends.	_____	_____	_____
_____ I might have to go against patterns that are prevalent and accepted in my family or ethnic group.	_____	_____	_____
_____ I might have to drop a lot of my present activities and school or work assignments in order to find time to make this change.	_____	_____	_____
_____ I might have to get some information that isn't readily available to me now.	_____	_____	_____
_____ I might have to talk to a friend, a religious leader, or a guidance counselor.	_____	_____	_____
_____ I might have to move to another dormitory/apartment/house.	_____	_____	_____
_____ I might have to change colleges/jobs.	_____	_____	_____
_____ I might have to move to another town/neighborhood.	_____	_____	_____

Will it be worthwhile to make these changes? The answer is up to you.

SUMMARY

1. A drug may be defined as any nonfood substance that is deliberately introduced into the body in order to produce some physical or psychological effect.

2. Prescription drugs can relieve symptoms, prevent illness, control chronic conditions, or treat certain diseases. Other drugs, available without prescription, are called over-the-counter (OTC) drugs.

3. Drugs can act on specific parts of the body because their molecules "fit" with certain receptor sites in the body. When a drug works adversely on parts of the body other than the intended receptor sites—and all drugs do to some extent—it produces side effects. Some drugs are likelier than others to produce side effects. Side effects may or may not be serious and may affect some people and not others. A prescribing physician must take into account the relative risks and benefits of any drug for each patient.

4. Drug allergies are one kind of side effect. They range in seriousness from mild to life-threatening. A person who is allergic to one drug may also be allergic to chemically related drugs, a tendency called cross-sensitivity.

5. Drugs may enter the body via a number of routes of administration: by mouth or other orifices, injection, inhalation, implantation, or skin contact. Drugs taken orally dissolve in the stomach and pass into the bloodstream through the intestinal walls. Injected (parenterally administered) drugs enter the bloodstream directly, or nearly so, and more rapidly than with other methods of administration. Inhalation also quickly introduces a drug, usually in the form of a gas or fine spray, through the lungs into the bloodstream.

6. Pharmacokinetics is the study of what happens to drugs once they enter the body—their distribution within the body, their biotransformation, and their excretion. As to distribution, most drugs first affect the body parts most richly supplied with blood vessels and then move to other organs and to muscles, fat tissues, and skin. Some drugs tend to end up in specific spots: iodine in the thyroid gland; lead in the bones; antianxiety drugs and many psychoactive drugs in the brain and central nervous system. The distribution patterns of drugs influence how quickly they take effect and how long their effects last.

7. Some drugs do not change chemically in the body, but others are biotransformed (metabolized) into chemically new substances, or metabolites.

8. Drugs and metabolites may be excreted in urine or feces, exhaled, or secreted in sweat, tears, saliva, or mothers' milk.

9. The relationship between how much of a drug is taken and the effects that drug has is different for every person. The threshold dose is the amount of a drug necessary to produce an intended effect. A dose that causes the intended effect in 50 percent of the population is called the Effective Dose 50 (ED 50). The lethal dose—LD 50—is the amount of a drug that could be deadly for 50 percent of the population. The safety margin between the lethal dose and the effective dose is known as the therapeutic index.

10. Drugs may act together in several ways. One drug may block the effects of another. One drug's side effects may intensify the side effects of another. Synergism may occur, meaning that one drug may potentiate another, intensifying its effects. A classic, and possibly deadly, synergistic combination is alcohol and sedatives.

11. An individual may become physically or psychologically accustomed to drugs. He or she may develop tolerance for a drug, needing larger and larger doses to produce the original effect. Tolerance may develop into dependence, a feeling that the person cannot function without the drug. An indication that a person has a physical, as opposed to a psychic, dependence on a drug is that deprivation of the drug produces a withdrawal syndrome.

12. *Addiction* refers to a pattern of compulsive drug use, marked both by tolerance and by psychic and physical dependence. *Habituation* is the term used to describe compulsive drug use that arises from psychic dependence but does not usually involve tolerance.

13. A person's level of nonmedical drug use may fall into one of a number of patterns, in rough order of increasing dependence: experimental, recreational, situational, intensified, or compulsive.

14. The legal control of drugs in the United States is the responsibility of the Food and Drug Administration (FDA). The FDA determines

whether drugs are to be sold by prescription or over the counter and whether a new drug can be marketed. It checks the accuracy of drug advertisements, recalls hazardous or misleadingly labeled drugs, and reviews the safety and effectiveness of drugs.

15. Of all the legal and moral issues related to drugs, most people agree on two: Some drugs are dangerous enough to be restricted to adults, and society must try to end organized crime's control over the distribution of illegal drugs.

GLOSSARY

addiction A compulsive pattern of drug use, marked both by tolerance and by psychic and physical dependence. Compare **habituation.**

allergy (hypersensitivity) An acquired overreaction to a specific substance by the body's immune system.

anaphylactic shock A life-threatening allergic reaction in which blood pressure can drop so low that the person dies.

biotransformation (metabolism) The process by which reactions inside the body change chemical substances, such as drugs, into different compounds.

cross-sensitivity A situation in which allergy to one drug warns of possible similar reactions to other, chemically related ones.

dependence A situation in which an individual becomes so accustomed to a drug that he or she cannot function without it; may be physical, psychic, or both.

drug A nonfood substance that is deliberately introduced into the body in order to produce some specific physiological or psychological effect.

habituation A pattern of compulsive drug use that arises from psychic dependence but does not usually involve tolerance. Compare **addiction.**

inhalation A route of administration that involves breathing a drug into the lungs.

metabolites The products of biotransformation.

molecule The smallest unit of a chemical substance such as a drug.

oral administration The introduction of a drug into the body through the mouth.

parenteral administration The introduction of a drug into the body in such a way as to bypass the digestive system, usually by injection.

pharmacokinetics The study of what happens to drugs once they are in the body.

receptor sites Specific spots within cells where the molecules of a specific drug "fit."

route of administration The method by which a drug is introduced into the body. See **inhalation, oral administration,** and **parenteral administration.**

side effects Effects of a drug that are unwanted and are not related to the essential purpose of the drug.

synergism A type of drug interaction in which two drugs, when taken at the same time or in rapid sequence, have more powerful effects than the two drugs would have if taken alone.

teratogenic drugs Drugs that, if taken by a pregnant woman, can interfere with crucial stages of a baby's prenatal development and are thus associated with birth defects.

therapeutic index The safety margin between the effective dose of a drug and the lethal dose.

tolerance A situation in which the body becomes adapted to a drug, so that increasingly larger doses are needed to produce the original desired effect.

withdrawal syndrome An unpleasant and possibly painful condition that an individual who is physically dependent on a drug experiences when deprived of the drug.

NOTES

1. Brent Q. Hafen and Brenda Peterson, *Medicine and Drugs,* 2nd ed. (Philadelphia: Lea & Febiger, 1978), p. 33.

2. Ibid., p. 28.

3. Brent Q. Hafen, *The Self-Health Handbook* (Englewood Cliffs, N.J.: Prentice-Hall, 1980), p. 77.

4. *FDA Consumer,* December 1980–January 1981, p. 14.

5. Jerome H. Jaffe, "Drug Addiction and Drug Abuse," in L. S. Goodman and A. Gilman (eds.), *The Pharmacological Basis of Therapeutics,* 6th ed. (New York: Macmillan, 1980), pp. 535–577.

6. National Commission on Marijuana and Drug Abuse, *Drug Use in America: Problem in Perspective, 2nd Report* (Washington, D.C.: U.S. Government Printing Office, 1973).

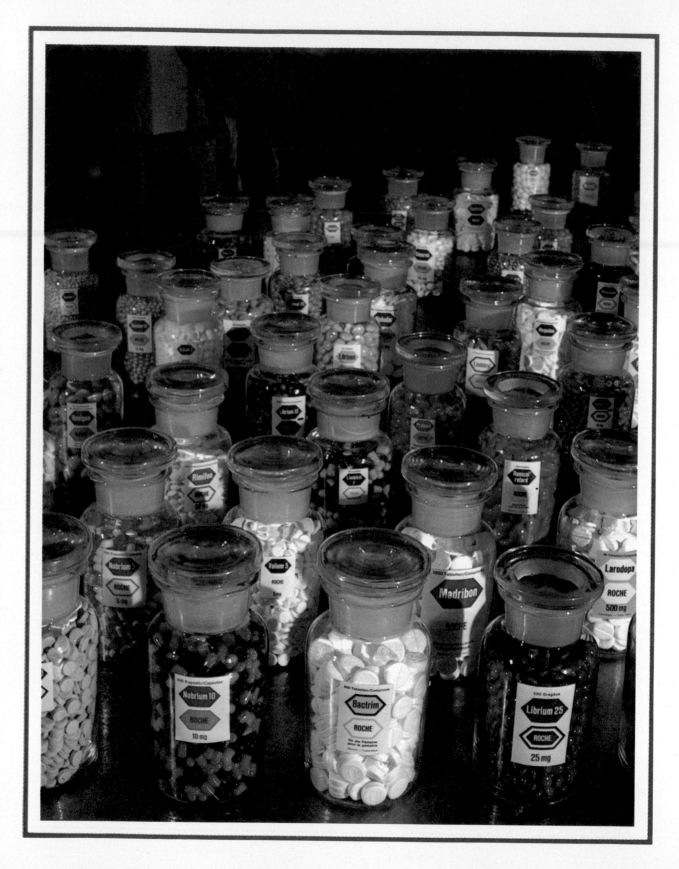

CHAPTER 4

Psychoactive Drugs

In Chapter 3 we mentioned a number of psychoactive drugs that have posed major problems. These drugs fall into eight broad categories. Two, alcohol and nicotine, create such pervasive problems that we shall devote separate chapters to each of them (see Chapters 5 and 6). In this chapter we'll take a closer look at the other six categories of psychoactive drugs. Some of these are prescription medications, used legitimately to treat a variety of ills but subject to abuse by patients—as well as by other people into whose hands they may fall. Others are illegally marketed versions of these drugs. Still others are strictly "street drugs": They have not been deemed to have a legitimate place in medicine, and their sale and use are wholly outside the law.

There are some psychoactive prescription drugs we shall *not* be examining in this chapter, simply because they have not posed a particular societal abuse problem. One group consists of the drugs known as "major" tranquilizers (the antipsychotics), powerful drugs used primarily to treat acute or extreme emotional and mental problems. The other is the antidepressants, covering two broad subclasses: monoamine oxidase (MAO) inhibitors and tricyclics. These two groups of drugs have proved extremely useful in treating severe psychoses and acute emotional difficulties, but they do not produce the general stimulation that invites recreational use.

So the six categories of psychoactive drugs with potential for abuse that we'll discuss in this chapter are: the narcotic analgesics, the hypnosedatives, the stimulants, the psychedelic/illusionogens, the volatile chemicals, and marijuana. Information about the uses and effects of these drugs is summarized in Table 4.1. The federal government's classification of these drugs according to their potential for abuse and dependence is presented in Table 4.3 at the end of this chapter (page 112).

HOW PSYCHOACTIVE DRUGS ACT ON THE BRAIN

Although there is no direct cause-and-effect relationship between a drug and a behavior, we do know that the chemical substances called **psychoactive drugs**, which we are discussing in this chapter, alter our moods, consciousness, and behaviors. The brain, it is believed, controls most of these functions. The human brain consists of several structures that are thought to be in control of different behaviors, feelings, and thoughts. Psychoactive drugs affect these different structures. However, some drugs are more specific to some structures than others. For example, biochemical studies have shown that certain brain structures contain higher levels of certain types of drug receptors than others (see Figure 4.1).

NARCOTIC ANALGESICS: DESCENDANTS OF THE POPPY

An **analgesic** is a substance that eliminates or reduces the sense of pain. The word *narcotic* comes to us from the Greek *narkoun*, "to make numb." The narcotic analgesics do, indeed, make the user numb in both mind and body. They act on the user's central nervous system, and are very effective in relieving pain without causing loss of consciousness.

94

Table 4.1 · Comparison Chart of the Major Psychoactive Drugs

Name of Drug or Chemical	Schedule	Trade or Other Names	Medical Uses	Physical Dependence
Narcotic Analgesics Opium	II, III, V	Dover's Powder, Paregoric, Parepectolin	Analgesic, antidiarrheal	High
Morphine	II, III	Morphine, Pectoral Syrup	Analgesic, antitussive	
Codeine	II, III, V	Codeine, Empirin Compound with Codeine, Robitussin A-C	Analgesic, antitussive	Moderate
Heroin	I	Diacetylmorphine, Horse, Smack	Under investigation	High
Hydromorphone		Dilaudid	Analgesic	
Meperidine (Pethicine)	II	Demerol, Pathadol	Analgesic	
Methadone		Dolophine, Methadone, Methadose	Analgesic, heroin substitute	
Other Narcotics	I, II, III, IV, V	LAAM, Leritine, Levo-Dromoran, Percodan, Tussionex Fentanyl, Darvon, Talwin, Lomotil	Analgesic, antidiarrheal, antitussive	High-Low
Hypnosedatives Chloral Hydrate	IV	Noctec, Somnos	Hypnotic	Moderate
Barbiturates	II, III, IV	Amobarbital, Phenobarbital, Butisol, Phenoxbarbital, Secobarbital, Tuinal	Anesthetic, anticonvulsant, sedative, hypnotic	High-Moderate
Glutethimide	III	Doriden	Sedative, hypnotic	High
Methaqualone	II	Optimil, Parest, Quaalude, Somnafac, Sopor		
Benzodiazepines	IV	Ativan, Azene, Clonopin, Dalmane, Diazepam, Librium, Serax, Tranxene, Valium, Verstran	Anti-anxiety, anti-convulsant, sedative, hypnotic	Low
Other hypnosedatives	III, IV	Equanil, Miltown, Noludar, Placidyl, Valmid	Anti-anxiety, sedative, hypnotic	Moderate
Stimulants Cocaine	II	Coke, Flake, Snow	Local anesthetic	Possible
Amphetamines	II, III	Biphetamine, Delcobese, Desoxyn, Dexedrine, Mediatric	Hyperkinesis, narcolepsy, weight control	
Phenmetrazine	II	Preludin		
Methylphenidate		Ritalin		
Other stimulants	III, IV	Adipex, Bacarate, Cylert, Didrex, Ionamin, Plegine, Pre-Sate, Sanorex, Tenuate, Tepanil, Voranil		
Psychedelic/Illusionogens LSD		Acid, Microdot	None	None
Mescaline and peyote		Mesc, Buttons, Cactus		
Amphetamine variants	I	2,5-DMA, PMA, STP, MDA, MMDA, TMA, DOM, DOB		Unknown
Phencyclidine		PCP, Angel Dust, Hog	Veterinary anesthetic	Degree unknown
Phencyclidine analogs		PCE, PCPy, TCP		
Other psychedelic/illusionogens		Bufotenine, Ibogaine, DMT, DET, Psilocybin, Psilocyn	None	None
Cannabis Marijuana	I	Pot, Acapulco Gold, Grass, Reefer, Sinsemilla, Thai Sticks	Under investigation (glaucoma, nausea of cancer chemotherapy)	Degree unknown
Tetrahydrocannabinol		THC		
Hashish		Hash	None	
Hashish oil		Hash oil		
Volatile chemicals Glue, gasoline, commercial solvents		Plastic model cement Hydrocarbons Toluene, acetone, naphtha	None	Unknown
Nitrous oxide	None	"Laughing gas"	Local anesthetic	
Amyl nitrite			Angina	
Butyl nitrite			None	

Psychological Dependence	Tolerance	Duration of Effects (in hours)	Usual Methods of Administration	Possible Effects	Effects of Overdose or Long-Term Use	Withdrawal Syndrome
High	Yes	3–6	Oral, smoked	Euphoria, drowsiness, respiratory depression, constricted pupils, nausea	Slow and shallow breathing, clammy skin, convulsions, coma, possible death	Watery eyes, runny nose, yawning, loss of appetite, irritability, tremors, panic, chills and sweating, cramps, nausea
Moderate			Oral, injected, smoked			
			Oral, injected			
High			Injected, sniffed, smoked			
		12–24	Oral, injected			
High–Low		Variable				
Moderate	Possible	5–8	Oral	Slurred speech, disorientation, drunken behavior without odor of alcohol	Shallow respiration, cold and clammy skin, dilated pupils, weak and rapid pulse, coma, possible death	Anxiety, insomnia, tremors, delirium, convulsions, possible death
High–Moderate	Yes	1–16	Oral, injected			
High		4–8				
Low						
Moderate						
	Possible	1–2	Sniffed, injected	Increased alertness, excitation, euphoria, increased pulse rate and blood pressure, insomnia, loss of appetite	Agitation, increase in body temperature, hallucinations, convulsions, possible death	Apathy, long periods of sleep, irritability, depression, disorientation
High	Yes	2–4	Oral, injected			
			Oral			
Degree unknown	Yes	8–12	Oral	Illusions and hallucinations, poor perception of time and distance	Longer, more intense "trip" episodes, psychosis, possible death	Withdrawal syndrome not reported
		Up to days	Oral, injected			
High			Smoked, oral, injected			
Degree unknown	Possible	Variable	Oral, injected, smoked, sniffed			
Moderate	Yes	2–4	Smoked, oral	Euphoria, relaxed inhibitions, increased appetite, disoriented behavior	Fatigue, paranoia, possible psychosis	Insomnia, hyperactivity, and decreased appetite occasionally reported
Minimal to moderate	Not known	Variable	Sniffed	Euphoria	Organic brain syndrome, nerve damage, liver and kidney disease, possible death	Withdrawal syndrome not reported
	Not known	−1		Euphoria, shortness of breath, nausea	Nerve damage, hearing loss, severe anemia	
	Yes	−1		Euphoria, headache, dizziness, perspiration, flushing, nausea, fainting	Not known	

Source: National Institute on Drug Abuse, adapted from *Health Management: Promotion and Self-Care* (Englewood, Colo.: Morton, 1982), pp. 162–163; (inhalants) Annabel Hecht, "Inhalants: Quick Route to Danger," *FDA Consumer*, May 1980, pp. 19–22.

Figure 4.1   The Effects of Psychoactive Drugs on Major Structures of the Brain

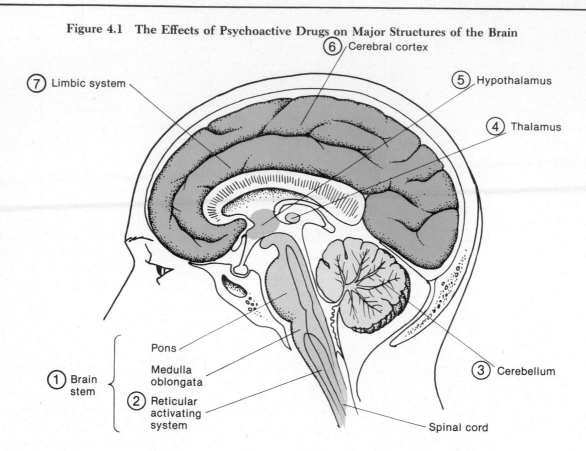

Brain Structure	Function	Effects of Drugs
1. Brain stem	Carries messages from spinal cord to brain	Depressants—such as anesthetics—can cause vasomotor, cardiac, and respiratory failure.
2. Reticular activating system (RAS)	Alerts the brain to stimuli *or* blocks out certain competing stimuli	Sedatives dampen RAS activity; stimulants are used to overcome RAS underactivity.
3. Cerebellum	Controls coordination, balance, and agility	Drugs such as alcohol produce uncoordinated movements.
4. Thalamus	Communication center, directing messages to and from the brain	Psychedelics disrupt transmission of impulses contolling cognitive, sensory, and motor functions.
5. Hypothalamus	Regulates hormone production, temperature, and fluid balance, feelings of hunger and fullness, pleasure and pain	Analgesics alter the pleasure-pain function.
6. Cerebral cortex	Controls learning and memory, integration of sensory impressions, inhibitions and emotions, time-space orientation, vision and hearing, and motor skills	Toxic solvents alter thought processes and behaviors.
7. Limbic system	Portion of the cerebral cortex that provides a connection between it and the thalamus and hypothalamus	Antianxiety drugs alter physiological responses to emotions.

The **narcotic analgesics** include what are often called the **opiates**—opium, morphine, and heroin —and the **opioids,** a group of synthetic drugs that are chemically similar to the opiates. **Opium,** the parent substance, comes from the juice of the opium poppy, which is native to Asia Minor; the word comes to us nearly unchanged from the ancient Greek *opion,* "poppy juice." **Morphine** is the active ingredient in opium. **Heroin,** which is in turn derived from morphine, is more than twice as potent as morphine. The opioids, which were first synthesized in the laboratory in this century, include methadone and meperidine, plus other drugs with similar dependence-creating potential.

DEPENDENCE AND TOLERANCE

All the narcotic analgesics have a strong potential to create both physical and psychological dependence. And tolerance—the need for higher and higher doses to obtain the original effect—typically develops when any of them is taken over a period of time.

Opium and the Opiates in History

If the only member of this drug family were opium itself, as it was first used, society's current "narcotics problem" would be nonexistent. Opium was taken orally for centuries in China, Egypt, Greece, India, and the Arab world; it was used for both medical and social purposes, and there is no record of its posing any problems for society. Only much later, with the introduction of opium smoking and its much swifter effects, did dependence become widespread. Then, in the mid-nineteenth century, came two other innovations: Morphine was refined from the raw opium, and the hypodermic needle was introduced.

Curious as it may seem now, it was at first believed that injected morphine, more potent than opium, would prove to be a "cure" for opium dependence. Later, at the turn of the century, when morphine dependence had become a clear reality, the error was repeated: It was expected that a new and still more potent derivative, heroin, would provide the cure for *that* problem. As we now know, this hope was tragically unfounded.

Potential Risks of Dependence

The nation's—indeed, the world's—major narcotics problem is heroin. Heroin is typically injected **intravenously** (into a vein). It is also sometimes injected **subcutaneously** (under the skin—a practice known as "skin popping") or sniffed ("snorted"). People sometimes mistakenly believe that these routes are somehow less likely than intravenous injection to lead to dependence.

Typically, the heroin user is seeking the drug's

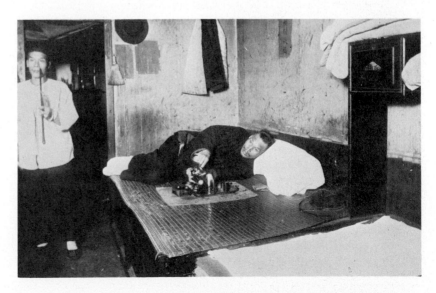

Opium use became a social problem when, instead of swallowing it, abusers began to smoke it, which enhanced its addictive properties. This is an opium den in San Francisco at the turn of the century. (Culver Pictures)

mind-numbing effect, its blurring of thought and feeling, which can include euphoria. Later, when the user has become dependent on heroin, it is also needed to avoid the distress of withdrawal. As the user becomes dependent on the drug, he or she is also likely to develop a tolerance to it: The usual initial dose of heroin, about 3 milligrams, can escalate to 1,000 milligrams within a matter of months—with hundreds of dollars required every week to support that need.

Treatment Programs: What Approach Works Best?

There is still no agreement on the ideal way to deal with people who are dependent on narcotics. Some experts feel that the dependent individual should simply be given the drug as often as he or she needs it. This approach would make it unnecessary for the drug-dependent individual to commit crimes to pay for increasing doses of the drug. Others advocate **methadone** treatment, in which methadone's cross-tolerance with heroin is used to "wean" the dependent individual from heroin. This approach is based on the idea that methadone removes the desire for heroin, blocks its effects, and has no serious side effects at therapeutic doses; taken orally, methadone does not produce euphoria.

How well do methadone programs work? Many participants have in fact reordered their lives, given up crime, and become productive citizens. But critics argue that substituting one dependence-producing drug for another is not exactly curing the patient: Methadone only allows stabilization; it does not bring about true change. (Some experts feel that true change occurs only in single and group psychotherapy.) Critics note, too, that some patients in such programs have turned to other drugs such as alcohol, barbiturates, or stimulants. Further, some ask whether the programs are really successful in the long run: One posttreatment study found that the relapse rate from certain treatment centers was 89 percent. Some individuals in that study had left the program early, against medical advice—but a follow-up six months later found that even among those who had completed the program, only 9.5 percent had remained drug-free.[1]

"DOWNERS": THE HYPNOSEDATIVES

Call them "downers," calmers, soothers, relaxers, tranquilizers, sleeping pills. Or use the term we've adopted, **hypnosedatives**. The term *hypnosedatives* implies that these drugs have both sedative (calming) and hypnotic (sleep-inducing) effects—the difference between them is really just a matter of dosage. Technically, all the hypnosedative drugs are depressants—slowers of central nervous system activity.

Classes of Hypnosedatives

The hypnosedatives include three major groups of drugs: (1) barbiturates, (2) anxiolytics, or antianxiety drugs, and (3) a number of nonbarbiturate agents used primarily as hypnotics. Let's take a quick look at the drugs in these categories—there are a lot of them, and it's easy to get them confused.

THE BARBITURATES

The **barbiturates** range from short-acting types, with effects lasting less than six hours—such as amobarbital (marketed under the brand name Amytal), pentobarbital (Nembutal), secobarbital (Seconal), and Tuinal (a combination of amobarbital and secobarbital)—to longer-acting ones such as butabarbital (Butisol), and still longer-acting types such as phenobarbital (Luminal and others) whose effects may persist up to twenty-four hours. (Even the shorter-acting agents may affect the user twenty-four hours after administration.) The barbiturates are used primarily to treat insomnia, less often for daytime sedation; certain barbiturates also have anticonvulsant properties.

THE ANTIANXIETY (ANXIOLYTIC) DRUGS ("MINOR TRANQUILIZERS")

The **anxiolytics,** or relaxants (which used to be called "minor tranquilizers"), include meprobamate (brand names: Equanil, Miltown), hydroxyzine (Atarax), and a host of others. A number of the anxiolytics—chlordiazepoxide (Librium), diazepam (Valium), chlorazepane (Tranzene), oxazepam (Serax)—are in the chemical group called benzodiazepines. Anxiolytics are widely used as anxiety reducers. Some, including meprobamate and the benzodiazepines, have significant muscle-relaxant properties as well, and a few have proved useful in controlling specific types of convulsive seizures.

NONBARBITURATES USED AS HYPNOTICS

A number of nonbarbiturate agents are used primarily as hypnotics. They include chloral hydrate (Noctec, Somnos), ethchlorvynol (Placidyl), gluthethimide (Doriden), methyprylon (Noludar), methaqualone (Quaalude, Optimil, Parest, and others), and flurazepam (Dalmane). (Flurazepam happens to be a benzodiazepine.)

Potential Risks of the Hypnosedatives

A variety of side effects may occur with hypnosedatives, including hangovers, nausea, headaches, dizziness, and drowsiness, and the user may be subject to accidents at home, at work, and while driving.

No one should drive or operate dangerous tools or machinery while using any hypnosedative.

Furthermore, the hypnosedatives are all potential killers via accidental or purposive overdose —a fact often ignored in media coverage, which tends to focus more on the narcotics situation with its related violence and death. According to the National Institute on Drug Abuse, barbiturates and other hypnosedatives are involved in nearly 25 percent of all drug-related visits to hospital emergency rooms and in 26 percent of all drug-related deaths.[2] It is true that the antianxiety drugs carry a lower risk of accidental overdose and death than, say, the barbiturates. But even they must still be used with care.

CAUTION: MAY BE FATAL IN COMBINATION

A special danger enters the picture with all the hypnosedatives: the concurrent use of one hypnosedative with another hypnosedative or with another depressant substance such as alcohol. In Chapter 3, we talked about potentiation (the enhancing of a drug's effects by the addition of another drug) and synergism (the phenomenon in which two drugs with similar effects produce a total effect greater than both drugs would produce if taken alone). The danger of synergism can arise in both medical and nonmedical use of hypnosedatives. In fact, aside from the problem of dependence, the most serious danger with the hypnosedatives is the unintentional or deliberate combining of the drug with another depressant— especially alcohol.

A person who is taking one of these drugs on physician's orders may be ignorant of that lethal potential or may dismiss a physician's or pharmacist's warning about drinking while taking the drug. Young people have been known to combine hypnosedatives with alcohol on purpose, seeking heightened intoxication. In either case, the depressant effects of both drugs on the central nervous system can be intensified: Amounts of either drug that might not do serious harm alone can combine to cause critical conditions, including coma and death.

Hypnosedatives and Dependence

Daily use of 500 milligrams or more of barbiturates, or equivalent doses of other hypnosedatives, usually produces classic physical dependence. Such users can rapidly develop tolerance for up to fifteen times the normal dose.[3] If the drug is removed, the person suffers withdrawal symptoms.

THE EXTREME DANGERS OF HYPNOSEDATIVE WITHDRAWAL

The acute withdrawal symptoms undergone by people who are dependent on barbiturates (particularly the shorter-acting barbiturates) or on other hypnosedatives are more severe than those associated with opiate dependence. The symptoms begin with nervousness, trembling, and weakness. If untreated, the person can suffer epileptic-like seizures or a toxic psychosis with delusions and hallucinations, and can lose consciousness. The most severe symptoms of untreated withdrawal last about four days *and can be fatal.* When a pregnant woman is dependent on any of the hypnosedatives, her baby will have to go through the withdrawal syndrome shortly after birth.

No one who has any degree of dependence on *any* hypnosedative should withdraw from the drug without medical supervision.

Are Hypnosedatives Prescribed Too Frequently?

The hypnosedative drugs are all twentieth-century products of the laboratory—many introduced only within the past two or three decades. Do they really mean better and calmer living through chemistry? There is reason to doubt it. Although accurate figures are hard to obtain, it is believed that dependency problems with hypnosedatives, particularly the barbiturates, exceed those of opiates. Patterns range from infrequent sprees aimed at gross intoxication to prolonged, compulsive, daily use of large quantities, where the user is preoccupied with securing and maintaining adequate supplies. In a medical patient, the problem may develop gradually. It may begin with prolonged use for insomnia and progress to larger and larger doses each night, plus a few capsules at particularly stressful times during the day. Eventually, the drug may become a major focus of the user's life.

Many observers have concluded that hypnosedatives, "minor tranquilizers" in particular, are vastly overprescribed. In 1979 alone, according to the National Prescription Audit, 62.3 million prescriptions for the latter were filled.[4] Until 1981, diazepam (Valium) was actually the most-prescribed drug in the United States. (That year, it dropped to fourth place, behind Tagamet, an ulcer medication; Inderal, a drug used for high blood pressure; and Motrin, an antiarthritic.)[5] Are

Americans really so beset by serious anxiety? If so, there is all the more reason for public concern.

Recent Trends in Hypnosedative Abuse

The barbiturates have long enjoyed a certain standing as recreational drugs, sometimes in alternation with stimulants ("uppers"), each countering the exaggerated effects of the other. They have been joined more recently by other hypnosedatives. The age group most likely to use hypnosedatives socially, according to government figures, is young adults (ages eighteen to twenty-five): 17 percent of this group admit nonmedical experience with hypnosedatives—although fewer than 3 percent report continuing use.[6]

Prominent among the hypnosedatives used recreationally in recent years is methaqualone, popularly known as "ludes," an abbreviation of "Quaaludes," one of its trade names. When it was first introduced, some people thought methaqualone was completely nonaddictive. But it does produce both physical and psychological dependence, with the same sort of withdrawal syndrome described for the barbiturates. There is also a notion in some circles that methaqualone is a sexual stimulant. In fact, it enhances neither sexual performance nor sexual pleasure. Like alcohol, it is likely to lower inhibitions and increase sexual desire while actually diminishing the ability to perform.

Another recent trend has been toward the use of "loads"—the combination of a prescription painkiller containing codeine, plus a prescription hypnosedative known as Doriden. The combination acts as a severe depressant to the nervous system and is extremely dangerous.

ON THE ALERT: STIMULANTS

The most widely used stimulant in America is, of course, caffeine. Drinking all those cups of coffee and cans of cola *can* cause harm. More harmful, perhaps, are two other kinds of stimulant—amphetamines and cocaine. Both, the amphetamines in particular, can be extremely dangerous.

Just what do stimulants do? Basically, **stimu-**

lants "rev up" a neural network known as the sympathetic division of the autonomic nervous system. The autonomic nervous system (ANS) relays impulses to those muscle tissues throughout the body that are not under voluntary control—the heart, the intestinal muscles, and so on. The sympathetic network is the part of the autonomic nervous system that readies us to cope with stress (discussed in Chapter 2). Once the emergency is past, another part of the system (the parasympathetic nervous system) reverses things and restores normality—slowing the heart rate, sending the digestive system back to work, and so on.

The stimulant drugs mobilize the body's fight-or-flight mechanism inappropriately, when it may not in fact be needed. Caffeine does so on a relatively low level. The more powerful stimulants do so on a larger scale and, as we shall see, may thereby be endangering the body rather than protecting it.

Caffeine

Most people who crave that extra mug of coffee, tea, or cola drink to pep up a slow day know that each swallow contains **caffeine** but few realize how potent a drug it is. Caffeine, sometimes found with chemically related stimulants known as *theophylline* and *theobromine,* is a drug that acts fast. In less than five minutes after you've downed that cup of coffee, caffeine has raced to every part of your body: it increases the flow of urine and stomach acid, relaxes involuntary muscles, steps up the intake of oxygen, and speeds up the basal metabolic rate by 10 percent. It also heightens the pumping strength of the heart; but too much caffeine can lead to an irregular heartbeat. Caffeine improves the user's physical coordination; for example, it improves the skills of typists and motorists. But it can also hinder your efforts: It can make a painstaking task, which needs a steady hand and accurate timing, more difficult.

Figure 4.2   The health hazards of caffeine have not been definitely established, but it is known to be a potent drug with a risk of physical dependence. Many people ingest much more caffeine than they realize because they are unaware that some of the beverages and over-the-counter medicines they consume contain caffeine. The caffeine content of beverages and OTC drugs varies widely, as this chart shows.

(*Sources:* National Coffee Association, Consumers Union, National Soft Drink Association, Food and Drug Administration)

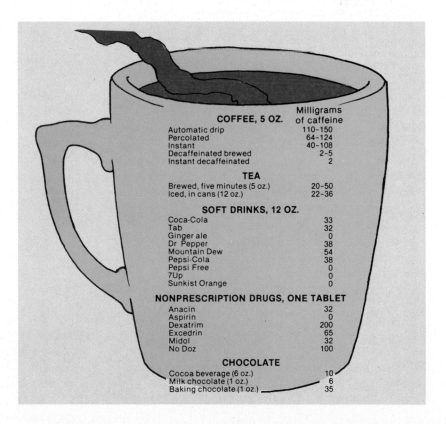

COFFEE, 5 OZ.	Milligrams of caffeine
Automatic drip	110–150
Percolated	64–124
Instant	40–108
Decaffeinated brewed	2–5
Instant decaffeinated	2
TEA	
Brewed, five minutes (5 oz.)	20–50
Iced, in cans (12 oz.)	22–36
SOFT DRINKS, 12 OZ.	
Coca-Cola	33
Tab	32
Ginger ale	0
Dr Pepper	38
Mountain Dew	54
Pepsi-Cola	38
Pepsi Free	0
7Up	0
Sunkist Orange	0
NONPRESCRIPTION DRUGS, ONE TABLET	
Anacin	32
Aspirin	0
Dexatrim	200
Excedrin	65
Midol	32
No Doz	100
CHOCOLATE	
Cocoa beverage (6 oz.)	10
Milk chocolate (1 oz.)	6
Baking chocolate (1 oz.)	35

Can caffeine hurt you? While cramming for final exams, you may stay up all night, and find—looking nervously at the sunrise—that your seventh cup of coffee has left you with quivering hands and a grinding headache. No wonder. For most of us, three to four cups of coffee, around 400 milligrams of caffeine, can bring on irritableness, headaches, tremors, and nervousness. If that dose is doubled, the jittery coffee drinker can suffer hallucinations, perhaps convulsions. The fatal dose is 10 grams (or 10,000 milligrams). But to die from a caffeine overdose, you'd need to polish off 67 to 100 cups in a brief sitting.[7] Luckily, our bodies metabolize this drug rapidly, so that a morning dose of caffeine leaves little trace in the bloodstream by evening.

Caffeine can create dependence. Those who drink at least five cups of coffee a day can suffer several days of withdrawal symptoms—including nausea, headaches, irritability, and lassitude—if they kick the habit. The person who drinks too much in a big way can experience "caffeinism," a syndrome characterized by rapid breathing, agitation, mood changes, and heart palpitations. A heavy coffee drinker may develop the habit over a period of time; when these symptoms occur, he or she may not realize that caffeine is the culprit. If you're troubled by anxiety and other symptoms, cut out the caffeine from your diet; even your physician may overlook this syndrome when treating your case of nerves and arrhythmia (irregular heartbeat).

And caffeine *may* pose other dangers. Although no proof has been found, studies have linked the drug in cola drinks and coffee to heart disease, benign and malignant tumors, pancreatic cancer, and birth defects. Still other studies refute these links.[8] Nevertheless, it's a good idea for pregnant women to avoid caffeine as they would avoid any other drug. Recently, researchers have expressed concern over children who get the caffeine habit. After all, even one cola drink gives an eight-year-old a hefty jolt of this drug, and many children consume much more than this every day.

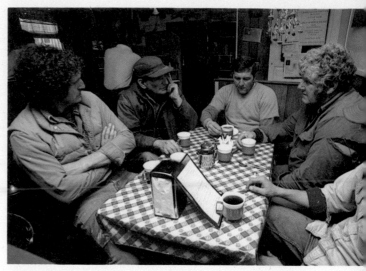

Caffeine is the world's most widely consumed drug. The coffee break is a social ritual in our society, as in many others. Coffee is so readily available and so popular that people who wish to reduce their consumption of caffeine may find it difficult to resist or avoid that cup of coffee with friends. (© Ulrike Welsch 1982/Stock, Boston)

among them. They include amphetamine (Benzedrine or "bennies"), dextroamphetamine (Dexedrine or "dexies"), and methamphetamine (Methedrine or "meth" or "speed"; the word "speed" is often used to refer to this entire group of drugs).

People have been using and misusing amphetamines for a variety of purposes since they were introduced almost fifty years ago. Dieters used them, thinking they were an easy route to weight loss; students used them to stay awake in all-night cramming sessions; truck drivers used them when they were struggling to stay awake during long overnight hauls. And the 1950s and 1960s saw the advent of the "speed freak," often a dually dependent individual seesawing between "uppers" (sometimes taken by injection) and "downers" in the form of barbiturates or other hypnosedatives.

The Amphetamine Family

The **amphetamines,** long known in nonmedical use as "pep pills" or "uppers," are a group of synthetic drugs with slight chemical differences

USES OF THE AMPHETAMINES

The amphetamines have only two legitimate uses in medicine. First, they are used in treating an extremely rare condition called *narcolepsy* (an uncontrollable need for short periods of deep sleep). Second, they, as well as certain other drugs with similar properties, have been used to treat *hyperkinetic* (uncontrollably overactive) children. Interestingly, the drugs' effects are paradoxical in hyperkinetic children: They seem to calm these children, rather than stimulating them.

WEIGHT CONTROL: MEDICAL MISUSE   Some amphetamines have been combined, with each other or with barbiturates or tranquilizers, in a variety of products marketed primarily for weight control. (Prominent brand names include Dexamyl, Appetrol, Eskatrol, Nobese, and Obetrol.) But it's unwise to use any of the amphetamines as an appetite suppressant. After two to four weeks they are no longer effective, and the risks are hardly worth it—many pep-pill dependents in our country started out by employing them as weight-loss aids. Amphetamines are frequently prescribed by "diet doctors" and "fat clinics," some of whose clients "make the rounds" of such sources to boost their supplies. Nevertheless, most thoughtful physicians no longer prescribe amphetamines for weight loss, and this use has been outlawed by some states and may be outlawed nationally.

It's a good idea to avoid "diet pills" and the doctors who prescribe them.

THE POTENTIAL RISKS OF AMPHETAMINES

SHORT-TERM USE   In the short term—with just a single, small dose—amphetamines often have unwanted side effects, which are essentially exaggerations of the drugs' basic impact. These side effects include nervousness, elevated blood pressure, and headache. These effects will be more annoying to some people than to others—and, obviously, amphetamines are more hazardous for some people (such as those with heart disorders) than others.

If the drug is used on a single occasion, say to help a student through an end-of-term cramming session, there may be no further detrimental effects. However, it should be noted that amphetamines do *not* improve intellectual function, and knowledge gained in a pill-driven night of study

may well be lost after the drug wears off. (It may be remembered only when the student is in the same state as when he or she learned it initially.) But if the drug is taken in a situation that is inherently risky—such as by a trucker traveling a superhighway—there is an additional peril. Amphetamine effects can often cease abruptly and unpredictably, and sleep or even death can be the consequence under such circumstances.

No one should drive or operate dangerous tools or machinery while under the influence of amphetamines.

LONG-TERM USE   In large doses or over prolonged periods, amphetamines have unpredictable effects, which may include insomnia, dizziness, agitation, confusion, delirium, and malnutrition. The user may develop wildly exaggerated feelings of confidence and power, which can lead to errors of judgment; the user may believe, for example, that he or she can cross a busy intersection with impunity or can leap, like Superman, above traffic. For some people prolonged use can lead to actual psychosis. Elevated blood pressure, continuing over a period of time, can put a strain on normal blood vessels—and a vessel may finally burst. (Intravenous use can also lead to death via burst blood vessels or stroke.)

AMPHETAMINES AND DEPENDENCE

Unlike alcohol or "ludes," or even heroin to some extent, amphetamines are not really recreational drugs. They tend to be used by individuals who want them or think they need them rather than to be shared in social situations. Thus the first two steps to drug dependence listed in Chapter 3 (page 86)—experimental and recreational use— are omitted. Individuals may proceed fairly quickly to situational, intensified, and compulsive use. Once users get into this pattern, they may find they need increased supplies of the drug. Tolerance does develop, requiring larger and larger doses, and psychic dependence is strong. Though the potential for physical dependence is not as great as with the narcotic analgesics or the hyp-

ACTIVITY: EXPLORING HEALTH

ASSESSMENT: Could Drugs Be Causing Problems in Your Life?

Most Americans use drugs regularly, although many of us do not realize that we do. In fact, even those people whose lives are seriously affected by drug use are often unaware of it. The following questions are designed to help you determine whether your medical and nonmedical use of drugs is a possible source of health risk.

DIRECTIONS: Fill in the substance in the blank spaces (such as alcohol, caffeine, nicotine, marijuana, cocaine, steroids, tranquilizers), and answer yes or no to the following questions. Remember that *any* drug (prescription, OTC, or substances used for social and recreational purposes) applies.

YES   NO

_____ _____ 1. Do you miss classes or lose time from studying because you use _____?

_____ _____ 2. Is _____ making your college life unhappy?

_____ _____ 3. Have you ever felt guilt or remorse after using _____?

_____ _____ 4. Does _____ impair your functioning or efficiency?

_____ _____ 5. Do you ever borrow money to buy _____?

_____ _____ 6. Have you ever sold any personal item in order to buy more _____?

_____ _____ 7. Are you reluctant to use your "_____ money" for essential personal and college expenditures?

_____ _____ 8. Does _____ make you careless or forgetful of the welfare of your family or friends?

YES   NO

_____ _____ 9. Do you ever use _____ to escape worry or trouble?

_____ _____ 10. Do you ever use _____ in larger amounts, or more frequently, or longer, than you had planned?

_____ _____ 11. Do disappointments (such as receiving a lower grade than you had hoped), arguments (such as a lovers' quarrel), or frustrations (such as an unavailable library book) make you want to use _____?

_____ _____ 12. Do you ever have an urge to celebrate any pleasant experience or good fortune by using _____?

_____ _____ 13. Have you ever been criticized for the amount of _____ you use?

_____ _____ 14. Have you ever committed an illegal or unlawful action while using _____?

_____ _____ 15. Have you ever lied about or minimized your _____ use?

Scoring: If you answered yes to two or three questions about any drug, you would be well advised to reexamine your decisions about this drug use. Answering yes to more than three questions may be an indication that you need help in resolving the problem.

Source: Adapted from J. Fort and C. T. Cory, *American Drugstore* (Boston: Little, Brown, 1975).

nosedatives, there is often *some* degree of physical dependence, evidenced by withdrawal symptoms when the drug is stopped: depression, an increased appetite, and an increased need for sleep.

Cocaine

Probably the fastest-growing illegal drug in popularity in recent years, despite its expense, is **cocaine,** a drug extracted from the leaves of the South American coca bush. Cocaine's "high" is a little different from that of amphetamines—it's more sociable, less agitated, but faster, more intense, and more euphoric. It is also shorter-lasting. The drug suppresses appetite and temporarily re-

The expense of cocaine and the elaborate rituals surrounding its recreational use—such as inhaling it through rolled-up high-denomination bills—have contributed to its mystique as a "glamorous" drug. However, many people are discovering the drawbacks of this kind of glamour: About 4 million Americans have problems with cocaine abuse, and a nationwide cocaine hotline (toll-free number: 800-COCAINE) received 18,000 calls in its first two weeks of operation in May 1983. (© Ken Love 1979/Black Star)

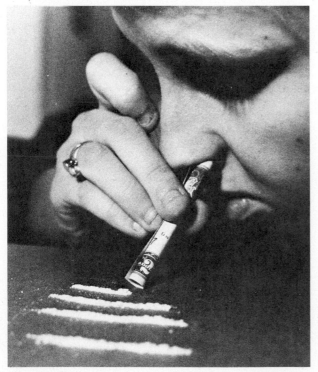

lieves depression. As a central nervous system stimulant, cocaine is closely related to caffeine, theophylline, and theobromine, but it is markedly more potent. Coca leaves have been chewed by workers in the Andes for centuries, primarily to prevent fatigue.

A federal survey on drug abuse in 1979 found that 27.5 percent of Americans between the ages of eighteen and twenty-five reported that they had tried cocaine at least once, up from 20 percent of that age group only two years before.[9] It is not completely clear why this increase has occurred, but it is possible that the expense of cocaine (it has been called "the champagne of drugs"), plus elaborate cocaine-taking rituals, are strongly reinforcing elements in some social circles. The price of cocaine may range from eighty dollars to several hundred dollars a gram, depending on purity.

USES OF COCAINE

MEDICAL USES   Medically, cocaine is used as a local anesthetic in certain types of surgery, numbing tissues; it also constricts blood vessels, so that local bleeding is reduced.

RECREATIONAL USE   Recreationally, a powdery form of the drug formerly known as "snow" and now more commonly called "blow," "toot," "flake," or just "coke," is sniffed or "snorted." Some individuals, seeking new thrills, switch to injecting the drug, often along with some other drug such as heroin; this combination is known as a "speedball" and is extremely dangerous. Another method of taking cocaine is known as "freebasing"—preparing a pure (almost 100 percent) extract of the drug (the usual street cocaine is 20 to 50 percent pure) and smoking it in a pipe; this method is also very risky.

THE POTENTIAL RISKS OF COCAINE

SHORT-TERM USE   Like the amphetamines, cocaine elevates blood pressure. It also raises body temperature and in large doses can be cardiotoxic (damaging to the heart).

The risk of toxicity is far higher when cocaine is injected or smoked than when inhaled, since extremely high levels in the blood are reached far more quickly; it can kill within minutes.

———————————————————————— ▣

The American College of Emergency Physicians, pointing to reports implicating cocaine in dozens of sudden deaths and a number of suicides (the depression after the high can be very severe), has flatly termed the drug "medically dangerous."[10]

LONG-TERM USE Repeated snorting of cocaine irritates the mucous membranes of the nose, so that individuals who use it frequently often have stuffy or runny noses and seem to have perpetual colds. The septum between the nostrils can also deteriorate after a time, although actual perforation is rare.[11] Chronic users may also experience restlessness, anxiety, and irritability, and some develop a characteristic cocaine psychosis, which may include tactile hallucinations of "bugs" crawling on the skin.

Repeated use can lead to problems similar to those that occur with amphetamines: depression, anxiety, and paranoid delusions.

COCAINE AND DEPENDENCE

At this time, it is thought that cocaine may produce physical dependence. Very strong psychic dependence is known to develop, however, and there have also been some reports of tolerance.

MIND-ALTERING SUBSTANCES: THE PSYCHEDELIC/ ILLUSIONOGENS

The **psychedelic/illusionogens** are drugs that create illusions, distorting the user's mind by creating moods, thoughts, and perceptions that would otherwise take place only in a dream state. These drugs are also called *hallucinogens, deliriants, psychotogens,* and *psychotomimetics,* among other terms. The use of such substances has a lengthy world history. The earliest forms were derived from plants native to various areas and have been employed sometimes in folk medicine but primarily as part of religious rituals.

In the late 1940s **LSD (lysergic acid diethylamide)** was synthesized by research chemist Albert Hofmann. Since then, similar agents have been synthesized, and the group now in recreational use includes a spectrum of substances—some natural plant derivatives, others concocted in the chemistry lab. Among them are LSD itself, **mescaline** (derived from the peyote cactus of the U.S. Southwest), **psilocybin** (a Mexican mushroom derivative), **PCP (phencyclidine,** an animal anesthetic), and a variety of other agents known chiefly by abbreviations of their lengthy chemical labels (*DMT, DET, DOM, STP,* and others).

None of these drugs causes physical dependence, and they involve little if any psychic dependence, although tolerance can sometimes develop with frequent use. The dangers of the psychedelic/illusionogens—and they are very real dangers—lie chiefly in their unpredictable and sometimes devastating effects during use, and occasionally long after.

LSD

An average dose of 50 to 100 micrograms of LSD, or "acid," produces slight dizziness, weakness, dilation of the pupils, and particularly such perceptual alterations as intense visual experience, distorted time sense, sharpened hearing, and **synesthesia**—the blending of two senses so that the person, for example, "hears" colors or "sees" sounds. Psychological symptoms include the flooding of consciousness with numerous thoughts in new combinations, rapid changes in mood, and a feeling that one's body is distorted. These effects usually occur in sequence. Physical changes come first, then the perceptual alterations, and finally the psychic changes. There is considerable overlap, however, among the three phases.

THE POTENTIAL RISKS OF LSD

"BAD TRIPS" Severe panic reactions ("bummers" or "bad trips") and other adverse effects sometimes occur with LSD. Users report having hundreds of pleasurable good trips, then for no apparent reason having a "bummer," complete with monstrous perceptions and delusions of being trapped forever in the drugged state. Such "bummers" are common with high doses and impure drugs. They sometimes occur accidentally

A Word to the Wise About Drug Identity

A drug purchased from a pharmacist is labeled, and one may be reasonably sure that the label accurately reflects the content. But a "street" drug—whether the seller claims it's a prescription medication, a plant substance, or a custom-made chemical—carries no such assurance; nor does the buyer have any legal recourse if the substance turns out to be, or contain, something other than claimed. Even a pharmaceutical manufacturer's name or logotype on capsules or tablets are suspect, since they can be counterfeited.

A purchaser faces several possible risks in these circumstances:

▶ A great deal of money may be expended on a cheaper look-alike.
▶ Since the strength of an unlabeled drug is unknown, *dosage* is difficult to calculate, and effects may be either greater or less than expected.
▶ The *effects* are, in fact, unpredictable, since the substance may be, or include, some other psychoactive drug—and of course adverse effects are similarly unpredictable.
▶ Treatment for toxicity or overdose may be made difficult or impossible.

because the purity of black-market LSD varies widely and because it takes much skill to measure the extremely small amounts needed for an acid trip.

PSYCHOTIC REACTIONS Both occasional and chronic users can experience acute (short-term) psychotic reactions and flashback phenomena. **Flashbacks** are brief, sudden, unexpected perceptual distortions and bizarre thoughts—similar to those experienced while on an LSD trip—that occur long after (perhaps months or years after) the immediate effects of the drug have worn off. In some people LSD can trigger serious depressions, paranoid behavior, or chronic psychoses. Fatal accidents and suicides have also occasionally been associated with the use of LSD.

PCP ("Angel Dust")

Phencyclidine, also known as **PCP** and deceptively as "angel dust" (as well as by many local and regional nicknames), had one legitimate medical use—as a veterinary anesthetic. It is no longer manufactured in the United States. Most PCP sold on the street is concocted illegally and may be combined with—or represented as—any of a number of other illegal substances (notably THC, the principal active ingredient in marijuana, which is not actually available on the street). It is sold in the form of water-soluble powder, liquid, or tablets and is taken orally, sniffed, injected, or—more often—sprinkled on marijuana, kitchen herbs, or tobacco and smoked. Strengths and dosages vary

considerably. The powder may be 50 to 100 percent pure; in other forms the concentration of PCP may range from 5 to 30 percent.

THE POTENTIAL RISKS OF PCP

PCP is a perplexing and alarming drug, with conflicting and paradoxical properties. It can act not only as a deliriant, but also—and variably—as a stimulant, a depressant, and an analgesic. Low doses (1 to 5 milligrams) may—depending on the dosage as well as the individual—produce a feeling of intoxication, euphoria, overall numbness, staggering, thought disorganization, slurring of speech, hostile and bizarre behavior, or any combination of these.[12] Among the additional effects of somewhat larger doses (up to 19 milligrams) may be nausea and vomiting, fever, loss of muscle control, or coma. Still larger doses may lead to any of the foregoing plus large increases in blood pressure, heart rate, disorientation, psychotic behavior (including violence), convulsions, or coma that may last for days. PCP is stored in the body for days after the last dose.

All of these reactions may vary from person to person as well as from one time to another in the same person. A number of PCP-related deaths have been reported.

Other Psychedelic/Illusionogens

MESCALINE AND PSILOCYBIN Mescaline—in the form of peyote buttons—is employed in ceremonies of the Native American Church. **Psilocy-**

bin, from the Mexican psilocybe mushroom, has played a part in religious lore since the days of the ancient Aztecs. When taken in connection with these traditional rituals, under the supervision of those who have long experience with the drugs and their effects, these substances probably do no lasting harm. But outside that highly controlled and structured setting, these drugs, although far less potent than LSD, are unpredictable and potentially hazardous.

CHEMICAL RELATIVES: DMT AND DOM   DMT is chemically related to psilocybin but is inactive when taken orally, so instead is sniffed or smoked. At low doses, DOM (STP) is somewhat less likely to cause illusions than certain other drugs in this class. But as it happens, almost all of these chemicals sold on the street, by whatever letters, turn out when chemically analyzed to be LSD; so, practically speaking, they carry the same risks.

JIMSONWEED   A recent fad among teenagers in some parts of the country is Jimsonweed *(Datura stramonium),* also known in various locales as Jamestown weed, stinkweed, thorn apple, devil's apple, or loco weed.[13] Taking Jimsonweed is extremely risky: All parts of the plant contain toxic levels of belladonna alkaloids, chemicals that can produce visual and auditory hallucinations, neurological problems, increased heart rate, elevated blood pressure, fever, urine retention, and liver dysfunction; deaths have been reported.

THE VOLATILE CHEMICALS

As with many drugs in recreational use, there are fads and fashions in **inhalants**—substances containing volatile chemicals that have psychoactive (and other) effects when inhaled. In the 1960s, the "in" substance in this category was model-airplane glue. More recently a variety of other substances have been sniffed in quest of a quick "high," including gasoline, furniture polish, insecticides, transmission fluid, paint thinners, and more. All are highly toxic and can cause damage to vital organs such as lungs, kidney, liver, and brain, and death.

Nitrous Oxide

Recreational use of **nitrous oxide,** discovered in 1773 and first used in dentistry in the 1840s, actually predates its medical use. Still employed as an anesthetic (it is also the propellant in whipped-cream dispensers), it is among the least toxic inhalants. It *is* toxic, nevertheless, and death can follow if it is inhaled with insufficient oxygen.

What happens if a person takes nitrous oxide over a long period? Repeated, long-term use can result in nerve damage, muscle weakness, hearing loss, changes in heart rate, impotence, or life-threatening anemia due to suppression of bone-marrow production (possibly through inactivation of vitamin B_{12}). A leading dental educator even warned in 1981 that dentists and their assistants should beware of long-term low-level exposure, checking their equipment for leaks and being sure to utilize efficient exhaust systems. A study of 60,-000 dental workers, published by the American Dental Association the previous year, had found that people occupationally exposed to nitrous oxide had increased rates of miscarriage, increased birth-defect rates in the children of both males and females, and increases in the incidence of certain types of cancers.[14]

Amyl Nitrite and Butyl Nitrite

Amyl nitrite is a prescription drug used in the treatment of angina (severe chest pain due to coronary insufficiency), although it is used less now than it was in the past. Its analog **butyl nitrite** has never been used medically to any significant extent. Both amyl nitrite and butyl nitrite have been employed recreationally as euphoriants and presumed sexual stimulants; butyl nitrite has been sold in "head shops" and other stores as a "room odorizer" or "liquid incense" under a variety of trade names (two of the most widely distributed, at this writing, are "Locker Room" and "Rush"). A more recent development has been the use of isobutyl alcohol, which has been advertised in sexually oriented publications. Inhalation of its vapors produces a similar but less powerful effect than butyl nitrite.

Immediate effects of nitrite inhalation include headache, dizziness, flushing, muscle relaxation, heightened heart rate, and lowered blood pressure, with possible nausea, vomiting, or fainting. The effects may be especially dangerous in persons with normally low blood pressure and in those who suffer from glaucoma. There is some tolerance to nitrites, although physical dependence has not been reported. Inhalation of substantial amounts of nitrites over a period of time can lead to a condition called methemoglobinemia, in which normal hemoglobin has been chemically converted and can no longer carry oxygen. There is also a long-term risk of heart and blood-vessel damage.[15]

MARIJUANA

Last we come to marijuana—the third most popular recreational drug in the United States (after alcohol and nicotine), possibly the most widely used of all the controlled substances, and the one controlled substance that has come closest to gaining acceptance among relatively conservative people in many spheres of American society. In some people's minds, "pot" or "grass" is almost on the same level as alcohol: Both alcohol and pot are relatively inexpensive and easy to obtain, both are relatively safe (some people *think*—we'll go into this question later), and both are somehow less taboo than drugs such as heroin or cocaine. To

these people's thinking, the only reason alcohol is legal and marijuana is not is that alcohol happens to have been part of our culture for a much longer time.

Marijuana laws are changing; sixteen states have sanctioned medical use of marijuana, and eleven states have decriminalized their marijuana laws. A 1980 Gallup poll showed that although a majority of Americans were not ready to support legalization of marijuana, opinion had shifted toward more liberal viewpoints.[16] It is expected that this liberalization trend will continue.

There is still much controversy about marijuana's effects on humans, and one can find physicians, scientists, law-enforcement officials, and legislators on both sides of the controversy. It is hard to decide who and what to believe about marijuana. The annual reports to the U.S. Congress by the Secretary of Health and Human Services serve as the basis for the material that follows.

What Is Marijuana?

Cannabis sativa is the botanical name for the hemp plant, which grows all over the world. Its chief products are **marijuana** (plant material that is dried and prepared for smoking) and **hashish** (a concentrated and more potent resin from the plant). While some 150 chemical compounds have

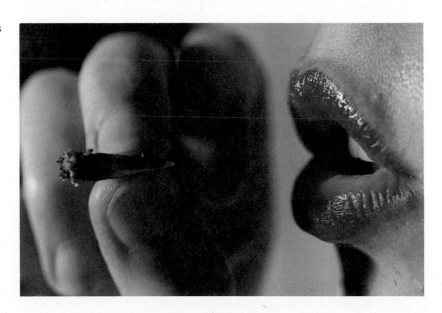

Young people are under tremendous peer pressure to experiment with marijuana—even though some researchers express concern that the drug may have greater potential for harm in younger users. (© Al Rubin/Stock, Boston)

been identified in cannabis, the chief psychoactive ingredient is **tetrahydrocannabinol (THC)**. The amount of this chemical in a given quantity of marijuana determines its potency. Potency varies, and marijuana sold recently (3 to 4 percent THC) has typically been more potent than marijuana available a few years ago (about 1 percent THC).

Cannabis has a 5,000-year history of medical use, mostly as an analgesic. It was largely superseded by aspirin and other pain-relieving drugs of which dosages could be standardized, but it remained an accepted drug in American medicine until the late 1930s. It appears to have therapeutic potential for relief or control of a number of conditions, most notably glaucoma and the gastrointestinal side effects of cancer chemotherapy.

Short-Term Effects of Marijuana

Marijuana doesn't fit neatly into any of the classes of drugs discussed earlier. In average doses, its effects are not much different from those of moderate quantities of alcohol, with some additions: There is a distinct distortion of time perception, some increase in heart rate, and dilation of blood vessels in the eyes (causing a reddened or bloodshot appearance); appetite and thirst are often increased slightly to markedly; and there is some degree of muscular weakness.

Other effects may vary with the individual as well as with the setting and may sometimes be like those of a mild sedative, sometimes like those of a mild stimulant. An individual who is emotionally unstable may react in an exaggerated manner, in almost any direction, as may someone who is anxious or under stress. With higher doses, there may be significant sensory distortion. The ability to think clearly and to learn is usually reduced by marijuana, as are short-term memory and psychomotor performance. Knowledge acquired under the influence of the drug is likely to be forgotten when it wears off—which means that a student using the drug during the school day invariably suffers diminished learning capacity.[17]

MARIJUANA'S EFFECT ON DRIVING ABILITY

A person who drives while under the influence of marijuana is running serious risks (see Table 4.2).

TABLE 4.2 · Drugs and Driving

Drug	Effect
Tranquilizers	In normal or larger doses or in combination with other drugs such as alcohol, tranquilizers may result in sedation to the point of dizziness or drowsiness.
Analgesics	These drugs affect judgment, produce drowsiness, interfere with concentration, impair vision, and may release inhibitions against reckless driving and other improper behavior.
Marijuana	Marijuana use, even at dose levels normally consumed in social settings, impairs to a significant degree visual perception and temporally controlled responses. Many users have found that marijuana often interferes with peripheral as well as central vision. It is a definite hazard to highway safety.
Psychedelic/ illusionogens	The use of these drugs can be dangerous, for it can produce distorted sensory perception, especially visual, disruption of thought processes, alterations in time and space perception, impaired memory, and feelings of unreality, to name just a few.

Source: Adapted from Brent Q. Hafen and Brenda Peterson, *Medicines and Drugs: Problems and Risks, Use and Abuse,* 2nd ed. (Philadelphia: Lea & Febiger, 1978), p. 186.

In one study the subjects who had taken pot suffered from an inability to make the swift decisions sometimes necessary on the road,[18] and in a 1982 study by the National Academy of Science's Institute of Medicine, drivers' perceptions and motor coordination were hindered if they were under the influence of marijuana.[19] Subjects could not follow a moving object or detect a flash of light. The combination of marijuana and alcohol may be especially hazardous on the road.

Even more crucial: Marijuana's effects may last from four to eight hours after the "high" begins—so there is a long time period in which the user *should not drive.*

Long-Term Effects

The distorted "Reefer Madness" depiction of marijuana as a drug that led its users to crazed mayhem helped banish it from medical use in the 1930s. This myth of course has long since been discredited, along with more recent assertions almost as irresponsible—that marijuana causes permanent brain damage, for example. But there are still some genuine concerns about marijuana's long-term effects.

TOLERANCE AND DEPENDENCE

Tolerance can develop with marijuana, but the reverse also occurs: The experienced user may require less of the drug to experience its effects than the beginner. Though the risk of physical dependence is probably insignificant, psychic dependence is entirely possible.

EFFECTS ON THE LUNGS

The major risk, since marijuana is usually smoked, is that of possible respiratory damage. As long ago as the 1890s, a report of a special commission in India that had investigated health problems of ganja smokers (*ganja* is a cannabis preparation intermediate in potency between marijuana and hashish) noted a "chronic bronchitis" among many of them. Marijuana may, like tobacco, decrease the efficiency of the lungs. There is also some evidence that marijuana smoke may impair antibacterial defense systems within the lungs, thus posing an increased risk of infection.[20] And although there is no direct proof that marijuana smoking is correlated with lung cancer, cannabis-smoke residuals, like tobacco-smoke residuals ("tar"), have been found to produce tumors in experimental animals. Benzopyrene, a known cancer-causing chemical in tobacco smoke, is also found—and at higher levels—in marijuana smoke.

EFFECTS ON THE REPRODUCTIVE SYSTEM

A second serious concern is marijuana's effect on the reproductive system, notably because of its proven impact on the secretion of certain hormones. The National Organization for the Reform of Marijuana Laws (NORML), which typically goes to great pains to discredit unjust accusations about

the drug, has singled out marijuana's effects on the reproductive system as something users should definitely be wary of. The organization has warned that these findings may be important for "individuals with already impaired fertility or other evidence of marginal endocrine function."[21] A number of studies have found lowered testosterone levels in males who are heavy marijuana smokers (although the levels were still within normal limits), and two studies of such groups have found abnormalities in sperm count and in sperm motility and morphology (structure). It is believed that these effects are reversible when the drug is discontinued.[22]

IS MARIJUANA PARTICULARLY DANGEROUS FOR YOUNGER USERS?

A third area of concern is marijuana's impact on the developing mind and body—that is, on the fetus and the growing child. This is hardly just a theoretical question. It is known that younger and younger people have been using the drug: According to surveys conducted by the National Institute on Drug Abuse (NIDA), in 1971, 10 percent of fourteen- and fifteen-year-olds reported having used it at least once, while by 1979, 32 percent of that age group reported some experience with it, as did 8 percent of twelve- and thirteen-year-olds.[23] These figures are, as in most such surveys, probably lower than the actual figures.

The concern is twofold. First, given the previously cited hormonal effects, what impact might marijuana have on the still maturing reproductive system? And second, what impact might it have, in the long or short term, on adolescents who are going through an emotionally shaky period of life? Most of the questions in this area remain unanswered. But even those who advocate the loosening of restrictions on marijuana generally agree that, like the use of alcohol, the use of marijuana should be limited to those over a certain age.

As to possible effects on the unborn: Again, there are no firm answers, but the rate of miscarriage has been found to quadruple in monkeys treated with THC in quantities equivalent to fairly heavy marijuana smoking in humans.[24] And since harmful effects on fetal development, evidenced by babies born with clear disorders, are known to occur with alcohol and other dependence-producing substances and are suspected with other drugs including tobacco, there is general agreement

TABLE 4.3 • Schedules of Psychoactive Drugs Under the Federal Controlled Substances Act

Schedule*	Types of Drugs and Examples (see also Table 4.1)	Comments
I	Certain opium derivatives and opiates (heroin) Some psychedelic/illusionogens (LSD, mescaline, psilocybin, PCP, STP) Marijuana, THC	High potential for abuse. No currently accepted medical use. Psychedelic/illusionogens included in Schedule I purely for regulatory purposes.
II	Opium Coca leaf derivatives (cocaine) Class A narcotics (methadone, morphine) Amphetamines	High potential for abuse and severe physical and psychological dependence. Have currently accepted medical uses; must be dispensed only on written prescription (except in emergencies), and may not be refilled without new written prescription.
III	Short-acting barbiturates (pentothal, Seconal) Class B narcotics (Empirin, codeine preparations) Paregoric	Less potential for abuse than drugs in Schedules I and II, but may lead to moderate physical and psychological dependence. May be dispensed on either oral or written prescription, but may not be refilled more than 5 times or more than 6 months after date.
IV	Certain major tranquilizers, antianxiety drugs, and long-acting barbiturates (barbital, phenobarbital, chloral hydrate, meprobamate)	Lower potential for abuse and more limited physical and psychological dependence than drugs in Schedule III. May be dispensed on either oral or written prescription, but may not be refilled more than 5 times or more than 6 months after date.
V	Exempt OTC narcotic preparations, usually for treatment of coughs and diarrhea	Lower potential for abuse and more limited physical and psychological dependence than drugs in Schedule IV.

*The federal government places drugs into schedules, or classes, on the basis of their degree of abuse potential and risk for psychological or physical dependence. In general, the lower a drug's schedule number, the more severe the penalties for possession or sale. No drug listed in Schedule I has a currently accepted medical use in the United States; the drugs in all the other schedules do have accepted medical uses, so the criteria for classifying drugs into the other schedules are relative to one another.

Source: Adapted from Brent Q. Hafen and Brenda Peterson, *Medicines and Drugs: Problems and Risks, Use and Abuse,* 2nd ed. (Philadelphia: Lea & Febiger, 1978), pp. 206–207.

that the use of marijuana (as well as other recreational drugs) in pregnancy poses possible risks that are best avoided. As we noted in Chapter 3, THC is also excreted in breast milk, and a nursing mother who smokes marijuana will pass THC to the infant; the exact consequences are unknown.

FINDING ALTERNATIVES TO DRUG USE

What choices are available to an individual if he or she decides that there might be times when some

other activity would be preferable to the use of drugs? What can a person do—other than take a drug of some sort—to obtain relief from anxiety, or become more alert, or experience a feeling of excitement, or get any of the other effects offered by drugs? (Note that when we talk about drugs here, we include alcohol and cigarettes—even coffee, a drug many people would like to avoid if they could find a better way to get the same effect.)

Obviously, the alternative would be some sort of activity that gives the individual an even better effect—not just one that's almost as good as the drug effect. It also has to be something that the individual can't do while taking the drug at the same time. A number of alternative routes and activities have been suggested. Some of the stress-reducing methods mentioned in Chapter 2 may help reduce anxiety; some counseling or even just private self-examination may help with emotional problems (as noted in Chapter 1); a healthy diet and a program of vigorous exercise can boost one's overall sense of well-being (see Chapters 13 and 15). Music, movies, dancing, games, laughs with friends, a trip to a beautiful outdoor spot can provide "natural highs."

But these decisions are very personal, and each of us must figure out an answer that works for us. In this society, people turn to drugs for different reasons; each person may have to develop not one, but a number of alternatives to the use of drugs.

SUMMARY

1. Certain chemical substances called psychoactive drugs affect parts of the brain that control mood, consciousness, and behavior.

2. Narcotic analgesics are addictive natural or synthetic substances—including opiates (morphine, heroin, and opium) and opioids (methadone, meperidine)—that relieve pain without causing loss of consciousness. Dependence on narcotics requires increasingly higher doses to produce the original "high" and to stave off withdrawal symptoms. The best way to cure addiction is debated, but among the possible approaches are sudden or gradual withdrawal, legal maintenance, and psychotherapy.

3. Hypnosedatives, or "downers," have both calming and sleep-inducing properties and include antianxiety drugs, barbiturates, and hypnotics. Each has valuable medical uses, but each is also subject to abuse. Hypnosedatives tend to act synergistically and so should not be combined. Sudden withdrawal can produce serious reactions, and dependent people need medical supervision in withdrawing from hypnosedatives.

4. Stimulants, or "uppers," include caffeine, amphetamines, and cocaine. They act by stimulating the sympathetic nervous system. Amphetamines have only two legitimate medical uses: control of narcolepsy and control of hyperactivity in children. Users can become physically and psychologically dependent on amphetamines. A cocaine high is more sociable and less agitated than an amphetamine high and is chemically related to, although more powerful than, a caffeine high. Cocaine is used medically as a local anesthetic. Physical and psychological dependence can develop from recreational use of cocaine.

5. Psychedelic or illusionogenic drugs create illusions and alter users' thoughts, moods, and perceptions. LSD distorts visual and auditory perception, causes synesthesia, and produces psychological changes. LSD can produce "bad trips" and flashbacks. "Angel dust," or PCP, produces intoxication but also numbness, slurred speech, and, in large doses, psychosis and coma. Mescaline, psilocybin, DMT, Jimsonweed, and DOM (STP) are other psychedelic drugs, with individually variable effects.

6. Volatile drugs, or inhalants, that have recently become popular as recreational drugs include nitrous oxide, medically used as an anesthetic, and the volatile nitrites, medically used to treat angina.

7. Marijuana, though widely used, is still an illegal drug. Its active ingredient is tetrahydrocannabinol (THC), with medical uses in treating glaucoma and the nausea of cancer chemotherapy. Psychological, but not physical, dependence may develop. Long-term marijuana use may have negative effects on the lungs and on male fertility.

GLOSSARY

amphetamines A group of synthetic stimulant drugs ("uppers," "pep pills").

amyl nitrite A prescription drug used in the treatment of angina; used recreationally as a euphoriant and presumed sexual stimulant.

analgesic A substance that eliminates or reduces the sense of pain.

anxiolytics (relaxants) Hypnosedative drugs used as anxiety reducers; some also used as muscle relaxants and to control specific types of convulsive seizures; formerly known as "minor tranquilizers."

barbiturates Hypnosedatives used primarily to treat insomnia and less often for daytime sedation; some also have anticonvulsive properties.

butyl nitrite An analog of amyl nitrite used recreationally as a euphoriant and presumed sexual stimulant.

caffeine A stimulant drug found in coffee, cola drinks, chocolate, tea, and other beverages as well as some OTC drugs.

cocaine A stimulant drug extracted from the leaves of the coca bush of South America.

flashbacks Brief, sudden, unexpected perceptual distortions and bizarre thoughts—similar to those experienced while on an LSD trip—that occur long after the immediate effects of the drug have worn off.

hashish A concentrated and potent resin of *Cannabis sativa* (the hemp plant).

heroin A narcotic analgesic derived from morphine and more than twice as powerful.

hypnosedatives A group of drugs that have both sedative (calming) and hypnotic (sleep-inducing) effects ("downers").

inhalants A group of substances containing volatile chemicals that have psychoactive (and other) effects when inhaled.

intravenous injection Injection of a substance into a vein. Compare **subcutaneous injection.**

LSD (lysergic acid diethylamide) A synthetic psychedelic/illusionogen drug used recreationally ("acid").

marijuana Material from *Cannabis sativa* (the hemp plant) dried and prepared for smoking; has a variety of mind-altering and physiological effects that may resemble those of a mild sedative or a mild stimulant, depending on the individual and the setting ("pot," "grass").

mescaline A psychedelic/illusionogen drug derived from the peyote cactus of the U.S. Southwest.

methadone An opioid used in treatment of heroin addiction.

morphine A narcotic analgesic that is the active ingredient in opium.

narcotic analgesics A group of drugs—including the opiates and the opioids—that act on the central nervous system to eliminate or relieve pain without causing loss of consciousness.

nitrous oxide An anesthetic gas sometimes used recreationally as an inhalant.

opiates A group of narcotic analgesics, including opium, morphine, and heroin.

opioids A group of synthetic narcotic analgesics, including methadone and meperidine, that are chemically similar to the opiates.

opium A narcotic analgesic that is the parent substance of the opiates; derived from the juice of the opium poppy.

PCP (phencyclidine) An animal anesthetic used recreationally as a psychedelic/illusionogen drug ("angel dust").

psilocybin A psychedelic/illusionogen drug derived from a Mexican mushroom.

psychedelic/illusionogens A group of drugs that create illusions, distorting the user's mind by creating moods, thoughts, and perceptions that would otherwise take place only in a dream state (also known as *hallucinogens, deliriants, psychotogens, psychotomimetics*).

psychoactive drugs Drugs that alter a person's moods, consciousness, and behaviors.

stimulants Drugs that activate the sympathetic division of the autonomic nervous system.

subcutaneous injection Injection of a substance under the skin. Compare **intravenous injection.**

synesthesia The blending of two senses so that, for example, a person using LSD "hears" colors and "sees" sounds.

THC (tetrahydrocannabinol) The chief psychoactive ingredient in marijuana and hashish.

NOTES

1. Brent Q. Hafen and Brenda Peterson, *Medicines and Drugs: Problems and Risks, Use and Abuse,* 2nd ed. (Philadelphia: Lea & Febiger, 1978), pp. 371–382.

2. National Institute on Drug Abuse, *Statistical Series I, No. 1: Data from the Drug Abuse Warning Network,* Annual Data, 1981, pp. 25, 49.

3. Robert Fink et al., "Sedative-Hypnotic Dependence," *American Family Physician* 11 (1974): 116.

4. National Institute on Drug Abuse, Research Monograph Series No. 33, *Benzodiazepines: A Review of Research Results, 1980.* DHHS Publication No. (ADM) 81-1052, 1981.

5. *FDA Consumer* 15, no. 1 (December 1981–January 1982): 24.

6. National Institute on Drug Abuse, *National Survey on Drug Abuse: Main Findings, 1979* (Washington, D.C.: U.S. Department of Health and Human Services, 1980).

7. David Duncan and Robert Gold, *Drugs and the Whole Person* (New York: Wiley, 1982), p. 71.

8. *Harvard Medical School Health Letter* 7, no. 9 (July 1982): 1–2.

9. National Institute on Drug Abuse, *National Survey on Drug Abuse.*

10. Robert Byck et al., "Cocaine: Chic, Costly, and What Else?" *Patient Care* 14 (September 15, 1980): 136–138.

11. Duncan and Gold, *Drugs and the Whole Person,* p. 130.

12. Jerome H. Jaffe, "Drug Addiction and Drug Abuse," in Alfred G. Gilman et al., eds., *Goodman and Gilman's The Pharmacological Basis of Therapeutics,* 6th ed. (New York: Macmillan, 1980), p. 567; National Institute on Drug Abuse, Research Monograph Series No. 21, *PCP: Phencyclidine Abuse: An Appraisal.* DHHS Publication No. (ADM) 79-728, 1979.

13. American Academy of Pediatrics, "New Form of Drug Abuse Popular, but Dangerous" (press release), April 16, 1979; "New 'Loco Weed' Fad Is Sending Teens to the ICU," *Medical Tribune Report,* February 21, 1979.

14. Annabel Hecht, "Inhalants: Quick Route to Danger," *FDA Consumer* 14, no. 4 (May 1980): 19–22; Sidney Cohen, "The Volatile Nitrites," *Journal of the American Medical Association* 241, no. 19 (May 11, 1979): 2077–2078; Phil Gunby, "Nitrous Oxide No Laughing Matter; Nerve Damage Seen," *Journal of the American Medical Association* 239, no. 23 (June 9, 1978; "Here's the Topper: Whipped-Cream Cans May Be Fatal for N₂O Abusers," *Medical World News* 20, no. 8 (April 16, 1979): 16; Michela Reichman, "Dentist Urges Colleagues to Cut Occupational Exposure to Nitrous Oxide," *News from SFGH/UC–San Francisco,* August 2, 1981.

15. Cohen, "The Volatile Nitrites."

16. "Legalization of Marijuana," Gallup Poll, September 14, 1980.

17. National Institute on Drug Abuse, Research Monograph Series No. 31, *Marijuana: Research Findings, 1980,* DHHS Publication No. (ADM) 80-1001, 1980.

18. Report from the Injury Control Research Laboratory of the Public Health Service, "Effect of Marijuana on Risk Acceptance in a Simulated Passing Test," HE 20.2859:71-3, March 1972; National Institute on Drug Abuse, *Marijuana: Research Findings, 1980.*

19. *Marijuana and Health,* Report of a Study by a Committee of the Institute of Medicine, December 1981 (Washington, D.C.: National Academy of Science Press, 1982), pp. 117–119.

20. AMA Council on Scientific Affairs, "Marijuana: Its Health Hazards and Therapeutic Potentials," *Journal of the American Medical Association* 246, no. 16 (October 16, 1981): 1823–1827.

21. George Farnham, Director, National Organization for the Reform of Marijuana Laws.

22. National Institute on Drug Abuse, *Marijuana: Research Findings, 1980.*

23. National Institute on Drug Abuse, "Drugs and the Nation's High School Students: Five-Year National Trends," *1979 Highlights,* HE 20.8202: D84/11/979 (Washington, D.C.: U.S. Government Printing Office, 1980).

24. AMA Council on Scientific Affairs, "Marijuana: Its Health Hazards and Therapeutic Potentials."

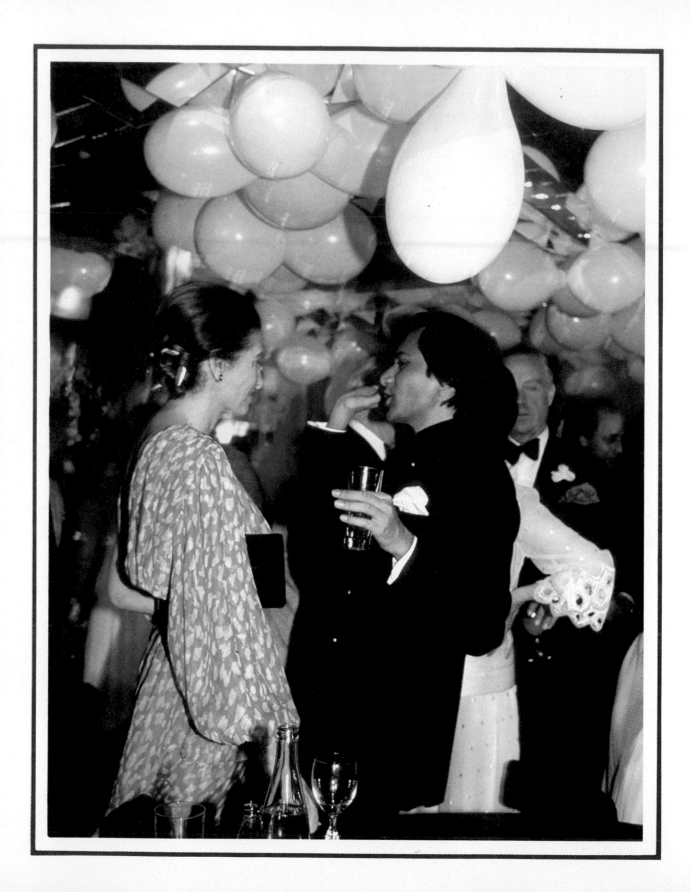

CHAPTER 5

Alcohol

Ethyl alcohol (the type of alcohol found in alcoholic beverages) is one of the most widely used, yet least understood, drugs in our society. Few of us even think of it as a drug. Many of us simply accept alcohol as part of our lifestyle; about one out of every three American adults has at least one alcoholic drink a week.[1] Many people think it's "harmless" to have a few drinks, and sometimes people think that having a drink or two is helpful in social situations. A little alcohol is often seen as a way to relieve tension and even improve one's sex life. Many people believe a drink will warm them up if they are cold.

Small amounts of alcohol, safely used, can indeed be pleasant. But many of the ideas people have about alcohol are myths—and our steadily increasing consumption of alcohol is causing some of the worst public health problems in our country. Alcohol consumption has doubled in the last twenty years and is expected to rise another 32 percent in the next decade.[2] The National Institute on Alcohol Abuse and Alcoholism has estimated that between 9 and 10 million adult Americans are either full-fledged alcoholics or problem drinkers.[3] The human costs of this abuse are staggering. Alcohol plays a leading role in highway accidents—some 25,000 Americans are killed each year by drunk drivers. Alcohol can also damage vital organs and may cause birth defects and infant deaths. Alcohol-related absences from work and school have reached alarming proportions, and there is a strong association between drinking and violent behavior, financial problems, family conflicts, criminal acts, and mental illness.

Experts now believe that the best way to combat alcohol abuse is to get rid of the myths and spread some solid information instead. People need to know how the body takes in alcohol and what changes occur as the alcohol is absorbed. Understanding these facts can help people regulate their consumption so it does not become a problem. People also need information about "problem drinking" and alcoholism; they can then tell when they are abusing alcohol or when someone close to them has a problem with alcohol—and they will know what steps to take to get help.

SOURCES AND TYPES OF ALCOHOL

Ethyl alcohol is the common active ingredient in such varied beverages as wine, beer, hard liquors (gin, whiskey, brandy, rum), and cordials. It is prepared from a number of natural plant products, including fruits and grains. Some methods for making it have been known since before the beginning of recorded history.

The different forms of alcoholic beverages vary greatly in strength, as measured by the concentration of alcohol they contain. The most common alcoholic beverages—beers, wines, and distilled spirits—are made by different processes.

- *Beer* and *ale* are derived from various grains by a brewing process; they generally contain from 3 to 6 percent alcohol.
- *Wines* are made by fermenting the juice of grapes or other fruits. Table wines, which are often served with meals, have a natural alcohol content ranging from 9 to 12 percent. Other varieties, such as sherry, port, and muscatel, are reinforced by the addition of distilled spirits to bring their alcohol content up to as much as 18 to 22 percent.

■ *Distilled spirits*—the strongest alcoholic beverages, such as *gin, whiskey, brandy,* and *rum*—are manufactured by distilling brewed or fermented products so that liquids containing from 35 to 50 percent alcohol are recovered. Ounce for ounce, the amount of pure alcohol in most distilled liquors is ten to twelve times greater than that in beer. *But* when a person has a beer, he or she drinks 12 ounces of beer (in contrast to the typical shot glass of whiskey, which contains about 1 ounce).

It's important to be aware that a person gets as much alcohol in one bottle or can of beer as he or she gets in a glass of wine or a shot of whiskey. (And "light " beer contains as much alcohol as regular beer; it's called "light" only because it has fewer calories.)

The term **proof** indicates the concentration of ethyl alcohol in a beverage. Proof can be converted to percent by dividing the proof number in half. Thus, 80-proof whiskey is 40 percent alcohol, and 100-proof whiskey is 50 percent alcohol. Every ounce of 100-proof whiskey, then, contains one-half ounce of pure ethyl alcohol.

Some alcoholic beverages also contain **congeners**—substances other than alcohol that are natural products of the fermentation and preparation process. Congeners alter the smell, taste, and color of the various beverages. The percentage of congeners in a beverage depends primarily on the fermentation process; it varies from 0.01 percent (in beer) to 0.4 percent in certain aged distilled spirits. Modern distilling processes have tended to reduce the amount of congeners in the various beverages, but some congeners still remain and can be toxic. A headache that develops after having a drink is sometimes an allergic reaction to the congeners the drink contains, not a reaction to the alcohol.

HOW ALCOHOL WORKS AS A DRUG

Alcohol takes a rather direct route into an individual's system (see Figure 5.1). It travels to the stomach and small intestine, and from there it is directly absorbed into the blood. Its absorption can be quite rapid, especially on an empty stomach. Since the stomach can absorb fully one-fourth of the total dose (the rest is absorbed in the small intestine), when a drink is taken on an empty stomach the maximum level of alcohol in the blood can be reached in as short a time as thirty minutes.

Dose Levels and Time Factors

As the blood races through the body, the alcohol travels with it and is distributed fairly uniformly throughout the body tissues and fluids. The more the individual drinks, the more his or her entire body becomes saturated with alcohol, and the more he or she will feel its effects.

A small amount of alcohol will be removed through the breath and sweat, but most of the alcohol must be processed by the liver before it is expelled from the body via the urine. Alcohol is made up of oxygen, hydrogen, and carbon atoms; they react with chemical substances in the cells and are eventually turned into carbon dioxide and water. This metabolic process takes place primarily in the liver.

HOW FAST IS ALCOHOL METABOLIZED?

The liver metabolizes pure ethyl alcohol at a constant rate of about two-thirds of an ounce per hour. This means that the average 150-pound man would maintain a constant level of alcohol in his bloodstream if, every hour, he drank one 12-ounce can of beer or one shot of spirits, or one glass of wine. Drinking more than these amounts in less than an hour would put alcohol into his bloodstream faster than his liver could remove it—and he would increasingly begin to feel its effects and would begin to behave differently.

If you wish to drink safely, a reasonably reliable rule of thumb is to take no more than two drinks the first hour, then one drink each hour following—or less, if you weigh under 150 pounds. (By "one drink" we mean 12 ounces of beer, one ounce of distilled spirit, or one four-ounce glass of wine.)

Figure 5.1   Alcohol in the Body

6. Alcohol reaches the brain last, but within minutes. Keeps passing through brain—and rest of body—until liver has had time to break down all alcohol consumed.

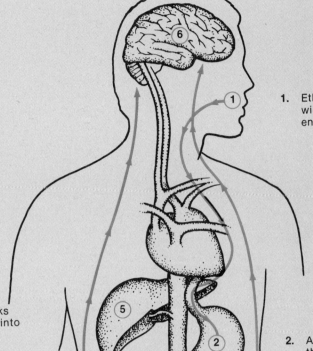

1. Ethyl alcohol (beer, wine, hard liquor) enters the body.

5. The liver breaks down alcohol into water, carbon dioxide, and sugar at a rate of about 2/3 oz. per hour.

4. Bloodstream carries alcohol to *all* parts of the body, including liver, heart, and brain.

2. Alcohol goes first to the stomach. Some enters the bloodstream directly; most goes to small intestine.

3. Most of the alcohol enters the bloodstream from the small intestine.

Source: Scholastic Science World 39, no. 1 (September 3, 1982): 13.

TEST YOUR AWARENESS

Alcohol: Facts and Fallacies

There are lots of myths about drinking alcohol. Most are based on inaccurate information about the action of ethyl alcohol. Which of the following statements are based on facts? (The answers are given upside down below.)

FACT/MYTH

_____ 1. Alcohol is a food: It contains calories that can quickly be converted into usable energy and nutrients for growth and repair of body tissues.

_____ 2. Alcohol acts as a stimulant: In low doses, it produces excitation of the central nervous system.

FACT/MYTH

_____ 3. If you mix your drinks (that is, drink several kinds of alcoholic beverages at once), you are more likely to have a hangover the next morning than if you just drink one kind of alcoholic beverage.

_____ 4. A cup of strong, black coffee will reduce an individual's recovery time from intoxication—that is, it will help the person sober up more quickly.

_____ 5. Alcoholic beverages can be used to warm the body when a person is exposed to very cold temperatures.

ANSWERS

None of these statements is based on fact. They are all myths!

1. The calories in alcohol can only be burned at a steady rate; therefore, they are not very useful as a source of *immediate* energy. Ethyl alcohol contains none of the nutrients (such as vitamins, minerals, proteins, fats) found in food. Furthermore, most heavy drinkers experience appetite suppression, which can lead to nutritional deficiencies.

2. Ethyl alcohol is a CNS *depressant* at all dose levels. Low doses cause a depression of the part of the brain that controls inhibitions; thus, the individual may have a *subjective* feeling of excitation—but this is not the true excitation caused by stimulants such as caffeine.

3. We do not have a complete explanation of the basis of "hangover." However, the symptoms associated with the syndrome (headache, thirst, fatigue, nausea, gastric distress) suggest that overindulgence can trigger a short-term withdrawal phenomenon. Mixing drinks does not result in a more severe hangover than drinking only one kind of beverage.

4. Ethyl alcohol is metabolized at a steady rate—it's impossible to induce the body to process it faster. Coffee has no effect on either the biotransformation or the elimination of ethyl alcohol in the body.

5. Ethyl alcohol dilates the peripheral blood vessels, causing increased heat loss in the body. A person may *feel* warmer, contributing to the notion that drinking alcohol is a good way to warm the body, but a cup of hot soup is a much better choice.

PEOPLE'S RESPONSES VARY

The effects of alcohol depend on a person's **blood alcohol level (BAL)**—how much of it is in the person's blood at any one time; and the BAL can fluctuate with body weight, stress, what's in the person's stomach, and other factors. If an individual is drinking a lot of liquor quickly and not eating anything, the alcohol will get into the bloodstream quickly. Many people find that after a hard day at school or work, when teachers or coworkers have been making demands on them all day, they are likely to get quite drunk on a single martini before dinner. Yet the very next day, when they are feeling relaxed and happy, they can put away two martinis while they eat snacks at a party and hardly feel any effects from the alcohol at all.

Two people of very different sizes—a large man and a small woman, for example—can drink the same amount with very different effects: The amount that the larger person can drink with little effect could cause intoxication in a smaller person. There are good reasons for the differences. A smaller, lighter person, with a correspondingly lower volume of blood and a smaller liver, would have a higher alcohol level in the blood that flows

Alcohol is one of the few drugs with a high potential for dependence that are legally and readily available to the general adult population. (© Hazel Hankin 1983)

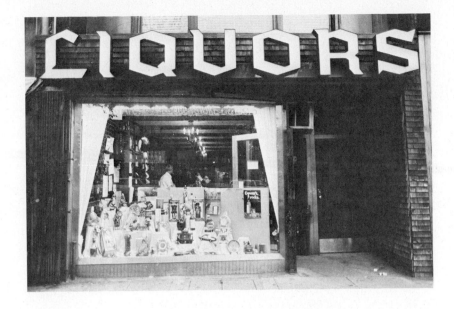

to the liver, and possibly an even higher level in the blood that leaves the liver. The blood alcohol level also depends on how quickly the alcohol is *removed* from the body, which can vary according to the individual's nutritional status, his or her previous drinking history, and even the time of day.

EFFECTS AT DIFFERENT BLOOD ALCOHOL LEVELS

Although the effects of different BALs vary among individuals, some generalizations are possible:

- Most people will experience little noticeable effect at a concentration of up to 0.02 percent alcohol in the blood (0.02 grams per 100 milliliters of blood, or 2 parts of alcohol per 10,000 parts of blood).
- Between the levels of 0.03 and 0.05 percent, the user will generally experience some recognizable sensations, including lightheadedness, a sense of relaxation and well-being, an elevation of mood, and a decrease in reaction time. There may also be a release of some personal inhibitions, so that the drinker may say or do things that are not in his or her normal behavior pattern.
- By the time the blood concentration reaches 0.1 percent, there is a loss of some motor coordination, a greater decrease in reaction time, and some impairment of judgment.
- At 0.15 percent blood alcohol there is significant impairment of motor coordination and

reaction time: The drinker may stagger slightly, fumble objects, and have some trouble saying even familiar words.
- If alcohol concentration reaches 0.2 percent, the drinker will usually be severely intoxicated, and both physically and psychologically incapacitated.
- At 0.3 percent the drinker is conscious but in limited control of functions.
- Concentrations above 0.4 percent lead to coma and, in fact, are lethal for about 50 percent of the population (LD 50; see Chapter 3).
- A concentration of 0.6 or 0.7 percent would cause suffocation and death in about 99 percent of the population (LD 99). Fortunately, such a high concentration rarely occurs: Most drinkers lose consciousness before they consume that much alcohol, and even if they do not, the alcohol is likely to irritate the stomach so that the drinker will vomit before absorption of a fatal dose occurs. However, fatalities *do* happen occasionally.

ALCOHOL'S SHORT-TERM EFFECTS

On every occasion that a person drinks, the alcohol produces physical, psychological, and behavioral effects.

Effects on the Central Nervous System

Alcohol is an anesthetic, a sedative, and a depressant. It is often valued at parties and weddings as a stimulant, because its sedating action on the highest cortical centers of the brain reduces social inhibitions. If enough alcohol is consumed, the result will be an easily measurable effect: the loss of motor coordination. The user will start to stagger, slur speech, and drop or spill things. An intoxicated person's vision may also be seriously affected by the alcohol, making it impossible to drive safely.

Small amounts of alcohol can also prolong glare recovery, making the drinker relatively blind in the face of bright lights at night, and a serious hazard on the road. People who have been drinking should avoid night driving, even if they have had just one glass of wine.

THE HANGOVER

The "hangover" that follows a few hours' intoxication is usually considered a state of mild withdrawal from alcohol. The sensations are caused in part by the toxic congeners in the drinks; as we noted, a person may be allergic to one of these substances. But part of the hangover pain may also be caused by nerve cells in the brain, which become dehydrated by the alcohol. The hangover's severity is related both to the amount and duration of the drinking and to the physical and mental condition of the drinker. Some people may feel weak and nervous, get nauseated, and vomit. The heart may beat faster, and the individual may have trouble concentrating.

No matter what you've read in popular magazines, there is no cure for a hangover except time. Neither coffee nor vitamins nor more alcohol ("the hair of the dog that bit you") can cure it, although aspirin, rest, liquids, and solid food will relieve the symptoms. Fortunately, hangovers usually last less than thirty-six hours.

INCREASED BRAIN AROUSAL

One of the hidden problems with alcohol—as with other depressant drugs—is that while the user gets an initial "glow" of relaxation, an underlying feeling of edginess and agitation also builds up at the same time. This increased brain arousal lasts longer than the feeling of relaxed well-being, and it makes the user want another drink to calm him or her down again—and that next drink will have its own "edge," possibly setting in motion a vicious cycle.

Most drinkers simply stop after the second or third drink, so the buildup of brain arousal doesn't present a problem. But this feature of alcohol's effects does give us an insight into a possible factor in alcoholism: It could be one of the reasons why some individuals are unable to stop after they have had just one or two drinks.

EFFECTS ON THE CARDIOVASCULAR SYSTEM

Earlier, we mentioned the myth that alcohol warms up the body. Where does this myth come from? Moderate amounts of alcohol can affect the cardiovascular system by increasing the heart rate and dilating blood vessels near the skin, and this vasodilation can give the drinker the illusion of feeling warmer. The truth is, however, that the person is actually losing heat from the body *more* rapidly than when alcohol is not present in the bloodstream.

Anyone drinking outdoors or in a cold room should be sure to be warmly dressed and should not stay in the cold air too long. It is possible to reduce your resistance to the common cold or even pneumonia if you drink while exposed to cold for long periods of time.

How to Drink Sensibly

How do you drink sensibly? Mostly by not allowing yourself to get intoxicated. To do that, you need to be aware of what alcohol is, what it does to you, and how to control its effects. Here are a few pointers:

1. Restrict your drinking, even on special occasions. Don't overdo it just because it's your best friend's wedding. A few extra drinks can put you out of commission and make you a danger or a nuisance to those around you.
2. Avoid drinking daily or regularly. If your drinking gets that steady, you're likely to develop a habit that can lead to dependence.
3. Know your limit and make sure you don't exceed it. Keep track of those drinks. If you aren't sure how much alcohol you can handle without losing control, test yourself at home with someone else observing. Then stay within that limit at parties.
4. Avoid mixed drinks that use two kinds of liquor, such as martinis and Manhattans. They are stronger and will get you drunk faster. Choose a drink that is mixed with a nonalcoholic beverage such as orange juice or club soda.
5. Drink slowly. Don't gulp down those drinks. The alcohol goes immediately to your stomach and is quickly passed to your bloodstream and circulated throughout your body. The faster you gulp, the drunker you'll get.
6. Never drink on an empty stomach—especially on a hot day. Food will slow down the absorption of alcohol. If your stomach is empty, the alcohol will pass into your bloodstream more quickly. On a hot day, drinking on an empty stomach can be especially harmful. It can produce hypoglycemia (low blood sugar), making you feel dizzy and weak and shifting your mood rapidly.
7. Find substitutes for alcohol that you enjoy at parties. Try one of the new mineral waters with a twist of lime or lemon, or sip some fruit juice. Break the habit of thinking that you need to drink to have a good time.
8. Make conversation while you're drinking. Get your attention away from the alcohol and be sociable. This can help reduce your alcohol intake.
9. Avoid bars and lounges when you are just killing time in an airport or train station. Buy a magazine or browse in the gift shop.
10. At parties or dinners, delay having your first drink as long as possible. If you cut down on the amount of time you spend drinking, you won't be able to consume as much—and you won't consume as much on an empty stomach.
11. Accept a drink only if you really want one. When you've reached your limit, politely refuse refills.
12. Think about your drinking. Is it getting out of hand? A bad habit can creep up on you if you don't monitor your behavior.
13. If a friend suggests that you have a drinking problem, take the comment seriously and get help.
14. When you eat out, have your drinks *with* dinner, not afterward. This rule is especially important if you must drive home.

Source: R. Engs, *Responsible Drug and Alcohol Use* (New York: Macmillan, 1979), pp. 67–72.

Dangers of Drug Interactions with Alcohol

People can experience serious complications when they drink while using other drugs (see Table 5.1). And they often find out the hard way that a drug interaction can happen even after just one drink, and even with seemingly harmless over-the-counter drugs such as aspirin. Alcohol itself is a powerful drug, and when two or more drugs are taken at the same time, they often produce a different, stronger effect than either one produces alone (see Chapter 3). If the two or more drugs affect the same systems in the body, their combined effect is often more powerful than might be expected.

ALCOHOL PLUS BARBITURATES   A case in point is the combination of phenobarbital, a barbiturate, with alcohol. Both are depressants. When taken together, even at doses that are well below the lethal level when taken alone, these drugs can kill.

ALCOHOL PLUS ASPIRIN   Alcohol tends to irritate the stomach lining; when taken in combination with aspirin, which also irritates the gastric system, it can cause internal bleeding.

TABLE 5.1 • The Effects of Combining Alcohol with Other Drugs

Drug	Effects
Analgesics Narcotic— methadone, morphine, Demerol	Depression of respiration and brain activity. Possible coma and death.
Nonnarcotic—aspirin	Stomach irritation and gastric bleeding.
Antialcohol Antabuse	Nausea, vomiting, headache, blood pressure rise, irregular heartbeat.
Antidiabetic Insulin and oral medication	Severe lowering of blood sugar, tremors, dizziness, shock.
Antihistamines	Increase in sedative action.
Antihypertensives Reserpine and others	Increase in sedative action; decrease in blood pressure; fainting; dizziness.
Anticoagulants Dicumarol, etc.	Decrease in anticoagulant effect.
Anticonvulsants Dilantin	Decrease in anticonvulsant effect.
Antidepressants monoamine-oxidase inhibitors	May increase blood pressure to a dangerous point and cause stroke.
Stimulants amphetamines, caffeine, nicotine	Euphoria and sense of well-being; also sense of security.
Diuretics	Reduced blood pressure.
Hypnosedatives barbiturates, etc.	Severe sedation, respiratory depression, possible coma, and death.
Anxiolytics	Severe sedation, slurred speech, impaired motor skills, possible coma, respiratory depression, and death.
B vitamins	Decreased absorption leading to deficiency diseases after heavy or prolonged drinking.

Source: R. Engs, *Responsible Drug and Alcohol Use* (New York: Macmillan, 1979), p. 70.

ALCOHOL PLUS OTHER MEDICATIONS Alcohol can produce problems when taken with almost any medication. Even common cold remedies sold at the corner drugstore, when they contain antihistamines, can have a tragic interaction with alcohol. These drugs tend to act as sedatives, further decreasing motor control and judgment (already lowered by drinking), which can mean serious trouble for a user who attempts to drive.

Everyone should know that *no* drug, even aspirin, is completely safe when combined with alcohol.

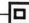

PEOPLE WITH SPECIAL CONDITIONS OR SPECIAL SENSITIVITY TO ALCOHOL

It is important to mention certain additional factors affecting the individual's response to alcohol, although these factors are perhaps the least understood. In some cases they may involve a permanent or temporary decrease in the efficiency of the individual's alcohol absorption or breakdown process.

- Some people are particularly sensitive to alcohol, and even small amounts produce unpleasant reactions.
- People with certain diseases—diabetes and epilepsy, for example—should not drink. Even more than other people, such individuals should not be encouraged or pressured to drink merely for the sake of conformity.
- Many people seem more susceptible to alcohol's effects when they are extremely fatigued or have recently been ill. Such people find they simply cannot drink the way they usually do without feeling uncomfortable effects.

DANGERS OF ALCOHOL IN PREGNANCY

Drinking alcohol during pregnancy has been known to be a danger to the fetus since biblical times. The Greeks and Romans believed that an alcoholic woman could conceive a deformed baby. In the 1700s, when the English government allowed a poor-quality gin to be widely distributed, medical literature of the time reported that drinking alcohol during pregnancy could cause birth

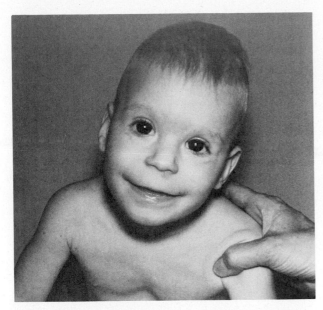

Among the characteristics of fetal alcohol syndrome are: mental retardation, smaller-than-normal body size, and physical defects such as a thin upper lip, lack of a philtrum (the shallow groove below the nostrils), eyes set far apart, and flattened bones. (From *The Journal of the American Medical Association*, 1976, Vol. 235, 1458–1460. Courtesy, James W. Hanson, M.D.)

defects. But interest in the issue died down, and modern medicine did not start to take such reports seriously until 1968, when a French researcher described malformations in babies born to alcoholic mothers.[4] Five years later other researchers reported similar findings, coining the term **fetal alcohol syndrome** to describe the phenomenon.[5] Physicians now realize that even mild drinking during pregnancy can produce severe adverse effects in the fetus.

The fetal alcohol syndrome consists of three main features—mental retardation, slow growth before and after birth, and a wide range of physical defects, ranging from cleft palates to hip dislocations. Mild to moderate mental retardation is characteristic of the syndrome: In fact, some researchers suggest that maternal alcoholism is the third leading cause of mental retardation in the United States.[6] The physical defects in babies born to alcoholic mothers are believed to be caused by a depletion of zinc in the mother's body, a depletion caused by alcohol.[7]

Some studies show that 74 percent of the in-

fants born to mothers who drink heavily—more than ten drinks a day—have the syndrome. Alcoholic mothers are also more likely to abort or give birth to stillborn children.[8]

There is no known safe level of alcohol that a woman can consume during pregnancy, and warning labels about the risks of fetal alcohol syndrome have been proposed for alcoholic beverages.

The Surgeon General recommends that women who are pregnant or are considering pregnancy drink *no* alcoholic beverages and be aware of the alcohol content of certain foods and medicines.[9]

Alcohol's Psychological Effects

Many studies have shown that alcohol, even in small amounts, can hamper an individual's ability to do certain simple tasks. The adverse effect of alcohol increases with the complexity and unfamiliarity of the task. It also increases with the individual's lack of experience with alcohol: A person who rarely drinks can have trouble performing simple household chores after only a small amount of alcohol.[10]

The irony of alcohol's effect on the mind is that it makes the drinker feel as if he or she is doing better, even when he or she is actually doing worse. Even at small concentrations—only about 0.1 percent—the drinker loses some dexterity and reaction speed; touch, sight, and hearing are also less acute. At the same time, however, the alcohol relaxes the drinker and gives the illusion of doing better. That false sense of well-being may lead the drinker to try things he or she cannot do safely, such as driving, or to make decisions that require more discriminating judgment than he or she has at the time.

The circumstances in which one is drinking, one's previous experience, the attitude of one's family, and society's customs and beliefs about alcohol—all these can make a difference in alcohol's psychological effects. Often, it is our expectation of alcohol's effects, rather than the alcohol itself, that reduces our inhibitions. In one study, people who were told they were drinking alcohol but

How to Host a Party Sensibly

When you are hosting a party, you can help your friends drink sensibly and avoid accidents on the way home. You need not be bossy or intrusive, just do a little planning. You'll be a good host, and your guests will enjoy themselves and get home safely.

1. Plan the party so that guests can move around and can't just stand in a corner and drink. If necessary, rearrange the furniture to make additional floor space, which encourages movement.
2. Pace the drinks. Serve drinks at reasonable intervals, but don't push them. If you have a bartender serving guests, tell him or her that it is not necessary to keep everyone's glass full at all times.
3. Make sure people get what they expect in their drinks. Don't serve doubles, or you'll have guests exceeding their limits. People who keep track of their intake tend to assume that there's a one-ounce jigger of liquor in each drink, and they may not appreciate getting twice as much as they bargained for.
4. Serve plenty of snacks. Make appetizing, hearty snacks and pass them around often so people aren't drinking on an empty stomach.
5. Serve some nonalcoholic beverages. Not everyone drinks alcohol, so don't force people to choose between doing so and going thirsty.
6. Don't end the party with drinks. Decide in advance when you want the party to end. When that time approaches, stop serving liquor and offer coffee, tea, and a good-sized snack. That gives your guests some nondrinking time before they go home, and the food will slow the absorption of alcohol.
7. As the slogan says, friends don't let friends drive drunk. If you do, you're putting your friend and others in serious danger on the road. Offer an obviously drunk guest a ride, call a cab, or let him or her spend the night on your couch.

Source: R. Engs, *Responsible Drug and Alcohol Use* (New York: Macmillan, 1979), pp. 67–72.

were actually drinking tonic water had the same sexual arousal levels as those given alcohol.[11]

Emotional Effects—and Their Consequences

As we've noted, mild doses of alcohol may make us feel less inhibited—but drinking does not generally promote social behavior. Quite often, drinkers act in antisocial and sometimes even violent and belligerent ways. Drinking is involved in a high percentage of violent crimes and accidents (see Table 5.2).

VIOLENCE

Alcohol is highly correlated with aggressive and violent behaviors, and the more alcohol consumed, the more aggressive and disruptive the behavior. Consider the criminal statistics: In just one year, 5 million Americans were arrested for alcohol-related offenses, ranging from disturbing the peace to public drunkenness to vagrancy.[12] Some 43 percent of inmates in state prisons in-

TABLE 5.2 · **Percentages of Crimes and Injuries Involving Alcohol in the United States**

Homicides	74 (70 on weekends)
Beatings	69
Stabbings	72
Shootings	55
Sexually aggressive acts against women	39
Sexually aggressive acts against children	67
Suicides	30
Fatal auto accidents	50
Fatal aircraft accidents (private)	20
Pedestrian accidents	36
Snowmobile accidents	40
Fire deaths	58
Accidental poisonings	71
Drownings	45
Fights or assaults in the home	56
Home accidents	22
Narcotic deaths	20
All arrests	55

Source: James T. Weston, "Alcohol's Impact on Man's Activities: Its Role in Unnatural Death," *American Journal of Clinical Pathology* 74, no. 5 (November 1980): 757.

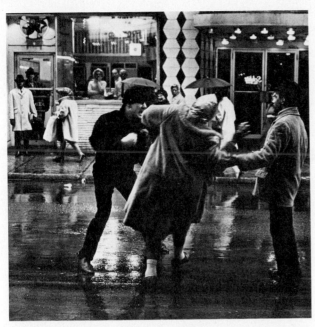

Drinking is often associated with aggressive and violent behavior. (© Jerry Berndt/Stock, Boston)

dicated that they had been drinking at the time they were arrested.[13] Delinquent adolescents held in state detention homes have also been shown to drink more frequently than other teenagers.[14]

Aggressive, disruptive behavior by intoxicated students on the nation's campuses is a serious problem. A study at Oregon State University found that students referred to the university or local police for discipline were often charged with "alcohol misconduct." Their actions ranged from property damage to harassment of police and other people.[15] It seems that alcohol may provide some people with an excuse to behave in a disruptive way, either verbally or physically.

ACCIDENTS

As most of us can attest, drunkenness is by no means limited to public offenders, locked up in jail. In fact, most intoxication today occurs among men and women who live with their families, hold jobs, and maintain stable community ties. With alcohol such a widely used drug, most of them have learned to mask the obvious signs of drunkenness. Their perception of time and space may be altered, their judgment faulty, and their reaction time slowed by alcohol, but they try to compensate.

Routine drinking in our society has become all the more ominous as life has become faster-paced and more technological. More and more jobs, such as jobs where the individual is required to operate machine tools, require exacting skill and judgment. Most people cannot avoid these everyday activities that are made impossible or at least extremely difficult by excessive drinking.

The most vivid evidence of this is the daily slaughter of men, women, and children on the highways in alcohol-related accidents. In less than eight years, intoxicated drivers have killed more than 200,000 people. At this writing it has been estimated that drunk drivers kill over 25,000 people a year—a figure representing about half of all traffic fatalities.[16] Automobiles are the leading cause of death among children between one and fourteen years of age.[17] Car accidents kill more people between the ages of fifteen and twenty-four than all other causes combined.[18] And intoxicated drivers have a habit of maiming people as well: One-third of all the people who suffer the loss of arms, legs, or other abilities can blame inebriated drivers for their condition.[19]

Not until the early 1980s did DWI (driving while intoxicated) really become a national issue. Before then, authorities in many localities had not been in the habit of sending drunk drivers to jail, even those with numerous convictions. Judges and juries, feeling "I could easily have been behind the wheel myself," had been reluctant to make drunk drivers suffer for their offense. But angered by the high death toll, citizens and state legislators in many areas began to push to have "slap-on-the-wrist" DWI laws toughened. By 1983 thirty-six states had passed harsher drunk-driving laws. Fourteen of these laws made having a blood alcohol level of 0.10 a crime in itself (rather than just "admissible evidence"). Most also mandated jail sentences for certain DWI offenses, and stipulated that drunk-driving incidents could no longer be removed from a driver's record.[20]

For guidelines on blood alcohol levels and impairment of driving ability, see Figure 5.2.

ALCOHOL'S LONG-TERM EFFECTS

While alcohol creates its characteristic effects each time it is used and affects people even the very

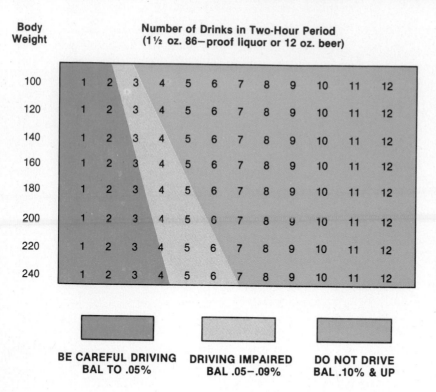

Body Weight	Number of Drinks in Two-Hour Period (1½ oz. 86—proof liquor or 12 oz. beer)											
100	1	2	3	4	5	6	7	8	9	10	11	12
120	1	2	3	4	5	6	7	8	9	10	11	12
140	1	2	3	4	5	6	7	8	9	10	11	12
160	1	2	3	4	5	6	7	8	9	10	11	12
180	1	2	3	4	5	6	7	8	9	10	11	12
200	1	2	3	4	5	6	7	8	9	10	11	12
220	1	2	3	4	5	6	7	8	9	10	11	12
240	1	2	3	4	5	6	7	8	9	10	11	12

BE CAREFUL DRIVING
BAL TO .05%

DRIVING IMPAIRED
BAL .05—.09%

DO NOT DRIVE
BAL .10% & UP

Figure 5.2 The best advice is not to drive when you've been drinking. But if you must drive, you should be aware of the approximate blood alcohol level (BAL) a given number of drinks produces in a person of your weight, and restrict your alcohol intake accordingly. For example, as this chart shows, if you weigh 140 pounds and have three or four drinks within two hours, your BAL is between .05 and .09 percent and your driving ability is impaired. With five or more drinks in two hours, your BAL is .10 percent or more; you are legally drunk and should not drive. (This chart shows *average* responses. You should get to know your own responses; younger people tend to become impaired sooner.)

(*Source:* National Highway Traffic Safety Administration)

first time it is consumed, it also has separate and damaging effects when it is used heavily over weeks, months, and years. Chronic, heavy alcohol use can not only damage the body, it can also tear apart the drinker's family life and work life.

Tolerance and Dependence

Alcohol is a drug; people can develop a tolerance to it and a psychological and physical dependence on it. When a person develops a tolerance to alcohol, he or she must consume more and more of it to achieve the same effects. A tense person who drinks to relax, for example, will gradually have to increase the dosage in order to feel relaxed.

While tolerance is most often thought to take months to develop, that is not always the case. Some research reveals that people can develop a tolerance after just two or three weeks of heavy drinking.[21]

Not everyone who develops a tolerance to alcohol develops a physical dependence on it. But it is not unusual for a person with a high tolerance to also have a physical need for alcohol, a chemical dependence that becomes evident when the person stops drinking. In such individuals an abrupt end to drinking will produce painful withdrawal symptoms—ranging from delirium tremens, often called the DTs or the "shakes," to seizures, hallucinations, and other signs of intense disturbance of the central nervous system. Persons going through alcohol withdrawal should be supervised so that they do not harm themselves or others during a seizure or hallucination.

Diseases and Long-Term Alcohol Use

Alcohol is linked with many serious illnesses that can destroy the body's most important organs and sometimes result in death.[22]

EFFECTS ON THE GASTROINTESTINAL (GI) SYSTEM

Alcohol stimulates secretion of digestive acid throughout the GI system, irritating the lining of

ACTIVITY: EXPLORING HEALTH

Are You Having a Problem with Alcohol?

There is a difference between people who drink irresponsibly at times and people who have a drinking problem. Irresponsible drinkers are a danger to themselves and others when they are drinking. People with a drinking problem are in serious trouble and need help. If you check *yes* to any *two* of the following questions, you may have a drinking problem.

	YES	NO
1. Do you gulp drinks for the effect that rapid drinking produces?	____	____
2. Do you start the day with a drink?	____	____
3. Do you drink alone to escape from reality, boredom, or loneliness?	____	____
4. Do you frequently overdose on alcohol or get drunk?	____	____
5. Do you drink to relieve a hangover?	____	____
6. Do you lose time from school because of drinking?	____	____
7. Do you drink to lose shyness and build up your self-confidence?	____	____
8. Is drinking affecting your reputation?	____	____
9. Do you drink to escape from study or home worries?	____	____
10. Does it bother you if somebody says maybe you drink too much?	____	____
11. Do you have to take a drink to go out on a date?	____	____
12. Do you ever get into money trouble over buying liquor?	____	____
13. Have you lost friends since you've started drinking?	____	____
14. Do you hang out now with a crowd where alcohol is easy to get?	____	____
15. Do your friends drink less than you do?	____	____
16. Do you drink until the bottle is empty?	____	____
17. Have you ever had a loss of memory from drinking?	____	____
18. Has drunk driving ever put you into a hospital or a jail?	____	____
19. Do you get annoyed with classes or lectures on drinking?	____	____
20. Do *you* think you have a problem with alcohol?	____	____

Source: Adapted from *Young People and AA* (New York: Alcoholics Anonymous, 1969), in R. Engs, *Responsible Drug and Alcohol Use* (New York: Macmillan, 1979).

---

the drinker's stomach and the linings in the esophagus and intestines. It is not unusual for alcoholics to develop bleeding ulcers in their stomachs and intestines and sometimes lesions in the esophagus. Alcohol can give "binge drinkers" diarrhea. It may inhibit the pancreas's production of enzymes that are crucial for the digestion of food. When heavily abused, it can also lead to **pancreatitis** (inflammation of the pancreas).

IMPACT ON NUTRITION

A common myth holds that alcohol, being made from fruit or grain, is food. It is not. Worse, alcohol actually starves the body of essential nutrients. It does consist of calories, so it produces energy; but it does not contain any of the chemical substances the body needs to build and repair tissue (see Chapter 13). Alcohol abuse has been reported as the most common cause of vitamin deficiency in this country. An alcoholic may undereat; or, because the digestive system is disrupted, he or she may be unable to process properly the nutrients that are eaten. Alcoholics may also suffer nutritional imbalances because of diarrhea, loss of appetite, and vomiting. In short, alcoholism can be a form of slow starvation.

LIVER DAMAGE

The liver is one of the organs most vulnerable to alcohol abuse. Alcohol changes the way the liver processes important substances; it can also contribute to infections and other disorders. If the liver is disturbed or infected, the body's immune system and ability to flush out poisons are affected. Damage to the liver can also harm other organs, because the liver is essential to the production and modification of many substances the body needs.

Many alcoholics suffer **cirrhosis of the liver,** a chronic inflammatory disease of this organ in which healthy liver cells are replaced by scar tissue. Cirrhosis of the liver caused more than 31,000 deaths in 1981; it was the eighth leading cause of death that year.[23] Drinking can also cause **alcoholic hepatitis,** in which the liver becomes swollen and inflamed. It may also lead to a "fatty liver" condition by changing the way the liver processes fats.

EFFECTS ON THE CARDIOVASCULAR SYSTEM

There is some debate in the medical community about whether small amounts of liquor, such as one drink a day, may actually lower the rates of some heart diseases. It may be some years before that question is answered. But there is no question that *excessive* drinking takes a toll on the heart and circulatory system, even causing heart failure in some cases. Most often, heart failure occurs in people who have been alcoholics for at least ten years. But cases of sudden, acute heart problems and of disease similar to coronary artery disease have been reported after shorter periods of heavy drinking.

EFFECTS ON THE GLANDULAR (ENDOCRINE) SYSTEM

Excessive drinking can damage the body's glandular system, which regulates such important functions as moods and sexuality. Men who drink too much may suffer impotence and reduced levels of the hormone testosterone: In one study, researchers found that the second most frequent reason for impotence among men was excessive drinking. Women may also throw their hormonal system out of balance through heavy drinking; recent studies indicate that alcohol abuse can lead to early menopause.

EFFECTS ON THE CENTRAL NERVOUS SYSTEM

As we mentioned earlier, alcohol's most visible and measurable short-term effects are on the central nervous system. Even small amounts of the drug can change the user's emotional picture and physical behavior. Prolonged abuse can have even more damaging and sometimes permanent effects on the CNS. Detoxified alcoholics, like people known to have brain damage, have been found to have difficulty remembering things and to have trouble with motor skills and perception. A number of studies have estimated that 50 to 70 percent of alcoholics who seek treatment suffer CNS problems: Alcohol has literally killed some of their brain cells.

Alcohol abuse is also associated with severe emotional problems. Alcoholics consistently score higher on items measuring depression in psychological tests. The risk of suicide among alcoholics runs thirty times higher than among the general population, according to some studies; it is well documented that a high percentage of people who commit or attempt to commit suicide are alcoholic.

ALCOHOLISM AND PROBLEM DRINKING

Although people may become intoxicated occasionally in private without undue harm, for millions of Americans alcohol creates serious and long-lasting consequences. It can disrupt their work and family lives, and it sometimes leads to alcoholism.

How Is "Alcoholic" Defined?

Debate lingers over the exact definitions of the terms *problem drinker* and *alcoholic,* but some authorities now make this distinction as follows:

THE PROBLEM DRINKER An individual is described as a **problem drinker** when he or she:

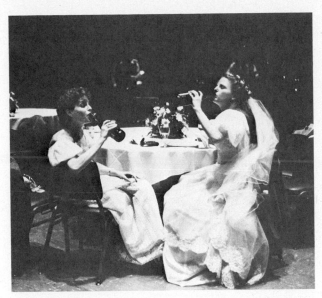

Many people feel that drinking lends an air of festivity and glamour to weddings and other special occasions. (© Gale Zirker/Stock, Boston)

1. Must drink in order to function or cope with life.
2. Frequently drinks to intoxication.
3. Often goes to work or class intoxicated.
4. Drives while intoxicated.
5. Sustains injury requiring medical attention as a consequence of intoxication.
6. Does something while under the influence of alcohol that he or she would never do otherwise.

Often the problem drinker will need to drink before facing stressful situations or even before eating breakfast; he or she will gradually increase alcohol intake and will experience difficulty with family, work, and other social relationships. Nearly one in eleven American adults is believed to be a problem drinker.[24]

THE ALCOHOLIC An **alcoholic** not only suffers from the serious personal and social disruptions and lack of behavioral control experienced by the problem drinker but has also developed *a preoccupation with alcohol and a physical and psychological dependence on it.* An alcoholic suffers memory lapses, develops a tolerance for alcohol, and generally makes drinking the central activity in his or her life.

Who Are the Alcoholics?

There are significantly more male than female alcoholics—about four men to every woman—but the gap is closing, with the number of female alcoholics on the rise.[25] (One estimate puts the number of female alcoholics in the United States at 5 million.[26]) The highest incidence of the disease is among men under the age of thirty. Alcohol is the preferred drug among American adolescents, with 77 percent of high school seniors reporting that they have tried alcohol at least once.[27] Alcohol is the most commonly used drug among college students, too. In a study of five American universities, researchers found that from 78 percent to 92 percent of students used alcohol.[28]

As these statistical observations indicate, alcohol use is widespread, and all types of people can become alcoholics. Scientists have learned that alcoholism does not affect only a small number of susceptible people; rather, they believe that *any* individual can become dependent on alcohol—given enough alcohol and an environment that condones drinking.

SIGNS OF ALCOHOLISM

The diagnosis of alcoholism is not something that can be precise, and it is often difficult for outsiders to make. The disease carries such a stigma that the alcoholic, friends, and family often postpone seeking treatment for as long as possible. Meanwhile, it's not unusual for the alcoholic to deny the problem and rationalize continued drinking. Yet if the problem can be pinpointed and dealt with early, years of anguish can be saved for all concerned.

What are the early warning signs of alcoholism? How can you tell if a person's drinking has turned into a serious problem that requires treatment?

SPOTTING POTENTIAL ALCOHOLISM

In addition to the signs of problem drinking listed above, certain changes in behavior, including the following, warn of possible alcoholism:[29]

▶ Surreptitious, secretive drinking.
▶ Morning drinking (unless that behavior is not unusual in the person's peer group).

► Repeated, conscious attempts at abstinence.
► Blatant, indiscriminate use of alcohol.
► Changing beverages in an attempt to control drinking.
► Five or more drinks daily.
► Two or more blackouts while drinking. (A blackout is an episode of temporary amnesia, in which the drinker continues to function but later cannot remember what happened; this is not the same thing as "passing out" when drunk.

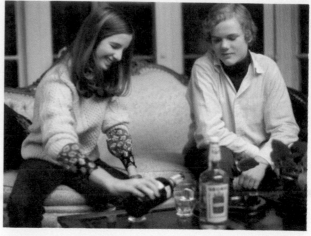

Teenagers who drink are flirting with danger. Alcoholism develops much more rapidly at this age than in older people. (© Mimi Forsyth/Monkmeyer Press Photo)

What Causes Alcoholism?

Most authorities now agree that alcoholism stems from a number of interrelated factors, ranging from family life to peer pressure to emotional upheavals. The significance of these factors may vary from person to person in determining whether that person will become an alcoholic.

Alcoholism does definitely run in families. Studies in the United States and Europe show that about 50 percent of the fathers, brothers, and sons of hospitalized alcoholics are also likely to become alcoholics.[30] Yet no study has yet turned up a genetic link, and researchers remain uncertain as to whether the family environment, heredity, or a combination of the two determines whether a person will develop alcoholism.[31]

A number of psychological traits have been closely associated with alcoholics: These drinkers tend to have more psychological problems than others, including deep-seated feelings of inadequacy, anxiety, and depression. Researchers also see drinking as a learned behavior that is reinforced by repetition: A person learns to take a drink to relax, for example, and then repeats the behavior in stressful situations until a pattern of heavy drinking has developed.[32]

Alcoholism can become a "family disease," with serious psychological effects on the drinker's spouse and children. Sometimes the nonalcoholic members of the family become so enmeshed in resentment, guilt, and feelings of helplessness that their lives are seriously disrupted. Marriages may be strained by problems relating to employment, finances, and sex. The alcoholic's family may become socially isolated.

Everyone should be aware that alcoholism poses a special threat to young people. When alcoholism develops early in life, it often occurs after only two or three years of heavy drinking. Among teenagers the process is so rapid that they can become alcoholics after only three or four months of heavy drinking. (Later in life it usually takes six to ten years of steady excessive drinking.) No one knows the reason for these differences among age groups.

How Alcoholism Is Treated

In the past three decades alcoholism has finally become accepted as an illness rather than a weakness or a simple failure of will power. Alcoholics Anonymous (discussed below) led the way in this attitude change, showing that most alcoholics *will* respond to treatment if it is offered.

DETOXIFICATION

Treatment is likely to start with **detoxification,** the process of weaning the person from his or her physical dependence and repairing the toxic effects of alcohol in the body. Many medical professionals rely heavily on the drug **disulfiram** (known under its trade name, *Antabuse*) in this process. Antabuse disrupts the alcoholic's ability to metabolize alcohol, so the individual will feel ill if he or she drinks. Use of Antabuse must be carefully supervised, since it can be highly toxic in combination with alcohol. In the early stages of treatment, the alcoholic's nutritional needs must also be addressed—as must other health problems created by drinking.

COUNSELING

After detoxification and attention to the alcoholic's medical needs, many treatment programs address the drinker's psychological and social problems. Some programs use a behavioral approach, in which the therapist concentrates on simply changing the person's behavior. The goal of this therapy is to get the alcoholic to associate drinking with unpleasant experiences. Other programs use counseling or in-depth psychotherapy. Sometimes other family members are encouraged to be part of the counseling, especially if the drink-ing seems tied to a family situation or a family conflict.

ALCOHOLICS ANONYMOUS (AA)

Alcoholics Anonymous (AA), founded in the 1930s, is among the most successful treatment programs. AA's basic approach involves a "Twelve-Step" program. Members start by admitting that they have lost control over alcohol. They are then encouraged to think about the spiritual dimension of their lives. Even if they are not "religious" in the formal sense, they are encouraged to think about the idea that there is some power higher than themselves. Then they take a hard look at themselves, taking inventory of where alcoholism has led them and where they can go in the future.

They are supported throughout the program by fellow members. Eventually, they themselves will work to help new members through the process. AA's combination of group support, behavior modification, and spiritually oriented thinking may not be for everyone, but it *has* helped many alcoholics recover.

MAKING HEALTH DECISIONS

Responsible Decisions About Alcohol Use

The drinking of alcoholic beverages has long been associated with college life. Many of the social events that are part of the college scene involve some ritualistic alcohol consumption, both on and off the college campus. It is not surprising that many college students frequently find themselves in situations that require decisions about alcohol use (picnics, dorm parties, campus bars, tailgate parties, fraternity or sorority dances, and so on). Although each person has the option of drinking or abstaining, the peer pressures are often so strong that free choices seem impossible for many college students. This has become a serious problem, especially for entering freshmen; many are living away from home for the first time and are being exposed to new stress-provoking situations.

Although the effects of alcohol are unpredictable, the fact is that even moderate amounts of alcohol may affect parts of the brain that control inhibitions, judgment, and feelings. The choices and decisions people make can be influenced by these alcohol-induced changes. Alcohol problems can be prevented by taking responsibility for your drinking behavior *before* your judgment is impaired.

The following exercise is designed to assist you in formulating decisions about drinking. Note the feelings and behaviors you would most likely experience or engage in for each situation described below.

1. You are invited to a fraternity or sorority party. After arriving, you realize that if you do not drink to the point of intoxication, you will probably never be invited back.

   a. How would you feel? _____

_____

b. What would you do? _____

_____

2. Several people arrive at the party with a variety of their own alcoholic beverages (whiskey, wine, brandy) in addition to the beer provided at the party. Your date starts to drink the other alcoholic beverages along with the beer.

a. How would you feel? _____

_____

b. What would you do or say? _____

_____

3. During the party, people begin to smoke marijuana while drinking, and you are told that it is rude to refuse a joint when it is being passed around.

a. How would you feel? _____

_____

b. What would you do or say? _____

_____

4. Several drinking games are being organized at the party (guzzling contest, lapping beer, shots-a-minute, Biz & Buzz, thumper, quarters, and the like). Your best friend implores you to join in on the games.

a. How would you feel? _____

_____

b. What would you do or say? _____

_____

5. Your date says that the more a person drinks, the better sex is.

a. How would you feel? _____

_____

b. What would you say? _____

_____

6. A friend who is also present at the party has become very intoxicated. He or she decides to drive into town (about ten miles) to pick up more beer.

a. How would you feel? _____

_____

b. What would you do or say? _____

_____

7. It has become apparent to you that your friend has a drinking problem. He or she can't remember much about the party the night before and shows up for class drunk on several occasions.

a. How would you feel? _____

_____

b. What would you do or say? _____

_____

8. In health class the next day, a student presents a report on alcohol and health hazards. The student states that in order to experience optimum health, alcoholic beverages should be completely avoided.

a. How would you feel? _____

_____

b. What would you do or say? _____

_____

9. An instructor in your sociology class the following day suggests that the alcoholic beverage industry, because it promotes drinking, is responsible for the medical, legal, and family problems associated with alcohol abuse.

a. How would you feel? _____

_____

b. What would you say? _____

_____

10. You attend services in the college chapel this

weekend. The chaplain asserts that drinking alcoholic beverages is sinful, according to the Scriptures.

a. How would you feel? _____

_____

b. What would you do or say? _____

_____

Now go back over your responses to these ten situations. Which do you think represent responsible decision making? Why are they responsible?

_____

_____

_____

Which answers do you think represent irresponsible decision making? Why are they irresponsible? _____

_____

_____

What would have been a more responsible decision in each case? _____

_____

_____

FINDING ALTERNATIVES FOR ACTION

Here are some decisions for things you might do or say in the above situations. You may think of other choices, too. It's up to *you* to find the response you're most comfortable with—no one else can tell you the best way to respond.

1. a. Stand on your principles—do not drink to intoxication.
   b. Make believe you're intoxicated—fake it.
   c. Go along with the crowd.

2. a. Lecture your date about the dangers of mixing drinks.
   b. Ask your date to stop, or end the evening early.
   c. Suggest that you dance, take a walk, play ping-pong, or get involved in some other activity that might be likely to reduce everyone's immediate drinking behavior.

3. a. Leave immediately.
   b. Decline on the basis of possible drug interaction effects.
   c. Smoke the marijuana to be sociable.

4. a. Join in enthusiastically.
   b. Decline without explanation.
   c. Decline with a reason, based on the information you have about how alcohol is absorbed in the body.

5. a. "Not so! Alcohol depresses sexual function."
   b. "Who wants sex when you're too drunk to enjoy it?"
   c. "What's wrong with the quality of our relationship that we need alcohol to make it better?"

6. a. Hide your friend's keys.
   b. Tell your friend that he or she is too intoxicated to drive safely.
   c. Suggest that you drive for the beer.

7. a. Find an excuse to break up the friendship.
   b. Try to talk your friend into seeking professional help.
   c. Send your friend some literature about AA.

8. a. Argue the other side of the issue.
   b. Say nothing.
   c. Suggest that the risks of alcohol consumption depend on a variety of factors and that individual responses differ.

9. a. "The professor knows more than I do on the subject, so I just agree."
   b. Argue that nobody forces people to drink to excess.
   c. Ask whether there has been any research that supports a causal relationship.

10. a. Walk out on the sermon.
    b. Ask for an interview to discuss the issue with the chaplain.
    c. Write an essay or letter to the editor of the school newspaper about the chaplain's views.

SUMMARY

1. Alcohol abuse is a major social and medical problem in the United States. About 10 million Americans have drinking and alcoholism problems. Excessive drinking is a factor in many fatal car accidents and in cases of birth defects.

2. Ethyl alcohol is the common active ingredient in beer, wine, and distilled spirits. All of these drinks are made by different processes from natural products like fruits and grains. The term *proof* indicates a drink's alcohol content. To derive the percentage of alcohol from the proof, divide the proof number in half. Congeners are natural substances other than alcohol that are products of the preparation process.

3. Alcohol travels to the stomach and small intestine and then into the bloodstream. Alcohol is fairly uniformly distributed throughout the body, but most of it must be processed by the liver before it is excreted from the body.

4. Blood alcohol level depends on the strength of the alcoholic drink consumed, body weight, amount of food in the stomach, rate of consumption, and rate of absorption.

5. The effect of alcohol on behavior is measured by blood alcohol level. Most people feel few effects with a BAL of up to 0.02 percent. At 0.1 percent, there is major depression of sensory and motor functions. Concentrations above 0.4 percent lead to coma and possible death.

6. Physically, alcohol acts on the central nervous system as an anesthetic, a sedative, and a depressant. It is *not* a stimulant.

7. A hangover is probably a state of mild withdrawal from alcohol. Symptoms may result from allergy to congeners and from dehydration of nerve cells in the brain. A hangover's severity is related to the amount and duration of drinking.

8. Alcohol increases brain arousal, generating feelings of agitation that underlie the initial feeling of relaxation. Alcohol also gives the illusion of body warmth, when actually the body is losing heat because of the alcohol.

9. Alcohol is a powerful drug. It should not be combined with other drugs, especially barbiturates, aspirin, and common cold remedies. The synergistic effects of alcohol combined with another drug can be extremely dangerous.

10. Certain conditions may make people especially sensitive to alcohol, including diabetes, epilepsy, recent illness, and fatigue. Pregnant women should avoid drinking alcohol, because there is no known level of drinking that is safe for the unborn baby. Women who drink heavily risk bearing children with *fetal alcohol syndrome*, a pattern of physical defects and mental retardation.

11. Psychologically, alcohol hampers the ability to perform tasks, yet makes the drinker feel that he or she is actually performing better. The circumstances in which one drinks, one's expectations, and social customs and beliefs influence the psychological effects of alcohol.

12. Emotionally, alcohol is highly correlated with aggressive and violent behavior and with the impaired judgment and reaction time that lead to traffic accidents.

13. The long-term effects of drinking alcohol can include tolerance and physical and psychological dependence. Prolonged, heavy use of alcohol can lead to central nervous system and gastrointestinal disorders, malnutrition, cirrhosis of the liver, hepatitis, cardiovascular disease, glandular disorders, brain damage, and severe emotional problems.

14. In addition to the serious personal and social disruptions and lack of behavioral control of the problem drinker, the alcoholic develops a preoccupation with alcohol and a physical and psychological dependence on it.

15. Anyone can become an alcoholic. Alcoholism does run in families, is associated with a number of psychological traits, and is a learned behavior.

16. The treatment of alcoholism usually involves detoxification, treatment of medical problems, and then counseling or therapy for social and psychological problems. Alcoholics Anonymous, or AA, is among the most successful treatment programs.

GLOSSARY

alcoholic A person whose drinking is associated with serious disruptions in his or her personal and social life and with loss of behavioral control *and* who has developed a preoccupation with alcohol and a physical and psychological dependence on it. Compare **problem drinker.**

alcoholic hepatitis An alcohol-related disease in which the liver becomes inflamed and swollen.

blood alcohol level (BAL) The concentration of alcohol in the blood at a given time.

cirrhosis of the liver A chronic inflammatory disease that causes scarring of the liver and impairs liver function; frequently associated with alcoholism.

congeners Substances other than alcohol that are natural products of the fermentation and preparation of some alcoholic beverages.

detoxification The process of weaning a person from physical dependence on alcohol and repairing the toxic effects of alcohol in the body.

disulfiram (Antabuse) A drug that disrupts the body's ability to metabolize alcohol; causes a person to feel ill if he or she drinks alcohol while taking it.

ethyl alcohol The active ingredient in alcoholic beverages (distilled spirits, wine, beer) prepared from natural plant products such as fruits and grains.

fetal alcohol syndrome Characteristic adverse effects (including mental retardation, slow growth before and after birth, and a wide range of physical defects) exhibited by children born to women who drink heavily.

pancreatitis Inflammation of the pancreas associated with heavy alcohol intake.

problem drinker A person whose drinking is associated with serious disruptions in his or her personal and social life and with loss of behavioral control. Compare **alcoholic.**

proof A number indicating the concentration of ethyl alcohol in a beverage; can be converted to percent by dividing by two (thus, 80-proof whiskey is 40 percent alcohol).

NOTES

1. *Third Special Report to the U.S. Congress on Alcohol and Health,* Department of Health and Human Services, Pub. No. (ADM) 78-569 (Washington, D.C.: U.S. Government Printing Office, 1978).

2. Charles Kaelber and George Mills, "Alcohol Consumption and Cardiovascular Diseases," *Circulation* 64, no. 3 (September 1981): III-1–III-6.

3. National Institute on Alcohol Abuse and Alcoholism, *Facts About Alcohol and Alcoholism,* DHHS Pub. No. (ADM) 80-31, 1980.

4. P. Lemoine et al., "Les Enfants des Parents Alcooliques," *Ouest Med.* 25 (1968): 477.

5. Claire Toutant and Steven Lippmann, "Fetal Alcohol Syndrome," *American Family Physician* 22, no. 1 (July 1980): 113–117; M. A. Pelosi et al., "Drinking and Pregnancy," *Journal of the Medical Society of New Jersey* 77, no. 2 (February 1980): 101–102.

6. Toutant and Lippmann, "Fetal Alcohol Syndrome."

7. Arthur Flynn et al., "Zinc Status of Pregnant Alcoholic Women: A Determinant of Fetal Outcome," *The Lancet,* March 14, 1981, pp. 572–574.

8. Toutant and Lippmann, "Fetal Alcohol Syndrome."

9. *FDA Drug Bulletin* No. 11, December 1981, p. 1.

10. Berton Roueché, *The Neutral Spirit* (Boston: Little, Brown, 1960).

11. G. Allan Marlatt and Damaris J. Rosenow, "Cognitive Processes in Alcohol Use: Expectancy and the Balanced Placebo Design," in Nancy K. Mello, ed., *Advances in Substance Abuse,* Vol. 1 (Greenwich, Conn.: JAI Press, 1980), pp. 159–199.

12. National Institute of Law Enforcement and Criminal Justice, Law Enforcement Assistance Administration, *Alcohol and Crime: Reference Services Statistics* (Washington, D.C.: U.S. Department of Justice, 1976).

13. W. E. Barton, "Deficits in Treatment of Alcoholism and Recommendations for Correction," *American Journal of Psychiatry* 124 (1968): 1679–1686.

14. Darwin D. Dennison et al., *Alcohol and Behavior: An Activated Education Approach* (St. Louis: Mosby, 1980), pp. 13–15.

15. Ibid., pp. 15–16.

16. *Report from the Committee on Public Works and Transportation to the 97th Congress, 2nd Session,* Report No. 97-867, September 23, 1982, p. 7.

17. James T. Weston, "Alcohol's Impact on Man's Activities: Its Role in Unnatural Death," *American Journal*

of Clinical Pathology 74, no. 15 (November 1980): 755–758.

18. Ibid.

19. Ibid.

20. *Hearings Before a Subcommittee of the Committee on Appropriations, U.S. Senate, 97th Congress, 1st Session,* Part 2 (Washington, D.C.: U.S. Government Printing Office, 1982), p.31.

21. Cited in Michael J. Eckardt et al., "Health Hazards Associated with Alcohol Consumption," *Journal of the American Medical Association* 246, no. 6 (August 7, 1981): 648–661.

22. The following discussion of the impact of alcohol on body organs, glands, and central nervous system is based on information and studies cited in Eckardt et al., "Health Hazards Associated with Alcohol Consumption."

23. National Center for Health Statistics, *Monthly Vital Statistics Report* 30, no. 13 (December 20, 1983): 22.

24. William R. Miller, "Problem Drinking and Substance Abuse: Behavioral Perspectives," NIDA Research Monograph No. 25, *Behavioral Analysis and Treatment of Substance Abuse,* 1979, Chapter 11.

25. W. B. Clark, L. Midanik, and G. Knupfer, *Report on the 1979 Survey* (Rockville, Md.: National Institute of Alcohol Abuse and Alcoholism, 1981).

26. Dennison et al., *Alcohol and Behavior.*

27. Ibid.

28. Ibid.

29. N. J. Estes and M. E. Heinemann, eds., *Alcoholism: Development, Consequences, and Interventions,* 2nd ed. (St. Louis: Mosby, 1982); George Vaillant, *The Natural History of Alcoholism: Causes, Patterns, and Paths to Recovery* (Cambridge, Mass.: Harvard University Press, 1983).

30. Cited in Marc A. Schuckit and Robert M. J. Haglund, "An Overview of the Etiological Theories on Alcoholism," in Estes and Heinemann, eds., *Alcoholism,* p. 21.

31. Ibid.

32. Jean Kinney and Gwen Leaton, *Loosening the Grip: A Handbook of Alcohol Information* (St. Louis: Mosby, 1978).

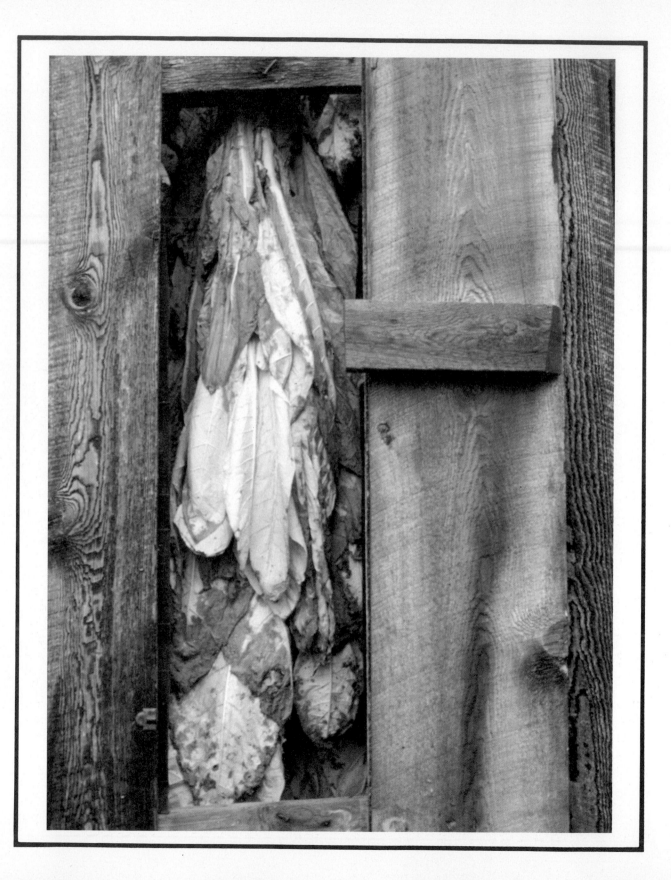

CHAPTER 6

Smoking

If people "knew" they could add eight years to their lives by taking one specific action, do you think they would do so? If that action could dramatically reduce their chances of having certain costly, painful, debilitating, and life-threatening illnesses—do you think they would be inclined to take it?

Most of us would probably agree that a rational human being would jump at the chance. Why then do 52 million Americans still smoke cigarettes?[1] Why are the millions of Americans who never took up smoking—or who have given up the practice—exposed to the chemical constituents of tobacco smoke in their daily living environment? Why must every pack of cigarettes still carry the warning, "The Surgeon General has determined that cigarette smoking is dangerous to your health"?

CIGARETTES IN AMERICAN CULTURE: THE POWER OF THE IMAGE

One reason smoking is so prevalent today is that it has become a well-established part of our culture. When cigarette manufacturing first became a major industry at the turn of the century, the typical smoker was a middle-class working man. But beginning in the 1920's, cigarettes came to seem fashionable and sophisticated. More women started to smoke. By the 1940s, advertising had started to build shining images for cigarettes. Smokers seemed to be the heroes of the day—

fighter pilots, soldiers in the foxhole, tank drivers, good-looking doctors, pretty nurses. In the 1950's, the "right" cigarette became a sexual lure, attracting sweater-girl pinup beauties into the waiting arms of handsome young men.

By the 1960s, advertising campaigns penetrated the youth market. Air travelers received complimentary cigarettes with their meals, and children memorized advertising jingles that glorified "good" cigarettes. As a result of this drumbeating, more and more people became smokers. By 1964, the year of the first report on smoking put out by the Surgeon General of the United States, more than one-half of American men and nearly one-third of American women smoked daily—a total of 50 to 60 million smokers. In the age group between twenty-five and thirty-four, nearly 60 percent of the men and 44 percent of the women smoked.[2]

More recently, however, a major shift in the general attitude toward smoking has taken place. Cigarette commercials have been legally banned from television and radio since 1970. Recent surveys have documented a pattern of steady decline in the proportion of smokers at most age levels: Decline has been most dramatic among health professionals, but it is detectable among other groups as well. Only one-third of adults smoke today—which represents a 42 percent decline from the 1965 figure.[3] In addition, most current adult smokers have either tried to quit smoking completely or want to try.[4] The 1982 Surgeon General's Report described smoking as "the most important health issue of our time" and identified the effects of cigarette smoking as "the chief preventable cause of death in our society."[5]

WHY DO PEOPLE SMOKE?

As we've noted, forty years of advertising have helped associate smoking with strength, attractiveness, or sophistication in some people's minds. But if you ask smokers why they smoke, you'll get a number of other answers, too: "Smoking relaxes me." "Smoking gives me a lift." "I need to smoke at parties. It gives me something to do with my hands."

Researchers have found that it isn't possible to lump all smokers into one category: For some people, the need to continue to smoke comes from an actual physiological craving; for others, psychological factors are more important. One study, for example, found six different types of smokers, ranging all the way from a group who had a strong physical craving for cigarettes to a group who had little or no physical craving and said they would not find it at all difficult to stop smoking. Interestingly, the importance of social pressure in the individual's smoking behavior varied from group to group. Among the group that had a strong physical craving, there were actually two subgroups: straight "high need" smokers, and a "high need–social" subgroup who had friends who smoked (and thus would probably feel pressure to keep smoking in order to be like their friends). Among smokers with a medium physical craving, some disapproved of smoking and wished they could

quit, but some said smoking made them feel more confident in social gatherings (these people were above-average beer drinkers too).[6] So, when we ask why cigarettes have such a strong hold on people, we can see that we are dealing not only with a drug but also with a social pattern.

Which Social Groups Influence People to Smoke?

Of course, advertising and high-powered public relations campaigns don't act on all of us equally. If they did, we would all be smokers. Other social pressures and our own psychological needs influence us as well, making some people more likely to smoke than others. Following are some findings about the role of peer pressure and other social pressures in smoking:

- Smokers tend to have mates who smoke. One study found, for example, that among young women smokers, 68 percent had boyfriends or husbands who smoke.[7]
- Blue-collar men have the highest smoking rates of all the social class/sex categories. Among women workers, however, it's the *white-collar* women who have high rates: More of them smoke than blue-collar women workers.[8]
- Although smoking among teenagers in general

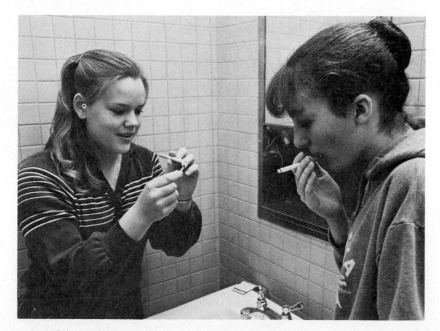

As with other forms of drug use, peer pressure is a strong influence on young people when it comes to smoking. (© Mimi Cotter/Int'l Stock Photo)

has decreased recently, smoking among teen-age girls has increased.[9]

It's risky to make broad generalizations about the meaning of these statistics, but they do underscore (1) how important some blue-collar men may feel it is to maintain a tough, "macho" image and (2) how rapidly women's behavior and self-image are changing in our society.

What Psychological Pressures Influence People to Smoke?

It's possible that some people use cigarettes, at least in part, as a drug to help them deal with psychological problems.[10]

- Among men, those who have more emotional problems and are less sociable are more likely to keep smoking.
- Smokers who are hard-driving, competitive, and overloaded with work are less likely to quit than those who are less driven.
- Some smokers show a tendency to use other drugs. One expert says, "Smokers consume more coffee, more alcohol, more psychotropic [mind-altering] drugs, more marijuana, and more aspirin than do nonsmokers."

Can Cigarettes Create Physical Dependence?

The answer to this question is "Probably yes—at least in some people." If a person smokes and has not been able to break the habit, he or she may have a true physical dependence. The probable culprit is **nicotine,** a toxic drug found in tobacco that acts as a stimulant and is responsible for many of the harmful effects of smoking, as we discuss below.

THE ACTION OF NICOTINE

Here's how nicotine works in the body when a person smokes a cigarette. Inhaling cigarette smoke brings nicotine directly to the lungs, where it is transferred through the thin membranes of the lung tissue into the bloodstream. From there, one-fourth of the nicotine soon passes directly into the brain, where it stimulates nicotine receptors.

As a result, the brain releases chemicals that, in turn, stimulate the cardiovascular system.[11] The heart beats faster and the blood pressure goes up.

Meanwhile, the remainder of the inhaled nicotine is carried in the bloodstream to the rest of the body, where it acts at a number of nicotine receptor sites in body cells. It stimulates the gastrointestinal tract and causes the adrenal gland to release epinephrine, causing the "fight or flight" reactions we discussed in Chapter 1. The heartbeat increases by fifteen to twenty-five beats per minute; the pupils of the eyes and the bronchioles of the lungs dilate, and the blood vessels in the fingers and toes constrict. (Thermograms, or heat pictures, of smokers' hands and feet clearly show the drop in temperature in fingers and toes after a cigarette is smoked.) Epinephrine also stimulates the breakdown of glycogen to glucose in the tissues.

HOW PHYSICAL DEPENDENCE MAY DEVELOP

Once a person smokes regularly, some experts believe, changes occur in the body. According to one theory, the brain actually starts to function differently. Whenever smokers are not actually smoking a cigarette, their brains seem to be in a state of **hypoarousal**—*less* aroused than normal—and they feel *less* stimulated than normal. Thus, these individuals have to smoke a cigarette to get their brain's stimulation or arousal level *back up* to normal. They think they're getting a lift—but actually, they're just getting a boost back up from drowsy to normal.[12]

Whether or not this particular theory is correct, researchers have observed that many people who quit go through what appears to be a true withdrawal syndrome. (As we noted in Chapter 3, true withdrawal symptoms are one indication that an individual has had an actual physiological dependence on a chemical substance.) Quitters often experience nausea, headache, constipation or diarrhea, and excessive hunger. Deprived of cigarettes, smokers may feel anxious, irritable, aggressive, and hostile—and in dire need of a cigarette. The most common symptom following withdrawal from tobacco is craving for tobacco.[13] All these symptoms appear while the body is going through more basic changes: Soon after a person stops smoking, his or her heart rate and blood

Smoking and Thinking

You've seen it countless times, and if you smoke, you've certainly done it: Students stand in the hall outside a classroom, smoking before an exam begins. Ask them why they do it, and many will say it makes them calm. Others will say that a cigarette helps them concentrate. In fact, though, smoking may actually interfere with a person's ability to think. That is the conclusion of a recent study in which a group of subjects were asked to recall a series of words they had had a chance to study before being tested. Those subjects who were smokers were not able to remember as many of the words from the list as the nonsmokers could; the difference was statistically significant. Furthermore, the smokers had less tendency to put the words from the list into logical categories as they wrote them down. So, if you know someone who smokes before taking an exam or facing any other situation that requires clear thinking, you might call attention to the fact that smoking reduces thinking. The person will do better *without* the cigarette.

Source: Mary Ann Gonzales and Mary B. Harris, "Effects of Cigarette Smoking on Recall and Categorization of Written Material," *Perceptual and Motor Skills* 50, no. 2 (April 1980): 407–410.

pressure drop, the level of adrenal hormones in the bloodstream drops, and the body's general arousal level drops.

Cigarettes and Psychological Dependence

Psychologists have drawn some insights from learning theory to help explain people's smoking habits. As they point out, the smoker may come to

People in high-pressure jobs may feel that smoking helps them relax. As smoking becomes a habit, however, they are likely to come to associate their work environment with smoking. The supposed relaxing effect becomes less important than the smoking ritual itself. (© Arthur Tress/Woodfin Camp & Assoc.)

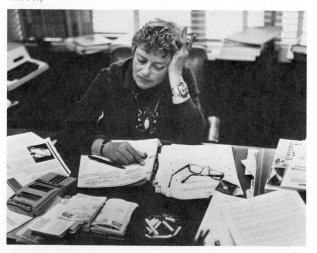

associate the action of smoking with reinforcers—pleasurable experiences or rewards that seem to result from the action. One writer points out,

A pack-a-day smoker takes more than 50,000 puffs per year and each puff delivers a rich assortment of chemicals into the lungs and bloodstream. Each puff stamps in the habit a little more and augments the establishment of secondary reinforcers, such as the sight and smell of cigarettes, the lighting procedures, and the milieu and context of a meal with a cup of coffee or a cocktail.[14]

This is not to say that the chemical factors—the effects of nicotine—aren't important. In fact, they may be part of the unique pleasure of the experience. (It's interesting to note that people *don't* seem to like cigarettes made of nontobacco materials such as dried lettuce.) But the chemical factors might not be quite so powerful if all those other "secondary reinforcers"—sights, smells, and agreeable surroundings—weren't there to help.

A Complicated Picture

Clearly, smoking is something people do for a variety of different reasons. Some may be doing it because it makes them feel better physically, at least temporarily. Some may also be doing it to satisfy psychological needs or in response to social pressures. Once they get into the habit, they may find it a hard one to break, not only because of the way their bodies may react physiologically, but also because of the millions of cues that subtly direct them to repeat the behavior ten, twenty, maybe forty times a day.

SMOKING AND HEALTH

Because smoking is extremely injurious to health, as we'll see in this section, the smoking habit is one that people should try hard to break.

How Cigarette Smoke Affects the Body

Smoking poses two basic health hazards. One is the drug-induced response the body makes to cigarette smoke. As we noted above, nicotine may be capable of creating a true physiological dependence; it also creates tolerance, and tolerance may also develop to the tar and carbon monoxide in cigarettes. The other hazard is the toxic substances—or poisons—that enter the smoker's body. Thus far, more than eighty major toxic substances have been identified in cigarette smoke, and the number is still growing.[15]

TOXIC GASES

Of all the compounds in cigarette smoke, 92 percent are gaseous—and many of these are toxic. **Carbon monoxide,** one of the gases found in tobacco smoke, is considered to be one of the most hazardous. Carbon monoxide affects our bodies in several ways, all related to oxygen deprivation:

- Carbon monoxide impairs the blood's capacity to carry oxygen, causing serious problems for people suffering from cardiovascular diseases.
- Some researchers believe that carbon monoxide is partly responsible for the heightened risk of heart attack and stroke among cigarette smokers: It may be the *combination* of carbon monoxide and nicotine that is at fault.[16]

SOLID MATTER

The remaining 8 percent of the smoke consists of solid (nongaseous) matter: ash, a tar-rich condensate, and a "wet particulate matter" comprising hundreds of different substances. **Tar** is a sticky residue from burning tobacco, consisting of more than 200 chemicals, which can be separated into three parts: acidic, basic, and neutral.

- In animal tests, the neutral part shows by far the highest *carcinogenic*, or cancer-causing, activity: It contains **benzopyrene,** one of the deadliest carcinogens known, and many other chemicals of the same family.
- The acidic part of the tarry condensate contains phenol and other materials that are not carcinogens but, some cancer researchers believe, could activate "dormant" cancer cells so that they grow and spread.
- The basic part of tar contains chemicals that have not been shown to pose a risk to human health.[17]

Smoking and Disease

Grim is the only word to describe the facts about the relationship between smoking and disease. About 340,000 deaths per year, or *nearly 18 per cent of all deaths* in the United States, are related to smoking.[18] Think of it—that's a huge number: 18 percent equals almost one-fifth of all deaths. These deaths are not due to old age, nor to car accidents, nor to any of the other common causes of deaths, but just to that one habit of smoking.

Cigarette smokers have a 60 percent greater chance of premature death than nonsmokers; of the ten leading causes of death, smoking is associated with six. And the reduction in a person's life expectancy increases with the number of cigarettes he or she smokes: A man who smokes one pack a day loses 4.6 years of life expectancy, but a man who smokes two packs a day loses nearly double that amount of time—8.3 years of life expectancy. Furthermore, the earlier a person begins smoking, the more years of life are lost: If a person starts before age twenty-five, for example, he or she loses four years on the average, but if he or she starts before age fifteen, as many as eight years are lost.[19]

The range of diseases that are involved is wide. Smokers have been shown to have greatly increased risks of premature coronary heart disease, arteriosclerosis, aortic aneurysms, peripheral vascular disease, thrombo-angiitis (Buerger's Disease), cerebrovascular disease, chronic bronchitis and emphysema, asthma, gastric problems, and

TABLE 6.1 • Sick Days Among Cigarette Smokers and Their Children: A Hidden Cost of Smoking

Sick Days	Number of Cigarettes Smoked Per Day			
	LESS THAN 15	15–24	25–34	35 OR MORE
Average number of days activity was restricted (per person, per year)				
Male smokers	23.9	22.8	20.3	20.6
Female smokers	25.6	21.0	27.2	20.6
Children whose parents smoke	8.7	9.2	11.2	10.1
Average number of days spent sick in bed (per person, per year)				
Male smokers	8.3	6.3	7.6	6.2
Female smokers	9.0	7.2	10.7	13.8
Children whose parents smoke	4.4	4.6	5.5	4.4
Average number of work days missed (per person, per year)				
Male smokers	8.5	9.6	6.8	7.0
Female smokers	7.5	7.7	9.3	12.3

Sources: Bureau of the Census, *Statistical Abstracts of the United States, 1981* (Washington, D.C.: U.S. Government Printing Office, 1981), p. 123; (children) G. S. Bonham and R. W. Wilson, "Children's Health in Families with Cigarette Smokers," *American Journal of Public Health* 71, no. 3 (March 1981): 291.

dental problems (including gingivitis, dental caries, and loss of teeth)—not to mention cancer of the oral cavity, esophagus, pancreas, larynx, lung, kidney, and bladder.

As Table 6.1 shows, smoking is associated with higher rates of illness in general. Smokers *and their families* are sick more often than nonsmokers.

SMOKING AND CANCER

"The evidence is now overwhelming." This is the way the Surgeon General describes the link between smoking and various cancers. "Cigarette smoking is the major single cause of cancer mortality in the United States."[20] If a man smokes, his risk of death by cancer is between 8 and 15 times higher than a nonsmoker's risk. If a woman smokes, her risk is 30 percent higher than a nonsmoker's risk. Of all cancer deaths, almost one-third can be linked to smoking.[21]

And if, after many years of smoking, an individual does not develop cancer, his or her risks are still not eliminated. Death from lung diseases is six times more frequent among smokers, and coronary artery disease is almost twice as great for smokers as for nonsmokers. In addition, when an

individual is exposed to tobacco and other carcinogens such as asbestos, there appears to be a synergistic effect—the combined effect is greater than the effect of each on its own. The risk of developing lung cancer increases sharply for those who

A heavily carbon-pigmented lung, at left, and a normal lung, at right. This discoloration is typical in the lungs of smokers and coal miners, and is more common among both smokers and nonsmokers in urban and industrialized areas. (Dr. Max E. Elliott/University of California, San Diego)

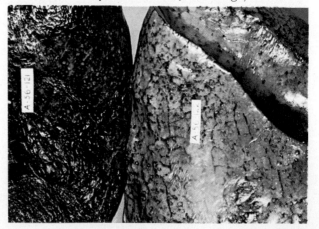

smoke *and* work with asbestos. Blue-collar workers face the greatest danger, because they are the group that is most exposed to toxic agents *and* they have the highest smoking rates, particularly among men.[22]

LUNG CANCER:
THE MANUFACTURED EPIDEMIC

About one hundred years ago, cigarettes were homemade and were smoked only by a few rugged individuals. But the invention of the cigarette-making machine in 1881 made them available to everyone. By 1981, one hundred years later, smokers were buying over 600 billion cigarettes a year.[23] And as more of us smoked, more of us developed lung cancer. (The early stages of lung cancer are diagramed in Figure 6.1).

Once a rare disease, lung cancer is now considered an epidemic. In 1982 it was estimated to have killed 111,000 people. Unlike other forms of cancer, lung cancer responds very poorly to treatment, and only 10 percent of people live five years after a diagnosis of lung cancer. The Surgeon General reported that 85 percent of those lung cancer deaths would not have happened if the people involved had never smoked. Lung cancer used to be a "man's disease," but women are catching up. "If present trends continue, [lung cancer] will be the leading cause of cancer death in women" by the early 1990s.[24]

The *way* an individual smokes influences his or her chances of developing lung cancer: The risk increases with the number of cigarettes smoked each day, how deeply the smoker inhales, and how high the tar and nicotine content of the cigarettes is. Smokers who started smoking early in their

Figure 6.1 The abnormal multiplication of cells (hyperplasia) that occurs in the early stages of lung cancer. Basal cells underlying the bronchial lining become irritated (by cigarette smoke, for example) and begin to increase in number. This is followed by loss of the ciliated respiratory epithelial cells that function to keep harmful materials out of the lungs. The remaining cells then take on a characteristic "squamous," or scale-like, structure. (Tom Lewis)

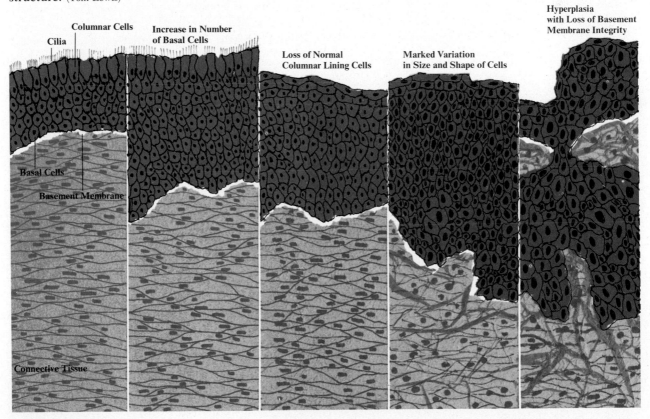

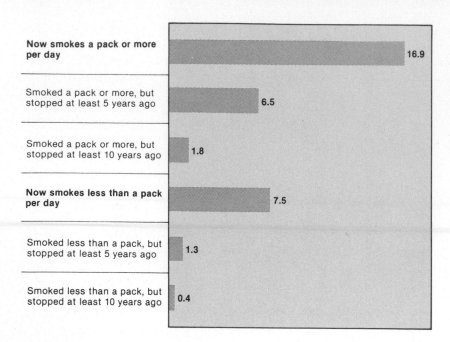

Now smokes a pack or more per day	16.9
Smoked a pack or more, but stopped at least 5 years ago	6.5
Smoked a pack or more, but stopped at least 10 years ago	1.8
Now smokes less than a pack per day	7.5
Smoked less than a pack, but stopped at least 5 years ago	1.3
Smoked less than a pack, but stopped at least 10 years ago	0.4

Figure 6.2 This graph shows the number of male heavy and light smokers, current and former, who die of lung cancer for every man who never smoked and dies of lung cancer. The picture improves considerably for both heavy and light smokers who stop smoking.

(*Source:* American Cancer Society)

lives are also at greater risk than those who have only smoked for a few years.

If a person stops smoking, will his or her chances of dying from lung cancer drop? Yes, but it takes ten to fifteen years for the smokers' mortality rate to drop back to the nonsmokers' rate.[25] Figure 6.2 shows how giving up cigarettes reduces the risk of dying from lung cancer.

SMOKING AND CARDIOVASCULAR DISEASE

HEART ATTACK   Is there a history of heart disease in your family? Do you have high blood pressure? People who answer yes to one or both of these questions and also smoke are putting themselves in a high-risk category for having a heart attack at some time in their lives. The more they smoke, the greater their risk of having a heart attack—and at a younger age than nonsmokers. The excess risk of heart disease will disappear within two years after they quit, but, as with lung cancer, it takes *ten years* after they quit smoking for their risk of heart attack to drop to that of nonsmokers![26]

ATHEROSCLEROSIS   Smokers also share a high risk of developing atherosclerosis, and smokers who have survived a heart attack face an increased possibility of suffering another one. (We

discuss atherosclerosis in more detail in Chapter 12.) The risk of coronary heart disease in cigarette smokers is 1.5 to 2 times that of nonsmokers.[27]

SMOKING AND THE PILL   If a woman uses birth control pills and smokes as well, she runs a much greater chance than a nonsmoker of suffering from a heart attack. (This combination *may* also be linked to strokes.) The risks increase with age, according to the Food and Drug Administration, and with heavy smoking (fifteen or more cigarettes a day).[28]

Since 1978, the FDA has required that birth control pills be labeled with the warning: "Women who use oral contraceptives should not smoke."

SMOKING AND OTHER HEALTH PROBLEMS

Heart disease and cancer are not the only diseases people may develop if they smoke. "Cigarette smokers have a higher prevalence of chronic bronchitis and emphysema than nonsmokers and *have an increased chance of dying from these diseases* compared to nonsmokers."[29]

Tobacco may also cause allergic reactions in some people, particularly those who are allergic to other substances and suffer from asthma or rhinitis (inflammation of the nasal mucous membranes).

SMOKING, PREGNANCY, AND INFANT HEALTH

The woman who smokes may endanger the health of her unborn child if she becomes pregnant. Several large studies, involving tens of thousands of pregnancies, reveal that mothers-to-be who smoke have twice as many spontaneous abortions (miscarriages) and stillbirths and two to three times as many premature babies as nonsmokers.[30] In one study, researchers calculated that one out of five babies who died would have been saved if their mothers had not been smokers.[31]

Furthermore, babies born to women who smoke during pregnancy are on the average nearly one-half pound lighter than babies born to nonsmokers, according to the 1979 Surgeon Gen-

Researchers have established a definite relationship between smoking during pregnancy and adverse effects on the health of the baby. (Courtesy, American Cancer Society)

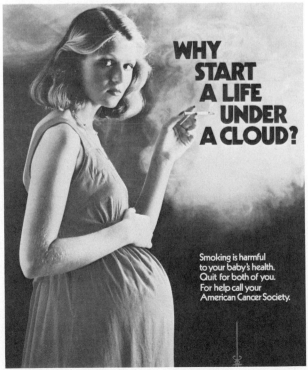

eral's Report. The importance of birth weight cannot be overstated. A newborn's weight is an important index of risk; the lower the weight, the greater the risk of death. The minimum weight for a healthy newborn is 2,500 grams (5 1/2 pounds). But among the infants of mothers who smoke, twice as many weigh less than 2,500 grams at birth as do babies of nonsmoking mothers. And, says the Surgeon General, "there is abundant evidence that maternal smoking is a direct cause of the reduction of birth weight."[32]

The precise way in which tobacco smoking affects the fetus is not known. It has been suggested that the oxygen supply to the fetus may be reduced by the carbon monoxide in cigarette smoke, which reduces the amount of oxygen in the red blood cells. Carbon monoxide has been found to concentrate in fetal blood; the higher the fetal carbon monoxide hemoglobin level, the smaller the baby. The oxygen supply to the fetus may also be reduced by the action of nicotine, which constricts the arteries and reduces the blood flow across the placenta.[33]

The effects of lowered birth weight don't end when the baby leaves the hospital. Studies of long-term growth and development have found that "smoking during pregnancy may affect physical growth, mental development, and behavioral characteristics of children *at least up to the age of 11.*"[34]

The Public Health Service says, "Stopping smoking is recommended during pregnancy."

Are There Any Safe Cigarettes?

Since the Surgeon General's first report on smoking and health in 1964, there has been a definite trend away from nonfilter cigarettes toward filtered ones, and away from high-nicotine, high-tar cigarettes toward low-nicotine, low-tar brands.

Does this change do smokers of the low-nicotine, low-tar cigarettes any good? According to a review of recent research in the Surgeon General's report, there is a problem with these cigarettes: Some people who smoke them intensify

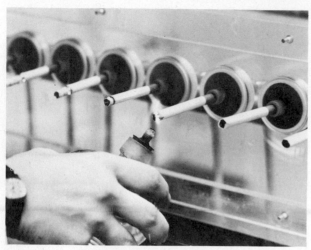

The search for a "safe" cigarette goes on—without much success to date. (© Jim Anderson 1982/ Woodfin Camp & Assoc.)

their smoking—smoke more cigarettes per day and inhale more deeply—in order to satisfy their craving for nicotine, and this means they take in more carcinogenic tar.

One researcher's data did show that in smokers who chose cigarettes with perforated filter tips, the level of nicotine in the blood was lower. But the smokers of these filter-tips may deliberately or unconsciously block some of the little ventilation holes in the filter with their fingers—which of course partly defeats the purpose of smoking these cigarettes in the first place.[35] Another study of patients who had been hospitalized for heart attacks showed that smokers of low-nicotine cigarettes had as great a risk of heart attacks as smokers of high-nicotine cigarettes did.[36] Reduced levels of nicotine and carbon monoxide did not reduce the risk of heart attack.

The smoker who uses "safer" low-tar, low-nicotine cigarettes may not actually gain much advantage from them.

QUITTING

Almost all smokers know the unpleasant truth about smoking. A 1978 Gallup Poll found, for ex-

ample, that 90 percent of respondents agreed that smoking was harmful to health; over 80 percent thought that smoking caused lung cancer; and nearly 70 percent identified smoking as a cause of heart disease. That knowledge may be having a positive effect: The proportion of smokers is declining in almost every age category. Another Gallup survey found that "almost all current adult smokers . . . have either tried or want to try to quit smoking completely."[37]

All told, about 30 million smokers have quit since 1964. The U.S. National Center for Health Statistics reported a decrease in the percentage of people seventeen years of age and older who currently smoked, from 36.7 percent in 1970 to 33 percent in 1979.[38]

What Are the Chances of Quitting Successfully?

Not everyone who tries to quit is able to do so. Researchers have summarized the situation this way:

1. Most smokers are unsuccessful in their initial attempt to quit smoking.
2. Although high proportions of smokers, especially middle-aged males, eventually do quit, many do not succeed in quitting until the negative consequences, especially the physiological effects, become very immediate and inescapable (for example, symptoms of chronic heart or lung diseases, or the more traumatic myocardial infarction).
3. Even if a smoker who is unable to quit unaided seeks formal treatment, the probabilities of his or her long-term success remain very discouraging.
4. People who smoke fewer cigarettes a day are more likely to succeed in quitting than those who are more dependent on smoking.
5. Many successful quitters know someone whose health was affected by smoking and who quit.
6. Men are more likely to quit than women.[39]

The psychologist Stanley Schachter has recently pointed out, however, that there may be a somewhat more hopeful side to this story. Schachter believes that more people may be able to quit successfully than the studies indicate. As he notes, there may be a lot of people who quit by themselves, without going into treatment programs. Because they never "stand up to be counted" by the researchers who study those programs, they are never recorded as having succeeded in quitting. Moreover, most studies of treatment programs only test the success of people who try to quit *once*. Smokers who try to quit more than once, all by themselves, may do better.

To test his idea, Schachter conducted a survey of smokers in the general population who were not necessarily in treatment programs. A good number of these smokers did quite well—more than 60 percent of those who tried to quit reported success. This figure is considerably better than the success rate reported in studies of treatment programs. How much faith should we place in Schachter's findings? Social scientists are still debating this question. But it is worth noting that Schachter's conclusions apply also to people who have other bad habits they need to break—such as people who overeat. In fact, Schachter studied overeaters who were trying to eat more moderately and found that they, like the smokers he had studied, also had a 60 percent success rate.[40]

It's important not to get too discouraged by the statistics. A number of people who try to quit succeed. If you are a smoker, you do stand a good chance of quitting successfully. If you are not a smoker, you can communicate this hopeful message to friends and relatives who may need some support in trying to quit. We'll look at methods of quitting in the section that follows; some tips on kicking the habit are given in the box on page 152.

Methods of Quitting

There are many ways to break the smoking habit, ranging from simply quitting "cold turkey"—which some authorities consider the most effective method—to elaborate, highly structured (and sometimes expensive) group programs that may taper off cigarette smoking over a period of many weeks. No one method is right for everyone.

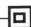

HOW TO BREAK THE SMOKING HABIT

If you are a smoker (if not, you may be interested in suggesting these pointers to a friend or relative

who is a smoker) and if you can figure out what *your* particular reasons are for smoking, you may be able to pinpoint the quitting method that's best for you.

▶ If you like cigarettes because they're a stimulant, try something else that will make you feel "revved up," such as moderate exercise.
▶ If you smoke to have something to do with your hands, doodle or twist a rubber band every time you get the urge to fidget.
▶ If the "habit" aspect of smoking is the one that seems strongest in your case, you may need to try some of the approaches psychologists have recommended for breaking habits of any kind—such as becoming more aware of the specific cues that lead you to take each cigarette out and light it. (We'll talk more about this later.)

Also, it may help to review in your mind the reasons you want to quit. Your own particular reason may be one or more of the following—or others not listed:

1. You want to take control of your life.
2. You have a problem with your respiratory system—shortness of breath, perhaps, or frequent colds. You want to beat these problems.
3. You want to set a better example for your children or younger siblings—they're much more likely to smoke if their elders do.
4. You are tired of having nonsmoking friends and loved ones comment on your smoking.
5. You are sick of smoking because it's dirty—it fouls furniture, clothing, your breath, the air, and so on.
6. You want to save the money you're now spending on cigarettes.[41]

PRODUCTS AND PROGRAMS

INDIVIDUAL PROGRAMS A number of products are offered on the market as aids for do-it-yourself quitting programs. These products include books, records and cassettes, over-the-counter tablets, and sets of graduated filters designed to reduce, over a period of weeks, a person's tar and nicotine intake. Since people carry out these programs on their own, the experts find it hard to evaluate their effectiveness.

GROUP PROGRAMS There is also a wide variety of group programs and clinics. Some are sponsored by nonprofit health organizations such as the

Tips on Kicking the Cigarette Habit—For Good

Have you ever tried to quit smoking? Do you know someone who wants to give it up but just can't?

It's tough to break the cigarette habit, but 30 million Americans *have* done it. The American Cancer Society has compiled a list of methods that some of these people have used to help them quit smoking for good. Here are a few that you can recommend to others—or try yourself.

1. Smoke an *excess* of cigarettes (three or four packs) for a day or two, to spoil their taste, then quit. Or quit when you have a cold or the flu and have no desire for cigarettes.
2. Imagine yourself smoking, and at the same time imagine some disgusting event (such as vomiting on the cigarette pack you're holding).
3. Write a list of your reasons for quitting. Read your list often and add new reasons when you can.
4. List a few things you would like to buy. Calculate their cost in terms of packs of cigarettes. Put the money you would have spent daily on cigarettes into a special piggy bank. Then splurge!
5. Bet a friend that you can quit. Bet with your cigarette money.
6. Never buy cigarettes by the carton. Finish one pack before you buy another.
7. Never carry cigarettes, matches, or a lighter.
8. Change brands every week. Each new brand must have less tar and nicotine than the previous one.
9. Smoke only during even- or odd-numbered hours.
10. Smoke only half a cigarette. Inhale only every other puff.
11. Say to yourself, "I don't want to smoke," not "I've quit smoking." That way, if you do have a cigarette, you won't feel that you've broken your resolution.
12. Help someone else to quit.
13. Always ask yourself, "Do I need this cigarette, or is this just a reflex?" If you really need the cigarette, go to a mirror and watch yourself light up.
14. If you crave a cigarette, take ten deep breaths. Strike a match while you hold the last breath. Exhale slowly, blowing out the match. Crush the match into an ashtray as if it were a cigarette. Get back to work immediately.
15. After you quit, use your lungs more: Increase your activities and exercise moderately.
16. Think about what the toxic elements in cigarette smoke are doing to your body internally—your lungs, your kidneys, your blood vessels.
17. Think about how smoking affects the odor of your breath . . . your clothes . . . your home.
18. Think about the damage you may be doing to members of your family—especially to young children, who are breathing the air you contaminate with tobacco smoke.
19. Imagine a clear day with blue sky, slowly turning gray from the smoke you exhale into the air.
20. Ask yourself whether your health is important to you and to those who love you—your family and close friends.

American Cancer Society, the American Heart Association, and the American Lung Association. Other stop-smoking programs are run as profit-making businesses. Group programs usually involve lectures, films, discussions, and practical tips on how to stop. Many use the "buddy system," pairing off participants so that they can bolster each other's determination. Some of these programs meet regularly over a period of weeks; others are concentrated five-day programs. Some hospitals even offer intensive, twenty-four-hour-a-day, live-in programs.

HYPNOSIS Some programs involve hypnosis, usually one or more sessions, where a practitioner puts the prospective quitter into a mild trance and then coaches him or her about how to stop.

AVERSION THERAPY Other programs rely on aversion techniques such as the administration of mild electric shocks, or having the person breathe stale cigarette smoke or smoke extremely rapidly, in an effort to associate smoking with an unpleasant experience. One form of aversion therapy that has gotten good results is rapid smoking. Once daily, the smoker sits down and chain-smokes as many cigarettes as possible, taking puffs every six seconds. No cigarettes are allowed between these sessions. Six months after this type of treatment is completed, 60 percent of clients report that they

Excuses for Smoking/Reasons for Quitting

For many smokers, smoking has become such a deeply ingrained habit and has worked itself so thoroughly into their daily behavior patterns that they have developed many excuses for continuing to smoke. Some of these excuses are in the smoker's conscious mind, some may be unconscious—and all have little or no basis in fact.

"IF I QUIT SMOKING, I'LL GAIN WEIGHT."

This is a common fear: According to the U.S. Public Health Service, 60 percent of women and 47 percent of men say they continue to smoke because they're afraid of gaining weight. Studies have indicated, however, that most smokers do *not* gain weight when they quit. "On the average, only about one-third of ex-smokers gain weight, one-third remain about the same, and one-third actually lose weight because they incorporate their quitting into a total self-improvement program."

"BUT I REALLY ENJOY SMOKING. I LIKE THE TASTE."

The question here is, how many moments are truly enjoyable—and how many are just so-so? Is it real enjoyment the smoker is getting—or just satisfaction for the physical craving? After a day of particularly heavy smoking, almost every smoker can remember cigarettes tasting terrible the next morning.

"IF I QUIT SMOKING, I'D BE TOO NERVOUS. SMOKING HELPS ME RELAX."

The truth here is that nicotine is actually a stimulant, not a depressant; it is not a substance that tends to make people relax. After the first few days of trying to quit, when ex-smokers may find themselves feeling nervous because they have nothing to do with their hands, most people find they have better self-control and are actually *less* nervous than they were when they smoked.

"I HAVE TO SMOKE IN ORDER TO PERFORM/PRODUCE/CREATE/STUDY."

Here we're looking at that problem of habit again. For a long time, the individual may have *associated* smoking with writing, studying, dealing with coworkers, or whatever the performance behavior in question is. Actually, once they quit, ex-smokers may find they spend more of their time productively. As a plus, their bodies will function more efficiently now that the excess carbon monoxide from inhaled smoke is no longer displacing oxygen in their bloodstreams.

"I'LL QUIT WHEN I HAVE TO—WHEN MY HEALTH IS THREATENED."

As we noted in our discussion of lung cancer, the symptoms of many smoking-related diseases don't show up until after the disease is well established. Moreover, many of those diseases result in a long, painful death.

"IT'S TOO LATE TO QUIT. I'VE BEEN SMOKING TOO LONG."

It's *never* too late, as long as you quit before a serious disease has developed. After you quit, your chances of dying from smoking-related diseases gradually decrease till they're close to those of people who have never smoked.

"THE AIR IS POLLUTED ANYWAY—I MIGHT AS WELL SMOKE."

In fact, even in a heavily polluted urban area, the concentrations of pollutants in the air are *tiny* in comparison with the concentrations in the cigarette smoke the smoker breathes in and out.

"I CAN'T AFFORD TO JOIN A STOP-SMOKING PROGRAM."

Most approaches to quitting cost nothing. But if you think paying to join a formal program is the only way you can succeed, you should take into account how much money you'll be saving by not buying cigarettes.

Source: U.S. Department of Health and Human Services, "Helping Smokers Quit: A Guide for Physicians" (NIH Publication No. 79–1825), June 1979.

are still not smoking. For this approach to succeed, a good relationship needs to exist between the smoker and therapist. You should also realize that rapid smoking can be hazardous.[42]

BEHAVIOR MODIFICATION Another approach applies the principles of behavior modification. The idea is simple. People who smoke generally do so at certain predictable times: with a cup of coffee, at a party, after a meal. Instead of smoking at those times, the person substitutes another behavior. At a party, the person walks around the room instead of lighting up. When having a cup of coffee, he or she reads a magazine instead of smoking. When this approach, known as *response substitution,* is combined with the "oversmoking" approaches outlined above, results are good.[43]

APPLYING LEARNING THEORY Rewards and punishments can be effective too. Researchers have reported good short-term results when smokers had to forfeit money every time they smoked. The support of a good friend when a person is trying to give up smoking can also have positive results.[44]

HOW TO CHOOSE A STOP-SMOKING PROGRAM

What basic things should you look for when you consider signing up for a stop-smoking program?

▶ *Cost:* Can you afford what you'll be charged to participate? Don't forget, of course, to take into account the cost of continuing to smoke. The average smoker spends more than $10,000 on smoking during his or her lifetime. The two-pack-a-day smoker spends over $500 per year on cigarettes.
▶ *Success Rate:* How good is the program's record? Ask the sponsors of the program what its success rate is *after one year.* (Many people find it relatively easy to give up cigarettes temporarily, but hard to *stay* off them for over a year.) Good stop-smoking programs have success rates of 30 to 40 percent at one-year follow-ups.

"PASSIVE SMOKING" AND THE RIGHTS OF NONSMOKERS

More and more, the signs are appearing: Nonsmokers are tired of **passive smoking**—breathing in air polluted by other people's tobacco smoke. Restaurants are reserving tables for nonsmokers, commuter trains have more "no smoking" cars than "smoking" cars, and pediatricians are cautioning parents against smoking to protect their *children's* health. Why all the fuss? How are nonsmokers affected by other people's smoking?

Smoking and Indoor Air Pollution

The series of reports from the Surgeon General on the health consequences of smoking suggests that tobacco smoke in enclosed indoor areas is an important air pollution problem. Carbon monoxide levels of **sidestream smoke** (smoke from the burning end of a cigarette) reach a dangerously high 42,000 parts per million. (For purposes of comparison, note that the Environmental Protection Agency sets 100 parts per million as the maximum allowed for air to be considered "clean.") True, the smoke can be greatly diluted in freely circulating air, depending on ventilation, size of the room, total amount of combustion, and other factors; but the 1 percent to 5 percent carbon monoxide levels attained in smoke-filled rooms, says the Public Health Service, can be sufficient to harm the health of people with chronic bronchitis or other lung disease or coronary heart disease.[45] These levels can also significantly reduce the exercise tolerance of some people with cardiovascular disease.

HOW SMOKERS' FAMILIES ARE AFFECTED

Recent evidence also links children's health to their parents' smoking habits. Children whose parents smoke have a higher incidence of respiratory problems than children whose parents do not smoke, and they demonstrate impaired respiratory function. More bronchitis and pneumonia during the first year of life occur among children whose parents smoke.[46] In Japan, studies have

TABLE 6.2 ▪ **Risk Ratio for Selected Causes of Death in Nonsmoking Women by Smoking Habit of Husbands**

| | *Husband's Smoking Habit* | | |
Cause of Death	NON-SMOKER	EX-SMOKER OR 1–19 CIGARETTES PER DAY	20 OR MORE CIGARETTES PER DAY
Lung cancer	1.00	1.61	2.08
Emphysema, asthma	1.00	1.29	1.49
Cancer of cervix	1.00	1.15	1.14
Stomach cancer	1.00	1.02	0.99
Ischemic heart disease	1.00	0.97	1.03

Source: T. Hirayama, "Non-smoking Wives of Heavy Smokers Have a Higher Risk of Lung Cancer: A Study from Japan," *British Medical Journal* 282 (January 17, 1981): 183–185.

shown that wives of men who are heavy smokers have a greater chance of developing lung cancer and other serious diseases than women whose husbands don't smoke (see Table 6.2).[47]

TOBACCO SMOKE AND ALLERGY SUFFERERS

While most people suffer some discomfort from heavy concentrations of tobacco smoke, people allergic to such smoke suffer the most. It's difficult to estimate exactly how many people suffer from allergies related to tobacco sensitization. But according to the 1979 Surgeon General's Report, "Substantial proportions of the population experience irritation and annoyance when exposed to cigarette smoke. . . . Such irritation increases with increasing levels of smoke contamination."[48] They suffer reactions ranging from mild eye irritation and upper respiratory congestion to life-threatening asthma attacks. Severe allergic reactions to tobacco smoke are more frequent than is commonly recognized, because attacks are typically delayed until an hour or longer after exposure.

Nonsmokers' Groups

Today, increasing numbers of militant nonsmokers are demanding their right to breathe air that is free of tobacco smoke. Individually, many nonsmokers are asking smokers not to light up in certain places. Some have established no-smoking rules in their cars and homes. In 1976 a New Jer-

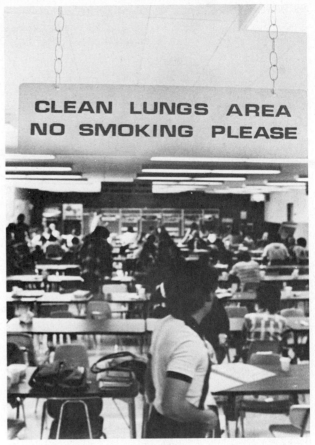

A growing awareness of the rights of nonsmokers has led to the prohibition of smoking in designated areas of restaurants and many other public places. (© Mimi Forsyth/Monkmeyer Press Photo)

sey woman who was allergic to tobacco smoke sued her employer, the telephone company, for the right to a smoke-free working place—and the New Jersey Superior Court set a precedent by ordering a ban on smoking in the office she shared with other workers.

Collectively, nonsmokers in many communities have organized groups such as ASH (Action on Smoking and Health) and GASP (Group Against Smokers' Pollution). These groups have succeeded in securing "nonsmokers' rights" laws that prohibit smoking in certain public places—usually those where people do not merely pass through but must spend some time, such as food markets, public waiting rooms, service lines, and elevators. Twenty-eight states have passed "clean indoor air" laws restricting smoking in public places and such facilities as hospitals and nursing homes. One of the most comprehensive state laws is Minnesota's Clean Indoor Air Act, which went into effect in 1975. It banned smoking in all public places—stores, buses, hospitals, schools, auditoriums, airports, restaurants, arenas, and meeting rooms—except in designated smoking areas. People who smoke in the prohibited areas can be fined up to $100.

Laws are not automatically obeyed, especially when they run counter to established traditions and habits. As substantial numbers of nonsmokers publicly express their support for these laws, however, a profound change is taking place not only in public smoking but in the social acceptability of smoking in general. This erosion of public tolerance of smoking may, in the long run, have a greater impact on this deadly and crippling habit than all the scientific and educational efforts combined.

MAKING HEALTH DECISIONS

Responsible Decisions About Smoking

Most smokers simply do not understand why they smoke. Finding out why they do may be the first step toward quitting. This activity is designed to help smokers identify the basic "reward" they are seeking when they smoke. It also suggests behaviors that the smoker can substitute to achieve a similar but healthier outcome.

If you are a smoker yourself, you may be interested in exploring this question by completing this self-test. If you are not a smoker, you may want to show the test to a family member or friend who does smoke but is thinking about quitting.

Directions: Following are eighteen statements about smoking. Read each statement and decide whether it is *always, frequently, occasionally, seldom,* or *never* a reason for your smoking. Circle the appropriate number for each statement. Be sure to respond to *every* statement.

Your total score in each category gives you a rough idea of how important that factor is to you. In addition, a high score in any category indicates a need that is being met by your smoking behavior. For each need, substitute ways to get satisfaction are suggested below; thus, this activity gives you an opportunity to decide on nonsmoking alternatives.

	Always	*Frequently*	*Occasionally*	*Seldom*	*Never*
A. Smoking keeps me from slowing down.	5	4	3	2	1
B. Handling a cigarette or pipe is part of the enjoyment of smoking.	5	4	3	2	1
C. Smoking is pleasant and relaxing.	5	4	3	2	1
D. I smoke when I feel angry about something.	5	4	3	2	1
E. I smoke automatically, without even being aware of it.	5	4	3	2	1
F. When I run out of tobacco, I find it almost unbearable until I get more.	5	4	3	2	1
G. I smoke to stimulate myself, to perk myself up.	5	4	3	2	1

	Always	Frequently	Occasionally	Seldom	Never
H. Part of the enjoyment of smoking comes from the steps involved in lighting up.	5	4	3	2	1
I. I find smoking to be a pleasurable activity.	5	4	3	2	1
J. When I feel uncomfortable or upset about something, I smoke.	5	4	3	2	1
K. When I am *not* smoking, I am very much aware of that fact.	5	4	3	2	1
L. I light up a cigarette without realizing that I still have one burning in the ashtray.	5	4	3	2	1
M. I smoke to give myself a lift.	5	4	3	2	1
N. When I smoke, part of the enjoyment is watching the smoke as I exhale it.	5	4	3	2	1
O. I want to smoke most when I am relaxed and comfortable.	5	4	3	2	1
P. When I feel blue or want to take my mind off cares and worries, I smoke.	5	4	3	2	1
Q. I get a real, gnawing hunger for tobacco when I haven't smoked for a while.	5	4	3	2	1
R. I've found a cigarette in my mouth and not remembered putting it there.	5	4	3	2	1

				"Need" categories
___ +	___ +	___ =	___	
A	G	M		Stimulation
___ +	___ +	___ =	___	
B	H	N		Handling
___ +	___ +	___ =	___	
C	I	O		Pleasure
___ +	___ +	___ =	___	
D	J	P		Crutch
___ +	___ +	___ =	___	
E	L	R		Habit
___ +	___ +	___ =	___	
F	K	Q		Craving

SCORING INSTRUCTIONS

Enter the number you circled for each statement in the corresponding space at left. For example, put the number you circled for statement A over line A, for statement B over line B, and so forth. Add the three scores on each line to tabulate the total score for each "need" category. Scores can vary from 3 to 15: 11–15 indicates a highly important reason; 7–10, a less important one; 3–6, a relatively unimportant one.

INTERPRETATION OF SCORES

A score below 8 in every one of the six "need" categories means that it should be relatively easy to give up smoking. A score higher than 7 in one category means that it may be necessary to use a substitute behavior to meet the need. A score higher than 7 in *more than one* category might require the use of several substitute behaviors to counteract the reward that smoking provides the smoker.

Stimulation: This person smokes for the energizing effect tobacco smoke has on the nervous system. Exercise (such as a brisk walk) is an excellent nondrug alternative.

List several activities that you would recommend for a person who scores high on this factor:

_____

_____

_____

Handling: This person enjoys the manual aspects of the smoking process. Activities that keep the hands busy (such as needlepoint) serve as useful alternatives.

List several activities that you would recommend for a person who scores high on this factor:

_____

_____

_____

Pleasure: This person simply enjoys smoking. He or she needs to weigh the pleasurable aspects against the potential health risks. Educational materials (such as American Cancer Society materials) can provide information; enjoyable activities with family, friends, or community groups (such as dancing) can provide pleasurable relaxation.

List several activities that a person who scores high on this factor could participate in with others. Also, identify several resources that he or she could use to obtain free or inexpensive factual information:_____

_____

_____

_____

Crutch: This person smokes as a way of calming down when feeling tension or stress. Relaxation techniques (such as progressive relaxation, discussed in Chapter 4) are useful ways to reduce

tension and are a much healthier means of managing stress than smoking.

List several stress-management techniques that a person who scores high on this factor could use:

_____

_____

_____

_____

Habit: This person scarcely realizes when he or she smokes. The alternatives are actually ways to make the smoker *aware* of each cigarette; an example is keeping a smoking diary.

List several ways in which a person who scores high on this factor can be reminded of the smoking behavior: _____

_____

_____

_____

Craving: This person has probably developed a dependence on nicotine. Research suggests that nicotine may be the primary incentive and reinforcer in smoking; carbon monoxide and tar components also play an important role in the development of tolerance to the effects of smoking. For people with a real craving for nicotine, tapering-off programs are often counterproductive, and stopping abruptly ("cold turkey") can produce a variety of adverse reactions. Therefore, such alternatives should be done only under the direction of a physician or other trained professional. Two pharmacological aids are commercially available: lobeline sulphate, a nicotine imitator, sold OTC in a buffered form as Nikoban or Bantron; and chewing gum containing nicotine, also available OTC. Note, however, that more is involved in quitting than just giving up, or finding substitute chemicals for, nicotine; so these OTC preparations are usually ineffective unless they are accompanied by other measures.

Source: Adapted from *A Smoker's Self-Teaching Kit* (Bethesda, Md.: National Clearinghouse for Smoking and Health, 1974).

SUMMARY

1. Some 52 million Americans smoke cigarettes, but people's attitudes toward smoking seem to be shifting. The percentage of people who smoke has declined since 1965.

2. People may smoke in response to various psychological and social pressures. Some form a psychological dependence on cigarettes, and a physiological dependence on the drug nicotine may also be involved. Nicotine enters the lungs in inhaled smoke, passes into the bloodstream, and from there goes to nicotine receptor sites throughout the body. When people quit smoking, they often experience a true withdrawal syndrome, the most common symptom of which is a craving for tobacco. Tolerance may also develop to tar and carbon monoxide in cigarette smoke.

3. Smoking is hazardous to health. Benzopyrene, a deadly carcinogen, occurs in cigarette smoke. Smoking is implicated in 18 percent of all deaths in the United States, and smokers have a 60 percent greater chance of dying prematurely than nonsmokers. Smoking has been linked to cancer, cardiovascular disease, respiratory disease, and allergic reactions.

4. Women who take birth control pills should not smoke, for the combination puts them at greater risk of heart attacks and possibly of strokes. Pregnant women who smoke have higher rates of miscarriage, stillbirth, and premature deliveries than nonsmokers. Their babies who survive weigh less and have higher mortality rates and poorer growth and development than other children.

5. There are no safe cigarettes, and the person who smokes low-tar, low-nicotine cigarettes gains little advantage from them.

6. The proportion of smokers is declining in almost every age category (except among teenage girls), and 30 million smokers have quit since 1964. Although most smokers are unsuccessful on their first try, many succeed on later tries. Methods of quitting include "cold turkey," individual programs, group programs, hypnosis, aversion therapy, behavior modification, and systems of reward and punishment.

7. Smoking can have adverse effects on nonsmokers. Carbon monoxide levels in smoky rooms can harm the health of nonsmokers with chronic lung ailments. Nonsmokers are increasingly militant about their right to breathe air unpolluted by tobacco smoke.

GLOSSARY

benzopyrene A chemical found in tobacco smoke; one of the deadliest carcinogens known.

carbon monoxide One of the most hazardous gases in tobacco smoke. It impairs the blood's capacity to carry oxygen and concentrates in the blood of the fetus of a pregnant woman who smokes.

hypoarousal A state in which the body is less aroused than normal.

nicotine A toxic drug found in tobacco that acts as a stimulant and is responsible for many of the harmful effects of smoking.

passive smoking Breathing in air polluted by the tobacco smoke of other people. Especially dangerous to children whose parents smoke.

sidestream smoke Smoke from the burning end of a cigarette.

tar A sticky residue from burning tobacco, consisting of more than 200 chemicals, many of which are hazardous.

NOTES

1. Bureau of the Census, *Statistical Abstracts of the United States, 1981* (Washington, D.C.: U.S. Government Printing Office, 1981), p. 123.

2. *Report of the Surgeon General* (Washington, D.C.: U.S. Public Health Service, 1964).

3. *Smoking and Health: Report of the Surgeon General,* 1979, p. 23.

4. Terry F. Pechacek, "An Overview of Smoking Behavior and Its Modification," *NIDA Research Monograph Series: The Behavioral Aspects of Smoking,* U.S. Department of Health and Human Services Pub. No. (ADM) 79-882, 1979, pp. 92–94.

5. *Cancer: Report of the Surgeon General,* 1982.

6. NIDA, *Behavioral Aspects of Smoking,* p. 10.

7. Ibid., p. 109.

8. Ibid., p. 110.

9. *The Health Consequences of Smoking for Women: Report of the Surgeon General,* 1980, pp. 12, 13.

10. NIDA, *Behavioral Aspects of Smoking,* pp. 112, 114–115.

11. Ibid., pp. 12–13.

12. Ibid., p. 23.

13. Ibid., p. 29.

14. Ibid., p. 10.

15. *The Changing Cigarette: Report of the Surgeon General,* 1981, pp. 33–34.

16. NIDA, *Behavioral Aspects of Smoking,* p. 12.

17. *Smoking and Health: Report of the Surgeon General,* 1979, pp. I-15–I-17.

18. Ibid., p. II-43.

19. *The Changing Cigarette: Report of the Surgeon General,* 1981.

20. *Cancer: Report of the Surgeon General,* 1982.

21. *The Changing Cigarette: Report of the Surgeon General,* 1981.

22. Ibid.

23. Ibid.

24. *Cancer: Report of the Surgeon General,* 1982.

25. *Smoking and Health: Report of the Surgeon General,* 1979, p. I-16.

26. Ibid., p. I-15.

27. *The Changing Cigarette: Report of the Surgeon General,* 1981.

28. *Smoking and Health: Report of the Surgeon General,* 1979, p. I-18.

29. *The Changing Cigarette: Report of the Surgeon General,* 1981 (emphasis added).

30. Ernest L. Abel, "Smoking During Pregnancy: A Review of Effects on Growth and Development of Offspring," *Human Biology* 52, no. 4 (December 1980): 593–625; Richard L. Naeye, "Influence of Maternal Cigarette Smoking During Pregnancy on Fetal and Childhood Growth," *Obstetrics & Gynecology* 57, no. 1 (January 1981): 18–21.

31. *Smoking and Health: Report of the Surgeon General,* 1979, p. I-22.

32. Ibid., p. I-21.

33. Abel, "Smoking During Pregnancy."

34. *Smoking and Health: Report of the Surgeon General,* 1979, p. I-21.

35. *Cancer: Report of the Surgeon General,* 1982.

36. D. W. Kaufman et al., "Nicotine and Carbon Monoxide Content of Cigarette Smoke and the Risk of Myocardial Infarction in Young Men," *New England Journal of Medicine* 308, no. 8 (February 24, 1983): 409–413.

37. "Smoking in America: Public Attitudes and Behavior," *Gallup Opinion Index,* Report No. 155 (June 1978): 1–26.

38. Cited in Bureau of the Census, *Statistical Abstracts of the United States, 1981,* p. 123.

39. NIDA, *Behavioral Aspects of Smoking; The Health Consequences of Smoking for Women:* Report of the Surgeon General, 1980.

40. Stanley Schachter, "Recidivism and Self-Cure of Smoking and Obesity," *American Psychologist* 37, no. 4 (April 1982): 436–444.

41. U.S. Department of Health and Human Services, "Helping Smokers Quit: A Guide for Physicians" (pamphlet) (National Institutes of Health Pub. No. 79-1825; reprinted June 1979).

42. J. Allan Best and Maurice Bloch, "Compliance in the Control of Cigarette Smoking," *NIDA Research Monograph Series* No. 17 (1977): 209.

43. Ibid., p. 213.

44. Ibid., p. 214.

45. NIDA, *Behavioral Aspects of Smoking.*

46. Steven L. Gortmaker et al., "Parental Smoking and the Risk of Childhood Asthma," *American Journal of Public Health* 72, no. 6 (June 1982): 574–578; D. M. Fergusson et al., "Parental Smoking and Respiratory Illness in Infancy," *Archives of Disease in Childhood* 55 (1980): 358–361.

47. Takeshi Hirayama, "Non-smoking Wives of Heavy Smokers Have a Higher Risk of Lung Cancer: A Study from Japan," *British Medical Journal* 22 (January 1981): 183–185.

48. *Smoking and Health: Report of the Surgeon General,* 1979, p. I-25.

PART THREE

Developing Intimacy: Health and Interpersonal Relationships

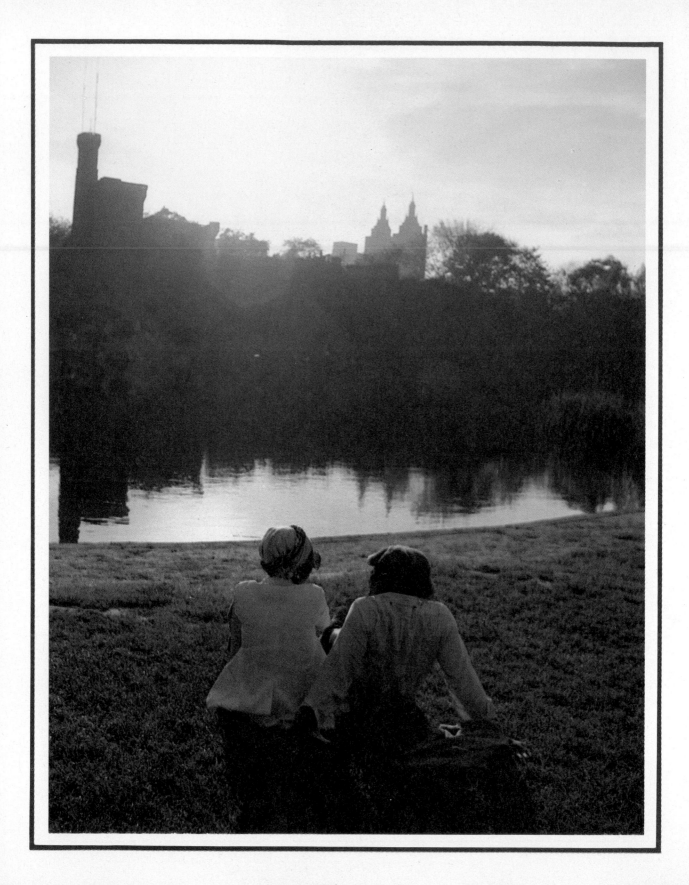

CHAPTER 7

Human Sexuality

From the commercials we see on television to the looks we get on the street, we are constantly bombarded by messages about our sex and our sexuality. We are influenced by society in the way we walk, talk, dress, flirt, and even mate—and these influences differ according to our sex. The messages start in the cradle, when our parents choose between pink clothing for a girl and blue for a boy. By adolescence we are fully aware there is something important, even explosive at times, about sex and sexuality. The way we think and feel about sex and our sexuality is woven into the fabric of our daily lives, starting with the clothes we don in the morning. Yet rarely do we take time to examine our attitudes about these issues. In this chapter we're going to explore this emotion-laden topic.

One quick question before we go on: What exactly is the difference between sexuality and sex? By **sex,** we usually mean either our gender (our maleness or femaleness), or the way we physically express affectionate or erotic feelings, from kissing and hugging to sexual intercourse. By **sexuality,** we mean our masculinity or femininity, the way in which our gender, male or female, is integrated into our personalities—what it means to be a man or a woman in our society. We express our sexuality in every situation, from deciding how to ask for a raise at work to deciding who will make dinner at home.

In this chapter, we're going to talk mainly about our sex—that is, about our sexual anatomy, how it works, and how we feel about it. At the same time, we will be discussing our sexuality, because the way we feel about being male and female in our society directly affects the quality of our sexual lives and the way we feel about ourselves generally.

SHIFTING VIEWS OF SEX, SEX ROLES, AND SEXUALITY

Americans have changed their views of sex, sex roles, and marriage in the last several decades—and many have also changed their sexual behavior.

New Attitudes Toward Premarital Sex

Premarital sex is more widely talked about than it was several decades ago. Among young people there's less belief in the "double standard" that says premarital sex is all right for men but not for women. More unmarried college women today say they've engaged in sexual intercourse—the number has moved from about 40 percent in the 1950s to at least 80 percent in the 1970s.[1] Teenagers, too, may be more likely to approve of premarital sex, and *some* may be more likely to engage in it *if* there is an emotional commitment between the partners—though the widespread notion of the "promiscuous teenager" is a myth.[2]

New Attitudes Toward Gender Behavior

Traditional expectations for "male" and "female" behavior have also begun to change, both in marriage and outside marriage. It is now more widely recognized that environment plays an important role in shaping each individual's identity as a male or a female, and more people now realize that if men and women are different, it isn't "because they're just born that way."

There *are* some inborn differences in the way

male and female babies behave that are noticeable shortly after birth, but these differences are not as great as people once assumed. Meanwhile, from the first announcement of a baby's sex, society imposes different expectations depending on which sex it is. The baby gets either a girl's name or a boy's name, either a pink blanket or a blue one. The parents tend to talk more with a baby girl and to roughhouse more with a baby boy. When a small girl flirts with her father, he may flirt back. When a small boy wants to play with a ball, Dad plays catch. These responses contribute to the child's growing sense of being male or female. Even by the age of three or four, most children have a strong gender identity and have begun to learn behavior appropriate to their gender.

Today the social conditioning that shaped the "typical man" and "typical woman" of yesteryear is changing. Little girls are now encouraged to be more physically active, even to join Little League teams. More mothers are working, and they provide different role models from the homemakers of several decades ago; children can now see that women have careers. Children also see that fathers are expected to pitch in and help with the housework; that fathers don't always have to fit the tough "macho" stereotype of the American male, but can be loving and tender.

These changes in the way men and women are conditioned to behave affect not only their approach to work and family but also their approach to sexual experience. Some women now feel more free to be sexually assertive, and some men feel more free to express their emotional needs in a sexual relationship. Among both men and women, sexual behavior is no longer an unmentionable topic.

Finding Our Own Values

Yet even with this new openness about sex, not everyone is—or necessarily should be—leaping into intimate relationships. Many people are still shy about sex and ambivalent about sexual intimacy. Each one of us grows up with different attitudes, born of our own experience at home and our relationships with other people. Each of us must decide for ourselves just what is comfortable and appropriate sexually, depending on our feelings, the setting, and our partner. Sex can be one

of the most pleasurable experiences in our lives, an intimate and special way of showing that we care about another person—but only if we are fully aware of our own attitudes about sex and our sexuality and can make choices based on our own individual needs.

SEX AND THE HUMAN BODY: OUR SEXUAL ANATOMY

Before we talk about sex in detail, we need to summarize the functions of our sexual anatomy and physiology. Basically, of course, we are talking about the mechanism that enables us to reproduce. This mechanism makes it possible for two special types of cells—a **sperm** cell, produced by the male, and an **ovum** (a Latin word meaning egg), produced by the female—to unite to form a **fertilized ovum,** or **fertilized egg,** the cell from which a new human being will eventually develop.

In sexual intercourse, the male's penis deposits millions of sperm in the female's vagina (the external opening of her reproductive tract). These sperm travel through the vagina up into the uterus and into the Fallopian tubes, which end in the abdominal cavity near the female's ovaries. (See Figure 7.1.) Once every 28 days or so, an ovum is normally released from one of the ovaries and travels into the Fallopian tube near that ovary. *If* a sperm happens to be in the Fallopian tube when the ovum arrives, the two *may* unite, resulting in a pregnancy. (We'll discuss these aspects of human reproduction in more detail in Chapter 8.)

When we talk about our sexual anatomy and physiology from the point of view of reproduction, we are telling only part of the story—and a small part at that. To most of us, the function of these parts of our bodies is interesting to us more because of their sexual aspects than because of their reproductive capacities. We are attracted to one another sexually because of the erotic qualities of our sexual anatomy and physiology. Our bodies have many **erogenous** areas—areas that excite sexual desire, or produce sexual arousal. Sexual pleasure and sexual behavior may follow that arousal in a multistaged cycle of sexual response.

TEST YOUR AWARENESS

Sex: Myths and Realities

Sex is a subject around which many myths have developed. How much do *you* know about "the facts of life"? Try this brief quiz and see. We'll talk about many sexual myths in this chapter.

True   False

_____   _____ 1. Men with large penises are better lovers.

_____   _____ 2. Women with large breasts are more sexually responsive than women with small breasts.

True   False

_____   _____ 3. Masturbation is a habit of the young and immature; it normally ends after marriage.

_____   _____ 4. Homosexuals are as emotionally stable as other segments of the population.

_____   _____ 5. Any sexual behavior is legal when the partners are mutually consenting adults.

ANSWERS

1. *False.* All penises are pretty much the same size when they are erect, and a woman's vagina can clasp a penis of any size tightly enough to give both partners pleasure.

2. *False.* Breast size is not necessarily an indication of sexual responsiveness.

3. *False.* Masturbation commonly continues throughout much of the adult lives of both men and women, whether married or single.

4. *True.* Recent studies have shown that the average homosexual is as emotionally well-adjusted as the typical heterosexual.

5. *False.* Most states have laws forbidding most forms of sex except penile-vaginal intercourse. These laws are most often used to prosecute sex offenders, but they can be invoked against anyone.

Erogenous Zones

Our external sexual structures, which we will describe below, are erogenous, but there are also many other so-called erogenous zones. Actually, the term *erogenous zone* isn't really very specific. No specific body part can be relied on to produce sexual arousal in everyone at any time. We are all different. Some of us respond sexually to erotic things that we see, while others react more strongly to touch. Most of us, however, react to a variety of stimuli that for us have an erotic quality. As far as our bodies are concerned, we can learn to associate virtually any part of our body—or any activity, even thought—with sexual arousal.

Most of us react to stimulation of our external sexual structures—the male's penis and scrotum, the female's vulva—and the areas near them, the perineum and the anus. But we also may experience sexual arousal from stimulation of our breasts, our ears, the inner sides of our thighs, or any other part of our skin. Our mouth areas are especially reactive; hence, the practice of kissing for sexual excitation in this society. In fact, any area of the body may serve as an erogenous zone. We all develop preferences for stimulation in particular areas in specific ways.

It is a mistake to think that we all have the same patterns of sexual arousal and that to have gratifying sex all an individual needs to do is learn the proper erogenous zone to stimulate. Sex isn't —and should not be—such a mechanical experience.

The Female Sexual Anatomy

FEMALE SEXUAL STRUCTURES

Sexual structures of the human female are shown in Figure 7.2; we'll discuss each of the major structures in this section.

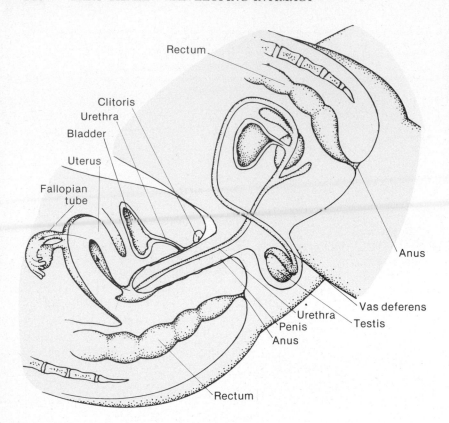

Rectum

Clitoris
Urethra
Bladder
Uterus
Fallopian tube

Anus

Vas deferens
Urethra
Penis
Anus
Testis

Rectum

Figure 7.1 Sexual intercourse, viewed from the side. The man's erect penis is inserted into the woman's vagina. When the man ejaculates, sperm manufactured in his testes travel through his vas deferens and out of his urethra into the woman's vagina. From the vagina, the sperm "swim" up the uterus and into the Fallopian tubes, where one may unite with an egg and begin a pregnancy unless effective contraception is used.

THE VAGINA The **vagina** is the canal-like structure that extends from the bottom of the uterus to the vulva (see below). The vagina receives the penis during sexual intercourse and acts as a passageway for a baby during birth. But it is much more than a simple receptacle: It is a responsive, muscular organ equipped to widen and clasp the penis during intercourse. Ordinarily, the vagina is shaped like a flattened tube of toothpaste, about four inches long. Its inner lining is a moist, elastic membrane, much like the inside of the mouth. The vagina has few sensory nerve endings, except near its opening, so the inner two-thirds of the organ is relatively insensitive to touch or pain.

THE VULVA AND THE MONS VENERIS Most of a woman's most sensitive sexual areas are located around the opening of the vagina in the external genital region called the **vulva** (which means "covering"). In this area, over the pubic bone, is the woman's **mons veneris** (Latin for "mound of Venus"), a cushion of fatty tissue, covered with skin and hair, that is extremely sensitive. Many women find stimulation of the mons to be one of the most pleasurable sexual sensations.

THE LABIA The two soft, sensitive folds of skin at either side of the opening of the vagina are called the **labia** (Latin for "lips"). The outer, broad folds of skin are called the *labia majora;* inside them are two hairless lips called the *labia minora.* The labia act as protection for the **urethra** (the tube from the urinary bladder through which urine is passed out of the body) and for the vagina. The labia have many sensitive nerve endings, and stimulation of them can add to a woman's sexual arousal.

THE CLITORIS The labia minora meet to form a hood over the **clitoris**, one of a woman's most sensitive sexual organs. Some people think of the clitoris as a miniature penis, since it is highly sensitive to sexual stimulation and is even derived from the same tissues in an embryo's anatomy. But the comparison is incorrect, for the clitoris has no reproductive or urinary function and though it swells during sexual excitement, it does not become erect in the same way the penis does.

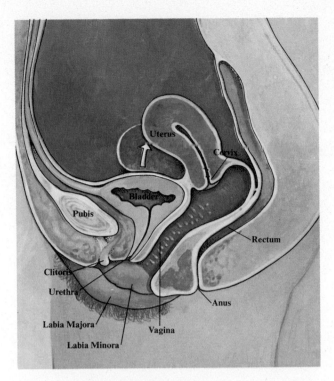

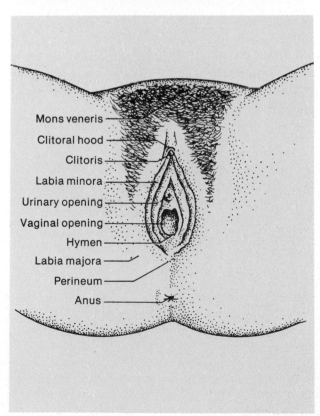

Figure 7.2   Female reproductive organs (*above*) and external genital structures (*below*).

THE PERINEUM   The hairless area of skin at the lower end of the labia near the anus is called the **perineum.** This area too is quite sensitive to touch, pressure, and temperature changes.

THE INTERNAL SEX ORGANS   A woman's internal sex organs can also add to her arousal and orgasmic sensations. Her **uterus,** or womb, is located at the internal end of the vagina. It is a hollow, muscular structure that shelters and nourishes the fetus during pregnancy. Its narrow lower end, the **cervix,** is a firm, smooth knob that can be felt at the upper end of the vagina.

THE BREASTS   A woman's breasts can also play a role in her sexual response. When a woman is sexually excited, her breasts may actually expand slightly, and her nipples may grow hard and erect.

The size and shape of women's breasts vary widely, just as other parts of people's bodies do. Contrary to popular myth, the size of a woman's breasts has little to do with her sexual response. Rather, her personal preferences, her experiences with her sexual partners and herself, and her biology determine her responsiveness.

MUSCLES ASSOCIATED WITH THE VAGINA

The vagina is remarkably elastic; after all, a full-sized baby can pass through it at birth. Yet it can also become very tight during sexual arousal, when the pubococcygeous muscles that surround it become tense.

After childbirth some women consider themselves "too large" or "too wide open." A woman can deal with this problem, at least in part, by learning to voluntarily contract and lift these muscles into the abdomen. Such voluntary contraction increases friction with the penis during intercourse, and thus can enhance enjoyment. Maintaining muscle tone in this area is also believed to help reduce pelvic difficulties in later life. If a woman's vagina is extremely stretched out, a physician may recommend exercises or surgery to restore muscle tone.

LUBRICATION OF THE VAGINA

Most women's vaginas begin to "sweat" when they are sexually aroused. Most of the fluid that appears at the vaginal opening comes from the vagina itself. Researchers do not yet completely understand this phenomenon, but it does seem that lubrication plays a helpful part—it makes penetration by the penis and intercourse easier, and makes the vagina a more appropriate environment for the movement of the sperm up into the uterus and Fallopian tubes.

WHAT IS THE HYMEN?

In infant girls, the vaginal opening is often narrowed by a circular membrane, which looks like the shutter of a camera and is called the **hymen.** It usually has a central opening large enough to admit an examining finger or a tampon.

It used to be believed that one could tell if a woman was a virgin by looking to see if her hymen was still intact. But it's now known that physical activity or just the passing of time can cause the hymen to tear, even when intercourse has not occurred. If it is still present in first intercourse, it normally stretches or tears a little to accommodate the penis. Only occasionally is the hymen so thick as to require a doctor's help to stretch it to allow intercourse.

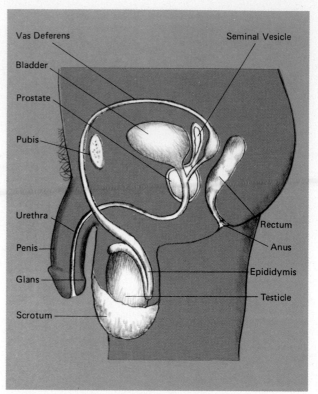

Figure 7.3   Male reproductive organs.

The Male Sexual Anatomy

The male's sexual anatomy, like the female's, not only functions as a reproductive system but also can give pleasure during sexual arousal. The external sexual structures, especially the penis, are easily stimulated.

MALE SEXUAL STRUCTURES

Sexual structures of the human male are shown in Figure 7.3; we'll discuss each of the major structures in this section.

THE PENIS Most visible and most important is the **penis,** the external male organ of sexual intercourse (and of urination). The penis is flaccid (limp) until sexually aroused. As a man becomes sexually excited, blood rushes to the arteries that supply the penis and surrounding tissue, and the increased blood flow and pressure in the area causes the penis to become erect. The head of the penis, called the **glans,** is particularly sensitive, as

are the rim of tissue (the **coronal ridge**) between the glans and the shaft of the penis and the triangular region (the **frenulum**) on the underside of the penis.

THE SCROTUM The **scrotum** is the loose pouch of skin that hangs behind and under the penis and contains the **testicles,** or **testes.** The scrotum acts as protection for the testicles, which produce the man's reproductive cells (the sperm). The testicles are so sensitive to touch that sometimes even light caressing can be irritating for some men. Other men find that gentle squeezing arouses them.

THE EPIDIDYMIS AND THE VAS DEFERENS When the sperm cells leave the testicles, they travel through a highly coiled network of tubing in the back of each testicle called the **epididymis.** Sperm cells may take several weeks to travel through the epididymis while they reach maturity. From there, the sperm travel through the **vas deferens,** long tubes that curve alongside the urinary bladder.

THE PROSTATE GLAND AND THE SEMINAL VESICLES The **prostate gland,** about the size of a chestnut, located just below the man's urethra, produces about 30 percent of the clear fluid called **semen** or **seminal fluid,** which is the liquid expelled from the penis during ejaculation. This liquid provides a medium in which the sperm can travel.

Two other small organs called the **seminal vesicles** produce the other 70 percent of the seminal fluid. The vesicles lie at the base of the bladder and join with the ends of the vas deferens to form the **ejaculatory ducts.** These ducts, in turn, join the urethra, forming one long tubing system from the testicles to the opening of the penis, through which the man can expel his semen.

COWPER'S GLANDS During sexual arousal, a few drops of fluid may appear at the end of the penis. The fluid is produced by **Cowper's glands,** two pea-sized organs just below the prostate gland. This fluid may reduce the acidity of the urethra before ejaculation, but researchers remain uncertain about this.

It is important to note that the fluid from Cowper's gland may contain viable sperm: A woman *can* become pregnant if any of this fluid finds its way into her vagina.

THE BREASTS Like a woman's breasts, a man's breasts can add to sexual arousal. Male breasts are less sensitive to touch than a woman's, but some men find that having their breasts stimulated by stroking or licking can increase their excitement.

DOES PENIS SIZE MAKE A DIFFERENCE?

Perhaps the oldest sexual myth of all is that the larger a man's penis, the better his sexual performance and the greater his partner's satisfaction. Research has not supported this myth. A small penis usually has a greater increase in size than does a larger one during erection, so that the two are likely to be about the same size once they are erect.[3] Also, a woman's vagina can open or close to clasp a penis of almost any size, large or small.

Therefore, penis size is believed to be an insignificant factor in sexual response.

DOES CIRCUMCISION MAKE A DIFFERENCE?

No. Contrary to popular belief, **circumcision,** the surgical removal of a flap of tissue called the **foreskin** from the head of the penis, has no apparent influence on sexual behavior. A comparison of circumcised and uncircumcised men showed no differences in ejaculatory control, difficulty in reaching an erection, or sensitivity of the penis.[4]

THE PHYSIOLOGY OF THE HUMAN SEXUAL RESPONSE

Many people find that one of their biggest problems in enjoying sex is the feeling that the opposite sex is alien, too "different" to be understood. Actually, although your partner's body may look different from yours, researchers have found that male and female physical sexual responses are quite similar. Both men and women have the capacity to experience four general stages (which we discuss in detail below), starting with excitement, moving into a plateau phase of sexual tension, resolving the tension in orgasm, and then returning to a normal, relaxed state. Both men and women also experience similar physiological changes when they are sexually excited. When a person is stimulated, muscles all over his or her body increase tension, in a generalized sexual response known as **myotonia.** Both men and women also experience increased blood flow, known as **vasocongestion,** to their genital organs during sexual arousal.

Despite these similarities, however, men and women do differ in their sexual wants and desires. And individual men and women may have very distinct sexual needs and distinct *feelings* about their sexual responses. It is important to remember that our thoughts and feelings about our sexuality play more important roles in determining our sexual behavior than our physiology does.

The Work of Masters and Johnson

Most of the physiology of the human sexual response was not understood until a few years ago, when William Masters and Virginia Johnson made extensive studies at their research institute in St. Louis. This research produced very specific descriptions of the typical physiological and behavioral responses involved in sexual activity. Masters and Johnson devised techniques for measuring body changes during different phases of stimulation. They placed electrodes inside the uterus to measure contractions there and used other instruments to measure respiration, blood pressure, and cardiac contractions. They studied changes in the vagina by using plastic penises that allowed direct observation and photographs of that organ.[5]

Stages of the Sexual Response

Following is a brief summary of the stages most human beings go through in their sexual response cycle. The general patterns of these stages in men and in women, as charted by Masters and Johnson, are diagramed in Figure 7.4.

THE FIRST STAGE: EXCITEMENT

Poets have written about the palpitating heart, and now scientists have confirmed it: When you are sexually stimulated, your heart beats faster, your blood pressure rises, and tissues and blood vessels in your pelvic region become congested with blood. Myotonia also begins, as muscles all over your body tense with excitement.

IN THE MAN If you are a man, as blood congests in your pelvic organs, spongy tissue in the penis fills with blood and an erection begins. In this phase the scrotum grows more sensitive and the testicles start to rise: Muscles in the **spermatic cords** (from which each testis is suspended within the scrotum) tighten and actually lift the testes, to prepare for eventual ejaculation. Late in this phase, the nipples may become erect, although not all men have this response. The intensity of all these responses varies depending on the circumstances, and these reactions can reverse themselves rather quickly if circumstances change.

IN THE WOMAN If you are a woman, your muscles will tense, and your heart will beat faster. Your vagina will begin to lubricate, which will make intercourse easier. The clitoris and the tis-

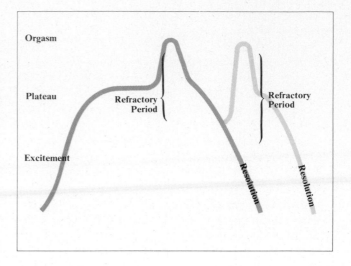

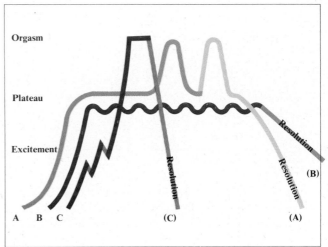

Figure 7.4 Masters and Johnson's graphs of sexual phases. *(Top)* The man's rise in sexual tension is shown diagrammatically. Once orgasm is achieved, there is a refractory period before he can have another orgasm. *(Bottom)* A woman can experience one orgasm and soon after experience another (line A). If she fails to experience orgasm, however, her resolution phase is longer (line B). Line C shows a rare kind of prolonged female orgasmic experience known as *status orgasmus.*

sues around it will swell as blood rushes into them. (This phenomenon is subtle; the difference may not actually be visible.) As sexual stimulation increases and continues, the vagina actually increases in size by two or three centimeters. The walls of the outer third of the vagina thicken to form what is called the "orgasmic platform." At this stage, the nipples may also become erect and slightly larger.

THE SECOND STAGE: PLATEAU

If sexual excitement continues, both partners will reach the next stage of response, which includes further muscle tension and even more blood flow.

IN THE MAN   The penis increases slightly in circumference, and as the testicles continue to rise, they also increase in size and may even double in size because of increased blood flow. It is at this stage that a small amount of fluid, which may contain viable sperm, may leak out of the penis.

IN THE WOMAN   At this stage, there is a marked change in the color of the tissue in the labia minora and the labia majora—so much so that these tissues are sometimes called "sex skin." Parts of the labia turn bright red, and others become a burgundy wine color. (The color depends on whether the woman has had children.) The vagina also continues to engorge with blood and expand. The uterus is elevated and moves back toward the spine. As the excitement continues, pulse, respiration, and blood pressure increase.

THE THIRD STAGE: ORGASM

Immediately before **orgasm,** the climactic stage of sexual response, the physiological reactions reach their most intense level in both men and women. The muscles are taut and will become more tense only in the contractions of the actual orgasm.

IN THE MAN   The man's orgasm begins with the contraction of the vas deferens, the seminal vesicles, and the prostate. These contractions release semen into the urethra, and the man reaches a point where ejaculation is about to happen and can no longer be controlled. The sense of impending orgasm is created as semen collects in the urethra before ejaculation. In **ejaculation,** contractions of the urethra, penis, and prostate force semen out of the tip of the penis. (At ejaculation, a band of muscle surrounding the exit from the urinary bladder contracts, making it impossible for urine to be expelled with the semen.) As the man ejaculates, muscle tension, heart rate, breathing, and blood flow reach their peak. Some men

(and women) learn to heighten their pleasure in this phase by voluntarily contracting the muscles in the buttocks, stomach, and anal area.

IN THE WOMAN   Women usually feel the orgasm for a longer time than men, starting with contractions in the uterus and vagina. As the contractions begin in the outer third of the vagina, an overwhelming sexual tension—a sense of total pelvic contraction—will be felt, and release of that tension is what most women identify as orgasm.

THE FOURTH STAGE: RESOLUTION

In this stage, the partners begin to relax and the tension throughout their bodies starts to dissipate. Blood flow and blood pressure begin to slow to normal, breathing becomes more regular, and muscles relax. The return to normal will be quickest if orgasm has occurred. Without orgasm, it usually takes longer.

IN THE MAN   The return to an unstimulated state occurs quickly in a man, and after orgasm most males experience a **refractory period.** The length of this period varies, and during it the male cannot be restimulated; in fact, efforts at renewed sexual stimulation may be irritating. The resolution of sexual tension begins even as the last contraction of the penile muscles completes the orgasm. Soon after orgasm, a normal heartbeat returns, muscles relax, and breathing slows to normal. In general, as men age, the refractory period lengthens.

The refractory period in men seems to include a strong psychological component. Some men experience extended refractory periods, perhaps because they consider ejaculation as "the end" of sexual relations. Others may think of an ejaculation as just one part of their "script" for a given sexual encounter, and may not experience an extended refractory period. Clearly, the key is sexual *desire.*

IN THE WOMAN   The tension fades more slowly in women. Because they do not have a refractory period after orgasm, as most men do, it is possible for a woman to have further orgasms soon after the first. But without further stimulation, the vagina will return to its normal size and position, muscles will relax, and breathing will slow.

Common Questions About the Human Sexual Response

CAN A WOMAN HAVE DIFFERENT KINDS OF ORGASMS?

It was long believed that orgasms that resulted from stimulation of the vagina—as in intercourse —were distinct from those that resulted from stimulation of only the clitoris, which might occur during masturbation or from stimulation by the hand alone. Freud's theories supported this view of different orgasms; Freud even claimed that in normal sexual development, women moved from an "immature" clitoral response to a "mature" vaginal one. However, Masters and Johnson's data refuted this view and revealed that orgasms are physiologically the same, regardless of the source of stimulation.[6] Thus, there is only one kind of orgasmic response in women.

DO ALL WOMEN REACT TO SEXUAL STIMULATION THE SAME WAY?

No. Each woman needs to discover what works best for her. The newly found properties of the clitoris do show that organ to be the focal point in a woman's pelvic area. It has the unique function of responding to and sending out neural messages of sexual stimulation.[7]

Some women do not need direct stimulation of the clitoris to reach orgasm. They can reach orgasm by stimulation of other sex organs such as the vagina and the vulva and need only indirect stimulation of the clitoris. Most women, however, need direct stimulation of the clitoris in order to become fully aroused. But the nature of that stimulation varies from woman to woman. Some find direct touching of the clitoris irritating rather than stimulating and prefer a more general stimulation of the clitoral area. Others respond well to contact between the penis and the clitoris during intercourse, although research shows that many more do not respond fully to this stimulation.[8] Each woman needs to try different approaches to find out what works best for her, and then let her partner know.

The size and position of the clitoris have *not* been found to affect the intensity of orgasm.

WHAT ABOUT SEXUAL ACTIVITY DURING MENSTRUATION?

There is a common myth that intercourse during a woman's menstrual period "hurts," or causes the woman other physical distress. Research has not proved this to be true; indeed, in some women, just the opposite may be true. In a recent study 10 percent of women reported that masturbation relieved the discomfort of the onset of menstruation: During orgasm the uterus contracts and expels blood clots that can contribute to cramps. About 40 percent expressed no particular like or dislike for sexual activity during menstruation. About half wanted sexual activity during menstruation, and only the remaining 10 percent objected to it on religious or aesthetic grounds.[9]

SEX AND THE WHOLE HUMAN BEING

Our sexual response is not based on physiology alone. We have what might be called a "psychosexual response," one that integrates both our physical and physiological reactions. The way we feel about sex, the way we have sex, the way we feel about ourselves as sexual beings—all these factors influence our sexual response. Those feelings are shaped by what we've learned—starting as young children and continuing throughout our entire lives—from our family, friends, previous sexual encounters, religious training, and even the mass media.

How We Learn About Sex

Most of us don't learn about sex or sexuality very directly. Instead, we receive indirect messages from other people, starting with our parents—the way they act toward each other and the way they feel about their own sexuality. We may feel shy about sex, for example, if our parents never showed affection in front of us. Or we may feel ashamed of our bodies if our parents were unduly strict about nudity, insisting that we keep our bodies well covered and hidden from others.

As we grow older, we also learn about sex and

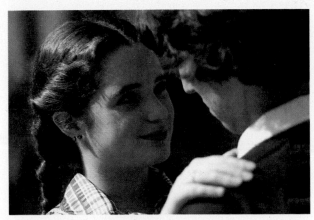

Mutually satisfying sex is one way for partners to communicate with each other—and effective communication is essential to sexual satisfaction.
(© Jeffrey Jay Foxx/Woodfin Camp & Assoc.)

our sexuality from our friends, from books and movies, from advertisements, and even from jokes. We begin to shape our own ideas of how men and women should handle themselves sexually, about what is right and wrong, and about the correct and incorrect way to handle sexual encounters and sexual feelings. We may learn the basic biological facts of sexual intercourse at school or from a manual, but we rarely talk about how we feel about our anatomy and our sexuality. Despite the fact that our feelings play a crucial role in sexual activity, we usually ignore them, almost pretending they don't exist.

People in our society often tend to feel guilty about sex. That is quite different from being shy, or feeling the need to be private about sex. Perhaps, unfortunately, sex is commonly thought to be "dirty," and some people even feel that they shouldn't have sex at all. Some people wonder if they are wrong to masturbate, and some feel so uncomfortable about having sex that their guilt prevents them from enjoying the experience at all. The unnecessary guilt may lead them to risk pregnancy by not planning for effective contraception and to feel bad about themselves and their partners.

Happily, however, many people see sex and their own sexuality in more positive terms. They recognize that sex can be a way of expressing affection and can add an important and satisfying dimension to a relationship when shared in a responsible way.

Sexual Fantasies

All of us have sexual fantasies that arouse us just as much as the real thing does. We spend time wondering, hoping, wishing, and even fearing different kinds of sexual experience. It's not unusual to dream of running off with your favorite singer or even to wish you were having a passionate affair with your best friend's brother. Fantasies are a safe way to explore feelings about ourselves and other people.

Our fantasies are usually harmless—in fact, healthy—even when they encompass what we normally consider to be bizarre behavior. Many people fantasize, for example, about having a sexual relationship with someone of their own sex; this does *not* necessarily mean they have homosexual tendencies. Others dream of having sex forced on them. These fantasies can even be repulsive or frightening at times, and the person having them begins to wonder: Is that what I really want? The answer is, probably not. Most people have the fantasy as a safe way of working out real-life fears or anxieties. They know the daydream is not real, and they don't want it to be.

The only time you need worry over sexual fantasies that frighten or repel you is when they linger for so long, or become so vivid and strong, that they interfere with what you do in your everyday activities. In such cases, it's a good idea to talk it over with a counselor or someone else whose advice you trust.

Masturbation

Masturbation is nothing new, of course, but different attitudes toward it are emerging. For centuries, people were discouraged from self-stimulation by myths about it. For example, many of today's adults were taught as children that masturbation was harmful to the body—that it would sap

Learning to Communicate in a Sexual Relationship

The best sexual relationship is one in which you feel close to your partner and are able to speak up about your feelings. Of course, it is not easy to talk about sexual needs and feelings, even to someone you know well and care deeply about. As a relationship grows more physically intimate, you may find yourself unable to say what you'd like to, for fear of hurting the other person's feelings, or of sounding too eager (or too prudish), or of just sounding "dumb." At romantic moments, for example, it may seem inappropriate to tell your partner that what he or she is doing is painful to you.

The most common sexual problems result from a lack of communication. You must tell your partner how you feel; you can hardly expect him or her to read your mind. Sex therapists often see couples who have had unsatisfying relationships for years because one or the other partner suffered in silence, unwilling to speak up about a sexual problem. Such cases testify to the extreme difficulty many people have in expressing themselves about what they like and don't like in sex.

It's not unusual for problems to arise from false assumptions about a partner's feelings. One person complains of feeling tired, for example, and the other assumes that this means "no making love tonight." In fact, the tired partner may not be rejecting sex altogether. He or she may simply be saying, "I may be slow to respond" or "I'd rather take a passive role tonight." Sexual reactions may also be misinterpreted, as when one partner mistakes the other's groans or grimaces of pleasure for pain and pulls away, much to the distress of the other. In other cases, one partner may very much want something from the other (a particular kind of stimulation, for example) and may grow resentful, wondering why it is never forthcoming.

Nearly all these problems can be helped if the partners simply communicate better. When one person says he or she is tired, the other should find out if that really means "I'm not interested in sex tonight." When a partner says he or she doesn't enjoy being touched in a particular place, the other partner should not interpret this as a rejection. Instead, he or she should try to find out what *is* pleasurable. Although speaking up about such matters may be difficult at first, it often happens that one partner's frank comments, if spoken in a loving way, may inspire the other to communicate better too, greatly enhancing the relationship. Indeed, it might almost be said that honest and intimate communication is the most important sexual skill of all.

Source: Louis R. Hott and Jacqueline Rose Hott, "Sexual Misunderstandings," *Medical Aspects of Human Sexuality* 14 (January 1980): 13–31.

a person's strength or that it was sinful. One man recalls that his grandparents gave him a book stating that only bad little boys masturbated, and when they were caught at it, their thumbs were cut off.[10]

But the truth is that masturbation is a harmless way of exploring your body and finding out how it works. We start this process when we are infants, touching ourselves all over to find out what feels good. In the same way, some adults find that masturbation can be a release for sexual feelings or can be a way to learn what is sexually pleasurable. Many people reach orgasm more quickly and easily in masturbation than in intercourse.

"Making Out"/Petting/Foreplay

There's a wide range of ways to show affection and enjoy sex with another person besides intercourse.

In our society most people start out with kissing and stroking each other, and then move on to other types of petting as they get more excited. The man may fondle the woman's breasts and genital area. The woman may caress the man's genital area as they hug and kiss. Petting techniques vary from person to person and from partner to partner, depending on what they both enjoy and feel comfortable with. Many couples enjoy the excitement of petting as much as intercourse, and use it as a substitute when they want to feel close but intercourse is impossible or inconvenient. Quite often, petting is also a form of *foreplay*—that is, sexual activity leading to intercourse.

Our society tends to emphasize intercourse as the most important sexual act, and many people behave as if all emotional and moral issues connected with our sexual behavior were linked to that single act. Yet petting is where most of us, usually as teenagers, first encounter the emotional

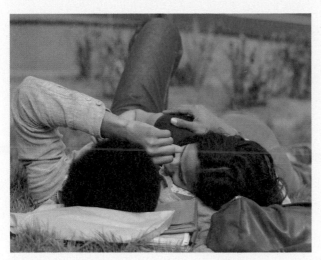

Petting is an important way for adolescents in our society to learn about sexual response. (© Timothy Eagan/Woodfin Camp & Assoc.)

issues and conflicts that arise in sexual relationships. Sex adds a new dimension to our relationships—a dimension that can add new joy or sorrow, depending on how well we communicate with our sexual partners, how we treat them, and how we treat ourselves.

Most of us, especially in our first sexual encounters, feel awkward and uncomfortable. Sexual feelings are exciting, even overwhelming at first, but acting on them can conflict with what our parents, friends, or religions tell us we should do. Some

Sexual relations can continue well into old age—and can continue to be a major source of satisfaction in a relationship. (© Hazel Hankin)

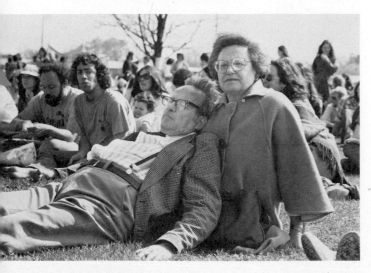

young people feel they must keep up with friends who brag about sexual exploits and experiences, even if they are not yet ready. It is a puzzling time: It's often hard to sort out what one feels about sex, about one's partner, and about oneself.

Sexual Intercourse

Sexual intercourse, when a man inserts his penis into the woman's vagina, is regarded by most people and most cultures as the culmination of a sexual relationship. Yet people rarely discuss the real experience of intercourse, which is as variable as the relationships themselves. It can be passionate, the expression of the deepest love between two people. But it can also be awkward, or playful, or even downright dull, depending on the two people involved, their feelings for each other, and the circumstances.

Many people are surprised to find, after all that they have been led to expect from intercourse, that the "first time" is rarely the best. It's frequently awkward and disappointing, with the two partners wondering what all the fuss was about. Although some people have an intense and satisfying experience the first time, it often takes practice to coordinate two inexperienced bodies into positions that give the most pleasure. And it also takes time to learn to be at ease with each other and find out just what is pleasing to each person.

Although there are many parallels between the sexual responses of men and women, there are also some significant differences. Men are usually more easily aroused and can engage in satisfactory intercourse more rapidly than women. The average woman simply needs more psychological and physical stimulation before she begins to respond. Men also tend to depend less on circumstances—such as romantic settings—to arouse them. Yet the differences between the sexes are not nearly so great as those between different individuals. There are women who respond very rapidly to sexual stimulation and men who respond quite slowly.[11]

Oral Sex

Oral stimulation of the female genitals *(cunnilingus)* or of the male genitals *(fellatio)* by a sexual partner is a matter on which people—and even

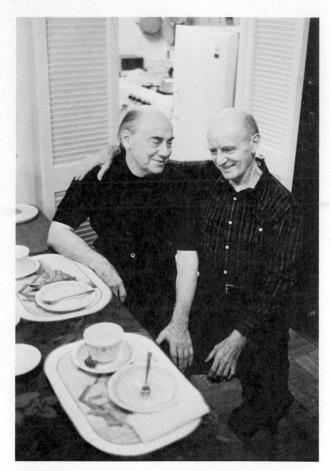

A homosexual relationship—like any other—can be stable, long-lasting, and affectionate. (© Richard Hackett)

cultures—differ markedly. In some cultures, oral sex is prevalent; in others, it is rare or regarded as unnatural or perverse. In the United States, oral-genital contact is common, occurring among more than half of all married couples.[12]

There is a wide variety of attitudes toward oral sex, ranging from pleasurable anticipation to disgust. In many ways, oral sex is one of the most intimate types of lovemaking, for it involves exposure of parts of the body that many feel most shy about to another person's view and touch. In some communities and families, religious beliefs forbid any type of sexual activity except intercourse. If that's true in your family, you may choose not to have oral sex now or ever. Other people mistakenly believe that only homosexual couples have oral sex, and an irrational fear of becoming homosexual keeps them from having oral sex.

So while oral sex can be pleasurable for some people, not everyone enjoys it. As with any kind of sexual activity, it's best to decide for yourself whether or not to engage in it and not to feel pressured or uncomfortable about it if you don't enjoy it.

OTHER PARTNER PREFERENCES

Homosexuality

Homosexuality is a sexual or emotional preference for persons of one's own sex. Few areas of human behavior have generated more theories or provoked more controversy than this one.

It is believed that both homosexual and heterosexual tendencies exist in everyone to some extent. A number of ancient societies, and some contemporary ones as well, have sanctioned homosexual behavior and at times even made it into an established practice. A comprehensive study by anthropologist Clellan Ford and psychologist Frank Beach, conducted several decades ago, revealed that forty-nine of seventy-six preliterate societies either accepted or actually prescribed homosexual activity, although none practiced it exclusively.[13] Modern Western cultures, however, encourage only the expression of **heterosexuality**—sexual or emotional preference for persons of the opposite sex. As a result, most of us learn to repress the homosexual component of our nature.

No one knows for certain what factors induce a person to pursue a predominately or exclusively homosexual behavior pattern. Some people may have a genetic predisposition to it; yet, like other behavior, it is also largely learned. Some researchers speculate that failure to identify with a parent of the same sex may lead to homosexuality.[14] Others suggest that it begins much earlier, with a faulty early identification with one's gender.[15]

HOW COMMON IS HOMOSEXUAL ACTIVITY?

Researchers agree that incidental, experimental homosexual activity is rather common, especially in adolescence. Alfred Kinsey surveyed the sexual behavior of American men in 1948 and American women in 1953; about one-third of the men and one-fifth of the women surveyed reported having at least one homosexual experience.[16] A 1970 questionnaire answered by the readers of *Psychology Today* revealed similar percentages.[17] Extensive or exclusive homosexual behavior, however, is far less common.

EMOTIONAL HEALTH AND HOMOSEXUALITY

Contrary to stereotypes, homosexuality is not proof of emotional or mental illness. A 1978 study by Alan Bell and Martin Weinberg revealed a wide diversity in the personalities of homosexuals, and refuted the widely held view that they are emotionally unstable.[18] Interestingly, the latest research shows that homosexuals tend to have more satisfying sexual encounters than heterosexuals. In interviews with 176 homosexuals, Masters and Johnson found that the homosexuals tended to communicate better with their partners about their sexual needs than the heterosexuals did, and thus tended to have better sex lives.[19]

Most homosexuals conceal their sexual preferences, although in recent years society has become somewhat more tolerant of homosexual lifestyles. Though discrimination against homosexuals persists at virtually every level of society, homosexuals have formed gay-rights organizations and demanded the right to live openly without being penalized for their sexual preferences.

SEXUAL PROBLEMS AND SEXUAL DYSFUNCTION

There are times when people become concerned about their sexual functioning. It happens to most of us once in a while. But for some people it is a recurring experience that becomes quite upsetting. Any problem that prevents a person from engaging in sexual relations or from reaching orgasm is known as a **sexual dysfunction.** (Note that the term applies only to problems in sexual *response,* not to sexual *preferences.*)

A key point is that while many forms of sexual dysfunction are emotional, others develop from organic causes. Anatomical variations, hormonal imbalance, and illness (heart disease, for example) may all be linked to sexual dysfunction.

The Broad Range of Sexual Dysfunctions

In everyday conversation, the term *impotence* is often used to describe all forms of male sexual dysfunction, and the term *frigidity* is applied to all types of female sexual problems. But neither term tells precisely what the problem is. The terms incorrectly suggest a permanent rejection of sexuality. They also incorrectly imply that a sexual problem is exclusively that of the female or the male.

The truth is that in most cases sexual dysfunction involves both partners, and both partners must work at solving the problems.

Many people have problems that arise from early sexual experiences. One of the most common complaints among male college students, for example, is **premature ejaculation,** the expulsion of semen before or immediately after insertion of the penis into the vagina. Premature ejaculation can be caused by a number of factors. Consider the case of a twenty-four-year-old man who went to a therapist after premature ejaculation had thoroughly disrupted relations with his wife. (In his case ejaculation occurred within fifteen to twenty seconds of penetration into his wife's vagina.) It turned out that before marriage his sexual encounters had taken place in locations such as the back seat of an automobile, where he had to hurry and had little privacy. Thus, he had never learned to slow his ejaculations down long enough to satisfy his partner. He needed therapy to overcome these early experiences.[20]

Many men troubled by premature ejaculation find that they can train themselves to delay ejaculation by using the "squeeze technique" developed by Masters and Johnson. In this procedure, the man or his partner gives a firm squeeze to the frenulum (the triangular area on the underside of the penis) just before he feels the urge to ejaculate. With repeated sessions of stimulation almost to ejaculation, followed by the squeeze technique,

When Is a "Sexual Problem" Really a Problem?

People inevitably compare their own sexual experiences with those they learn about in popular fiction or the media. As a result, many pick up distorted ideas about their own sexuality and about what constitutes a sexual problem.

NONPROBLEMS

Many people believe that a man should be able to achieve an erection and maintain it as long as he likes without ejaculating, that women should always have orgasms during intercourse, that all women should have multiple orgasms at least some of the time, or that neither a man nor a woman can be sexually satisfied without orgasm. Others believe that touching, holding, and kissing should always be foreplay for intercourse, or that sexual arousal without orgasm is somehow physically or emotionally unhealthy. Such beliefs are mistaken, and can themselves cause problems.

Each person needs to learn that he or she is the best judge of his or her own sexual experience. Simply touching, holding, and kissing, for example, may be quite satisfying and even exciting without any other sexual activity. Orgasm need not be the single goal of sexual arousal, and it is perfectly normal for some people to dislike some sexual practices or methods of stimulation that others enjoy.

REAL PROBLEMS

A couple may have a real problem, however, if both partners find lovemaking consistently unsatisfying, painful, or even distasteful. Similarly, if sex is being forced on one partner or used by one partner to exploit the other, the couple has a problem. One person need not always dominate the experience, and while lovemaking may not be sensational every time, both people should desire sexual activity and get pleasure from it. Consistently withholding sex can be a form of hostility or a sign of an unconscious power struggle in the relationship. Serious sexual problems also arise when one partner constantly makes the other feel inferior, unattractive, or unsexy.

When such problems persist, they can undermine a relationship. If the couple can't resolve them by talking to each other, a therapist may be able to help. The therapist may get to the root of lingering unconscious difficulties that one or both partners may be having related to earlier experiences, or may see unnoticed problems in the current relationship.

Sexual love can be a celebration of a relationship, but only when the partners are truly in tune, communicating their needs and expressing their affection for each other within the context of a healthy relationship.

Source: Mary S. Calderone and Eric W. Johnson, *The Family Book About Sexuality* (New York: Harper & Row, 1981), pp. 166–171.

---

the man can often learn to control his ejaculation satisfactorily.

WHAT IS TRUE IMPOTENCE?

Psychologists reserve the term **impotence** to describe a man's inability to achieve or maintain an erection long enough to reach orgasm with a partner. In the rare condition known as **primary impotence,** the man has never been able to achieve an erection. In most cases, however, the man has been able to have an erection in the past but is now unable to do so in some or all sexual encounters; this condition is termed **secondary impotence.** Men may also experience a **nonemissive erection**—that is, an erection with no ejaculation.

At one time or another in their lives, nearly all men have experienced one of these conditions.

SEXUAL DYSFUNCTION IN WOMEN

A very few women suffer from **vaginismus,** involuntary muscle spasms that cause the vagina to shut so tightly that it's impossible or painful for a penis to penetrate. There are other women who engage in and enjoy intercourse but never experience an orgasm. Women who have never experienced an orgasm by any method are described as having a **primary orgasmic dysfunction.** Women who frequently have trouble having an orgasm are said to have a **secondary,** or **situational, orgasmic dysfunction.**

Sexual problems are rarely the result of physiological problems. More often, they are the result of

SEXUAL VIOLENCE: Rape and How to Cope with It

Most states legally define rape as "sexual intercourse that occurs under actual or threatened forcible compulsion that overcomes earnest resistance of the victim." Though most rape victims are women, some are men—victims of homosexual rape.

FACTS ABOUT RAPE

What causes rape? Contrary to popular belief, rape is:

- *not* usually caused by the rapist's "uncontrollable sex drive," but rather by a desire to feel powerful and to express hostile and aggressive impulses;
- *not* usually committed by men who are mentally ill;
- *not* always committed against young, attractive single women (older women and married women—in fact, all types of women—have similar statistical chances of being raped);
- *not* committed because the victim secretly "wants" to be raped.

Most rapes *are* acts of violence, perpetrated against a victim who is often quite arbitrarily selected. The only quality in the victim that may make her more vulnerable to rape *may* be culturally conditioned attitudes. Women are less accustomed to using physical force and running hard to escape danger. According to one report, "women who are attacked often believe their only choices are to be killed, seriously injured, or raped."

COPING WITH RAPE

Here are a few important points about ways to cope with rape:

If Someone Threatens to Rape You

1. Run away if humanly possible.
2. If you cannot run, some authorities recommend that you resist by screaming, shouting, arguing, and/or fighting back physically. (You may want to consider taking self-defense classes to learn effective ways of fighting or resisting physically.)
3. Vomiting or "acting crazy" may help: such tactics may surprise or disgust the attacker.
4. You may be able to stall by talking to the attacker long enough to think out your next move; you may eventually spot an opportunity to escape.

If You Are Raped

1. Despite what you may have heard about police skepticism, *you should report the attack*—even if it was an unsuccessful attempt. The information you provide may help safeguard other women. Give as much detail as you can. Describe the attacker's physical appearance, voice, clothes, car.
2. Call the police immediately; do not take a bath or change your clothes. Semen, hair, and other materials may be aids to identification.
3. Most important: Do not blame yourself for what happened. You haven't committed a crime—the man who raped you has. If there is a rape counseling center in your area, contact the center as soon as possible; or talk to a friend, guidance counselor, psychologist, or member of the clergy. It is essential that you get a chance to work through the emotional trauma of the experience with a supportive listener.

Source: Robert Crooks and Karla Baur, *Our Sexuality* (Menlo Park, Calif.: Benjamin/Cummings, 1980), pp. 256–263.

previous unhappy or unsatisfying sexual experiences or the product of current communication problems between partners. Most can be resolved if both partners get involved in the treatment.

Sex Therapy

During the 1970s sex researchers developed a number of ways to treat people with sexual problems. In Masters and Johnson's original program, couples traveled to their treatment center in St. Louis, stayed in a motel, and went through an intensive, highly structured two-week program with two therapists (one a man and the other a woman, and at least one of them a physician).

Since then, other therapists have devised more flexible and less expensive approaches. Some therapists have the couple visit a sex clinic once a week. In one case, a twenty-two-year-old woman and her husband were referred to a clinic because the woman greatly disliked sexual activity. A brief history revealed that the couple's first sexual encounter had been disastrous, with both partners anxious, inexperienced, and uncomfortable. The woman said her husband had tried to penetrate after only a few minutes of foreplay, leaving her unsatisfied and disappointed. After several such experiences, she said, she began to think of sex as "nauseating," even though she very much wanted to enjoy marital intercourse.[21]

In her case, as in others, treatment included seven basic principles:

1. Both partners are included in treatment, since the sexual dysfunction affects both people.
2. Therapy often includes education on sexual anatomy; people are often misinformed about sexual organs, sexual response, and how to arouse their partners.
3. Negative attitudes about sex are explored;

however deeply buried, they often emerge as part of the problem.
4. The role of anxiety in the dysfunction is also explored. Often, people are so worried about how well they are "performing" that they take on a spectator role while engaged in sex and don't let themselves spontaneously enjoy the experience.
5. Therapy also aims to reduce the anxiety by redefining sex as a pleasure instead of a test of skill.
6. Tensions in the couple's overall relationship are also explored, since they often contribute to a sexual problem.
7. Finally, sex therapists offer the couple ideas on how to change their sexual behavior.[22]

At the beginning, couples are often urged to forget about intercourse altogether for a while and to learn to enjoy simply caressing each other again. In the case of some dysfunctions, such as premature ejaculation and vaginismus, specific sexual exercises may be prescribed.

MAKING HEALTH DECISIONS

ASSESSMENT: What Are Your Attitudes About Sex?

Carefully read each of the statements below. Indicate your reaction to each statement by putting a check mark in the appropriate space.

	STRONGLY AGREE		CAN'T DECIDE		STRONGLY DISAGREE
1. Homosexuals should be put in a place where the rest of society does not have to put up with them.	___	___	___	___	___
2. Masturbation by a married person is a sign of a poor marriage.	___	___	___	___	___
3. Mouth-genital contact can provide more effective sexual stimulation than intercourse can.	___	___	___	___	___
4. Premarital intercourse between consenting adults is acceptable.	___	___	___	___	___
5. Only young, white, middle-class people live together without being married.	___	___	___	___	___
6. Sexual intercourse is a kind of communication.	___	___	___	___	___
7. Homosexuals should not be employed in occupations where they might serve as role models for children.	___	___	___	___	___

	STRONGLY AGREE		STRONGLY DISAGREE		CAN'T DECIDE
8. Masturbation is acceptable when the objective is simply to attain sensory enjoyment.	___	___	___	___	___
9. Mouth-genital contact should be regarded as an acceptable form of sexual play.	___	___	___	___	___
10. Sexual intercourse should take place only between married partners.	___	___	___	___	___
11. Masturbation is generally unhealthy.	___	___	___	___	___
12. Communication barriers are the key factors in sexual problems.	___	___	___	___	___
13. Homosexuality should be regarded as an illness.	___	___	___	___	___
14. Relieving tension by masturbating is a healthy practice.	___	___	___	___	___
15. Women should be as willing as men to participate in mouth-genital sex play.	___	___	___	___	___
16. Women should experience sexual intercourse prior to marriage.	___	___	___	___	___
17. Many couples live together because the partners have a strong sexual need for each other.	___	___	___	___	___
18. The basis of sexual communication is touching.	___	___	___	___	___
19. Homosexuality repels me.	___	___	___	___	___
20. Mouth-genital contact repels me.	___	___	___	___	___
21. Men should experience sexual intercourse prior to marriage.	___	___	___	___	___
22. Masturbation should be encouraged under certain conditions.	___	___	___	___	___
23. Homosexuality is all right between two consenting adults.	___	___	___	___	___

INTERPRETATION OF RESPONSES

Now that you have noted your reactions, look over the pattern of your responses in each of the following categories:

- Masturbation: Items 2, 8, 11, 14, and 22 refer to masturbation.
- Premarital intercourse: Items 4, 5, 10, 16, 17, and 21 refer to premarital intercourse and attitudes toward it in our society.
- Homosexuality: Items 1, 7, 13, 19, and 23 indicate your attitude toward homosexuals and homosexual behavior.
- Sexual communication: Items 6, 12, and 18 deal with communication patterns and sexual functioning.
- Oral-genital sex: Items 3, 9, 15, and 20 refer to attitudes toward oral sex.

1. According to your response patterns, toward which of the themes listed above do you have the strongest (positive or negative) attitudes?

_____

_____

_____

2. How did you develop your attitudes toward these themes and toward other aspects of sexuality? _____

_____

_____

_____

3. Do you think that you would be able to cope with sexual matters better if any of the attitudes you expressed here were to be changed? Which ones? _____

_____

_____

_____

4. Now think about your sexual *behaviors* as they reflect or contradict your sexual *attitudes*.
   a. Do you consciously make decisions about your sexual activities?_____

_____

_____

_____

b. Do your attitudes toward sex influence any of your decisions about sexual behaviors? Explain. _____

_____

_____

c. Are you ever inconsistent? Do you make decisions about sexual behavior that are contrary to your sexual attitudes? _____

_____

_____

Source: Adapted from R. F. Valois, *The Effects of a Human Sexuality Program on the Attitudes of University Residence Hall Students* (Master's thesis, University of Illinois at Urbana-Champaign, 1980), in S. G. Cox, K. Doyle, S. Kammerman, and R. F. Valois, *Wellness R.S.V.P.* (Menlo Park, Calif.: Benjamin/-Cummings, 1981).

SUMMARY

1. Americans' sexual attitudes towards sex, sex roles, and marriage have changed in the last several decades. Their sexual behavior has changed to a lesser degree. There is a new openness about sexual topics, although many people remain shy or ambivalent about sexual intimacy.

2. Humans reproduce when a sperm cell, deposited in a woman's vagina by a man's penis, fertilizes an egg cell that is floating through the woman's Fallopian tubes toward her uterus. If the egg implants in the lining of the uterus, a pregnancy has begun.

3. Erogenous zones are areas of the body that excite sexual desire or produce sexual arousal. Erogenous zones include many parts of the body besides the external sexual structures.

4. Female sexual anatomy includes the vagina, hymen, vulva (mons veneris, labia majora and labia minora, and clitoris), perineum, internal sex organs (uterus and cervix), and breasts. The vagina is a very elastic, muscular organ; it becomes lubricated during sexual arousal, which makes penetration and intercourse easier.

5. Male sexual anatomy includes the penis, scrotum, epididymis and vas deferens, prostate gland, seminal vesicles, Cowper's glands, and breasts. Neither the size of a man's penis nor circumcision significantly affects sexual functioning.

6. Although male and female bodies look different, their patterns of sexual arousal and response are very much alike. During arousal, the muscles tense and blood fills the genital organs. Largely from the observations of William Masters and Virginia Johnson, sex researchers know that arousal in both sexes takes place in four stages: excitement, plateau, orgasm, and resolution.

7. Women have only one kind of orgasm, not separate "vaginal" and "clitoral" kinds as was once widely believed. Few women object to sexual intercourse during menstruation.

8. Sexual response is more than a matter of physiology. How people feel about sex, how they behave sexually, and how they feel about themselves as human beings all influence their psychosexual response. People learn about sex and sexual attitudes from parents and, later, from friends, books and movies, advertisements, and even jokes.

9. Most people have sexual fantasies. They are usually harmless, even when their content seems bizarre or frightening. Only if they interfere with everyday activities should they be considered cause for worry.

10. Many people masturbate. Such exploration of one's body is harmless, although negative attitudes toward masturbation are still not uncommon.

11. Petting is an important form of sexual behavior for many people, either as a prelude to sexual intercourse or as an end in itself. For many teenagers, petting is the first experience of sexual activity and its associated emotional issues.

12. Many people regard sexual intercourse as the culmination of a sexual relationship. It usually takes time for people to learn how to make intercourse an intensely pleasurable experience. In general, males are more quickly and easily aroused than females. People's responses to intercourse vary with circumstances.

13. Attitudes toward oral sex vary widely in the United States. It is common among married couples.

14. Homosexual activity is fairly common among American adolescents. A later, predominantly or exclusively homosexual preference is less common in the population. Homosexuals are not necessarily emotionally unstable, and they tend to have more satisfying sexual experiences than heterosexuals.

15. Any problem that prevents a person from having sexual relations or from reaching orgasm is called a sexual dysfunction. Some forms of sexual dysfunction are emotional in origin, and others are physical. Most cases of sexual dysfunction involve both partners and require the cooperation of both for their solution. Males may be troubled by premature ejaculation or by primary or secondary impotence. Females may suffer from vaginismus or from primary or secondary orgasmic dysfunction. Various forms of therapy are available for these dysfunctions.

GLOSSARY

cervix   The narrow lower end of the uterus, at the upper end of the vagina.

circumcision   Surgical removal of the foreskin.

clitoris   Extremely sensitive external female sexual organ located under a hood formed by the upper joining of the labia minora.

coronal ridge   The rim of tissue between the glans and the shaft of the penis.

Cowper's glands   Two pea-sized organs that sometimes produce a few drops of fluid at the end of the penis during sexual arousal.

ejaculation   Contractions of the urethra, penis, and prostate gland that usually accompany orgasm in the male, forcing semen out of the tip of the penis.

ejaculatory ducts   Two structures formed by the ends of the seminal vesicles and of the vas deferens that, in turn, join the urethra.

epididymis   Highly coiled network of tubing in the back of each testicle through which sperm cells travel as they mature.

erogenous   Exciting sexual desire or producing sexual arousal.

fertilized ovum (fertilized egg)   A cell formed by the union of a sperm cell and an ovum, from which a new human being eventually develops.

foreskin   The flap of tissue at the head of the penis.

frenulum   The triangular region on the underside of the penis.

glans   The head of the penis.

heterosexuality   Sexual or emotional preference for persons of the opposite sex.

homosexuality   A sexual or emotional preference for persons of one's own sex.

hymen   Circular membrane that narrows the opening of the vagina in some females who have never had sexual intercourse.

impotence   Sexual dysfunction in which a man is unable to achieve or maintain an erection long enough to reach orgasm with a partner. See **primary impotence, secondary impotence.**

labia   Two soft, sensitive folds of skin at either side of the opening of the vagina. The outer, broad folds are called the *labia majora;* the inner, hairless lips are called the *labia minora.*

mons veneris   A sensitive cushion of fatty tissue

covered with skin and hair, located in the female vulva over the pubic bone.

myotonia   Generalized sexual response in which muscles throughout the body increase tension.

nonemissive erection   Sexual dysfunction in which a man is able to achieve an erection but not to ejaculate.

orgasm   The climactic stage of sexual response.

ovum   Female reproductive cell.

penis   The external male organ of sexual intercourse and urination.

perineum   Hairless area of skin at the lower end of the labia, near the anus.

premature ejaculation   The expulsion of semen before or immediately after insertion of the penis into the vagina.

primary impotence   Sexual dysfunction in which a man has never been able to achieve an erection.

primary orgasmic dysfunction   Sexual dysfunction in which a woman has never experienced an orgasm by any method.

prostate gland   Male organ located just below the urethra that produces about 30 percent of the seminal fluid.

refractory period   A temporary state following orgasm during which most males cannot respond to renewed sexual stimulation.

scrotum   The loose pouch of skin that hangs behind and under the penis and contains the testicles.

secondary impotence   Sexual dysfunction in which a man who has previously been able to achieve an erection is now unable to do so in some or all sexual encounters.

secondary (situational) orgasmic dysfunction   Sexual dysfunction in which a woman frequently has difficulty achieving an orgasm.

semen (seminal fluid)   Sperm-carrying liquid expelled from the penis during ejaculation.

seminal vesicles   Two small structures located at the base of the bladder that produce about 70 percent of the seminal fluid.

sex   (1) gender (maleness or femaleness); (2) physical expression of affectionate or erotic feelings. Compare **sexuality.**

sexual dysfunction   Any problem that prevents a person from engaging in sexual relations or from reaching orgasm.

sexuality   Masculinity or femininity; the way in which one's gender is integrated into one's personality. Compare **sex.**

sperm   Male reproductive cell.

spermatic cords   Muscular structures from which the testicles are suspended within the scrotum.

testicles (testes)   Male organs that produce sperm.

urethra   The tube from the urinary bladder through which urine is passed out of the body; in males, the urethra is also the canal through which semen is discharged.

uterus   The womb; a hollow, muscular internal female sex organ that contributes to sexual response and that shelters and nourishes the fetus during pregnancy.

vagina   The canal-like structure of the female body that extends from the bottom of the uterus to the vulva; it receives the penis during sexual intercourse and acts as a passageway for a baby during birth.

vaginismus   Sexual dysfunction involving involuntary muscle spasms that cause the vagina to shut so tightly that penetration by a penis is impossible or painful.

vas deferens   Long tubes that carry sperm from the epididymis to the seminal vesicles.

vasocongestion   Increased blood flow, as to genital organs during sexual arousal.

vulva   The external genital region surrounding the opening of the vagina.

NOTES

1. Morton Hunt, *Sexual Behavior in the 1970s* (New York: Dell, 1975).

2. Ibid.

3. William H. Masters and Virginia E. Johnson, *Human Sexual Response* (Boston: Little, Brown, 1966), p. 191.

4. Ibid., p. 190.

5. Ibid., p. 21.

6. Ibid., p. 6.

7. Ibid., p. 45.

8. Ibid., pp. 58–60.

9. Ibid., p. 125.

10. Ruth Bell, *Changing Bodies, Changing Lives* (New York: Random House, 1980), p. 80.

11. Masters and Johnson, *Human Sexual Response,* pp. 4–8.

12. W. H. Masters, V. E. Johnson, and R. C. Kolodny, *Human Sexuality* (Boston: Little, Brown, 1982), p. 302.

13. Clellan S. Ford and Frank A. Beach, *Patterns of Sexual Behavior* (New York: Harper & Row, 1951).

14. Irving Bieber, *Homosexuality: A Psychoanalytic Study* (New York: Basic Books, 1962).

15. C. A. Tripp, *The Homosexual Matrix* (New York: New American Library, 1976).

16. A. C. Kinsey, W. B. Pomeroy, and C. E. Martin, *Sexual Behavior in the Human Male* (Philadelphia: Saunders, 1948), and A. C. Kinsey, W. B. Pomeroy, C. E. Martin, and P. H. Gebhard, *Sexual Behavior in the Human Female* (Philadelphia: Saunders, 1953).

17. R. Athanasiou, P. Shaver, and C. Tavris, "Sex," *Psychology Today,* January 1970, pp. 37–52.

18. A. P. Bell and M. S. Weinberg, *Homosexualities: A Study of Diversity Among Men and Women* (New York: Simon & Schuster, 1978).

19. William H. Masters and Virginia E. Johnson, *Homosexuality in Perspective* (Boston: Little, Brown, 1979).

20. C. D. Tollison and H. E. Adams, *Sexual Disorders: Treatment, Theory, Research* (New York: Gardner Press, 1979).

21. Ibid.

22. Ibid.

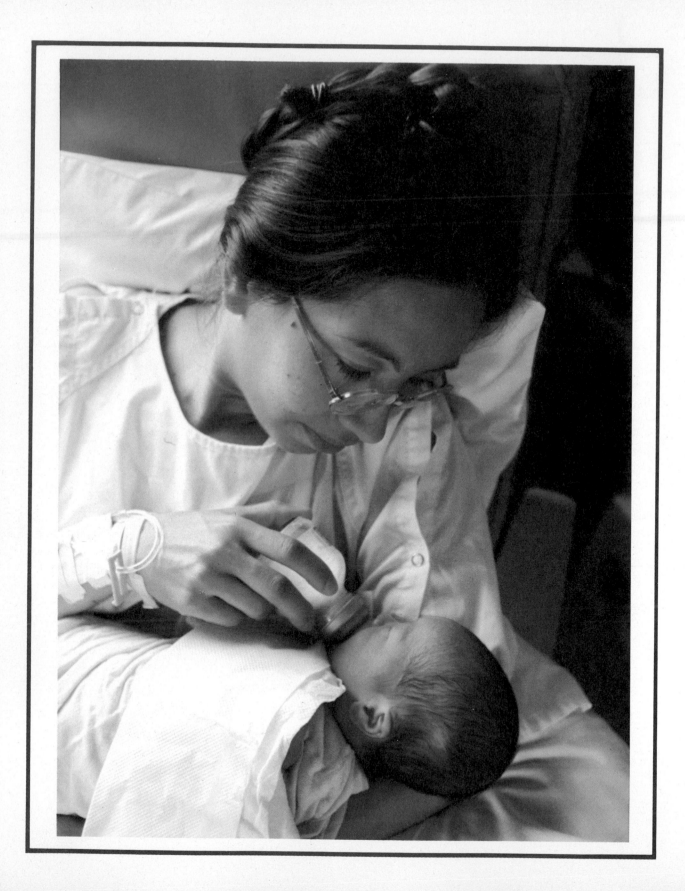

CHAPTER 8

Reproduction and Birth Control

As we noted in Chapter 7, people have long misunderstood how the male and female reproductive systems work. Centuries of inhibitions about the "private parts" of the human body have allowed myths and misconceptions to flourish. People are often reluctant to talk about the menstrual cycle, for example; they're not sure about the best ways to keep the male and female genitals clean; and even today, many people—particularly adolescents—have unwanted pregnancies just because they're ignorant of the biological facts of life. Yet we all can be comfortable with our own bodies, including our reproductive systems, if we learn a few basic facts about them.

In the last chapter we looked at male and female sexual anatomy from the point of view of sexuality, especially in regard to the social, emotional, and psychological issues that surround our sexual lives. In this chapter we will take a somewhat more practical view. We will be concerned with how human sexual anatomy works in reproduction—with what is involved in our truly awesome ability to create a new human life. Since the essential reproductive event takes place within the woman's body, it is with the female reproductive system that we will begin.

THE FEMALE REPRODUCTIVE SYSTEM

The female reproductive system has three basic functions. The woman's body produces egg cells, or *ova* (singular: *ovum*); it positions them where they can meet incoming sperm from the male; and it provides a hospitable environment where an egg, if fertilized, can develop into a fetus. All these functions are carried out in a woman's body in an efficient way. The organs that take part in this process are the ovaries, the Fallopian tubes, and the uterus.

The Ovaries

If you are a woman and plan to use birth control, or if you want to conceive a baby, it's particularly important for you to know about the ovaries and what they do. The **ovaries** are two small ovum-producing organs, each about the size and shape of an almond, that lie low in the woman's abdomen. Each ovary is positioned close to the end of a Fallopian tube, which, as we shall see, is the route the ovum takes when it leaves the ovary. Every normal woman is born with hundreds of thousands of unripened ova already present in her ovaries.

OVULATION

After the woman reaches puberty, ova ripen periodically and leave the ovaries in a process known as **ovulation.** It's important to know *when* ovulation occurs, since unless you ovulate in a given month, you simply are not fertile that month. In theory, ovulation takes place at about the midpoint of a woman's menstrual cycle—somewhere around thirteen to fifteen days before the first day

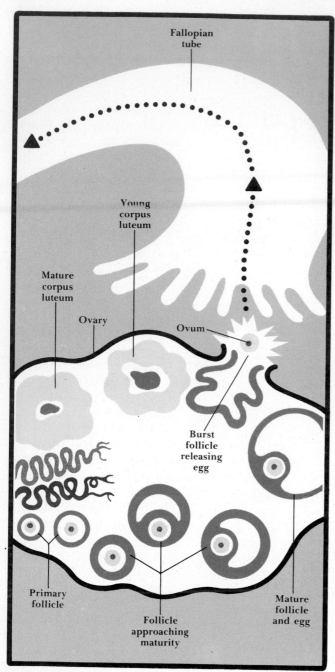

Figure 8.1   The process of ovulation. Every woman is born with anywhere from 200,000 to 500,000 unripened ova, or eggs, in her ovaries—her lifetime supply. Typically, about once a month in women of menstruating age, hormones induce one ovum to ripen inside what is known as a Graafian follicle. The ripe ovum bursts out of the ovary and is swept into the Fallopian tube, down which it travels to the uterus. (Edward Allgor)

of menstrual flow. But in prolonged cycles, ovulation occurs later than the midpoint. In short cycles, ovulation can occur earlier, even during menstruation—an important thing to know if you want to practice effective birth control.

You can't always tell when you are ovulating. Some women feel they can, however: Their pelvis feels heavy, or they feel a mild ache on one side of their abdomen or the other for a few hours or a few days.

OVARIAN HORMONES

Besides producing ova, the ovaries secrete a number of natural chemicals called *ovarian hormones*, which regulate the menstrual cycle. One of these hormones is **estrogen,** which helps a girl's body develop secondary sex characteristics (body hair, enlarged breasts, waist and hips) during puberty. Production of this hormone declines sometime during the woman's middle-age years, resulting in the process known as menopause: Her menstrual periods will gradually cease. The other hormone the ovaries secrete is **progesterone,** which stimulates the uterus each month to get ready to receive a fertilized ovum if one is present.

The Fallopian Tubes

The **Fallopian tubes,** or **oviducts,** are tiny, muscular tunnels that connect the ovaries and the uterus. But they are not just passageways for the ovum; they are actually the meeting place for the ovum and the sperm, and thus the spot where fertilization takes place. When a mature ovum has entered the Fallopian tube on either side, it begins to move slowly down the tube toward the uterus. If sperm are present in the tube, one of these sperm may penetrate the ovum, resulting in fertilization. If this happens, the fertilized ovum, an ever-multiplying mass of cells, continues to move down the tube into the uterus, where it will implant itself in the lining of the uterus. Implantation means that pregnancy has begun. In the uterus the fertilized ovum develops into an **embryo,** then a **fetus** (at eight weeks), and ultimately (after about nine months) a fully developed baby ready to be born.

The Uterus

The uterus, or womb, is quite an amazing organ. Pear-shaped in appearance, and resting on its small end (the *cervix*) in the center of a woman's pelvis, it houses and protects a fetus from implantation until birth. As the fetus grows during pregnancy, the uterus expands tremendously—from the size of a fist into a huge, muscular bag filling the woman's entire abdomen. That bag can hold not only a full-term baby, but a quart of fluid and a one-pound placenta besides!

THE MENSTRUAL CYCLE

Every month, if the woman is not already pregnant, the inner lining of the uterus (the **endometrium**) goes through a process of renewal and preparation known as the **menstrual cycle.** Basically, the menstrual cycle is the way the woman's uterus prepares to receive and nourish a fertilized ovum. The inner lining of the uterus thickens and grows, and the structure of its blood vessels changes. If an ovum does become fertilized that month and implants in the uterine lining, the uterus keeps its lining to nourish the growing fetus. But if pregnancy does not occur, the uterus sloughs off its entire inner lining. The blood and tissue pass through the cervix and the vagina in a discharge known as **menstruation**—a term that comes from the Latin word *mensis,* meaning "month." A woman's menstrual flow generally lasts from three to six days, and the typical menstrual cycle lasts twenty-seven to thirty days.

THE PHYSICAL EFFECTS OF THE MENSTRUAL CYCLE

Many women experience some physical effects related to bodily changes immediately preceding or during their menstrual periods. They may feel bloated, their breasts may be tender, or they may have backaches, leg pains, or changes in energy level. A few women have abdominal pains, or "cramps," that are severe enough to keep them in bed—or at least on a restricted schedule—for a day or so. Other women experience no physical discomfort during menstruation. In any case, these effects are the result of a normal physiological process: A menstruating woman is not "sick."

THE PSYCHOLOGICAL EFFECTS OF THE MENSTRUAL CYCLE

Some women find that their emotions are not affected by their menstrual cycles. Other women experience mood changes at some point in their menstrual cycle, typically just before their menstrual flow begins. This is not surprising, since the menstrual flow is brought on by the ebb and flow of hormones in the body, and hormones act on the whole body—including the brain.

The facts about the psychological effects of menstruation are still being established. Researchers have identified a condition known as **premenstrual syndrome** (PMS), which *some*—though not all or even most—women experience, and which can cause its victims great distress. PMS can involve one or more physiological symptoms (breast and abdominal swelling, food cravings, headaches, and acne) as well as irritability, lethargy, and depression. An English physician, Katharina Dalton, has even asserted that these symptoms can be so extreme as to make some women prone to violent behavior. Although other clinicians have disputed Dalton's accounts of patients driven to violence by PMS, most doctors and researchers seem to agree that such a syndrome does exist *in some women.* The syndrome is currently thought to be the result of a lack of the hormone progesterone, and some patients have been successfully treated for PMS with doses of progesterone.[1]

Further research will probably help clarify our picture of the psychological changes that can accompany the menstrual cycle. It is interesting to note that some women may actually perform *better* in their premenstrual days: One study, for example, found that typists were more accurate then.[2] Other research has found that women's senses of taste and smell, their identification of musical pitches, and the strength and steadiness of their hands vary slightly over the menstrual cycle.[3]

However, since so many periodic and situational factors affect our day-to-day moods, it is surely a mistake to focus exclusively on the role of women's hormones in producing emotional variability. For example, our mood and work performance may be low because we have a cold or a hangover, because we've slept poorly, because we don't like the hot (or cold) weather, because we

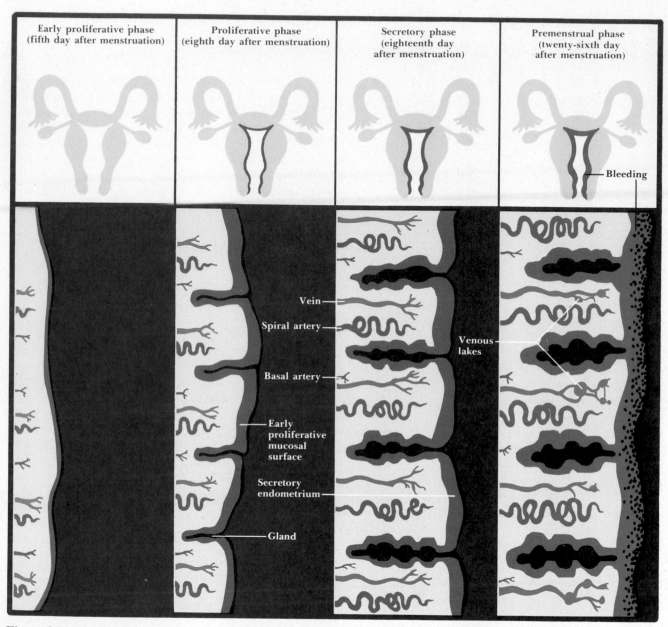

Figure 8.2   Changes in the uterine wall during one monthly menstrual cycle. On the fifth day after menstruation (early proliferative phase), the denuded surface is fed by short basal arteries. During the proliferative phase, estrogen causes glands and arteries to proliferate, and the uterine wall thickens. After ovulation, during the secretory phase, the lining swells as arteries corkscrew to the surface and the glands begin to secrete mucus. At the premenstrual phase (if fertilization has not occurred), the spiral arteries constrict, causing the surface layers to disrupt in preparation for the sloughing off of the menstrual blood.   (Edward Allgor)

have a family or financial problem, or simply because it's Monday. Those are factors that can affect either sex.

WHAT YOU CAN DO TO COPE WITH MENSTRUAL PROBLEMS

Menstrual problems are common. It has been estimated that as many as 50 percent of all women have them at some time in their lives. Among the common problems are painful menstruation, excessive bleeding, premenstrual syndrome (PMS), and *amenorrhea* (cessation of periods). Menstrual problems can be dealt with in a variety of ways.

First of all, don't let anyone try to convince you that your discomfort doesn't exist. (Menstrual problems were once thought to be primarily psychological, and women were often given tranquilizers or told to go home and relax.) *You* are the best judge of how you feel.

1. You may be able to cope with your problem by yourself, if it is mild.
   ▶ Keep a chart of your menstrual cycle, and plan a light schedule of activities for days that you're likely to have discomfort.
   ▶ For minor pain, take aspirin, use a heating pad, or try mild exercise.
   ▶ If you tend to feel bloated around the time of menstruation, eat less salt during your period and for a week before.
   ▶ If you have headaches or feel irritable, try eating frequent small meals, which will help keep your blood sugar at a stable level.

2. *See your doctor* if you have any of the following signs:
   ▶ An unusually heavy menstrual flow, or a heavy flow that lasts more than four or five days.
   ▶ Severe cramps or pain that lasts more than three days each month.
   ▶ Sudden irregularity of periods that cannot be explained by sickness, travel, weight gain or loss (see below).
   ▶ Bleeding in the middle of your cycle or at any time of your cycle other than your period.
   ▶ Severe cramps at times other than when your period is due.
   ▶ Lasting amenorrhea.

Recently it has been discovered that women with severe menstrual pain often have an excess of hormonelike substances known as *prostaglandins* in their bodies when they menstruate, and drugs are available to reduce prostaglandin levels.[4] Other medication may be appropriate for your particular problem.

TAMPONS AND MENSTRUAL HYGIENE

Many women choose to use tampons rather than sanitary napkins during their menstrual periods for reasons of comfort and convenience. Despite the popular misconception about this, most women—even young women—can use tampons safely. Although a young woman's vagina may be partly blocked by the hymen, it generally has an opening large enough for the menstrual flow to escape—and for a small tampon to be inserted.

One key point, though: It is a good idea for a woman to use tampons of varying size, depending on her anatomy and the heaviness of her menstrual flow. It is *not* wise to use superabsorbent tampons except on days of heaviest flow: If used on light days, they may absorb the vagina's natural moisture and cause irritation.[5] Women should not use tampons continuously; sanitary napkins should be used at night. In addition, use of superabsorbent tampons has been associated with toxic shock syndrome, a potentially life-threatening disease.[6] (We discuss toxic shock syndrome in Chapter 10.)

If you are using tampons and develop a high fever, nausea, diarrhea, dizziness, or a skin rash, you *may* have toxic shock syndrome. You should remove your tampon immediately and seek care from a physician or hospital emergency room as soon as possible.

Problems and Diseases of the Female Reproductive System

IRREGULAR PERIODS

Many women have cycles that vary considerably in length; this is normal. When does irregularity become abnormal, then? Menstruation that's so irregular that it seems not to be a cycle at all is considered abnormal, as is bleeding that occurs at intervals of less than eighteen or more than forty-two days.[7] Either of these patterns may mean that the woman's system is not functioning correctly.

If a woman's ovarian hormones become deficient or out of balance in relation to one another, a disturbance in her pattern of menstruation often follows. Her menstruation may be either too scant or too excessive, or it may stop altogether for a few months. Often, the hormone disturbance can be corrected with artificial hormone preparations, or at least an artificial balance can be achieved until the natural balance returns.

PROBLEMS WITH THE FALLOPIAN TUBES

The Fallopian tubes can become diseased or inflamed with a severity that's out of proportion to their small size. Inflammation in the tubes *(salpingitis)* may leave scars and constrictions that prevent egg cells from passing through, making it hard for the woman to become pregnant. Occasionally the tubes are only partially blocked, and the tiny sperm cells can wriggle past the constriction, but then the much larger egg cell cannot get down to the uterus. In this case, a pregnancy in the tube may result. This condition, an **ectopic pregnancy,** is relatively rare but always serious, for it is very difficult to detect. Eventually, the tube ruptures, and immediate surgery is necessary to stop internal hemorrhage.

FEMALE HYGIENE: BASICS WOMEN SHOULD KNOW

The vagina of a healthy woman secretes sufficient fluid to keep it moist. Cells are constantly being shed from the lining of the vagina, and these cells, mixed with fluid, produce a nonirritating secretion. This secretion is unremarkable unless it is allowed to collect in the folds of the skin surrounding the vaginal opening. Careful daily bathing of this area will prevent unpleasant odor from developing, since odor usually comes from the labia and outer folds rather than from the vagina itself. Soap and water are perfectly adequate for cleaning. To prevent irritation, however, you should use a minimum of soap and wash it away with plenty of clean water.[8]

When the normal vaginal secretion becomes excessive enough to stain clothing, or if it is yellow, irritating, watery, bloody, or bad-smelling, then it is called a vaginal discharge, or *leukorrhea.* This type of discharge may mean infection in some part of the genital tract. It is a warning signal that should send you to a physician for examination without delay. One way to prevent such infections is to avoid contaminating the genital area with bacteria from the anus. Toilet paper, for example, can spread germs unless it is used properly (wiping should always be done from front to back). Many women also find that wearing cotton underpants helps: a fabric that breathes, like cotton, allows

moisture to evaporate, making it more difficult for germs to breed.

Douching seems to be a popular practice among many American women, but it is not necessary for good health. The normal vaginal environment is acid, which keeps it free from undesirable bacteria. Douching does no particular harm, provided a mild acid solution such as vinegar and water is used; but it's not a good idea to use alkaline or commercial chemical douches, because they may neutralize the vagina's protective acids, allowing harmful bacteria to multiply.[9]

THE MALE REPRODUCTIVE SYSTEM

Unlike women, who are born with a full set of ova already in their ovaries, men are not born with *sperm,* or *spermatozoa* (the male cells that must travel up the woman's Fallopian tubes in order to fertilize an ovum). Instead, their bodies produce new mature sperm cells every day—at the rate of about 200 million daily in the normal man! This process of continual sperm production, called **spermatogenesis,** begins when a boy reaches puberty and can continue well into old age.

To accomplish their journey inside a woman's body to an ovum, the sperm cells need a fluid in which to travel. As we saw in Chapter 7, this fluid is known as the *seminal fluid,* or *semen.* It is produced in the prostate gland and the seminal vesicles. The sperm themselves are stored in another organ, the epididymis.

When the man is about to ejaculate, the sperm travel through a tube called the *vas deferens,* combining with the seminal fluid in the ejaculatory ducts. When the man ejaculates, a huge number of sperm—several hundred million—are discharged through the urethra and out of the penis. If a couple is having sexual intercourse, the semen is deposited in the woman's vagina. Only a small percentage of the sperm, however, can survive within the woman's body and actually find their way up through the cervix and the uterus and into the Fallopian tubes. Even then, fertilization may not take place; it may happen that none of the sperm succeeds in penetrating the egg.

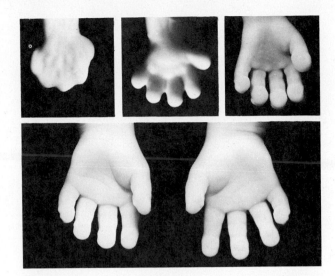

Development of the hands in the embryonic stage of pregnancy. In the fifth week, hands are a "molding plate" with finger ridges. In the sixth week, finger buds have formed. In the seventh and eighth weeks, the fingers, thumbs, and fingerprints form; note the prominent touch pads. In the third month, the pads regress, and the hands are well formed.

(Carnegie Institution of Washington, Department of Embryology)

MALE HYGIENE

One of the principal advantages of circumcision is that it makes it easier to clean the penis. Historically, it is thought that this was the major reason for circumcision. As it turns out, however, uncircumcised males can easily clean the glans of the penis by gently turning back the foreskin and washing with soap and water, being careful to rinse thoroughly. Should fluid accumulate under the foreskin, odor may develop. This can be remedied by careful cleaning.

PREGNANCY AND PRENATAL DEVELOPMENT

A pregnancy officially begins when a fertilized egg implants itself in a woman's uterine lining. Soon thereafter, the woman's entire body undergoes general changes that can be detected by pregnancy tests (see below). Meanwhile, spectacular changes are occurring in the uterine lining itself: Certain special cells from the uterus, plus some from the now-forming embryo, begin to develop into a structure known as the **placenta**—a mass of tissue, attached to the uterine lining, that for the next nine months will absorb lifegiving nutrients from the mother's bloodstream and transfer them to the bloodstream of the developing baby, and will carry away fetal wastes.

The events during the rest of the pregnancy constitute one of the truly amazing phenomena of life. What starts out as a single cell, a speck barely visible to the human eye, grows in a very short time into a complete and individual human being, equipped with miniature versions of all the necessary internal organs and external equipment.

The Stages of Development

As an embryo, the organism is less than an inch long and looks something like a curved fish. After two months, at which point it is called a fetus, it has developed arms and legs with perfectly shaped fingers and toes. By the end of the third month, although it is only about three inches long and weighs a mere ounce, the fetus can kick its legs, close its fingers, turn its head, and open and close its mouth. Also, by this time most of its internal organs are able to function, so that the remainder of the **prenatal** period (the period before birth) can be spent in the process of growth and in putting on the finishing touches. Throughout its prenatal life, the developing baby is attached to the placenta via the **umbilical cord** and is enclosed in a fluid-filled sac (the **amnion**, or **amniotic sac**), which primarily provides protection.

At birth, the average full-term infant weighs anywhere from five to twelve pounds and may be from seventeen to twenty-two inches long. The average length of pregnancy is 280 days, but babies born as early as 180 days or as late as 334 days after conception may be able to survive.[10]

Pregnancy: Diagnosis and Testing

Usually, the first sign of pregnancy in a woman is that an expected menstrual period does not occur. The woman may have a feeling that menstruation is about to begin but "can't get started." This is not a positive sign that she is pregnant, since it is not unusual for many women's periods to be delayed fourteen to twenty-one days, particularly in women who are normally somewhat irregular or who are under stress. The woman may also notice that her breasts are congested and tender, or that she's more irritable or has a tender or heavy feeling in her pelvis; sometimes she may be a little nauseated.

About three weeks after the missed period, a physician can usually, by pelvic examination, be fairly certain of the existence of a pregnancy. The woman's pelvic tissue will be slightly softened, the vaginal opening will be slightly purplish, and the uterus will have begun to enlarge.

Diagnostic tests may also be used to confirm the pregnancy. A pregnant woman's system produces a hormone known as *HCG (human chorionic gonadotropin);* tests of the woman's blood or urine can show whether this hormone is present. Blood testing is available in most cities at low cost; it often requires no more than a brief visit to a clinic to leave a blood sample and a follow-up phone call for the results. Referrals for this service are available through local chapters of the Planned Parenthood Federation of America, local health departments, and county medical societies. There are two commonly used urine-type pregnancy tests. One takes 2 1/2 minutes to show results and is done forty-two days after the first day of the last menstrual cycle. The other test takes one hour to show results and can be performed right after the missed period.

A woman may also want to use one of the do-it-yourself pregnancy testing kits that have been on the market for several years. Most of these are based on the same principles as physicians' urine tests—they are designed to detect HCG if it is present in the woman's body. If they are not used very carefully, however, these tests may produce inaccurate results.

Prenatal Health

Pregnancy, like menstruation, is not a disease! Under ordinary circumstances, the pregnant woman can do almost all the things she did before she became pregnant, including working, exercising, participating in recreational activities, and having sexual intercourse. She should, however,

take extra care of her health. For nine months, a baby will be depending on her for all its body-building materials. Ideally, she should be in excellent health *before* she starts the pregnancy, including being immunized against rubella (German measles), which can cause birth defects if the mother contracts it early in pregnancy.

It is to the woman's (and her baby's) advantage if she is well nourished, getting regular exercise, and of fairly normal weight before she begins to nourish a developing fetus. A woman in pregnancy should think of herself as an athlete in training, building up her body to the highest level of physical fitness, so that the childbirth that lies ahead will be more of a joy than an ordeal.

Prenatal Care

Prenatal care, or medical supervision of the pregnancy, requires visits to the doctor at regular intervals to guard against complications such as diabetes and *toxemia* (a potentially fatal condition involving high blood pressure) and to ensure that the baby's requirements are being met.

BLOOD EXAMINATIONS

Sometime during early pregnancy, the woman should have a series of blood tests. These tests include hemoglobin and red-cell counts to detect anemia; a white-cell count to reveal or rule out infection or other disorders; and a blood test for syphilis, required by law. In addition, an Rh test is always done to assess the risk of Rh hemolytic disease *(erythroblastosis fetalis)*, a genetically determined blood disorder. In most cases, both mother and father have a substance known as **Rh factor** in their red blood cells; if the mother lacks this substance and the baby inherits the factor from the father, the mother's blood could react against her baby's. The first pregnancy is usually not affected, but subsequent babies are at risk. (See Figure 8.3.) Today, all mothers with Rh disease can be immunized against this problem.

GENETIC COUNSELING

Genetic diseases, of which there are more than 2,000, affect 3 to 5 percent of all babies born in the United States.[11] Sickle-cell anemia, phenyl-

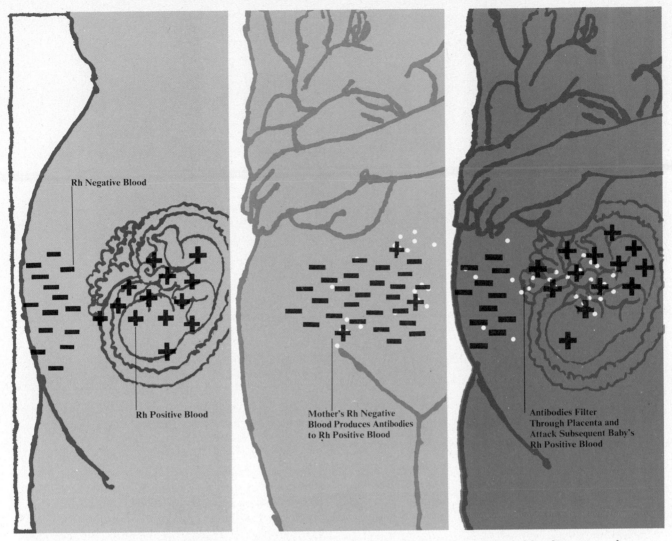

Figure 8.3   The Rh factor. The Rh-positive blood of the baby may get into the mother's bloodstream at the time of birth. Her body reacts by creating antibodies that may attack any subsequent Rh-positive children, destroying their red blood cells. (Tom Lewis)

ketonuria (PKU), Tay-Sachs disease, hemophilia, a type of muscular dystrophy, cystic fibrosis, Down's syndrome, and two forms of diabetes are among the conditions that may be avoided through genetic counseling.

Parents naturally want to have healthy children, and most would prefer to know in advance if they are likely to pass on a serious disease to a child. For this reason, genetic counseling can be most valuable to a couple *before* they make the decision to have a child at all. People who are carriers of Tay-Sachs disease, for example, which condemns a child to an early death, may decide not to risk having children at all, lest the children be afflicted with the disease.

A genetic counselor can explain to the prospective parents how a particular disorder is transmitted from generation to generation, what the odds are that the disease will recur in their family, and what the disease itself is like. If the risk of passing on a disease is slight, or if an effective treatment is available, parents may decide to go ahead with a pregnancy, despite the risks. Otherwise, adoption may be an alternative.

Some genetic disorders, unfortunately, cannot be identified before pregnancy. But many can be

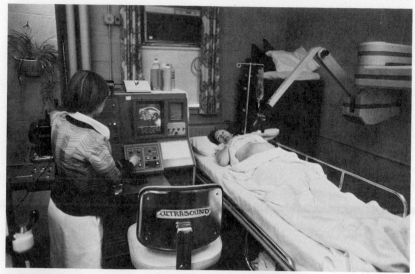

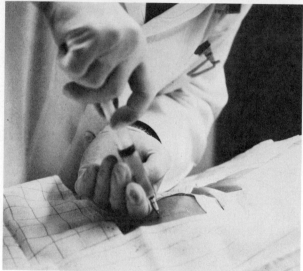

A sonogram, or "ultrasound" *(top)*, is a procedure in which sound waves from the fetus are electronically transformed into an image on a screen as a way of checking the baby's development and position within the womb. In amniocentesis *(bottom)* some amniotic fluid containing fetal cells is drawn from the uterus to be analyzed for the presence of certain genetic disorders in the baby. This procedure is not painful, and, because a sonogram is taken beforehand to determine the fetus's position, the risk of injury is slight for both the baby and the mother. (© James Holland/Stock, Boston; © William Hubbell 1980/Woodfin Camp & Assoc.)

identified while the fetus is still in the mother's uterus. It is now possible to test a developing fetus directly for about one hundred genetic disorders as early as the fourth month of pregnancy. In a procedure called **amniocentesis,** a doctor can withdraw some of the amniotic fluid that surrounds a fetus in the womb. Laboratory tests of the sloughed fetal cells contained in this fluid can then determine whether the fetus has one of these diseases.

Such tests are usually performed only if there is some reason to suspect that the unborn child may have a particular disease—that is, if the parents have already had one defective child or are known to be carriers of the disease. In the case of a few of these diseases, treatments can begin before birth. Otherwise, the prospective parents have the option of considering a therapeutic abortion to prevent the birth of the defective baby.

WHICH COUPLES SHOULD CONSIDER GENETIC COUNSELING AND AMNIOCENTESIS?

If a woman is over thirty-five, or if there is a history of hereditary disease in her or her husband's family, the couple may want to get genetic counseling, ideally before or shortly after a pregnancy begins.

Doctors generally recommend that any pregnant woman over the age of thirty-five—whether or not she has any other reason to suspect the presence of a genetic disease in her family—consider amniocentesis and possible therapeutic abortion if the tests are positive for Down's syndrome or other major genetic disease.

Maternal Behavior and Fetal Health

It has been estimated that fully 20 percent of all birth defects are caused by environmental factors.[12] And that means the mother-to-be must exercise great caution. Since she largely controls the fetus's environment, she is the one who must protect the developing infant from as many environmental hazards as she can.

INFECTIOUS DISEASE AND RADIATION

One such hazard, as we've already mentioned, is rubella. A woman who comes down with this illness early in pregnancy—even if she gets a mild case—may have a multiply handicapped baby. Other diseases, particularly sexually transmitted diseases, may also pose hazards to the developing fetus. Exposure to radiation, as in X-rays, can be dangerous too.

It's best for women to be immunized against rubella at least three months before becoming pregnant. At the least, pregnant women should avoid coming into contact with anyone who is known to have German measles. A pregnant woman should not be X-rayed unless it is absolutely necessary.

ALCOHOL, TOBACCO, CAFFEINE, AND DRUGS

The most common threats to fetal health come from substances the mother may ingest: alcohol, tobacco, caffeine, and drugs.

ALCOHOL A woman who drinks alcohol during pregnancy is in effect giving her baby a drink, too: alcohol will cross the placenta and act on the fetus's body as it does on the mother's. In the 1970s the term *fetal alcohol syndrome* (FAS) was coined in recognition of the fact that babies born to heavy-drinking mothers are often born with a predictable set of abnormalities.[13] (We discussed FAS in more detail in Chapter 5.)

Pregnant women, the Surgeon General has stated, should drink *no* alcoholic beverages because there is no known level of alcohol intake that is safe for the unborn baby.

TOBACCO Tobacco, like alcohol, is known to affect fetal development. Women who smoke have a higher than normal rate of miscarriage and stillbirth. And when their babies survive, the babies are smaller than average and are more likely to be irritable and hyperactive. Smoking has also been associated with a higher risk of cleft palate, crossed eyes, and hernias in the newborn.[14] (We discussed these problems in more detail in Chapter 6.)

Pregnant women should not smoke.

CAFFEINE Caffeine, which is present in coffee, tea, chocolate, and cola drinks, is another potential hazard to the fetus. A high caffeine intake has been associated with increased risk of miscarriage and birth defects.[15]

Pregnant women should not smoke.

The pregnant woman should think seriously about reducing or eliminating her intake of caffeine.

DRUGS In recent years doctors have become increasingly aware of the potential hazards to the fetus posed by drugs—prescription drugs and over-the-counter medications as well as illegal drugs.

Since most prescription drugs have not been proved safe for pregnant women (and several are known to cause birth defects), most physicians avoid prescribing any new medication for the pregnant patient.[16]

Not everyone realizes that over-the-counter drugs, which are often taken by pregnant women, are also risky. According to current medical knowledge, aspirin is dangerous to the baby and may pose risks to the mother, particularly if she takes it near the time of labor and delivery. (Aspirin is known to decrease the blood's clotting ability, and it may cause either mother or baby to bleed excessively.)[17]

The best course is to take *no* medication during pregnancy.

Diethylstilbestrol (DES), a synthetic hormone once given to pregnant women to help prevent miscarriage, has been linked with abnormalities (especially cancer) of the reproductive organs in children of mothers who have taken it.

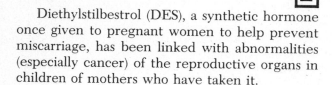

DES was given to mothers between 1945 and 1970, most frequently in the years between 1945 and 1955; children of such women should be aware that they are at increased risk of developing specific types of reproductive-tract cancers. If your mother took DES, be sure to tell your doctor.[18]

Spontaneous Abortion

In 10 to 20 percent of pregnancies—and perhaps even more—the woman has a **spontaneous abortion** (commonly called a "miscarriage").[19] The spontaneous abortion happens either because the developing organism was not implanted correctly or because the egg or sperm was defective to begin with. The woman's body simply gets rid of something that has no ability to survive. The woman starts to have vaginal bleeding and cramps, which continue until the uterus expels the defective fertilized ovum.

Contrary to some old wives' tales, spontaneous abortions are *not* caused by automobile trips, falls, or emotional shocks. They may be related to general glandular or body disorders—one of the reasons for having a thorough medical examination before starting a pregnancy.

CHILDBIRTH

Near the end of pregnancy, clear fluid will normally drain spontaneously from the woman's vagina. This means that the amniotic sac, or "bag of waters," has broken. True labor is about to start. The contractions usually begin at intervals of fifteen to twenty minutes and gradually become more frequent. In some cases, however, labor sets in abruptly, with contractions coming every three to five minutes.

How Birth Takes Place

To understand what happens during a contraction, it helps to picture the uterus as a big muscular bag that is upside down, with its open end emptying into the vagina. At first, the opening is almost closed by an elastic ring, the cervix. As the walls of the bag contract during labor, the baby's head is pressed firmly against the cervix, and the cervix begins to dilate (get wider). Finally, the cervix opens wide enough for the baby's head to pass through into the vagina.

When the baby's head is through the cervix and in the vagina, the woman feels a compulsion to bear down and expel the baby through the vaginal opening. First, the crown of the baby's head appears; then, with succeeding contractions, the head gradually slides out, usually face down. Once the head is out, the body usually follows easily, because the head is larger in diameter than the body. At this point, the attendant ties off and cuts the umbilical cord connecting the baby's navel to the placenta, and the newly breathing baby is welcomed into the world. Soon afterward, the uterus contracts again and expels the placenta, or "afterbirth."

More and more mothers-to-be are choosing prepared childbirth. Unmedicated childbirth—also known as "natural childbirth" or "the Lamaze method"—is one approach to prepared childbirth. The basic purpose is to reduce or eliminate the mother's need for pain-relieving drugs (which also affect the baby) during delivery by training her in ways of managing the pain of labor. Pregnant women and their husbands or other "coaches" attend a series of classes in which they learn exactly what to expect in the delivery room and practice special exercises in controlled breathing and relaxation. The mother is alert and in control of her responses during labor and delivery, and the father is able to be present and to play an active role in the birth of the child. (© Kenneth Karp)

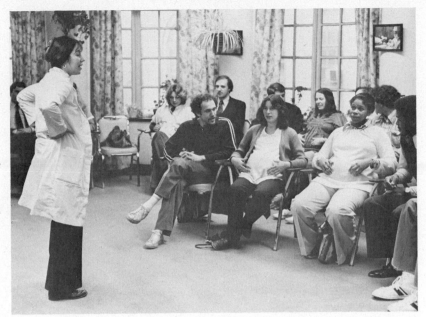

PROCEDURES SOMETIMES USED DURING DELIVERY

EPISIOTOMY   In the United States, a surgical incision called an **episiotomy** is commonly made between the mother's vaginal opening and the anus to prevent undue tearing of the tissues. Immediately after the delivery, this incision is repaired with sutures.

ANESTHESIA   Some women have general anesthesia, in which they are lightly asleep, during the delivery. Some have a regional anesthetic that blocks pain in only part of the body; others are given only local anesthesia or a pain reliever such as Demerol.

CAESAREAN SECTION   Sometimes it becomes necessary to perform a **Caesarean section.** Instead of being delivered through the birth canal, the baby is removed through surgical incisions in the mother's abdomen and uterus.

PROCEDURES AFTER DELIVERY   Whatever the method of delivery, after the birth the physician uses a suction apparatus to remove mucus from the infant's nose and mouth, to make breathing easier. The newborn's breathing, muscle tone, heart rate, reflexes, irritability, and color are then quickly assessed to determine whether the baby needs further medical help.

Alternative Approaches: Midwifery and Home Delivery

Today, some women are choosing to have their babies delivered by nurse-midwives, who are legally certified professionals trained to manage normal pregnancies and deliveries and to spot complications in time to call in an obstetrician.

Other women have recently been choosing to deliver their babies at home with the assistance of unlicensed "lay midwives." Those with high-risk pregnancies—women under fifteen or over thirty-five and those with a history of problem pregnancies, other illnesses at the time of birth, or abnormal fetal positioning—should consult with competent medical services about the advisability of home birth.

During labor and delivery, many things can go wrong with little warning: The woman may start hemorrhaging, the baby's heart rate may drop dangerously before it is born, the newborn may fail to breathe. And in many such cases, a physician's skills and a hospital's elaborate equipment are needed *within minutes* to save the life of the

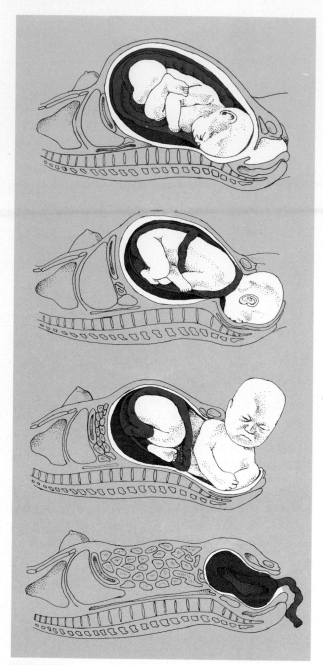

Figure 8.4 Stages of childbirth, shown diagrammatically. The baby's head lies close to the cervix, which becomes fully dilated. Strong uterine contractions begin to force the head into the birth canal (vagina). After the head appears, the shoulders rotate in the birth canal, and the rest of the body is expelled. In the last stage of delivery, the placenta and umbilical cord (sometimes called "afterbirth") are expelled. (John Dawson)

mother or baby or to prevent serious brain damage to the baby.

INFERTILITY AND ITS TREATMENT

In the United States today, approximately ten to fifteen of every one hundred couples try to have a baby without success.[20] Usually, it's impossible to predict whether a given couple will have difficulty achieving pregnancy; however, infertility often increases with age, especially with the mother's age—a factor to consider in family planning.

There are many causes of infertility, and a number of tests and procedures must be carried out by a physician before all possible causes have been identified and corrected. Both the man and the woman must be involved in the process, and the procedures often take many months—even a year or more.

In 1983, one study reported that one-third of all childless couples at a major infertility clinic were suffering from a common bacterial infection identified as *T. mycoplasma,* and that when the infection was treated with drugs, 60 percent of these couples became fertile. Researchers continued to debate these findings; possibly, the bacterium might be only one of a number of risk factors.[21]

Male Infertility

In the past there was a tendency to blame infertility on the woman. But in 40 to 50 percent of infertile matings, the man has an anatomical or physiological defect that is either wholly or partially responsible, and more and more specialists are recognizing this today.[22]

A man's fertility can be tested relatively easily, through microscopic study of a specimen of his semen: A low sperm count indicates low male fertility. This condition can be treated with medication.

Female Infertility

Infertility in a woman may be caused by some minor condition that is easily corrected, but sometimes it is difficult to tell what is causing the problem. General bodily disorders, glandular disorders, and a host of other conditions outside the pelvis can help make a woman sterile; thus, tests must be carried out not only in her pelvic area but in other parts of her body as well.

First, the specialist may run gas through her Fallopian tubes to find out whether they are open. Next may follow a microscopic examination of mucus obtained from the woman's cervix, at the time when she ovulates and several hours after she has had intercourse; the object is to see whether the sperm are still alive after intercourse. (Some women's vaginas seem to contain an unknown factor that kills sperm.) Sometimes a small sample of the woman's uterine lining is also taken, to find out whether it is favorable for nourishing a fertilized ovum.

A major advance was made toward overcoming blocked Fallopian tubes, one of the major causes of female infertility, when the world's first "test-tube baby" was born in England in 1978. Since then, many more such babies have been born. In this amazing technique, known as "in-vitro fertilization," a ripe ovum is surgically removed from the woman's body and mixed, in the laboratory, with the father's sperm. After the sperm fertilizes the egg, the embryo grows in an incubator for a few days and then is implanted into the mother's uterus for the normal nine months of pregnancy.

MENOPAUSE: MYTHS AND REALITY

We noted earlier that **menopause** is the gradual, permanent cessation of a woman's menstruation and of her cyclic reproductive activity. On the average, menopause begins at about age fifty-one, but may begin as late as age fifty-five.[23] The woman's menstrual periods usually falter for a few months and then cease altogether, at which point she is said to have "gone through" the menopause or had her "change of life." This change is also known as the *climacteric,* the time that marks the end of the reproductive phase of her life.

What has happened is that her ovaries, after thirty or forty years of activity, have lost their ability to produce mature eggs. The menopausal woman may welcome the end of fertility, but the reduced production of female hormones in her body can create other problems. Subtle and undesirable changes may occur in her body after menopause as the result of hormone deficiency. Her skin may gradually become drier and more wrinkled. Her vagina may tend to become drier and its lining thinner and more tender. Later, blood vessels may harden and bones may lose calcium and become more brittle.

It is not true, however, that a woman's sexual interest and activity decline after menopause. In fact, many menopausal and postmenopausal women, no longer concerned about becoming pregnant, actually feel more sexual desire and satisfaction.

CONTRACEPTION: METHODS AND THE "HUMAN FACTOR"

Men and women do not always want a child to be conceived when they have sexual intercourse. Obviously, intercourse can be a pleasurable experience and an expression of love as well as a reproductive act; the earth would undoubtedly be completely overpopulated by now if every mating produced offspring! Throughout history people have recognized this fact, and both sexes have tried to find ways to prevent conception. Despite recent technological advances, no 100% effective method of contraception (except for sterilization) has yet been discovered; but some of the methods currently available are much more effective than others, as we'll see below.

How People Use and Misuse Contraception

In the past, workers in the field of birth control thought that the ultimate answer to effective family planning was to be found in good, easy-to-obtain contraceptive methods. But this idea was only partly true. What the family-planning experts were ignoring was the human factor—the question of whether people would learn about contraceptive methods and then apply them correctly every time. It now turns out that human error has a great deal to do with the effectiveness of any

TABLE 8.1 · Contraceptive Methods: Failure Rates and Other Points to Consider

	Theoretical Failure Rate	*Actual Use Failure Rate*	
	(NUMBER OF PREGNANCIES PER YEAR PER 100 COUPLES USING THE METHOD)		*Points to Consider*
Methods Not Requiring Medical Care			
Withdrawal	Alone: 16	Alone: 23	Requires great will power. Penis must be withdrawn completely—pregnancy can result from ejaculation into or on the woman's labia. May cause anxiety or dissatisfaction in one or both partners.
Condoms	2	10	Especially effective when used in combination with vaginal spermicides. Readily available in drugstores (one size only). All condoms made in U.S. must meet government standards, so effectiveness is unrelated to price. Only water-soluble lubricants, if any, should be used (not petroleum jelly—causes condom to deteriorate and may turn rancid in the woman's vagina). Should not be carried in wallet—heat causes deterioration. One-half inch of space must be left at tip of condom to collect ejaculate; to prevent spilling, hold condom firmly against base of penis during withdrawal.
Vaginal spermicides (foams, creams, jellies)	3–5	15	Foam: Shake container well. Apply twice, no more than 15 minutes before each intercourse. Apply all spermicides before *each* intercourse, and against the cervix, not close to the vaginal opening. Douching less than 6 to 8 hours after intercourse is likely to wash away the protection.
Douching	(same as chance)	40	Not recommended.

birth control method. As Table 8.1 shows, for many methods there is a significant difference between how effective the contraceptive method may be in theory and how effective it is when people are actually using it.

Why *don't* people use their contraceptive methods effectively all the time? What are some of the psychological factors involved? Many people have ambivalent feelings about sexuality and reproduction, which may be operating consciously or unconsciously. Some also may be misinformed, or have naive beliefs about conception. They may believe that only the first ejaculation in any one sexual encounter can cause pregnancy, or that pregnancy cannot occur unless the woman has an orgasm, or that intercourse with the woman on top is safe. Such mistaken ideas have resulted in a great many unwanted pregnancies.

Researchers have found that the effectiveness of a contraceptive method is related to the motivation of the couple who are using it. Couples who are trying to *limit* the size of their families appear to have greater success in the use of contraception than those who are trying to *space* their children.

EFFECTIVE CONTRACEPTION: POINTS TO REMEMBER

If you wish to avoid unwanted pregnancies, it may be valuable for you to consider the following guidelines.

TABLE 8.1 · Contraceptive Methods: Failure Rates and Other Points to Consider (continued)

	Theoretical Failure Rate	*Actual Use Failure Rate*	*Points to Consider*
	(NUMBER OF PREGNANCIES PER YEAR PER 100 COUPLES USING THE METHOD)		
Methods Requiring Nonsurgical Medical Care			
Oral contraceptives (the Pill)	Combination pill: less than 1.0	2	Must be taken exactly as directed. If a pill is missed, two pills must be taken the following day and backup method should be used for the rest of that menstrual cycle.
Intrauterine device (IUD)	1.5	4	Effectiveness can be increased by using a vaginal foam around the time of ovulation. IUD should be removed if pregnancy is suspected, to reduce risk of miscarriage and uterine infection.
Diaphragm (with spermicide)	2	10	Insert no more than 2 hours before intercourse, and leave in place until 6 to 8 hours afterward. When the diaphragm is inserted correctly, the cervix can be felt through the rubber dome as a small bump an inch or so in diameter. For each additional intercourse, the diaphragm must be left in place and additional spermicidal jelly or foam inserted with an applicator.
Natural family planning	Calendar method: 2–20	20–30	Couple should abstain from intercourse for about a week in mid-cycle to allow time for ovulation, viability of sperm and ovum, and margin of error. Still, backup method should be used around the time of expected ovulation, if there is no religious objection.

Source: R. A. Hatcher et al., *Contraceptive Technology 1982–1983*, 11th ed. (New York: Irvington, 1982), p. 5.

1. No matter how effective birth-control methods are in theory, in order for them to be effective in practice you must use them *every time* you have intercourse.
2. It's important for you to understand how and why the method you are choosing works, and how to use the method correctly. Ask all your questions, and keep asking until you get the answers you need.
3. Know yourself. How do you feel about the various contraceptive methods that are available? Which method seems the best for you? Is this a method you *can* and *will* use, exactly as instructed, for all sexual intercourse?
4. Be prepared to select alternate methods as your life changes—as with the birth of a child, a change in partners, or the approach of menopause.

Methods Requiring No Medical Care

Of the various contraceptive and birth-control methods available, those that do not require medical prescription or supervision are: withdrawal; condoms; spermicidal jellies, creams, and foams; vaginal suppositories and sponges; and douching.

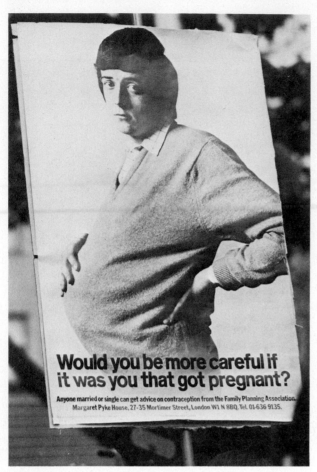

Would you be more careful if it was you that got pregnant?

Anyone married or single can get advice on contraception from the Family Planning Association. Margaret Pyke House, 27-35 Mortimer Street, London W1 N 8BQ. Tel. 01-636 9135.

This poster from a British family-planning advertising campaign is a reminder that men as well as women should take responsibility for the possible consequences of their sexual behavior. (© Julian E. Caraballo/Monkmeyer Press)

WITHDRAWAL

Withdrawal, or *coitus interruptus,* is an ancient method. As the name implies, the man withdraws his penis from the woman's vagina before he ejaculates. The idea is to prevent pregnancy by ejaculating outside the woman's body. The advantage of this method is that it is readily available and costs nothing. The disadvantage is that a few sperm are usually present in the lubricating fluids emitted from the penis during sexual arousal, prior to ejaculation. One of these may accomplish fertilization. One sperm is all it takes!

CONDOMS

A **condom** is a thin rubber or natural skin sheath that is placed over the erect penis just before intercourse. It captures and holds the man's seminal fluid, so that sperm will not be deposited in the vagina.

The condom has been widely used throughout the world for centuries. Condoms cause no harmful physical side effects, and they are the only form of contraception that definitely helps prevent the spread of sexually transmitted diseases. With the present epidemic of these diseases (see Chapter 10), this is an important consideration for sexually active men and women.

The condom is the leading mechanical method of birth control in the world. The importance of its easy accessibility and great effectiveness, especially when used in combination with vaginal foam, should not be underestimated; when used with foam, it is as effective as the IUD.

FOAMS, CREAMS, AND JELLIES

The nonprescription foams, creams, and jellies are **vaginal spermicides** that the woman inserts in her vagina, against the cervix, with a plastic applicator; they act by destroying sperm. Like the condom, vaginal foam is especially useful for individuals who require a portable, simple, inexpensive, nonmedical method, that can be used as often or as seldom as intercourse takes place. There are no harmful side effects with this method, with the possible exception of rare allergic reactions that can usually be avoided by changing brands.

OTHER PRODUCTS

In addition to vaginal foams, creams, and jellies, drugstores carry vaginal suppositories and tablets containing spermicides. However, these are considerably less effective than the foams, creams, and jellies, and they have been found to irritate and cause infection of the vagina in some women with continual use.

A new contraceptive method is the sponge, containing a spermicidal chemical, that the woman places against her cervix. It can be inserted up to twenty-four hours before intercourse and must be left in place for at least six hours before it is removed and discarded. The sponge is

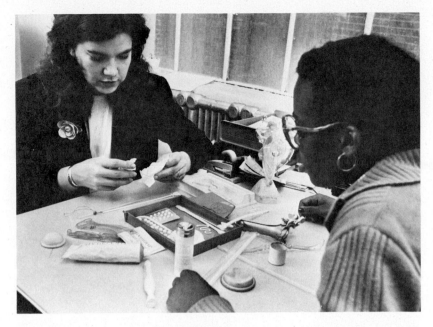

A variety of safe and effective methods of contraception are now available. Sexually active people who wish to avoid pregnancy should obtain complete and accurate information and then choose a birth-control method that they can use comfortably and consistently. (© Ann Chwatsky)

so easy to use that some researchers are calling it the "woman's condom." It was approved by the FDA in April 1983 for over-the-counter sale.

 ─────────────────────────────

Douching is the least effective method of birth control and cannot be relied on. It should also be noted that feminine hygiene products, often advertised to help with "intimate problems," are useless as contraceptives.

─────────────────────────────

Methods Requiring Nonsurgical Medical Care

Among the available birth-control methods that require some medical care are oral contraceptives, intrauterine devices, diaphragms, and the rhythm method.

ORAL CONTRACEPTIVES

Since 1960, when the Food and Drug Administration first approved **oral contraceptives** ("the Pill") for use with a doctor's prescription, millions of prescriptions for them have been written in the United States alone. Most forms of the Pill introduce into the body certain synthetic equivalents of the natural sex hormones, in such a way that the hormone cycle that leads the woman's body to ovulate is altered and ovulation is prevented.

Through the years, investigation has shown that ovulation can be effectively prevented with much smaller doses of hormones than were originally used, which is fortunate because side effects are directly related to the amount of hormone in the Pill. Most brands on the market today are "combination" pills; that is, each tablet contains both progestin (a synthetic progesterone derivative) and estrogen. The "mini-pill," not widely used, contains no estrogen.

RISKS AND BENEFITS The Pill does have many serious side effects, including: blood clots, which can impair circulation; increased risk of heart attack; and, for users between the ages of fifteen and thirty-four, about 8 times greater risk (about 1 in 12,000) of death due to circulatory disorders compared to those who do not use the Pill. All these risk factors are greatly increased if the woman smokes.[24]

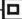 ─────────────────────────────

The Food and Drug Administration now recommends that *women who use oral contraceptives should not smoke.*

─────────────────────────────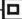

Pill users also run a greater risk of gall-bladder disease requiring surgery; benign liver tumors, which can be fatal if they rupture; and high blood pressure. And if a woman takes oral contraceptives by mistake when she is pregnant, her baby may have birth defects involving the heart and the limbs.[25] On the brighter side, some recent studies suggest that Pill users have a decreased risk of cancer of the ovaries and uterus.[26]

Whatever the risks and benefits of oral contraceptives, they are the most effective method of birth control other than surgical sterilization, and the overall risk of death is low—below that of pregnancy and childbirth itself—except for women who smoke. With all oral contraceptives, continuing medical supervision is necessary in order to minimize these risks and to prescribe the appropriate pill for each woman.

INTRAUTERINE DEVICES (IUDs)

Intrauterine devices (IUDs) are devices made of soft, flexible plastic, molded into various sizes and shapes; some are coated with copper. They are inserted into the uterus by a physician. Exactly how IUDs work is still not completely understood. They do not prevent ovulation, but it is thought that they interfere in some way with the implantation of a fertilized egg in the lining of the uterus. One variety, the Progestasert, contains progesterone, which is slowly released into the body.

Some types of IUDs must be replaced every year or so; other types can be left in place indefinitely. Some women select the IUD because it is long-lasting, it need not be put in place every time before intercourse, and it does not alter body chemistry.

PROBLEMS WITH IUDS IUDs may cause more discomfort in women who have not borne children than in those who have; about 15 percent of IUDs have to be removed because of persistent bleeding or cramps.[27] Another major disadvantage is that the device may be expelled from the uterus without the user's noticing. Although expulsion usually occurs during the first few months after insertion, there is a continuing, although low, incidence of loss. This is particularly true of women who have had many babies and in whom the cavity of the uterus is large.

The most common major complications of the IUD, however, are cramping and increased uterine bleeding. Nevertheless, IUDs are very effective contraceptive devices, with a failure rate of one to six pregnancies per hundred women per year.[28]

DIAPHRAGMS

The **diaphragm** is a shallow rubber cup, consisting of a circular metal spring covered with a fine latex rubber. The spring can be bent so that the woman can easily compress the entire device and pass it into her vagina. She then releases it, and it rests in the upper, large portion of her vagina, where it covers her cervix completely.

The diaphragm works as a mechanical barrier to prevent sperm from passing into the woman's uterus. Spermicidal jelly or cream, which the woman must apply to the diaphragm before she inserts it, adds to its effectiveness.

PROBLEMS WITH THE DIAPHRAGM When a diaphragm is inserted properly, it causes no discomfort and neither partner will notice it. The diaphragm does have a small failure rate. But improper insertion and use, along with forgetfulness, probably account for many pregnancies with this method, as they do for many other methods.

NATURAL FAMILY PLANNING

To use the method known as **natural family planning,** the couple avoids intercourse during the time when the woman may be ovulating. A number of variables are involved, including the length of time the sperm remain viable (stay alive) in the woman's reproductive tract and the length of time the released ovum is available for fertilization. Scientists don't know how to pinpoint these variables exactly, so there is about a 10 to 20 percent theoretical failure rate built in to this method.[29]

A key variable is the timing of the woman's ovulation. This can be determined *fairly* accurately, though not precisely, in a number of ways:

1. Utilizing the *temperature method,* a woman may try to pinpoint the time of ovulation by charting her basal body temperature every day. Ovulation will be followed by a slight temperature rise (one-half degree Centigrade) that will last until the start of her next

menstrual cycle. This method is not foolproof: Although the temperature change is a fairly good indication that ovulation has occurred, a slight rise in temperature may also be caused by minor colds and infections. Only pregnancy is true proof of ovulation.

2. The *calendar method* is based on the observation that most women usually ovulate around the fourteenth day before their next period. A woman must accumulate about a one-year record of her menstrual periods in order to be able to determine her fertile period with a reasonable degree of accuracy. Women vary considerably in the length of their menstrual cycles. To use the calendar method effectively, the woman needs to get the advice of a doctor, at least at the beginning, in order to learn how to chart her menstrual periods and daily temperatures, and to calculate the days it is "safe" and "unsafe" for her to have intercourse.

    The temperature and calendar methods, used together, are sometimes referred to as the "rhythm method."

3. A third method is known as the *mucus evaluation technique.* It has long been known that the consistency of the mucus in the vagina changes with the menstrual cycle: At certain stages of the cycle, it becomes more viscous—that is, thicker and of a more gluey texture (somewhat comparable to raw egg white). It is possible to learn to predict ovulation by examination of the consistency of the cervical mucus. The method has a fairly high dependability, but it is complicated. Couples who wish to use it must obtain special training and information from a physician or other trained health-care professional.

Methods Requiring Surgery: Permanent Sterilization

Millions of men and women have undergone surgical sterilization. How does this method work? In the man the standard technique is **vasectomy**—cutting and tying off the vas deferens—a minor surgical procedure that can be performed in a doctor's office. In the woman, the standard technique is **tubal ligation**—dividing or tying off the Fallopian tubes—an abdominal procedure often re-

quiring hospitalization. A new technique, **laparoscopy,** is now being used to divide the woman's Fallopian tubes with a small electrode; this method requires only a small incision in the woman's abdomen, and it is sometimes done under local anesthesia as an outpatient procedure. Another new technique utilizes a small plastic lip placed around each Fallopian tube.

For individuals who are certain that they no longer wish to conceive, voluntary sterilization provides the closest thing to an ideal alternative available today. It is virtually 100 percent effective. (The only failures are those due to improper technique or failure to use alternate means of contraception for six weeks following surgery.) Sterilization seems to have few side effects. The popularity of vasectomy, in particular, is growing, especially among educated professional families. The effects of sterilization are usually permanent, so it's crucial for the individual to think it over carefully before deciding on the procedure.

Contraceptive Methods of the Future

Scientists continue to search for better and safer methods of contraception.

METHODS FOR WOMEN

For women, some researchers are looking at implants of long-lasting contraceptive substances known as *progestogens.* Such implants might last five years, unless they were removed to restore fertility. Other researchers are working on the possibility of a tampon or suppository containing *prostaglandins,* which could be used to induce the woman to menstruate each month.

Another new device is a thimble-shaped rubber "cap" that fits snugly around the cervix and requires no spermicide. It can be left in place continuously until the woman wishes to become pregnant; a one-way valve lets menstrual blood and cervical mucus pass through. The cap is currently being tested, and may be available around 1985.

A more controversial method, currently under debate, is the use of injected drugs such as Depo-Provera, a contraceptive substance containing a synthetic hormone that prevents ovulation for at least ninety days. Depo-Provera has serious side effects, including weight gain, headaches, heavy bleeding, and depression; it may even cause a permanent loss of fertility. The FDA has forbidden its distribution in the United States for contraceptive purposes.

METHODS FOR MEN

Research is also under way on chemical contraceptives for men. There are many substances known to suppress sperm production but also to have unacceptable side effects. For example, *gossypol* (a cottonseed derivative) has had some success in China, but it has serious side effects, including difficulty in restoring fertility when a user stops taking the drug. Some male chemical contraceptives tend to reduce potency and sexual desire, and some are incompatible with alcohol. Nevertheless, some progress is being made. Various combinations of male and female sex hormones and other compounds are being tested in human volunteers, and a male Pill may be on the market within the next ten years.

ABORTION

Abortion is not a contraceptive method and should not be considered as one. Medically, **abortion** means ending a pregnancy before the embryo or fetus can survive on its own. Abortion is vigorously opposed by some people in the United States. But among others, attitudes are markedly different. Some assert (1) that abortion is now a relatively safe medical procedure, (2) that early abortion involves fewer risks than pregnancy, (3) that even under optimum conditions of correct and consistent use, most birth-control methods can fail on occasion, and (4) that millions of dangerous illegal abortions have been taking place, with the poor suffering the worst physical consequences. Some people also feel the issue of personal rights is involved: They believe a woman should have the right to decide not to bear an unwanted child.

In 1973 the Supreme Court ruled that a woman's right to privacy prevailed, and that in the first three months of pregnancy the decision whether to have an abortion should be left to the woman and her physician. The Court specified

further that in subsequent months of pregnancy, each individual state should be permitted to "regulate the abortion procedures in ways reasonably related to pregnancy" until the last ten weeks; in the last ten weeks, abortion should be prohibited except when necessary to preserve the woman's life or health. In 1977, under tremendous pressure from the antiabortion lobby, Congress passed legislation severely restricting the use of Medicaid funds for abortions.

Attitudes Toward Abortion

The issue of abortion is fraught with controversy over attitudes toward life and death, religion, and morality. For a variety of personal reasons, individuals often have mixed feelings about whether they would choose abortion, even when they are in favor of the option in principle. Similarly, there are those who oppose abortion in principle but nevertheless choose it when faced with the specific personal implications of undesired pregnancy. And there are others who absolutely oppose abortion under any circumstances.

Even the staunchest supporters of abortion as a free choice advocate the use of other birth-control methods as a first course of action, with abortion available as a backup measure so that no one is compelled to continue an unwanted pregnancy.

How Is Abortion Carried Out?

Therapeutic abortion during the first twelve weeks of pregnancy is a relatively safe procedure when performed by a qualified physician. One simple procedure, used during the first two weeks after a missed menstrual period, is *vacuum aspiration* (sometimes called *suction curettage*). It is an office procedure and does not require hospitalization. In cases where conception results from rape or incest or must be terminated for the safety of the woman, a "morning-after pill," containing ethinyl estradiol or horse estrogens, may be used.

An operative procedure known as *D and C*—dilation of the cervix and curettage (scraping) of the uterine cavity—is also used up to about the twelfth week. During the past few years, most abortions have been done by dilating the cervix and then aspirating the uterine contents with a vacuum suction apparatus. This procedure is usually followed by a D and C to make sure that all products of the conception are removed.

After the twelfth week of pregnancy, abortion is done either by a *hysterotomy,* an operation that is similar to a Caesarean section and requires an abdominal incision, or by inducing contractions by introducing a salt solution into the uterus via a catheter inserted through the abdominal wall. This latter procedure is called a *saline abortion.*

Illegal nonmedical—and dangerous—abortions have been performed by a variety of techniques employing the insertion of a foreign object into the uterus—rubber catheters, soap solutions, irritating pastes, and various chemicals. Although these agents initiate contractions of the uterus and the expulsion of part of the products of conception, the uterus is usually not completely emptied and infection is common. Soap solutions and pastes used in these procedures may cause immediate death if particles enter the bloodstream and travel to the lungs or brain. The mortality rate from legal medical abortions was 2.2 deaths per 100,000 abortions during 1972 to 1978, according to the Centers for Disease Control. But the mortality rates from nonmedical abortions are estimated to be much higher.

MAKING HEALTH DECISIONS

Which Contraceptive Method Would Be Best for You?

Listed below are several of the basic questions people ask themselves about contraception and contraceptive methods. If you use a method of contraception regularly, answer the items with reference to your method. Otherwise, answer in terms of the method that you would be most likely to use.

YES   NO

_____ _____ 1. Are you afraid of using this method of contraception?

_____ _____ 2. Would you really rather not use this method?

_____ _____ 3. Has pregnancy ever occurred while you were using this method?

_____ _____ 4. Do you (or would you) have trouble using this method correctly?

_____ _____ 5. Do you still have unanswered questions about this method?

_____ _____ 6. Does this method make menstrual periods longer or more painful?

_____ _____ 7. Does this method cost more than you can afford?

_____ _____ 8. Does this method have possible serious health complications that might affect you?

YES   NO

_____ _____ 9. Are you opposed to this method because of your religious beliefs?

_____ _____ 10. Are you using this method without your partner's knowledge?

_____ _____ 11. Did your partner participate in choosing this method?

_____ _____ 12. Does (or would) use of this method embarrass your partner?

_____ _____ 13. Does (or would) use of this method embarrass you?

_____ _____ 14. Do you (or would you) enjoy intercourse less because of this method?

_____ _____ 15. Do you (or would you) have trouble using this method because it interrupts lovemaking?

INTERPRETATION OF ANSWERS

Look over your answers, paying particular attention to the yes answers. Do you think that your yes answers, if any, indicate potential trouble with contraception for you now or in the future?

_____

_____

What factors led (or would lead) you to choose your method of contraception? _____

_____

_____

_____

If you were to change methods, what would be your principal reason(s) for changing? _____

_____

_____

_____

Are you satisfied with the role that your partner plays in your current contraceptive practices? What changes would you like to see occur?

_____

If another person asked you for advice about contraception, which of the following factors would you emphasize? Rank the factors in order of importance, beginning with 1 for the most important.

_____ safety   _____ embarrassment involved in use

_____ cost   _____ shared responsibility

_____ effectiveness   _____ (other) _____

_____ interruption of lovemaking   _____ (other) _____

Source: Adapted from R. A. Hatcher et al., *Contraceptive Technology, 1982–1983,* 11th ed. (New York: Irvington, 1982).

SUMMARY

1. The female reproductive system produces egg cells (ova), positions them to meet sperm from the male, and provides a hospitable environment for a fertilized egg to develop in.

2. The ovaries produce egg cells and hormones and are positioned near the Fallopian tubes. Ova travel through these tubes into the uterus. Ovulation is the release of an egg from the ovary. It usually takes place at about the midpoint of a woman's menstrual cycle. During pregnancy, the uterus houses the growing fetus.

3. The menstrual cycle is a process involving hormonal changes, egg maturation, and buildup of the lining of the uterus to prepare a woman's body for pregnancy. If no pregnancy occurs, the uterine lining is shed as menstrual flow, and the hormonal cycle begins anew. Some women experience physical discomfort and mood changes during menstruation, and some women suffer from premenstrual syndrome. Menstrual problems can be successfully treated medically.

4. The vagina is normally self-cleaning and moist and needs no special hygiene. Unpleasant discharges or irritations can mean infection and should be treated medically.

5. Sperm production in males is a constant process. Sperm are produced within the testes and travel out of the penis in seminal fluid.

6. Pregnancy begins when a fertilized egg implants in a woman's uterine lining. A missed period is one sign of possible pregnancy. Laboratory pregnancy tests can detect pregnancy very soon after conception. Early in pregnancy, the placenta develops, which transmits nutrients from the ma-

ternal bloodstream to the fetus's bloodstream and carries away fetal wastes.

7. A pregnant woman must get good prenatal care in order to ensure her own and her baby's well-being. Genetic counseling is available to determine (often through amniocentesis) whether a couple is at risk of having a defective baby and to provide advice on alternatives.

8. Radiation, German measles, alcohol, caffeine, tobacco, and certain prescription and over-the-counter drugs are extremely dangerous to the fetus.

9. Ten to 20 percent of pregnancies end in spontaneous abortion. A miscarriage does not mean that future pregnancies are inadvisable.

10. Childbirth is a process in which strong uterine contractions widen the cervix and push the baby out through the vagina. In a Caesarean section, the baby is removed through surgical incisions in the mother's abdomen and uterus.

11. Infertility has many causes. Its incidence increases with age. Both females and males can have anatomical or functional problems that cause them to be infertile. Specialists can successfully treat many, but not all, infertile couples.

12. Menopause is the gradual, permanent cessation of a woman's menstruation and of the reproductive phase of her life. Menopause brings decreases in hormone production, but does not signal the end of a woman's sexual life.

13. Contraceptives are devices and methods for preventing conception. Their effectiveness depends on the motivation of the users as well as on the nature of the particular method used. Methods available without medical supervision include: withdrawal, condoms, and vaginal spermicides (foams, jellies, creams, and sponges). Methods available with medical supervision include: oral contraceptives, intrauterine devices, diaphragms, and natural family planning.

14. Sterilization is an effective, permanent, surgical form of contraception. Vasectomy (for males) and tubal ligation (for females) can now be reversed surgically in a few cases, but must still be considered permanent.

15. Abortion is the ending of a pregnancy, not actually a form of contraception. The stage of development of the fetus determines the abortion technique used; the earlier in pregnancy an abortion is performed, the simpler and less risky it is to the mother.

GLOSSARY

abortion The termination of a pregnancy by removal of the uterine contents before the embryo or fetus is developed enough to survive on its own.

amniocentesis Procedure in which a doctor withdraws some amniotic fluid from a pregnant woman's uterus to test for certain genetic disorders in the fetus.

amnion (amniotic sac) Fluid-filled sac within the uterus that encloses and protects the developing baby.

Caesarean section Delivery of a baby through surgical incisions made in the mother's abdomen and uterus.

condom A thin rubber or natural skin sheath that is placed over the erect penis just before intercourse to prevent conception.

diaphragm A shallow rubber cup that is inserted into the vagina, where it completely covers the cervix, forming a mechanical barrier that prevents sperm from entering the woman's uterus.

ectopic pregnancy Condition in which a fertilized egg implants and begins to develop in the Fallopian tube rather than the uterus.

embryo A developing baby in the uterus during the first two months following conception.

endometrium The inner lining of the uterus.

episiotomy A surgical incision made between a mother's vaginal opening and anus to prevent undue tearing of the tissues during delivery of a baby.

estrogen An ovarian hormone that helps to regulate the menstrual cycle.

Fallopian tube (oviduct) One of two tiny, muscular tunnels that transport ova from the ovary to the uterus.

fetus A developing baby in the uterus from the beginning of the third month of pregnancy until birth.

intrauterine device (IUD)   A soft, flexible plastic device that is inserted into the uterus by a physician to prevent pregnancy.

laparoscopy   Surgical sterilization technique for women, in which a small electrode is used to sever the Fallopian tubes.

menopause   Gradual, permanent cessation of a woman's menstruation, and therefore of the reproductive phase of her life; also known as the *climacteric.*

menstrual cycle   The monthly cycle in which the lining of the uterus thickens and prepares to receive a fertilized ovum, then is discharged in menstruation if a pregnancy does not occur.

menstruation   The sloughing off of the thickened lining of the uterus that occurs about once a month if the woman is not pregnant.

natural family planning   A method of contraception in which a couple avoids intercourse during the time when the woman may be ovulating.

oral contraceptives ("the Pill")   Synthetic equivalents of natural sex hormones that are medically prescribed to prevent ovulation and thus prevent conception.

ovaries   Two small internal female sexual organs that produce ova (egg cells).

ovulation   The process by which ova periodically ripen and leave the ovaries.

placenta   A mass of tissue attached to the uterine lining that, during pregnancy, absorbs nutrients from the mother's bloodstream and transfers them to the bloodstream of the developing baby, and carries away fetal wastes.

premenstrual syndrome (PMS)   A pattern of physiological symptoms, irritability, lethargy, and depression that precedes menstruation in some women.

prenatal   Before birth.

progesterone   An ovarian hormone that helps to regulate the menstrual cycle, stimulating the uterus each month to prepare to receive a fertilized ovum if one is present.

Rh factor   A substance in the red blood cells which, if lacking in the mother and inherited by the first baby from the father, can cause the mother's blood to produce antibodies that result in a blood disorder called erythroblastosis fetalis in second and later children.

spermatogenesis   The process of continual sperm production.

spontaneous abortion   Expulsion of an improperly implanted or defective embryo or fetus from the uterus; commonly called a *miscarriage.*

tubal ligation   Surgical sterilization technique for women, in which the Fallopian tubes are severed or tied off.

umbilical cord   A ropelike tissue that connects the developing baby to the placenta.

vaginal spermicides   Nonprescription foams, creams, or jellies that a woman inserts in her vagina, against the cervix, to prevent conception by killing sperm.

vasectomy   Surgical sterilization technique for men, in which the vas deferens are cut and tied off.

withdrawal   A method of contraception in which the man withdraws his penis from the woman's vagina before he ejaculates; also known as *coitus interruptus.*

NOTES

1. Robert L. Reid and S. S. C. Yen, "Premenstrual Syndrome," *American Journal of Obstetrics and Gynecology* 139, no. 1 (1981): 85–104; "Premenstrual Syndrome: An Ancient Woe Deserving of Modern Scrutiny," *Journal of the American Medical Association* 245, no. 14 (April 10, 1981): 1393–1396.

2. Mary Brown Parlee, "New Findings: Menstrual Cycles and Behavior," *Ms.,* September 1982, pp. 126–128.

3. Ibid.

4. H. L. Judd and D. R. Meldrum, "Physiology and Pathophysiology of Menstruation and Menopause," in S. L. Romney et al., eds., *Obstetrics and Gynecology: The Health Care of Women,* 2nd ed. (New York: McGraw-Hill, 1981), p. 890.

5. Penny Wise Budoff, *No More Menstrual Cramps and Other Good News* (New York: Penguin, 1981), pp. 277–279.

6. Ibid., pp. 285–290.

7. L. N. Martin, *Health Care of Women* (Philadelphia: Lippincott, 1978), p. 98.

8. Budoff, *No More Menstrual Cramps,* pp. 279–285.

9. Ibid.

10. E. C. Sandberg, *Synopsis of Obstetrics,* 10th ed. (St. Louis, Mosby, 1978), p. 307.

11. H. K. Nadler and B. K. Burton, "Genetics," in E. J. Quilligan and N. Kretchmer, eds., *Fetal and Maternal Medicine* (New York: Wiley, 1980), pp. 59–107.

12. T. H. Shepard and R. J. Lemire, "Teratology," in ibid.

13. David W. Martin, "Alcohol and Drug Abuse in Pregnancy: Information for Patients," in Paul Ahmed, ed., *Pregnancy, Childbirth, and Parenthood* (New York: Elsevier, 1981), pp. 141–142; G. D. Zike, "Maternal Alcohol Use and Its Effects on the Fetus," *Physician Assistant and Health Practitioner,* February 1981, pp. 86–94.

14. Martin, "Alcohol and Drug Abuse," p. 142.

15. Ibid., p. 143.

16. Ibid., pp. 144–151.

17. Ibid., pp. 140, 145.

18. Mahnood Yoonessi et al., "DES Story: Review and Report," *New York State Journal of Medicine* 81, no. 2 (February 1981): 195–198; Donna M. Glebatis and Dwight T. Janerich, "A Statewide Approach to Diethylstilbestrol—the New York Program," *New England Journal of Medicine* 304, no. 1 (January 1, 1981): 47–50.

19. Nadler and Burton, "Genetics," p. 69.

20. R. A. Hatcher et al., *Contraceptive Technology 1982–1983,* 11th ed. (New York: Irvington, 1982), p. 218.

21. A. Toth, M. L. Lesser, C. Brooks, and D. Labriola, "Subsequent Pregnancies Among 161 Couples Treated for T-Mycoplasma Genital-Tract Infection," *New England Journal of Medicine* 308, no. 9 (March 3, 1983): 505–507.

22. Hatcher et al., *Contraceptive Technology,* p. 216.

23. A. B. Little and R. B. Billiar, "Endocrinology," in Romney et al., *Obstetrics and Gynecology,* p. 122.

24. H. W. Ory, A. Rosenfield, and L. C. Landman, "The Pill at 20: An Assessment," *Family Planning Perspectives* 12 (1980): 278.

25. Ibid.

26. D. A. Grimes, "Birth Control Pills: A Reappraisal of the Pros and Cons," *Medical Aspects of Human Sexuality* 16, no. 8 (August 1982): 32J–32Y.

27. Hatcher et al., *Contraceptive Technology,* p. 84.

28. W. H. Masters, V. E. Johnson, and R. C. Kolodny, *Human Sexuality* (Boston: Little, Brown, 1982), pp. 128–129.

29. Ibid., p. 137.

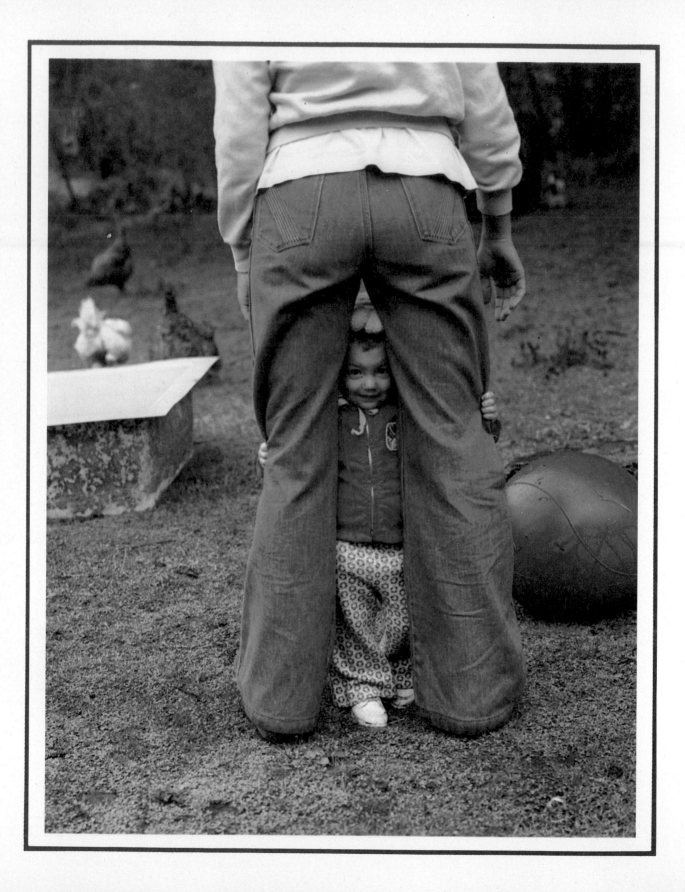

CHAPTER 9

Marriage, Parenthood, and Other Close Ties

Our culture values "rugged individualism" and "going it alone"; our need for warm human relationships is sometimes denied or viewed as a sign of weakness. Nevertheless, most of us try to achieve close personal ties with relatives, friends, and sexual partners, and some of us choose to have children as well. Such relationships can help give us a sense of our own value as human beings. They can also help satisfy a number of emotional needs. Each of us needs *intimacy:* A close, loving relationship allows us to express our thoughts freely and to feel that we can trust another person with our deepest feelings. Each of us needs *reassurance of worth*—the feeling that we are valued and considered special by the meaningful people in our lives. Each of us needs a sense of *support*—the knowledge that there are people to whom we can turn for help. And each of us needs *nurturance*—we need both to care for others and to be cared for by others.

No one relationship can fill all of a person's emotional needs. Regardless of whether a person is married or single, he or she also needs the special closeness and sense of sharing that can develop between friends, siblings, parents and children, and other relatives—sometimes even between coworkers. In this chapter we are going to focus on marriage and parenthood, because they are options that are selected by many people in our culture who want to share their lives with others. But we will also devote attention to other phases of long-term relationships, including courtship and cohabitation ("living together"). And we will discuss the single lifestyle: Today, not everyone assumes that the heterosexual married couple is the only natural and vital adult lifestyle, and the United States has a larger, more vocal, and more politically influential population of single people than ever before.

THE DECISION TO MARRY

Marriage has traditionally been—and often still is—an economic arrangement, in which the husband provides a home for his wife and children and supports them financially, while the wife provides him with a sexual outlet, cares for the children, and runs the home. Today, however, many Americans expect and get more from marriage: A successful marriage can provide intimacy, sharing, nurturance, comfortable dependency, and support. In this rapidly changing world of mobile people, a steady partner can be a sustaining factor in personality development: Happily married people often identify their spouse as their best friend—a person whose company they thoroughly enjoy, who is there in times of need, and who shares their joys and sorrows. If you're a man, marriage can even help promote physical health. Though single women experience lower rates of illness and have a longer life expectancy than married women, married men have a lower incidence of disease than single men, and outlive single men by an average of three to five years.[1]

Why Do People Get Married?

Because marriage is our society's norm, pressures to marry can be enormous. This pressure often comes explicitly from parents and other relatives, and implicitly from the media, romantic literature, and school.

- Despite recent changes in our society, many people still decide to marry for economic reasons.
- Marriage is still viewed by many people as the only acceptable framework in which people can freely enjoy sex.
- Sometimes, members of the family—or the ethnic or religious group—pressure the individual to marry so that property can be passed down to the younger generation in an orderly way, and so that the new generation can be raised in the teachings and values of that group.

Besides dealing with these external social pressures, people who are contemplating marriage must also grapple with their own motivations. Many marry for reasons that have little to do with the desire to develop a meaningful long-term relationship with another person. They may be trying to forge a sense of identity by picking a spouse who represents what they would like to become (secure, popular, well-read, or whatever). They may also be escaping from an unhappy home life, marrying "on the rebound" to get even with a former lover, avoiding loneliness, or looking for the security of a rich spouse. And many couples, especially young ones, feel forced into marriage when the woman becomes pregnant.

If you're thinking about getting married, be sure to ask yourself: Am I getting married for the right reasons? Am I marrying because other people want me to or because I want to? Many people marry who are not ready for the commitment that marriage requires; their personalities, values, and lifestyles are simply not geared toward living with another person. A person has a much better chance of long-term happiness if he or she thinks about these issues before jumping into marriage.

Selecting the Right Mate

When we are looking for a mate, we tend to zero in on those whose ethnic, religious, economic, and educational background closely approximates our own; size and other physical attributes are also significant factors.[2] Where we're *least* likely to match up with a similar person is in the area of compatibility. And this can lead to trouble. Personality factors are not as easy to observe as height and hair color, and people don't usually reveal their "true selves" until after the honeymoon. (They're usually on their best behavior during courtship.) People of opposite personalities often attract each other in relationships: the initial thought is that one personality rounds out the other. Unfortunately, the outcome is often to the contrary: In time, one person begins to try to change the other.

WHAT CAN YOU DO TO PICK THE RIGHT PERSON?

How can you make sure you're marrying someone truly compatible? One way is to take plenty of time to get to know the other person. Social scientists have noted that courting couples seem to go through three stages. First, in what's called the "stimulus stage," each person tries to measure his or her own good and bad qualities against those of the other; people tend to be drawn to others who seem to have about the same assets and liabilities as themselves (for example, people who are about equally good-looking or popular). Next, in the "value stage," the couple look for compatible beliefs, attitudes, and interests to support their initial attraction. But it isn't until they get to the "role stage" that they reveal to each other how they handle responsibility, react to disappointment, and cope with a wide variety of life situations.[3] The key to compatibility is to be sure you've arrived at this last stage before you think seriously about marrying each other. Those who marry during this stage are less likely to be unpleasantly surprised than those who impulsively marry on short acquaintance.

Women's Changing Attitudes Toward Marriage

Today, increasing numbers of women are no longer willing to take the traditional steps from

The wedding day is a landmark in the intimate process of mutual discovery through communication. (©Hazel Hankin)

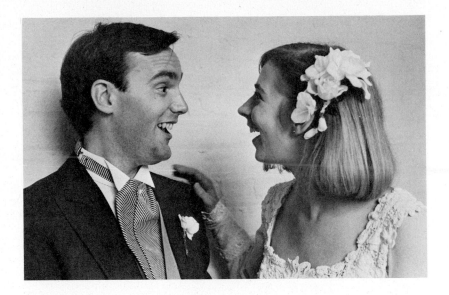

daughter to student to wife. Freed from sitting at home waiting for the phone to ring, they are focusing less energy on finding a husband and more energy on developing their talents and learning about themselves. A worldwide trend toward later marriage has been documented.[4] And the increasing numbers of career-oriented women are no longer seen as frustrated spinsters or mothers who are neglecting their children; now they are viewed as important role models for young women aspiring to fulfilling jobs.

To be sure, many women are not totally emancipated from age-old fears and pressures; nor have all women rejected the benefits that marriage can offer. Most women do want marriage and children, and some research suggests that, in comparison to men, women are less inclined to throw themselves wholeheartedly into a romance unless marriage is a possibility. According to other studies, women are more likely to end—or threaten to end—a relationship if marriage seems unlikely.[5] Often, the need for a lasting relationship combines with and clashes with the need for room to grow and realize one's full potential. Both women and men have had to adjust accordingly, and today both sexes are in transition.

SKILLS FOR A HAPPY MARRIAGE

There is no simple formula for a happy marriage. Successful couples ultimately find their own solu-

tions to the challenges that marriage offers. There are, nevertheless, certain qualities that one must bring to a marriage in order to make intimacy and emotional satisfaction possible:[6]

- A strong sense of identity. Lasting relationships are built by people who know, "This is who I am, this is what I need, and this is what I have to offer."
- An ability to be mutually supportive and to leave room for oneself and one's partner to grow emotionally and intellectually.
- A knowledge of how to give love and an understanding that love must be worked for and earned.
- An accurate and realistic perception of one's spouse.
- A willingness to loosen ties with one's original family.
- A capacity to take criticism, to express and share emotions, and to argue fairly and effectively.
- A commitment to work—with determination, flexibility, and spontaneity—toward resolving differences and keeping lines of communication open.
- An ability to play. This does not mean that marriage is "childhood revisited": One should not marry unless one is mature enough to consider the needs of others. Nonetheless, adult responsibilities can become oppressive if the spouses are unable occasionally to retreat together into fun, fantasy, and laughter.
- Respect for and commitment to the other person. This requires a shift in focus from "me" to "we."

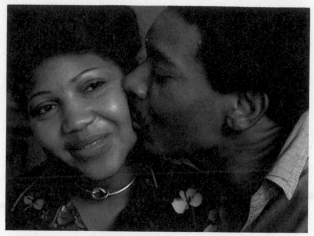

Among the requirements of a successful marriage are the respect and affection that the partners feel for each other. (©Edward L. Miller/Stock, Boston)

■ The ability to resolve power struggles. Like other relationships, marriage requires that the partners resolve the issue of power between them. A continual power struggle is unhealthy, as is a situation in which one partner is oppressively dominant or neither partner is able to make a decision. A relationship in which power is shared, in a setting of cooperation, relaxation, and good humor, creates an atmosphere in which love and trust can thrive.

Coping with Problem Areas

Unmet emotional needs, and problems in expressing affection and understanding, are among the most common difficulties in marriage. Other potential sources of friction are children (which we will discuss below); in-laws; choice of friends; differences in personal interests; and disagreements over how to spend leisure time. There are also problems inherent in sharing living space; partners often expend considerable energy in determining what is "yours," "mine," and "ours."

Money can be an explosive issue—symbolically as well as practically. Do the spouses make budget and spending decisions cooperatively? Does the wife feel devalued or controlled if she is financially dependent on her husband? Does the husband feel threatened if his wife's income exceeds his? Surprisingly, the acquisition of a large sum of money can put as much strain on a marriage as a devastating financial loss.[7]

Sex, too, can cause serious problems. Recently, researchers have found that tremendous changes have taken place in the sex lives of American married couples. Because sex is discussed more openly today and there are more sex education courses in schools—not to mention the frequent references to sex in the media—men and women usually know something about human sexuality when they get married, and sex is more likely to represent the desires of both partners rather than of the husband alone. Safe, effective birth-control methods have freed couples to enjoy sex as a means of giving and receiving pleasure. But this new emphasis on sex is putting its own strains on marriage: the couple may feel unconscious conflicts caused by traditional standards they may have learned long ago, while at the same time both feel pressured to "perform" sexually as frequently and as satisfyingly as they believe other couples are performing. Happily, in stable marriages individuals have an opportunity to work through sexual problems. (We discuss sexuality in detail in Chapter 7.)

Another area where serious disagreements often arise is the division of labor in the marriage. Nowadays, more and more women are working outside the home, and increasing numbers of men are taking on greater domestic responsibilities. For some men, the transition has not been smooth: Some feel that their masculinity is threatened by the breakdown in strictly segregated sex roles. Meanwhile, many working wives still bear the major responsibility for taking care of the home and the needs of the family: Studies show that women employed full-time spend an average of 4.8 hours a day on housework, while their husbands spend only 1.6 hours a day.[8]

THE DUAL-CAREER MARRIAGE: IS IT FOR YOU?

During the past decade, there has been a sharp increase in **dual-career marriages**, in which the wife doesn't just work full-time but pursues a professional career as seriously as her husband does. As many as half of today's college women want a small family (one or two children at most) *and* meaningful, satisfying jobs with opportunities for

Effective Communication in Marriage

To resolve any of the tricky issues in a marriage—power, sex, work roles, and others—it's absolutely vital to communicate well with each other. Researchers have noted that happily married couples tend to:

► Share power and converse frooly. Their conversation is peppered with pauses, laughter, interruptions, and questions, which indicate spontaneity, flexibility, and interest in what is being said.*
► Work together to solve mutual problems.
► Be assertive (some say aggressive) when necessary. One psychologist observed: "The danger for a marriage is much greater from apathy than it is from aggression."†
► Criticize each other constructively—or refrain from criticism.
► Deal with problems and difficult issues on their own merits, not as signs that the entire relationship is crumbling.

Many of the skills people need to make a marriage work are not innate. For instance, we are not born with the ability to communicate effectively with another human being. We must learn to communicate—and the sooner the better. This means learning what to say, what *not* to say, when to listen, how to listen, and when to be silent. We are always communicating something when we are in the company of another person; gestures, silences, and body language all have meaning. It takes skill to decode what is being conveyed and to reply in a way that can be understood.**

Sources: *Patricia Morgan Hurley, "Communication Patterns and Conflict in Marital Dyads," *Nursing Research* 30, no. 1 (January–February 1981): 38–42; †Arthur Burton, "Marriage Without Failure," in B. J. Chesser and A. A. Gray, eds., *Marriage: Creating a Partnership,* 2nd ed. (Dubuque, Iowa: Kendall-Hunt, 1979), pp. 81–86; **R. A. Hunt and E. J. Rydman, *Creative Marriage,* 2nd ed. (Boston: Allyn & Bacon, 1979), p. 25.

advancement—along with egalitarian relationships with their husbands.[9]

This introduces some new and potentially difficult issues. What happens, for instance, when the wife—but not the husband—is offered a promotion that involves moving to another city? Does she refuse the promotion, or does the husband quit his job and go with her? Conversely, should the wife be expected to leave a lucrative, exciting job if her husband's firm is relocated? These are some of the questions you need to think about if you're contemplating a dual-career marriage.

Learning to Fight—the Right Way

Most marriage counselors consider the statement "we never fight" to be a sign that a marriage is in jeopardy. All couples have to experience some conflict. It is both human and healthy to disagree occasionally. The key is to do it fairly and constructively, sticking to the issue at hand and avoiding the temptation to dig up past hurts. This way, each partner asserts his or her individuality, and the couple can learn about each other and deepen

their relationship. Strong relationships are built by working through these difficulties, not by trying to avoid them.

HOW YOU CAN GUARD AGAINST DESTRUCTIVE FIGHTING

Researchers have identified three basic types of marital quarrels: acute, progressive, and habituated.[10] These aren't just empty categories—they have practical implications for learning how *not* to fight.

► *Acute quarrels*—which are usually sharp and loud—are most common in new marriages, when each partner is jockeying for position within the union. Among the problems that must be worked out are personal habits, how money is spent, in-laws, sex, and family planning. Ominously, when the partners are genuinely in love, they may hide their anger and resentment to avoid hurting each other. Then, suddenly, the built-up resentments explode with the force—and unpredictability—of a volcanic eruption. The point here is: Try to ventilate your anger early, when it will do less damage.
► Quarrels become *progressive* when couples fail to focus on their differences and make the necessary adjustments. Conflicts blend into one another, ulti-

ACTIVITY: EXPLORING HEALTH

Your Attitudes Concerning Household Tasks

Whether we like it or not, certain household tasks must be performed regularly. Which marriage partner do *you* think should have responsibility for the following tasks? Check the response you feel is appropriate for each task.

Legend:
OW: only the wife
MW: mainly the wife
SH: shared between husband and wife
MH: mainly the husband
OH: only the husband
OP: another person other than either marital partner

TASK	OW	MW	SH	MH	OH	OP
Budgeting						
Shopping						
Household Repairs						
Automobile Maintenance						
Paying Bills						
Banking						
Child Care						
House Cleaning						
Meal Preparation						
Laundry						
Garbage Disposal						
Income Earning						
Disciplining Children						
Gardening and Lawn Care						
Pet Care						
Other Tasks (list them)						

Which tasks did you assign to "only" or "mainly" husbands? Why? _____

_____

Which tasks did you assign to "only" or "mainly" wives? Why? _____

_____

Which tasks did you assign to "shared" responsibility? Why? _____

_____

People who share in the necessary daily activities of living are more likely to be able to share in resolving the more significant and complex issues of their married life.

Source: Adapted from John Dorfman et al., *Well-Being: An Introduction to Health* (Glenview, Ill.: Scott-Foresman, 1980), p. 110.

mately snowballing into a verbal brawl in which the combatants zero in on each other's weaknesses. Even after the quarrel ends, scars remain. If you want to safeguard your marital happiness, try to keep fights from festering this way.

▶ *Habituated conflict* is what results after couples recognize that there are some issues on which they will never agree, and where accommodation is the best they can hope for. They learn to sidestep "problem" issues as often as possible, and they strive to avoid investing these issues with too much emotion when they do surface. This category of conflict may not imply as much danger to a marriage as the others; just be sure you don't shove too many issues under the rug this way.

PARENTHOOD

Parenthood: the ultimate responsibility. Twenty-four hours a day, seven days a week, fifty-two weeks a year, a small, weak, vulnerable, impressionable human being looks to his or her parents for food, clothing, shelter, love, and encouragement. It's more than a job—the parents can't quit. It's more than a marriage—the parents can't divorce the child. It's the supreme commitment. And, in some parents' experience, it's the supreme joy—if you're ready for it.

The Decision to Have a Child

In the past, it was to people's economic advantage to have children. Sons could become hands on the farm or apprentices in a trade; daughters could relieve some of the drudgery of the mother's housework and marry men who could provide additional help and income to the family. Today, however, children are anything but an economic asset. Every few years some organization or another calculates the cost of raising a child. The amount can be staggering, especially if college tuition is part of the package. Clearly, a child does not enhance a couple's financial status. Sometimes, people also have negative emotional and physical reactions to becoming parents—depression, resentment, guilt, fatigue, marital difficulties.

Yet people do have children—and, in fact, the birth rate has increased somewhat in the past decade (see Figure 9.1). Why do people in our culture have children? Some make the decision for the wrong reason—to try to bring stability to a shaky marriage, for example. But many decide to become parents because they have developed a strong, secure relationship with each other and they would like to extend and enrich it with a child. In the end a couple's decision about having a child should be most strongly influenced by each

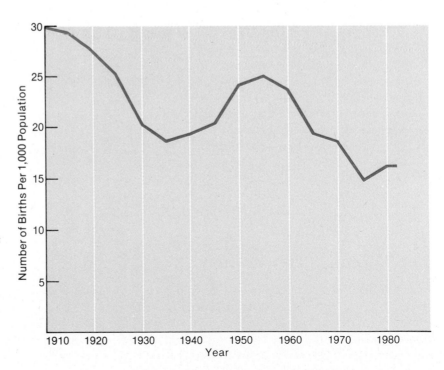

Figure 9.1 The birth rate—the number of births per 1,000 people —in the United States between 1910 and the present. The birth rate dropped after World War I as effective methods of contraception were introduced in the 1920s and 1930s. It soared during the post–World War II "baby boom," between about 1945 and 1957. In the 1970s that generation began to have children, producing a "mini-boom."
Sources: U.S. Bureau of the Census, *Statistical Abstracts of the United States, 1981* (Washington, D.C.: U.S. Government Printing Office, 1981), p. 58; National Center for Health Statistics, *Monthly Vital Statistics Report* 31, no. 12 (March 14, 1983): 1.

partner's willingness to accept the responsibilities of parenthood. Are they willing to give the time it takes to raise a child? Can they meet a child's physical and emotional needs? If they can answer yes to these questions, they will probably be happy with the decision to have a child.

Meeting Children's Health Needs

The health problems of today's young people are different from what they were a generation ago. In the first year of life, the leading causes of death are problems associated with low birth weight—especially respiratory distress syndrome ("crib death")—followed by birth defects and infections. In childhood, accidents are the major cause of death, followed by cancer (including leukemia). (Accidents are, in fact, the major cause of death among people up to age forty.) During the teenage years, major problems are suicide, drug abuse, and sexually transmitted diseases.[11]

Parents can make a difference in their children's growth and development: Children have a better chance of becoming healthy adults if they receive optimal care beginning before birth—before conception, if genetic counseling is considered—and continuing throughout infancy, childhood, and adolescence. The first consideration is to prevent retarded growth, especially in the first year of life: Too-slow growth may produce lifelong developmental deficiencies that may never be completely overcome in the adult years. Good prenatal care of the expectant mother (see Chapter 8) will give the newborn an excellent chance at birth; a well-balanced diet, with restricted sugar and food additives, are important in the childhood and teenage years. Parents also need to provide the child with opportunities for exercise, rest, and relaxation; and they need to restrict harmful substances.

The Parent–Child Relationship: The Parents' Contribution

Every child's primary need is for love and acceptance; only if a child feels deeply, basically loved can his or her *emotional development* proceed. Meeting this need begins as parents help their baby develop what the psychoanalyst Erik Erikson

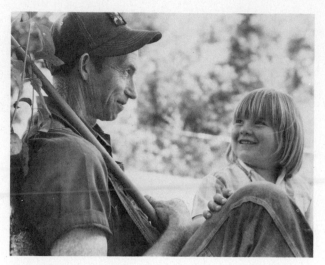

A feeling of trust in her or his parents is essential to a child's healthy emotional development. (©Harvey Wang)

has called "basic trust." If the adults can convey a sense of relaxation and enjoyment—rather than anxiety—as they feed and hold the baby, the baby will get the idea that the world is a friendly place and will begin to feel that he or she can depend on the parents. Sometimes a grandparent or in-law cautions the parents against spoiling the baby—"you mustn't pick the baby up every time the child fusses." In fact, however, theorists now believe the opposite is true: Studies have found that

> when the mother is responsive to the child's crying between three months and six months of age, this leads to a *lessening* of crying between six months and nine months. Responsiveness to the six- to nine-month-old leads to a *reduction* in crying from nine to twelve months.[12]

When early dependency needs are met, the child is free to grow toward security and independence. Eventually, just as the parents freely gave the child love, so they must freely let him or her go—love that is too possessive may prevent the child from becoming autonomous.

Parental care is also crucial for the child's *intellectual development*—and the key period is the child's first five years. One expert believes that about half of an individual's intellectual capacity has developed by age four, about three-fourths by age eight, and the remainder by age seventeen.[13]

Parents are needed to provide stimulation—by singing and talking to an infant; by decorating the child's room with toys and mobiles; by offering choices (red or green shirt? peas or carrots today?) to even very young children; by explaining family rules; by rewarding children for what they do right (*not* just scolding them for what they do wrong); by encouraging them to try new experiences and tasks even though they may fail the first few times. The best home environment for intellectual development is one in which parents are warm and loving, take time to explain their actions, let the children participate in decisions, try to answer questions, and show concern for the development of their children's competence.

Last but not least is the crucial input of **socialization**—the process by which people learn the ways of a given society or social group so that they can function within it.[14] The socialized child is the child who knows how to behave with other people. Children become socialized in part by modeling themselves on their parents; and in part through discipline—the process by which parents communicate rules to the child. Discipline sometimes involves an angry confrontation, sometimes just a quiet conversation—about issues that grow more complex as the child grows up. How much television is permitted? When is the child supposed to go to bed? What about household chores? As the child gets older, the parents' values may clash with those of the child's friends, and conflicts may become frequent. Parents may also find that they themselves disagree on methods of discipline; they may need to work these conflicts out in private so that they can present the child with a "united front."

The Parent–Child Relationship: The Child's Contribution

Guiding and disciplining a child may seem at times to be an awesome task. And it has been made even more formidable by the widespread belief, which gripped parents for many years, that the child's mind and personality were like a blank slate, on which the parents could write anything they wanted. If the child were like a blank slate—or, to make another comparison, like an empty bowl waiting to be filled—parents would find themselves in a position of terrifying responsibility. One false move, it seemed, and the child would be ruined!

Lately, however, psychologists are beginning to see parent–child interactions in another way. Researchers now think that during the first two months, infants actually use signals—such as gazing eye-to-eye with the parent, smiling, crying, thrashing around, cooing, or appearing particularly helpless—to guide their parents in giving them the care they need.[15] They can often induce the adult to play with them when they are in the mood for amusement, or to help them when they are hungry, wet, or uncomfortable. Tiny as they are, they can exert a tremendous amount of power over the adult. One expert has even noted that with a first baby, the infant knows more about infant care than the parent; the parent learns by interacting with the baby.[16]

A number of studies have demonstrated that the same behavior on the part of the parent can have different results, depending on the individual child's sex, temperament, needs for sleep, food, and stimulation, and personal likes and dislikes.[17] Thus, parents need to remember that although they can influence their children, they are also reacting constantly to the individual needs and dispositions their children are born with.

Smart parents learn to work with their children's temperaments, not fight against them. They learn to "read" their children's signals, and don't expect them to match their friends' or even their siblings' emotional responses.

Who Cares for Children, and How?

Does one have to be a biological parent to a child to effectively carry out the thousands of day-to-day interactions it takes to enable a child to develop into a mature, responsible, independent human being? Is it important for just *one* parent to be the primary adult in the relationship? Is there anything special or magical about having the *mother* as the primary caregiver, especially when the child is very young? With the women's liberation movement and the rapid escalation of the cost of living, many mothers are now at work outside the home; so these questions are now of practical importance.

CAN THE MOTHER'S ROLE BE SHARED?

Recent studies have shown that secure bonds *can* be formed with a small number of caregivers who become familiar figures in a child's life.[18] In fact, children may be better off with substitute caregivers than with mothers who would rather be working. As one psychologist has recently pointed out, educated mothers who remain at home full-time may "over-invest in [their] children, bringing an excess of worry and inadequate encouragement of independence."[19] The working mother, in contrast, tends to be more satisfied with her life than the mother who feels she must stay at home with her child; and satisfaction with one's life enhances one's effectiveness as a mother.

Researchers are particularly interested in the effects of shared mothering on preschool children. In one study of middle-class preschoolers, there was *no difference* in the amount of one-to-one mother–child contact among working and nonworking mothers.[20] Full-time mothers may not spend all their time talking or playing with their children; they may spend more time doing housework. Another study found that four-year-olds whose mothers had worked outside the home since the children were babies showed *better* social adjustment than the children whose mothers had not worked.[21]

And what about school-age children whose mothers work? They may get a boost in independence. These children have more responsibility for household tasks than the children of nonworking mothers have, and they are likely to see greater sharing of housework by their parents.

THE FATHER'S ROLE

Traditionally, fathers left for work in the morning and mothers stayed home and took care of the children. In those days, theorists inferred that "mothers were exclusively important influences on children's personality development."[22] The importance of the father's role in raising emotionally well-adjusted children was largely ignored. Recently, though, researchers have begun to study

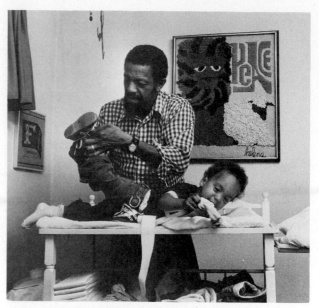

When the father participates actively in child care, both he and the child benefit. (©Michal Heron, 1981/Woodfin Camp & Assoc.)

that role more closely and they are finding out that fathers play an important role in parenting. Fathers tend to be playful and stimulating with their infants. Eventually, active play and physical games shift to more complex sports that require greater agility and coordination. Fathers needn't teach their children to be star athletes—much athletic ability is innate—but active play does help children to develop their kinetic senses of movement and balance, self-confidence, and social awareness. In many families, fathers also represent a link to the outside world. Through their fathers, children learn about working and life outside their homes. (As more mothers work, of course, this role is being shared by both parents.) Fathers are also important in the processes by which children develop their sex-role identifications.[23]

Today, while most fathers still do not share parenting equally with their wives, many are very different from the fathers who raised them. More and more, new fathers are changing diapers and bathing and feeding their babies, while grandfathers look on amazed. Comparing modern fathers to those of older generations, one expert has commented: "Many [of today's] fathers are more genuinely motivated to meet the individualistic needs of their children, are less likely to impose their own ambitions and hopes on their children, are less authoritarian and arbitrary, and are much less austere and unapproachable than fathers of the recent past."[24]

OTHER CHILD-CARE POSSIBILITIES

Not long ago, the question many new mothers asked was, "Should I go back to work?" As Figure 9.2 suggests, more and more women are answering "yes," and the question now is, "When should I go back to work, and who will care for my child when I do?"

The question of child care can come up even if the mother doesn't go back to work. Some researchers believe that a substitute parent is essen-

Figure 9.2 About 60 percent of the women in the American labor force are single. Almost half of all married women—with or without children—also have jobs outside the home. This graph shows the percentages of married, separated, and divorced women in the labor force according to the presence and age of their children. For example, 45 percent of married women who have children under the age of six work outside the home.

Source: U.S. Bureau of the Census, *Statistical Abstracts of the United States, 1981* (Washington, D.C.: U.S. Government Printing Office, 1981), p. 388.

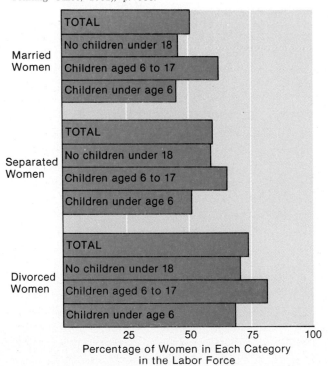

tial from time to time—no matter what—to give the mother some relief. A day off gives a new mother a chance to enjoy adult company. It can be even more welcome when babies become toddlers: The constant attention to their needs and activities can wear out even the most energetic parent.

WHAT'S THE BEST WAY TO SET UP A CHILD-CARE ARRANGEMENT?

A number of questions are asked by parents who are thinking of arranging for outside child care. Following are some of the most important.

When can the child be left with someone else? Some families wonder if there is a "right" age for a child to be left with a substitute parent. But regarding this question, no expert or research study can tell parents what they must do. Many women return to their jobs just days after giving birth. Others wait six months or a year, and others wait until their youngest child enters school. Often, decisions are based on what a woman feels will be best for herself. During the first few months of life, an infant will not get too upset if he or she is left with a competent substitute. If the baby has already formed an attachment with the caregiver, the transition is easier. After the first six months, most babies develop "stranger anxiety"; they become upset if the mother leaves. From about the age of one year, though, fear of strangers declines.

Which is better: group care or private care? There *are* some research findings about this question. If you do leave your child with a substitute parent during the first year of life, some experts believe that one adult caregiver is best. That way, the child can form a close attachment with the caregiver. Group care, in the opinion of some authorities, isn't appropriate until the child is two and a half to three years old. At this point, the child needs to be around other children of his or her own age and is able to play more independently. If a younger child must be placed in a group-care setting, it is best if the same adult cares for the child every day.

How can parents choose the right caregiver? Other important concerns are the kind of person who will help take care of the child and the kind of place in which the child will be cared for. Here are some things to look for:

▶ Will the child receive affection and mental stimulation?
▶ How many other children is the caregiver caring for?
▶ What is her or his philosophy about child discipline?

Is it all right to let the child come home to an empty house? Many working mothers make no after-school provisions for their children. A growing population of "latch-key" children may be getting too much independence before they are mature enough to cope with it. As the child development researcher Urie Bronfenbrenner has remarked:

> If parents begin to drop out as parents even before the child enters school, you then begin to get children who become behavior problems because they haven't been "socialized." . . . They haven't learned responsibility, consideration for others. You learn that from adults. There's no way that you can learn it from kids of your own age. So you begin to have problem kids. . . . In its most extreme form, kids who haven't had a chance to work and play with adults show a drop in competence—that is, in the capacity to use concepts and to think.[25]

Supervised after-school activities may be preferable to letting a child return home to an empty house each day.

FAMILY VIOLENCE

Domestic violence affects an alarming number of American families. There are indications that as many as 50 percent of married couples use physical force on each other at some time during their marriage, and as many as 10 million children are abused by their parents each year. Amazingly, statistics show that a married person is more likely to be killed by his or her spouse than by any other person![26]

Battered Spouses

Family violence cuts across all racial, religious, and socioeconomic lines, frequently affecting other-wise "normal" people who are able to control their behavior at work and in other public settings. Although some women regularly bite, kick, and scratch their husbands, the typical spouse abuser is a man, who uses his superior size and strength to maintain power in the marital relationship. A clinical social worker who has interviewed over 120 battered women says, "What seems to be occurring is fear of role reversal. The man feels called upon to defend his 'maleness,' and is socialized to use violence to do so."[27]

Several other factors may contribute to physical violence between spouses:

- The abusive spouse may be a person who feels he or she has a *right* to control others in his or her orbit.
- The family may be one that keeps to itself, so that there are fewer outside social controls on the behavior of individuals within the family.
- The wife may be unable to leave a violent husband because there are children involved or because she has nowhere else to go. The typical battered wife is a woman with a poor self-image who believes that she cannot alter her situation. Lacking marketable skills and financial resources, afraid or ashamed to confide in friends or relatives, she may view periodic beatings as the price she has to pay for the "security" of a home and a husband.
- The people involved may have previously learned to associate family life with physical pain. (Children who witness or are victims of physical abuse are more likely to grow up to abuse their own spouse and children.)[28]

With the help of a professional counselor, abusive spouses can learn to express anger in a way that is not destructive, and couples can be taught to work out their differences in a nonviolent fashion. More often, however, it is just the wife who seeks help. Some communities have set up twenty-four-hour telephone hotlines. In emergencies, there are volunteer shelters (usually in private homes) where women can go with their children.

There are other services a battered wife can turn to. She can join a support group made up of other battered wives. She can seek legal advice if she wants to file a formal complaint, seek a restraining order against her husband, or arrange for custody of children and property. And there are agencies that offer vocational counseling, assist-

Spouse battering and child abuse are social problems of increasing public concern. (©Elizabeth Hamlin/Stock, Boston)

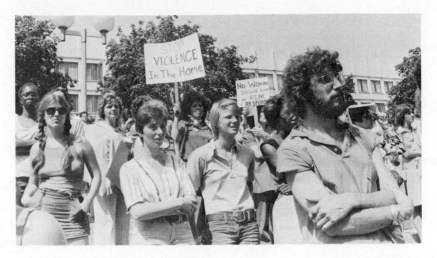

ance in finding a job and a place to live, and referrals to other appropriate social service agencies.

Child Abuse

"Spare the rod and spoil the child," goes the old saying about child rearing. Although it would be hard today to find a child development specialist who advocates spanking children, many parents discipline their children by hitting them. In one national survey, "45 percent of the sample hit their children regularly."[29] Does one slap when tempers are short make a parent a child abuser? No, but for some parents, one slap can lead to a beating of such violence that children are injured or even killed. Physicians and hospital emergency rooms often see children who have been beaten, burned, or otherwise battered; who have been starved or sexually abused; or whose X-rays show many broken bones that have healed without being set.

What separates the parent who, from time to time, smacks a misbehaving child from the one who loses control? While child abusers can be found in all social classes, most of those that are reported to authorities have low incomes and low occupational status. More mothers than fathers abuse their children, and "abuse occurs more frequently in larger families."[30]

The most common characteristic of abusive parents is that they were usually abused or neglected themselves when they were children. Abusing parents are often people who lead lonely, isolated lives; who have a strict, disciplinarian attitude toward child rearing; and who do not com-

municate well with their children. A stress within the family—say, the loss of a job or a household accident—frequently precipitates abuse. In fact, one study found that parents who had severely punitive parents themselves were least able to cope with a rapid series of life changes. Too much stress triggered violence toward their own children.[31]

DEALING WITH CHILD ABUSE

All states now have laws that require physicians and other health professionals to report suspected cases of child abuse to child welfare authorities. Many communities have crisis intervention hotlines, where parents who realize that they are getting out of control can get immediate help. There is also a national organization, Parents Anonymous (analogous to Alcoholics Anonymous), where abusive parents themselves help one another to overcome their tendencies toward violence.

But, warns one researcher, people who work with child abusers must be careful to avoid stigmatizing those who need their help. The label "child abuser" may be so terrifying that many parents who need help will refrain from seeking it.[32] It's not useful to call child abusers "crazy" or "sick," either—a wide variety of people end up abusing their children when the stresses in their lives become intolerably painful.

CHILDREN AND SEXUAL ASSAULT

Sexual assault has long been a topic surrounded by secrecy and taboos; yet before they reach the age of eighteen, from 30 to 46 percent of all children are sexually assaulted in some way. Traditionally, parents warn their children to stay away from strangers, yet studies show that only 10 to 15 percent of sexual assaults involve strangers. The most common incidents are those in which a person already known to the child takes advantage of the child's trust and dependency on adults for protection. Many involve incestuous relationships between parent and child; the most common form is between father and daughter. It is believed that as many as 50,000 children each year are sexually abused by parents or guardians.[33] The myth is that most assaults are isolated, extreme incidents, violent attacks that take place suddenly, "out of the blue." But the reality is that most assaults involve a situation that develops gradually over a period of time, with frequent incidents; usually, the adult uses bribery or threats rather than extreme physical force.

The basic point here is that children are extremely vulnerable psychologically; they may not understand that their bodies are their own and that no one has a right to touch them in a way that makes them uncomfortable—that they *can* say no. Today, there is an increasing number of groups and organizations dedicated to making the public more aware of this problem and giving parents reassuring, common-sense guidelines for protecting children from sexual abuse and for dealing with it if does occur.

DIVORCE

In 1970 there were 47 divorced people for every 1,000 married people in the United States; today there are 109—more than twice as many.[34] About one marriage in three ends in divorce, and this may be because people today are much less willing to remain in unsatisfactory marriages. Studies show that the most common complaint from both husbands and wives is "mental cruelty," followed by "neglect of home and children." Wives are far more likely than husbands to complain about financial problems, physical abuse, drinking, and verbal abuse. Husbands are more likely to complain of sexual incompatibility and in-law trouble. About one-quarter of the wives and one-fifth of the husbands complain of infidelity.[35]

Divorce is financially difficult. To ease problems of division of property, child custody and support, and alimony, all but two states had by 1983 instituted some provision for "no-fault" divorce, eliminating the need for separate attorneys and substantially reducing costs. In some very recent settlements, compensation has been awarded to one spouse for having put the other through school. Changes have also taken place in the area of child custody, which is currently determined according to the best interests of the children involved. The laws in most states have been rewritten so that fathers now have an equal opportunity to gain custody of their children.

No matter what the law, though, the dissolution of a marriage is a painful experience for everyone involved. Divorced people are suddenly on their own, attempting to deal with feelings of loneliness, anger, rejection, and failure. Panic and self-doubt are common; but there is optimism, too. Divorce *can* represent a new beginning, a chance to rebuild one's life, and an opportunity to seek a more fulfilling relationship than the one left behind.

What effect does divorce have on children? For most children, the experience is very traumatic. Extreme anger, regression to earlier forms of behavior, and physical symptoms such as asthma are not uncommon. Younger children especially seem to blame themselves; older adolescents are more often angry or ashamed. For the first few months most children wish the separation could be repaired; they want the father or mother to rejoin the household. It helps if parents can explain that the child did not cause the divorce; often, children feel that something they did divided their parents. When very young children are involved, they may benefit from special preschool programs designed to help ease the trauma of divorce. Such programs enable the remaining parent to reorganize family routines without having a preschooler at home for a full day.

ALTERNATIVES TO MARRIAGE

Is it necessary to be married to be happy? How well do alternatives to marriage work? What steps can one take to make them work?

Single Living

With increasing numbers of people choosing to remain single or becoming single through divorce or the death of a spouse, there has been a new social acceptance of singlehood as a fulfilling lifestyle. No longer do people tend to assume that single individuals have been condemned to "bachelorhood" or "spinsterhood" because of family problems, personal inadequacies, or financial limitations. The new view accepts the right of people to pursue a life outside of marriage.

Statistics on single people show how quickly this change has come about. In 1980 there were 34 million singles in the United States; the number of adults under thirty-five who have never married has jumped by 50 percent since 1960. Both men and women are marrying later, and the divorce rate has more than doubled—from 2.2 per 1,000 population in 1960 to 5.3 two decades later.[36] There are 1.5 million people under thirty-five who are divorced but have not remarried—double the number in 1960.[37] A closer look at one detail offers a revealing insight: Studies of college women have shown that 40 percent of the seniors did not know whether or not they would ever marry; many of these young women said that they thought traditional marriage was obsolete.[38]

Who are the new singles? Some are men and women who have a new awareness about marriage and value their freedom and independence. This trend is perhaps most striking among women, who—with better jobs available to them—no longer see marriage as the only route to economic security.

The single state can be comfortable and fulfilling for many. But it does have disadvantages for some people. It is difficult for those who live alone to satisfy their needs for intimacy, interdependence, sexual gratification, and parenthood outside of marriage. They may have to make extra efforts to put together these "building blocks" of a full, satisfying life.

Single Parents

As the divorce rate grows, so does the number of families headed by a single parent. And when we add in the number of families affected by separation, desertion, or death of a spouse, plus the number of women who decide to have children without marrying, the number of single-parent families represents a large segment of America's population. About 20 percent of all children under age eighteen live with one or no parents.[39]

All single parents face the normal difficulties of raising children, but they also face some unique problems. Most must work full-time and somehow also juggle both household responsibilities and day-care arrangements for small children. They face the impossible task of trying to be both

More divorced fathers are becoming single parents, as most state laws now offer them an equal opportunity to gain custody of their children. (©Barbara Alper/ Stock, Boston)

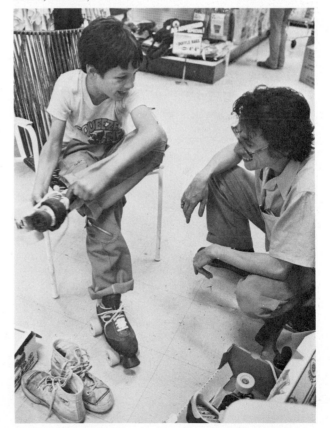

mother and father to the children. They must also make social lives for themselves in a world that still tends to be geared to married couples. And not least, single parents must cope with the everyday problems of childrearing without the help and emotional support of a spouse.

Cohabitation

The openness with which young people live together these days suggests that a new social institution is in the process of developing: **cohabitation,** an arrangement in which an unrelated man and woman live together without marrying. Today, with improved contraception and a decline in the emphasis on female virginity, moral objections to cohabitation are on the wane in many parts of the country, especially in the big cities. Some young people, aware of the complexities of marriage and alarmed about the increase in divorce rates, prefer to try living together first. This way, they hope, they can find out whether they are mature enough to engage in a lifelong caring relationship with another person. Often, they also want to find out if living together will interfere with the personal and professional development of either partner. One researcher has estimated that one-quarter of the college population have had a cohabitation experience and another 50 percent would cohabit if the situation presented itself.[40]

Cohabitation is not limited to young people. Because single, divorced, or widowed people who are retired sometimes lose their pension or social security benefits when they marry or remarry, a number of senior citizens are apparently also living together without formal marriage ties for economic reasons.

People who have been watching the trend toward cohabitation are eager to know the answers to a number of questions: Are people who cohabit able to sidestep the problems they expect to encounter in marriage? Are sex roles more equal among cohabiting partners? Will cohabitation erode the institution of marriage? Are those who cohabit free to come and go as they please, with no legal or emotional entanglements? We now have some answers to these and other questions.

First, available data suggest that the similarities between cohabitation and marriage are far more striking than the differences.[41] Cohabiting couples *aren't* more "liberated." The way they divide up labor closely mirrors the sex-role behavior of married couples their age, and there is no evidence that cohabitants are less monogamous than married couples.

Second, cohabitation is not necessarily a "free and easy" lifestyle. Though cohabitants are generally more likely than married couples to end an unsatisfactory relationship, they may have been just as deeply involved emotionally, and the breakup may be as painful as a divorce.

Nor has cohabitation displaced or eroded the institution of marriage, as many feared it would. Rather, cohabitation has been incorporated into the courtship phase for many young people, most of whom ultimately hope to marry. There is no evidence that cohabitation increases the likelihood of a successful marriage.

IS COHABITATION RIGHT FOR YOU?

If you're thinking about cohabiting, you should remember that living together often means different things to different people. For some, it is an arrangement of convenience without any commitment to a continuing relationship. Others regard cohabitation as a prelude to marriage. To avoid confusion and heartache, you should be careful to determine that the other person's goals are the same as yours. Don't forget: "Palimony" suits suggest that the dissolution of a living-together relationship is not without its difficulties.

MAKING HEALTH DECISIONS

Relating to Each Other: Plan Ahead to Prevent Problems

Many situations in daily living can cause conflict between wife and husband, between parents and children, or between other people in close relationships. These conflicts can be a source of irritation to all concerned, and they can result in more friction than is really necessary.

How can people living in intimate relationships avoid undue tension? One good way is to develop "anticipatory skills" for relating to each other, to reduce the chance that entangled problems will grow out of annoying everyday conflicts. The goal is to find a way of acting in the situation that will meet *everyone's* needs—not just yours. The process involves several steps: (1) Take a good look at your own feelings before you react. (2) Think about the feelings/attitudes you *believe* the other person has. (Often, you will find you don't really have evidence to support your assumptions—the other person may feel quite differently than you expected.) (3) Think through your goals in the situation—remembering that you are trying to find a way of meeting everyone's needs in this situation, at least partially. (4) Make a mental list of the various actions you could take that would make the situation worse—leading to later arguments and hidden grudges. (5) Finally, make a mental list of the various actions you could take that would make the situation better.

Following are five typical situations that might arise among people in close relationships. We'll go through the first situation in detail; in the remaining four, you will be able to supply your own detail.

SITUATION 1

You are attempting to talk to your spouse and you notice that the spouse is continuing to read a magazine while you are attempting to communicate.

a. What are your feelings? (These might include feeling angry, hateful, alone, hurt, ignored, pugnacious, upset, inferior, frustrated—*or* you might feel accepting, empathetic, loving, intimate, amused—*or* you might have other feelings.) Your feelings might well be mixed. Write *all* the feelings you think you would have in this situation: _____

_____

_____

_____

b. How do you interpret your spouse's behavior? What feelings and attitudes do you *think* he or she has? These might include one or more of the following:

_____Spouse is trying to avoid you.

_____Spouse is unaware of your intent.

_____Spouse is not interested in what you have to say.

_____Spouse is angry at you.

_____Spouse is too interested in himself or herself.

_____Spouse has a hearing defect.

_____Spouse is bored with you.

_____Spouse is no longer in love with you.

_____Spouse is having an affair.

Check *all* the feelings you *think* your partner has, and write any additional ones: _____

_____

_____

_____

Now ask yourself: do you have evidence that your spouse really feels this way? How realistic are your assumptions about your spouse's feelings?

c. Your goal: What would you try to accomplish in this situation? (Don't forget: you are trying to find a way to meet the needs of both people in the situation.)_____

d. Undesirable actions you could take: There are a number of things you could do in this situation that might turn the minor conflict into an entangled, ongoing problem. They include:

_____Yell/scream (e.g., "I feel ignored!")

_____Throw something (e.g., a pillow)

_____Physically shake spouse

_____Pull away the magazine roughly

_____Leave the room (loudly)

_____Sulk (openly)

_____Sulk (privately)

_____Set the magazine on fire

_____Spill water on spouse

Or you might do other equally nonconstructive things. Indicate any undesirable actions you think you might take: _____

e. Desirable actions you could take: There are a number of things you could do in this situation that could help prevent further problems from developing, and that might meet the needs of both you and your spouse. They include:

_____Gently touch spouse to gain his or her attention

_____Pull away the magazine (slowly and gently)

_____Leave the room (silently)

_____Ask for spouse's attention

_____Sit next to spouse and start reading too

Or you might do other constructive things. Indicate the actions you think would be most positive and responsible in this situation: _____

SITUATION 2

Your ten-year-old child regularly comes to the table with dirty hands.

a. What are your feelings? _____

b. What do you *think* the child's feelings and attitudes are? (Don't forget: after you list them, ask yourself whether you have evidence for your assumptions.) _____

c. What are your goals in this situation? _____

d. What undesirable actions might you take? _____

e. What desirable actions might you take that could help meet the needs of everyone in this situation?_____

_____

_____

_____

SITUATION 3

A close friend repeatedly telephones you while you are at work or school. She has a tendency to talk about her personal affairs for half an hour at a time. You are really too busy to talk to her, but it will be several weeks before you can see her for lunch or after hours.

a. Your feelings: _____

_____

_____

_____

b. The feelings and attitudes you *think* the other person has (don't forget to ask yourself how realistic your assumptions are): _____

_____

_____

_____

c. Your goals in this situation: _____

_____

_____

_____

d. Undesirable actions you might take: _____

_____

_____

_____

e. Desirable actions you might take: _____

_____

_____

_____

SITUATION 4

Your partner refuses to do any housework or yardwork. You seem to be doing all the work around the home.

a. Your feelings: _____

_____

_____

_____

b. The feelings and attitudes you *think* the other person has: _____

_____

_____

_____

c. Your goals in this situation: _____

_____

_____

_____

d. Undesirable actions you might take: _____

_____

_____

_____

e. Desirable actions you might take: _____

_____

_____

_____

SITUATION 5

You are the parent of a twenty-year-old college junior who has been placed on academic probation. His or her grades have gotten continually worse since midway through the sophomore year.

a. Your feelings: _____

_____

_____

_____

b. The feelings and attitudes you *think* your child has: _____

_____

_____

_____

c. Your goals in this situation: _____

_____

_____

_____

d. Undesirable actions you might take: _____

_____

_____

_____

e. Desirable actions you might take: _____

_____

_____

_____

Source: Adapted from Judith S. D'Augelli and Joan M. Weener, *Communication and Parenting Skills* (State College, Pa.: Pennsylvania State University, Division of Counseling and Educational Psychology, 1977), pp. 47–59.

SUMMARY

1. Intimate relationships can fulfill important human needs for a closeness, love, sharing everyday experiences, reassurance about one's worth, nurturance, and support. Marriage has traditionally been an economic arrangement, but today many people expect marriage to fulfill other needs.

2. People get married in response to external social pressures—economic advantage, legitimization of sex, and pressure from family or social group—as well as for personal reasons. People improve their chances for long-term happiness in marriage if they examine their motives before they marry.

3. People usually choose mates who are similar to themselves in ethnic, religious, economic, and educational background. Physical appearance and compatibility of personalities are other important factors in mate selection.

4. Many women today are marrying later and devoting less energy to finding a husband.

5. People in happy marriages are likely to have certain skills. They know how to be intimate, to communicate, to share power, and to resolve differences rather than letting them fester. Unhappy marriages tend to be plagued by communications difficulties. Money, sex, and division of labor are common problem areas in marriage.

6. Quarrels between spouses are of three basic types. Acute quarrels are sharp and loud and tend to occur in new relationships as the partners jockey for position. Progressive quarrels never really end the conflict between partners, and arguments tend to blend into one another. Habituated conflict is the situation when partners agree to accommodate each other on issues about which they will never agree.

7. Couples choose to have children for a variety of reasons, some better than others: for example, to stabilize a marriage or to enrich a strong relationship.

8. Parents have a responsibility to safeguard the health and growth of their children and to help them develop emotionally, intellectually, and socially.

9. Infants and older children are not passive beings. They contribute actively to social exchanges with their parents and others. Children are born with distinct temperaments.

10. For a long time, it was believed that only mothers could adequately care for their children. But many women who left home to work and so-

cial scientists interested in child development have challenged that assumption. It is now believed that consistent, loving care from mother, father, or other caretaker is healthy for children. Children need their fathers to be active parents, from whom they derive certain important qualities. Working mothers and nurturant fathers can produce well-adjusted children, and good child-care arrangements can be very healthy for all family members.

11. Violence occurs in as many as half of all American marriages, cutting across all racial, religious, and socioeconomic lines. Husbands abuse wives more than the reverse. Factors that correlate with violence between spouses include: a husband's belief that he has a right to control family members; isolation of the family from outsiders; a wife who is unable to leave; and early association of family life with physical pain.

12. Child abusers who come to the attention of authorities tend to have low incomes and low occupational status and to have been abused or neglected themselves as children.

13. Sexual abuse of children is more common than was once assumed. Sexual assault usually involves not a stranger, but someone the child already knows. Children often do not understand that they have the right to say no to anyone whose attentions make them feel uncomfortable.

14. One in three marriages ends in divorce. Because divorce is so painful, most states have instituted "no-fault" divorce laws to reduce the hardships of ending a marriage.

15. Alternatives to traditional marriage are being pursued by more people. These include remaining single, single parenthood, and cohabitation.

GLOSSARY

cohabitation An arrangement in which an unrelated man and woman live together without marrying.

dual-career marriage A marriage in which both partners seriously pursue a professional career.
socialization The process by which people learn the ways of a given society or social group so that they can function within it.

NOTES

1. L. M. Vebrugge, "Marital Status and Health," *Journal of Marriage and the Family* 4 (1979): 267.

2. Bernard I. Murstein, "Mate Selection in the 1970s," *Journal of Marriage and the Family* 42, no. 4 (November 1980): 777–792.

3. Bernard I. Murstein, ed., *Theories of Attraction and Love* (New York: Springer, 1971).

4. Murstein, "Mate Selection."

5. C. T. Hill, Z. Rubin, and L. A. Peplau, "Breakups Before Marriage: The End of 103 Affairs," *The Journal of Social Issues* 32 (1976): 147–168.

6. Arthur Burton, "Marriage Without Failure," in B. J. Chesser and A. A. Gray, eds., *Marriage: Creating a Partnership,* 2nd ed. (Dubuque, Iowa: Kendall-Hunt, 1979), pp. 81–86; Edward Waring et al., "Dimensions of Intimacy in Marriage," *Psychiatry* 44 (May 1981): 169–175; W. R. Beavers, "A Theoretical Basis for Family Evaluation," in J. M. Lewis et al., eds., *No Single Thread: Psychological Health in Family Systems* (New York: Brunner-Mazel, 1976), pp. 46–82.

7. Burton, "Marriage Without Failure," p. 84.

8. Julia A. Ericksen, William L. Yancey, and Eugene P. Ericksen, "The Division of Family Roles," *Journal of Marriage and the Family* 41, no. 2 (May 1979): 301–312; Karen P. Goebel, "Time Use and Family Life," *Family Economics Review,* Summer 1981: 22, 24.

9. G. R. Leslie and E. M. Leslie, *Marriage in a Changing World* (New York: Wiley, 1977), p. 279.

10. Ibid., pp. 154–156.

11. John M. Last, *Maxcy-Rosenau's Public Health and Preventive Medicine,* 11th ed. (New York: Appleton-Century-Crofts, 1980), pp. 1756–1757, 1087–1088, 252.

12. Ira Gordon, "Parenting, Teaching and Child Development," *Young Children,* March 1976, p. 179.

13. Benjamin S. Bloom, *Stability and Change in Human Characteristics* (New York: Wiley, 1964), p. 68.

14. F. P. Rice, *Marriage and Parenthood* (Boston: Allyn & Bacon, 1979), p. 567.

15. Jerome Kagan and Howard A. Moss, *Birth to Maturity* (New York: Wiley, 1962).

16. Richard Q. Bell, "Parent, Child, and Reciprocal Influences," *American Psychologist* 34, no. 10 (October 1979): 821–826.

17. Ibid.

18. Peter Smith, "Shared Care of Young Children: Alternative Models to Monotropism," *Merrill-Palmer Quarterly* 26, no. 4 (1980): 371.

19. Lois Hoffman, "Maternal Employment: 1979," *American Psychologist* 34, no. 10 (October 1979): 859.

20. R. J. Goldberg, "Maternal Time Use and Preschool Performance," paper presented at the Meeting for Research in Child Development, New Orleans, March 1977.

21. Hoffman, "Maternal Employment: 1979," p. 861.

22. Michael Lamb, "Paternal Influences and the Father's Role," *American Psychologist* 34, no. 10 (October 1979): 938.

23. James Henderson, "On Fathering (The Nature and Functions of the Father Role), Part II: Conceptualization of Fathering," *Canadian Journal of Psychiatry* 25 (1980): 419–421, 425.

24. David Lynn, "Father and America in Transition," in Arlene S. Skolnick and Jerome H. Skolnick, eds., *Family in Transition,* 2nd ed. (Boston: Little, Brown, 1977), pp. 380–384.

25. Urie Bronfenbrenner, "Liberated Women: How They're Changing American Life," interview conducted for *U.S. News and World Report,* June 7, 1975, p. 49.

26. R. A. Hunt and E. J. Rydman, *Creative Marriage,* 2nd ed. (Boston: Allyn & Bacon, 1979), pp. 309–310.

27. Quoted in *Redbook,* May 1979, p. 100.

28. Hunt and Rydman, *Creative Marriage,* pp. 313–314, 316.

29. Richard J. Gelles, "Demythologizing Child Abuse," in Skolnick and Skolnick, *Family in Transition,* p. 391.

30. Ibid., pp. 390–391.

31. Rand Conger, Robert Burgess, and Carol Barrett, "Child Abuse Related to Life Change and Perceptions of Illness: Some Preliminary Findings," *The Family Coordinator,* January 1979, p. 75.

32. Gelles, "Demythologizing Child Abuse," p. 393.

33. D. Finkelhor, "Psychological, Cultural, and Family Factors in Incest and Family Sexual Abuse," *Journal of Marriage and Family Counseling* 4, no. 4 (October 1978): 41–49; A. W. Burgess et al., *Sexual Assault on Children and Adolescents* (Lexington, Mass.: Heath, 1978); R. Summit and J. Kryso, "Sexual Abuse of Children: A Clinical Spectrum," *American Journal of Orthopsychiatry* 48 (1078): 237 251.

34. "Marital Status and Living Arrangements," *Current Population Reports,* Series P-20, No. 372 (March 1981): 1, 4.

35. Leslie and Leslie, *Marriage in a Changing World,* pp. 300–301.

36. National Center for Health Statistics, "Births, Marriages, Divorces, and Deaths for 1982," *Monthly Vital Statistics Report* 31, no. 12 (March 14, 1983): 1.

37. P. J. Stein, "Singlehood: An Alternative to Marriage," in Skolnick and Skolnick, *Family in Transition,* p. 518.

38. Carol C. Nadelson and Malkah T. Notman, "To Marry or Not to Marry: A Choice," *American Journal of Psychiatry* 138, no. 10 (October 1981): 1352–1356.

39. Rice, *Marriage and Parenthood,* p. 570.

40. Eleanor D. Macklin, "Nonmarital Heterosexual Cohabitation," in Chesser and Gray, *Marriage: Creating a Partnership,* pp. 63–76.

41. Ibid., p. 67.

PART FOUR

Reducing Health Risks: The Struggle Against Disease

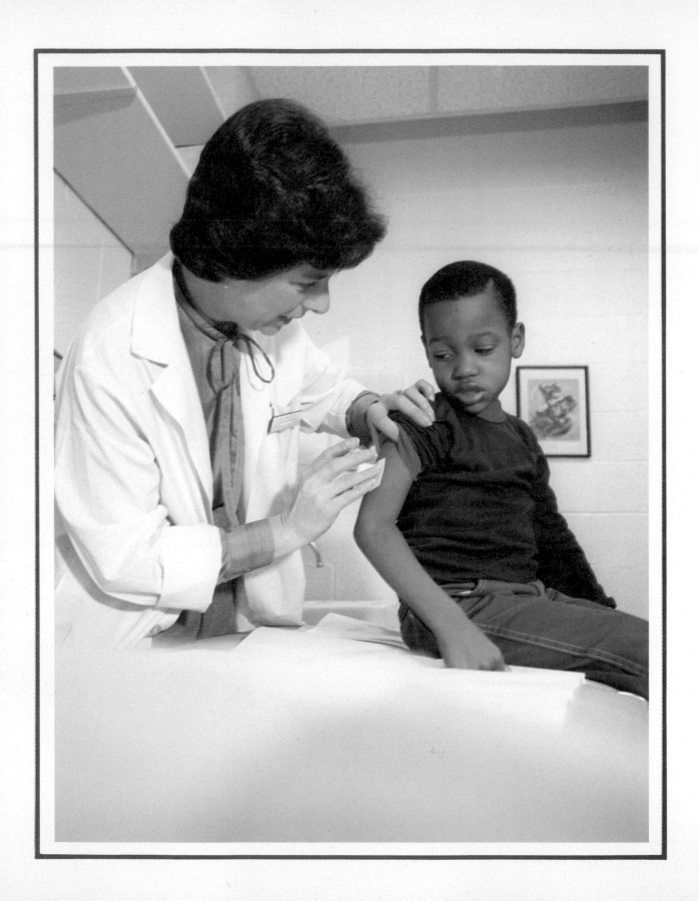

CHAPTER 10

Infectious Diseases

Did you know that there are about 15 million *million* microorganisms living on, and in, your body right now? There are billions in your mouth alone, perhaps 100 billion on your skin, and billions more in other parts of your body, particularly your intestines. As Anton van Leeuwenhoek, the first person ever to see bacteria, wrote in 1683, "there are more animals living in the scum on the teeth in a man's mouth, than there are men in a whole kingdom."[1] These microscopic organisms with which people live most intimately and harmoniously are called **endogenous,** or "resident," microorganisms, meaning that they normally reside within the human host. They are so small that the billions of them in your body combined probably would not take up much more than one and one quarter measuring cups. Most of them are quite compatible with the health of the human body, and in fact may contribute to its welfare.

Yet endogenous microorganisms cannot be regarded as completely or permanently harmless. If you are tired or in poor health, or in certain other circumstances, these microorganisms can cause serious disease. Disease can also be caused by **exogenous microorganisms**—microscopic organisms that are not normally residents of the human body —such as those that cause plague, cholera, influenza, tetanus, and sexually transmitted diseases. If you look in a medical textbook, you'll find a thick section on infectious disease: Modern medicine recognizes over five hundred infectious diseases, each caused by a different microorganism.

An **infection** is the invasion of the body by disease-causing organisms and the reaction of the body to their presence. Everyone knows what it feels like to contract an infectious disease, or have an infection. If you have a local infection, the site of the infection may become sore, hot, and swollen; if the infection spreads to other parts of your body, you may have fever, nausea, vomiting, or other uncomfortable symptoms. But what actually happens inside your body while this is going on? What do the unfriendly microbes look like? How do they get in and start to work their damage, and how does the body try to fight them off? This is the topic we're going to look at in this chapter. We'll discover that infectious disease, though mysterious and perhaps frightening, isn't always something that just "happens" to a person; there are many levels on which human behavior can make a great difference.

AGENTS OF INFECTION— AND SOME DISEASES THEY CAUSE

Like the natural world around you, your own body is part of the environment. You're the host to countless tiny animal organisms and plantlike organisms, plus some that are neither animals nor plants—all living together in your body and carrying out their own basic life functions of respiration, metabolism, excretion, growth, and reproduction.

Six categories of these organisms can become **pathogens,** or agents of infectious disease: bacteria, viruses, rickettsiae, fungi, protozoa, and worms (see the photographs on p. 240).

Bacteria

Most plentiful of the microorganisms endogenous to humans are the various kinds of **bacteria** (singu-

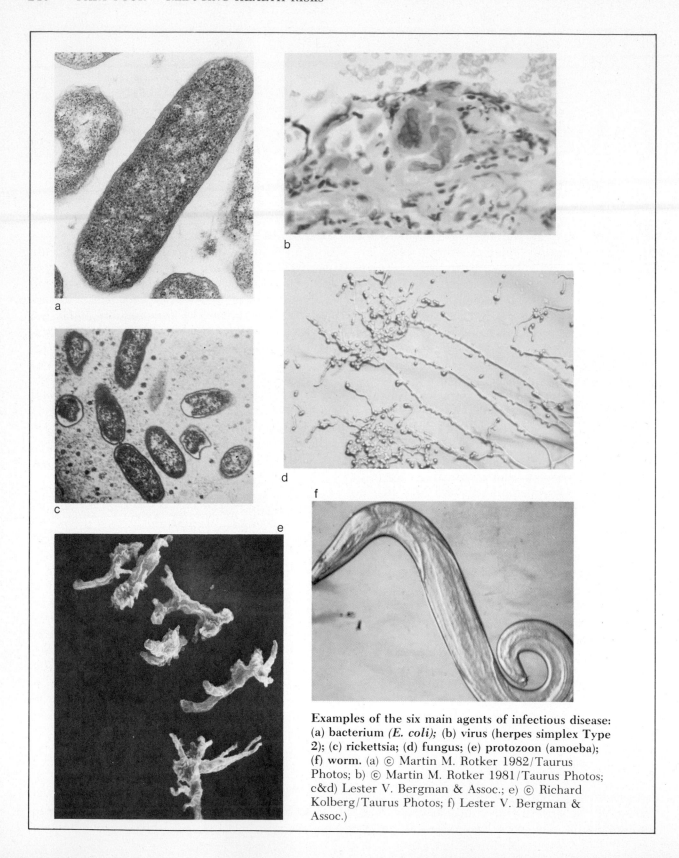

Examples of the six main agents of infectious disease:
(a) bacterium *(E. coli);* (b) virus (herpes simplex Type
2); (c) rickettsia; (d) fungus; (e) protozoon (amoeba);
(f) worm. (a) © Martin M. Rotker 1982/Taurus
Photos; b) © Martin M. Rotker 1981/Taurus Photos;
c&d) Lester V. Bergman & Assoc.; e) © Richard
Kolberg/Taurus Photos; f) Lester V. Bergman &
Assoc.)

lar: *bacterium*). Each of these tiny organisms consists of just one cell, with a protective cell wall and all the structures it needs to carry out its life functions. The bacteria fall into the category of *flora,* or plantlike organisms.

ENDOGENOUS BACTERIA AND DISEASE

Most kinds of endogenous bacteria are not harmful, and some, in fact, are vital to our existence. The bacterium *Escherichia coli* (often called *E. coli*), for example, lives in our intestines and is essential to the synthesis of the B vitamins; others help to kill off foreign infectious organisms. But our own endogenous bacteria can cause disease if for some reason they get out of hand. Skin bacteria sometimes cause acne; mouth bacteria sometimes help cause pyorrhea, a serious gum disease; intestinal bacteria may get into the urethra, particularly in a woman, and cause urinary tract infections. Different strains of *E. coli,* which we may be exposed to through travel, may cause diarrhea until our system adjusts to their presence.

STREPTOCOCCAL INFECTIONS Streptococcal bacteria, small dotlike organisms that grow in long chains, usually inhabit our mucous membranes, particularly those of the nose, mouth, throat, and intestines. If our resistance is lowered, they may cause disease such as "strep throat" (a severe throat infection), peritonitis (severe inflammation within the abdomen), scarlet fever (an acute fever with sore throat and rash), or rheumatic fever (an infection that primarily affects the joints and the heart). Streptococcal infections often produce spreading inflammation throughout the body.

Other streptococci may be introduced from outside the body, and this was once the cause of many cases of "childbed fever," which killed many new mothers in centuries past. The streptococci in this instance were introduced by the infected hands of the doctor or other attendant at childbirth.

WHAT YOU CAN DO: STREP THROAT

It's extremely important that a person with strep throat see a physician as soon as possible. If left untreated, a strep throat can lead to rheumatic

fever, heart valve disease, or other dangerous complications. How can you tell if a sore throat is probably caused by strep? Using a flashlight or other strong light, look for white or yellow patches, caused by pus, at the back of the throat. If these patches are present, see a doctor for diagnosis and treatment.

STAPHYLOCOCCAL INFECTIONS Staphylococci, which grow in small clusters, are normally present on our skin, and most of the time they live there harmlessly. Occasionally, however, if there is a scratch or other small opening in the skin, the staphylococci will get in. They usually produce a localized infection—in contrast to the widespread infections often caused by streptococci. All of us who have had pimples on the skin have had minor staphylococci ("staph") infections, and staphylococci are also the cause of more serious infections, such as boils (in which the organisms penetrate the skin more deeply) and styes (infections on the eyelids). When a cut or wound becomes infected, the invading organisms are likely to be staphylococci. The redness and soreness around the cut are the results of the body's defense against the infection. (We'll talk more about these defenses later.)

TOXIC SHOCK SYNDROME In 1980 and 1981, the public was made aware of a new and dangerous infectious disease—toxic shock syndrome, or TSS. The victim of TSS usually experiences headache, sore throat, high fever, pain in the abdomen, diarrhea, vomiting, and sometimes a skin rash. Blood pressure may drop suddenly and drastically, and shock and death may follow if the disease is not treated.[2]

News reports stressed that the disorder was most likely to occur in menstruating women, particularly those who used high-absorbency tampons. The culprit apparently is *Staphylococcus aureus* ("golden staphylococcus"), a strain named for its color when grown in colonies in the laboratory. Although staphylococcal infections are usually local, they can sometimes spread through the body, and this is what happens in TSS. TSS and menstruation seem to be connected because blood-soaked tampons offer the bacteria a fertile haven in the vagina. From this initial infection,

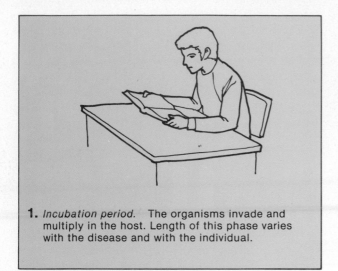

1. *Incubation period.* The organisms invade and multiply in the host. Length of this phase varies with the disease and with the individual.

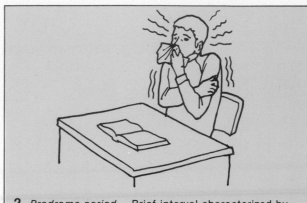

2. *Prodrome period.* Brief interval characterized by general symptoms such as headache, fever, runny nose, irritability, and general discomfort. Disease is highly communicable now.

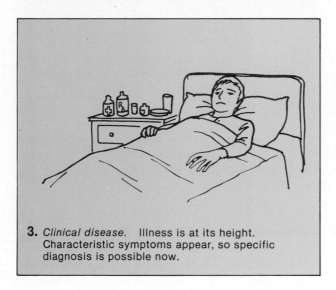

3. *Clinical disease.* Illness is at its height. Characteristic symptoms appear, so specific diagnosis is possible now.

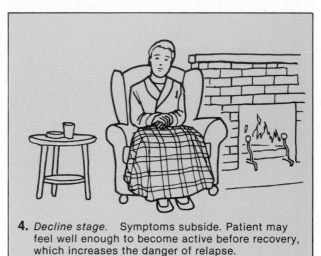

4. *Decline stage.* Symptoms subside. Patient may feel well enough to become active before recovery, which increases the danger of relapse.

Figure 10.1   Stages in the Course of an Infectious Disease

All infectious diseases depend on essentially the same mechanism: invasion by foreign organisms and the reaction of the invaded body to them. Therefore, infectious diseases have a common pattern, marked by the five phases summarized here.

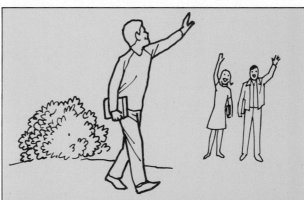

5. *Convalescence.* The recovery period. Disease may still be communicable. Patient who recovers but still gives off disease-causing organisms becomes a *carrier* of that disease.

the bacteria seem to produce a powerful toxin that produces a number of serious symptoms.

Although most cases of TSS reported in the United States occur in menstruating women (about 85 percent of all cases in 1981), the disease was first identified in 1978 in a group of children, and it continues to be reported in men, children, and nonmenstruating women (see Figure 10.2).[3] The nonmenstrual TSS is also thought to be caused by *Staphylococcus aureus,* in this case usually growing in a wound, a surgical incision, or some other body opening. Although researchers are still studying the link between tampon use and TSS, the connection is not yet clear.

WHAT YOU CAN DO:
TOXIC SHOCK SYNDROME (TSS)

Everyone should know the symptoms of TSS: headache, sore throat, fever, abdominal pain, diarrhea, vomiting, sometimes a rash. Millions of women have used tampons for years without developing the disease, but women who want to avoid even the small risk of developing TSS may

want to avoid tampons or to use them during only part of their menstrual periods.

EXOGENOUS BACTERIA AND DISEASE

A number of major diseases are caused by exogenous bacteria—gonorrhea, meningitis, tetanus, and syphilis, to name just a few. Some of these are being brought under control, thanks to **antibiotics** —a group of drugs that destroy or inhibit the growth of disease-causing bacteria. The bacterium

Figure 10.2   Confirmed Cases of Toxic Shock Syndrome in the United States, January 1970–March 1982

During the period shown, 1,660 cases of toxic shock syndrome were reported, mostly among white women of menstruating age. (The colored areas within the bars indicate cases among men, children, and non-menstrual women.) The incidence of TSS began to decline in 1981, possibly because more women heeded warnings to stop using superabsorbent tampons and to alternate tampons with sanitary napkins during their periods, to discourage the growth of bacteria.

Source: Centers for Disease Control, *Morbidity and Mortality Weekly Report* 31, no. 16 (April 30, 1982): 201.

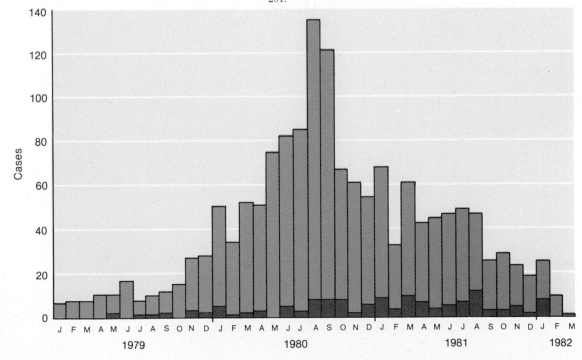

that causes tuberculosis is an example: in the 1930s about 80 percent of all Americans became infected with it before they were twenty years old, but today less than 5 percent become infected in most parts of the U.S., though there has been an upsurge of the disease in some metropolitan areas.[4] *Legionella pneumophila* is another example: Once experts figured out the link between this microbe and Legionnaire's disease, they determined that it could be controlled with the antibiotic erythromycin.

But there is an ominous new trend: Many bacteria have now developed resistance to antibiotics. About forty times as much penicillin is needed now to treat some infections as was needed when the drug was first used during World War II. Ominous, too, is the recent upsurge in certain bacterial sexually transmitted diseases, some of which are resistant to antibiotics. (We'll discuss sexually transmitted diseases in more detail later in this chapter.)

BACTERIAL TOXINS

As we mentioned, the symptoms in TSS are caused by **toxins** (poisonous substances) that the bacteria produce. Certain other bacteria also produce dangerous toxins. Diphtheria and tetanus are caused by bacterial toxins. The tiny botulinus bacterium is another example. This organism is harmless when it's eaten; it's often present on food. But if it is growing in a place where there is low acidity and little or no oxygen (inside a sealed can, for example), it starts to produce a toxin. One-millionth of a gram of this toxin can kill a person—and just one pint of the toxin would be enough to kill everyone on earth.

Viruses

When students took college biology twenty-five years ago, they were taught that one-celled animals and plants were the simplest living things that existed. But more recently, scientists realized that there is an even simpler form of life—viruses. Viruses cause mumps, measles, rubella (German measles), smallpox, and a number of other diseases. Viruses have a mysterious ability to exist and proliferate without carrying out the life functions of respiration and metabolism as we usually think

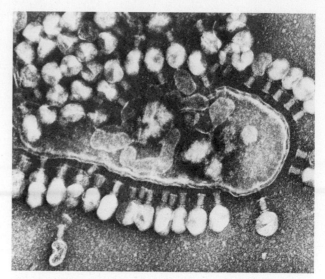

Viruses attacking a cell. This is an *E. coli* bacteria cell, but the process of viral infection is similar for human beings. Some of the viruses (those whose heads show white) have injected their DNA into the cell. The DNA is the genetic material that "takes over" the cell's machinery, instructing it to manufacture and release more virus particles. This cycle of virus infection takes only about 20 minutes to complete. (© Lee D. Simon/Photo Researchers, Inc.)

of these functions. Viruses are parasites of cells and live within the cells themselves. Some scientists doubt that they should even be considered totally living things.

What viruses *do* is reproduce. A single virus is nothing more than a bit of nucleic acid within a protein coat. Nucleic acid is the biochemical substance that carries genetic information—the information an organism needs in order to produce more organisms just like itself. (There are two kinds of nucleic acids, RNA and DNA: a virus contains one of these, but never both.) Thus, a virus is really just a machine designed to duplicate itself. In fact, a **virus** is best defined as a microorganism that can reproduce only in living cells of a person or animal.

Once inside a cell, a virus takes over the cell's machinery and directs it to produce many hundreds of new viruses. The cell, thus engorged with new viruses, breaks apart and spews its contents in all directions. Each new virus can enter another cell, capture its machinery, and start the cycle again.

Viruses don't seem to be affected by antibiotics: Once an individual has contracted a viral infection, drugs will not help fight the infection, nor will they cure it. But there is a brighter side to the picture: When exposed to *some* viruses, the body produces its own protective substance to help ward the virus off. This substance is called interferon, and we'll discuss it in more detail later in this chapter. Thanks to interferon, our bodies can develop a long-lasting immunity to the original virus we "caught." Unfortunately, not all viruses stimulate the body to produce interferon.

VIRAL INFECTIONS: THE COMMON COLD

The common cold is practically a universal nuisance; it contributes heavily to the amount of time lost from school and work each year. One theory suggests that healthy people carry cold viruses in their noses and throats all the time, but they exhibit cold symptoms only when something like fatigue or lowered resistance produces favorable circumstances for the viruses to proliferate. Be this as it may, colds are "catching." Cold viruses seem to survive in the air, beginning their journey to another person either in the spray of droplets

Cold viruses can travel over three feet from one person to another in the droplets from a sneeze, unless they are caught in a handkerchief or tissue. (© Alec Duncan 1982/Taurus Photos)

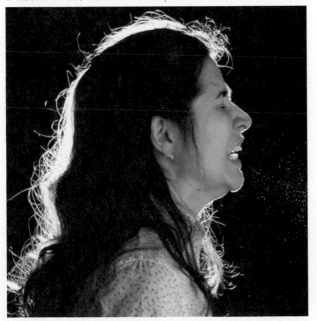

from a sneeze or in the air exhaled when a cold victim talks or breathes. They are also transmitted by skin contact, as when an infected person shakes another person's hand. The period of time between first exposure to the virus and the appearance of symptoms—the **incubation period**—is short, usually about eighteen to forty-eight hours.

Scientists know frustratingly little about cold viruses. They do know that a large number of different viruses can cause colds—and more may still be discovered. Also, cold viruses seem to differ from other viruses in that they do not cause the body to produce interferon or any other substance that could give long-lasting immunity. It may be that cold viruses mutate (change their genetic information) rapidly. If so, each successive cold could be caused by a different virus, resulting in an endless series of apparently similar diseases.

WHAT YOU CAN DO
TO HELP PREVENT COLDS

There is little you can do beyond avoiding people with "new colds" (colds are most communicable during the first twenty-four hours) or staying away from others when you yourself have a new cold. It is probably useful to keep your resistance up through adequate nutrition, rest, control of stress, and exercise. (Experts don't agree on this, though.) We discuss home care for colds in more detail in Chapter 16.

INFLUENZA

Influenza, or "flu," is not usually a serious disease unless it is complicated by secondary infection. When bacteria become involved, or when the flu virus spreads to the lungs, the condition may be lethal—particularly for the very young, the elderly, and those with heart or respiratory disease. The flu has killed more than half a million Americans in the last twenty years.[5]

According to recent research, the flu virus is "packaged" in a distinct way. In other viruses the strands of nucleic acid are strung together in one line, but in the flu virus the strands are in eight separate pieces—which makes it easier for a strand to become detached and change places with a strand from another virus.[6] Thus, the genetic information in the virus can change rapidly. Not surprisingly, there are not only three major varieties of flu virus—A (the most virulent), B, and C—but numerous changing strains within each type. Those who have immunity against one variety or strain do not necessarily have immunity against any other.

There is a fascinating possibility that flu viruses may actually "go south for the summer"! Sometimes, at the end of one winter epidemic, there is a cluster of flu cases caused not by the viral strain in *that* epidemic, but by another strain; this second strain often turns out to be the one that will cause the epidemic of the next winter. What happens to this new strain of viruses over the summer? One researcher believes they may actually migrate to another geographic location (possibly in the Southern Hemisphere), and return later.[7]

WHAT YOU CAN DO TO HELP PREVENT FLU

► There are vaccines against specific strains of flu virus, but they are not effective against other strains. Nevertheless, people over sixty-five, pregnant women, and people with chronic cardiovascular disease and certain other diseases should be vaccinated.[8] The components of the vaccine are changed periodically, so individuals must be revaccinated each year.

► Beyond that, at this point, you can only take the precautions you would take against colds: Stay away from people with the disease, and try to keep your resistance up.

Eventually, scientists may be able to offer more in the way of concrete help. Experiments are currently under way with two new drugs—amantadine and rimantadine—that may have some effectiveness. A vaccine that will give a longer period of immunity is also being worked on.[9]

OTHER VIRAL DISEASES: HEPATITIS AND MONONUCLEOSIS

HEPATITIS   Hepatitis (viral inflammation of the liver) has increased significantly in recent years, particularly among young people. Hepatitis A, commonly called infectious hepatitis, is the more common type (and, fortunately, usually the less dangerous); hepatitis B (which used to be called

serum hepatitis) is not common but is far more dangerous. The two types have similar symptoms —fever, headache, nausea, loss of appetite, and pain in the upper right abdomen. The urine becomes deep yellow, and the individual may become jaundiced. Researchers are working on vaccines for both types.[10] Immunization is now available for hepatitis A.

Both types of hepatitis may be prolonged illnesses, and both may damage the liver. In only one out of ten cases is the liver so badly damaged that the illness becomes clinically identifiable, but that one case may be extremely dangerous. If the liver failure is serious enough to cause a coma, the patient has only a 10 to 20 percent chance of surviving.[11]

WHAT CAUSES HEPATITIS? THINGS TO WATCH OUT FOR

Hepatitis Type A is generally transmitted by fecal contamination of food or water. Type B is transmitted through the blood and other body secretions; it is passed on from an infected person through blood transfusion or by improper sterilization or disposal of needles. It may also be sexually transmitted, particularly between male homosexuals who have had many sexual partners. Drug users, people who get tattoos, and hospital workers may become exposed very easily.

INFECTIOUS MONONUCLEOSIS   Infectious mononucleosis, or "mono," is common among high school and college students. Its short-term symptoms, which can be severe, can include fever, sore throat, nausea, chills, and general weakness; the individual may sometimes have a rash, enlarged and tender lymph glands, jaundice, and/or enlargement of the spleen as well. Other symptoms may mimic more serious diseases such as polio, meningitis, TB, diphtheria, and leukemia. Fortunately, mono can be diagnosed with a simple blood test.

The longer-term symptoms of mono are the frustrating ones: though permanent disability is unusual, the general weakness and feeling of fatigue can last for weeks or months. As one person who had had mono put it, "Every time I climbed one flight of stairs to my bedroom I had to lie down and take an hour's nap." Happily—for no one who has had mono ever wants to have it again—experts generally agree that the disease confers fairly long, if not permanent, immunity.[12]

What causes mono, and how is it spread? Research in the late 1960s identified a virus known as the Epstein-Barr virus as the cause of the most common form of infectious mononucleosis.[13] Though the disease is often teasingly referred to as the "kissing disease," kissing is probably only one of several ways it is spread. Strangely, however, it does not spread easily by ordinary contact; in fact, it is rare to have more than one case in a household.

Other Agents of Infection

RICKETTSIAE

Rickettsiae are considered to be intermediate between bacteria and viruses. Most of these organisms grow in the intestinal tracts of insects and insectlike creatures. The insect may serve as a **vector,** or carrier, of the infectious agent, transferring the organism to a human host.[14]

If you've ever tried to pick a tick off your ankle with a tweezer or get it to back out of your skin by covering it with oil, you've had first-hand experience with how a rickettsia vector operates. Ticks can transmit Rocky Mountain spotted fever; be very careful with them. Typhus fever is another major disease that's transmitted this way—the vectors are fleas, ticks, and lice.

FUNGI

Fungi are another type of infectious agent that many of us have had first-hand experience with: Athlete's foot is caused by fungi, and so is ringworm. The **fungi** are many-celled organisms (the mushrooms are a member of this family). Specifically, they're a type of plant that lacks chlorophyll and must therefore obtain food from organic material—in some cases, from humans. They tend to invade areas where these is much body hair, such as the scalp and the groin.

ANIMAL PARASITES

Last are the animal parasites; these include some single-celled animals (**protozoa**) and certain **para-**sitic worms, which of course are many-celled animals. An **animal parasite** is an organism that has developed the capacity to live in or on the body of another animal, known as the **host.** Animal parasites obtain food from the host; thus they live at the host's expense, weakening it and causing disease. Most animal parasites have acquired a remarkable ability: They spend part of their lives in one host (a human being) and the rest of their lives in another host (which can range from a mosquito to a cow; fish are particularly common hosts). Some major tropical diseases, including amoebic dysentery and malaria, are caused by protozoan parasites. There are some worms that make their homes in humans, including pinworms, tapeworms, and flukes.

HOW DOES THE BODY DEFEND ITSELF AGAINST INFECTION?

Suppose a pathogenic agent (an organism that is capable of causing an infection) does invade the body. The threat is that it will cause disease—either because it is present in great numbers or can multiply to great numbers (as in pneumonia) or because it can release toxins (as in botulism, TSS, tetanus, or diphtheria). What can the body do to fight off the pathogen?

The Outer Defenses

The skin and mucous membranes are the body's first line of defense. An invading microbe must find its way through the skin or the mucosae, the mucus-coated membranes that make an "inner skin" for the body by lining the respiratory, digestive, and urogenital tracts. Here are also secretions, such as tears, perspiration, skin oils, and saliva, that contain chemicals that can kill bacteria. In addition, the respiratory passages are lined with fine, short, moving hairs called *cilia.* Beating in a synchronized fashion, the cilia move a carpet of sticky mucus. The mucus works like fly paper to trap inhaled microbes and foreign matter and carry them to the back of the throat, where they are removed by sneezing, coughing, or nose-blowing, or are swallowed and disposed of by digestive fluids.[15]

Besides the cilia, other body hairs (the eyelashes, for example) may fend off invading microorganisms. Our reflexes (coughing, blinking, vomiting) are also part of our body's first line of defense. High acid levels in the stomach and vagina also help destroy invaders.

The Inflammatory Response

Microorganisms sometimes get beyond the body's outer defenses—through a cut in the skin, for example. They then face a second line of defense in the blood and the tissues—**inflammation,** or the **inflammatory response.** This response is a general one: It is aimed at helping to ward off any irritant or "foreign body"—whether it's a relatively large physical object (such as a splinter), a chemical substance, or a microbe.

As you may know, we have both red blood cells and white blood cells in our bloodstream. The red blood cells have an important function: They transport oxygen to all the cells in the body. But it's the white blood cells that we're interested in here. Some of them are of a type known as **phagocytes**—a term that literally means "cells that eat." Phagocytes sometimes come along and literally engulf foreign substances, so that they are no longer dangerous. Each individual phagocyte is made up of a semiliquid, jellylike substance, with a cell wall holding it together; it can come along and actually flow right around the foreign object, surrounding it. Then the cell can take the object apart chemically and digest it.

What happens in the inflammatory response is this: The supply of blood to the endangered area increases, and at the same time the *flow* of blood through that area slows down. As a result, some blood plasma (the fluid that transports the red and white blood cells) can leak through the walls of the blood vessels into the spaces between the cells in that area, bringing with it special proteins that can help destroy bacteria and toxins. Meanwhile, phagocytes rush to the area too; there they set to work engulfing bacteria and foreign particles.

FEVER

If the infection is localized in one part of the body, the patient usually shows the signs of inflammation in just that area—redness, local warmth, swelling, and pain. All indicate that the invaders are being counterattacked. But if the battle is being waged throughout the body, the patient will usually have a generalized fever. Fever is caused, at least in part, by toxic materials that are produced by the invaders or are released by the invaders while they are being destroyed. These toxins interfere with the regulatory mechanisms that normally control the temperature of the body, and the resulting elevated temperatures may be harmful to normal body functions. Nevertheless, fever can be helpful too: It stimulates the body to produce more white blood cells, and it may even kill off the invading organism—most pathogens cannot survive in above-normal body temperatures.

THE OUTCOME OF THE BATTLE

Will the inflammatory response be sufficient to knock out the infection? This depends on how many invading organisms there are and how strong they are, and also on how well the body is able to defend itself. Sometimes the battle comes to a standstill while it's still at the local level: As more and more of the local tissue is destroyed, the body may form a cavity, or **abscess,** filled with sticky, yellow-white **pus,** which consists of fluid, battling cells, and white blood cells that have died in the battle. The problem is resolved when enough of the invading organisms have been killed or inactivated to halt the infection.

But in more severe cases, this line of defense folds, and the invaders begin to spread through the tissues and even into the bloodstream. The infection then becomes generalized and highly dangerous.

Natural Immunity

The body's third line of defense against disease is **immunity,** a group of mechanisms that help protect the body against specific diseases. Immunity is the body's most efficient disease-preventing weapon; it may be called on to help fight either a viral infection or a bacterial one.

In our earlier discussion of viruses, we saw an intriguing pattern—an invader attacks the body but then turns around and helps bring about its own destruction. Natural immunity works in somewhat the same way. When an invading mi-

ACTIVITY: EXPLORING HEALTH

Charting Your Immunity History

We can prevent many communicable diseases through vaccination. And we may be immune to certain other diseases if we've actually had these diseases—they produce immunity for varying lengths of time through their actions on our bodies.

What diseases are *you* now immune to? Look at the communicable diseases listed below. Have

effective vaccines been developed for all of them? Check those that have vaccines, then write the dates when you had the disease or were vaccinated for it. Then answer Questions 1–5. (Note: You may need to consult your parents, your family physician, or some other source to obtain some of this information.)

	HAD THE DISEASE	INITIAL VACCINATION	MOST RECENT VACCINATION	LENGTH OF TIME THIS IMMUNIZATION WILL LAST
1. Ordinary ("red") measles				
2. German measles				
3. Mumps				
4. Flu				
5. Polio				
6. Whooping cough				

QUESTIONS

Your personal immunity

Which of the diseases are you protected from through immunity? When will you need a "booster"?

DISEASE	DATE WHEN "BOOSTER" WILL BE NEEDED
_____	_____
_____	_____
_____	_____
_____	_____

Do you know?

1. Which of the diseases listed above are considered "childhood" diseases? Are they dangerous to children? to adults? _____

_____

_____

_____

2. Rubella (German measles) can cause serious birth defects if the mother gets the disease during the first part of pregnancy. Did you know that if the woman is *vaccinated* for rubella during the early part of her pregnancy—or too soon before pregnancy occurs—the same birth defects may occur?

    If you are a woman: Have you had rubella? **YES** ☐ **NO** ☐

If not, you need to be sure that you are protected—vaccinated if necessary—at least three months before you conceive.

3. Which of the diseases listed above can you get vaccinated against, if you aren't already? Are you allergic to the vaccines for any of those diseases? _____

_____

_____

_____

croorganism (here called the **antigen**) enters the body, it stimulates the body to produce certain chemical substances called **antibodies** that can inactivate the microorganisms. Antibodies work only on the specific antigens that trigger them: Measles antibodies work only on the measles virus that triggers them, mumps antibodies on the mumps virus that triggers them, and so on. There

Figure 10.3 Antigen-antibody reaction. Research indicates that an antibody molecule has two identical halves, each with one large and one small component. Each antibody has only one antigen that fits with it. The two surfaces of the antibody molecule fit against the surface of two antigen molecules, thus deactivating both of them.

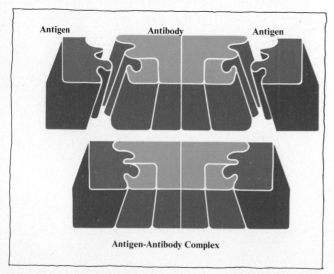

Antigen Antibody Antigen

Antigen-Antibody Complex

are over a million different specific antibodies—each capable of fighting just *one* antigen! That means there are over a million different foreign or invading substances—antigens—that can stimulate the body to take action in this way.

THE ROLE OF LYMPHOCYTES

In the immune mechanism, as in the inflammatory response, white blood cells come to the rescue. But here the protective white blood cells are of a type known as **lymphocytes**. Within this category are a number of key subtypes; we'll describe the most important ones here.[16]

B LYMPHOCYTES The substances we call antibodies come from B lymphocytes, which can be stimulated to produce them if certain foreign or invading substances are present in the body. When an antibody is sent out by the B lymphocytes into the fluid surrounding the cells of the body, it locks onto the enemy antigens, jigsaw-puzzle fashion. If the invaders are viruses, the antibody locks onto them and prevents them from entering their target cells. If the invaders are bacteria, the antibody locks onto them and causes them to clump together, making it easier for phagocytes to engulf and digest them. The bacteria-plus-antibody clumps also activate certain bactericidal (bacteria-killing) substances in the blood. In addition, antibodies can lock onto bacterial toxins to help make them less harmful to the body.[17]

T LYMPHOCYTES T lymphocytes fight infection in more ways than we have space to describe, but

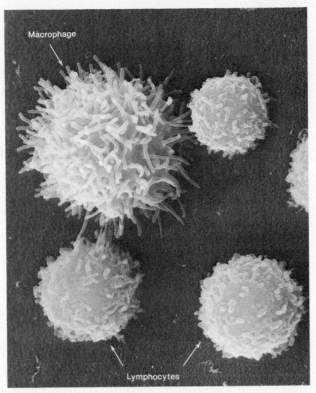

Electron microphotograph of a phagocyte (the large, loosely formed cell at top left) and lymphocytes. (E. Shelton/Dr. Don Fawcett/Photo Researchers, Inc.)

we can highlight three major mechanisms. First, some T lymphocytes spur the phagocytes to eat up foreign substances faster. Second, some help stimulate the B lymphocytes to produce antibodies. And third, some can attack foreign cells (such as cells in tissues that have been transplanted from another human body—as in a kidney transplant), cells that have been killed by viruses, and possibly also cancer cells.[18]

Currently, physicians are experimenting with a drug that can help counteract the effects of T-cell action in transplant surgery. Called cyclosporine, this drug can suppress the production of T lymphocytes so that the body is better able to accept the transplanted tissue.[19]

MALFUNCTIONING OF THE IMMUNE SYSTEM

Experts suspect that disorders of the immune system may be involved in many puzzling medical problems. At times, the body's defense mech-anisms seem to act against the body's own best interests.[20]

ALLERGIES   In response to dust, pollen, bee or wasp venom, and certain other substances, some people produce antibodies in such large quantities that they are harmful. The overabundant antibodies attach themselves to a type of cell called mast cells that are located in certain body tissues. The mast cells can release toxins that cause the individual to cough, produce large amounts of mucus, and suffer other allergic symptoms.[21]

DISEASES OF THE CONNECTIVE TISSUE   A number of still-mysterious diseases center around the various kinds of connective tissue in our bodies, such as the cartilage that holds our joints together. In the disease known as lupus, the immune system somehow attacks the body's own connective tissue. In rheumatoid arthritis, certain antibodies actually behave like antigens: They cause the body to put out *other* antibodies, which lock onto them and cause inflammation in the joints.[22]

ACQUIRED IMMUNE DEFICIENCY SYNDROME (AIDS)   In recent years, there has been an increase in a puzzling condition known as acquired immune deficiency syndrome (AIDS): In this syndrome, the immune system grows weak, leaving the individual vulnerable to viruses, bacteria, and other problems, including an extremely dangerous form of pneumonia *(Pneumocystis carinii)* and a rare skin cancer, Kaposi's sarcoma. Certain categories of people seemed to be more prone to the syndrome—male homosexuals, drug abusers, people suffering from hemophilia, and people of Haitian origin. At the time of this writing, it also seems possible that the syndrome is spreading to children, mainly the offspring of high-risk parents, and to a few women who have had regular heterosexual relations with male AIDS victims. Though some patients appear to have contracted AIDS from blood transfusions, researchers do not yet know whether it is transmitted by an infectious organism. There is not even a specific therapy for the syndrome at this point.[23]

Vaccination: Acquired Immunity

Not many years ago, having a disease was the only way people could develop immunity to it. (Immunity is acquired naturally when one develops a disease; in the course of the illness antibodies develop, and the body is able to fight off subsequent infection.) Today, however, immunity may also be induced artificially by means of a **vaccine,** which consists of killed or weakened viruses that are taken orally or by injection. Several days or weeks after the individual receives the vaccination, the body starts to produce specific antibodies, which circulate in the bloodstream, ready to attack the initiating antigen.

TYPES OF VACCINES

Some vaccines contain living infectious agents; included in this group are those used against yellow fever and measles, as well as the Sabin oral polio vaccine. These living agents have been weakened in the laboratory but still provoke the formation of specific antibodies. Other vaccines contain killed infectious agents; included in this group are the whooping cough and Salk polio vaccines. The killed microbes will not produce the disease, but they will stimulate production of specific antibodies against the same organism, thereby protecting the body from future infection.

Along similar lines, acquired immunity can be induced against certain microbial toxins that produce disease. Diphtheria and tetanus produce disease through their toxins. Modified toxins, called toxoids, which are no longer poisonous, are used to induce the production of antibodies that will inactivate the poisons if the invading organism strikes.

ACTIVE VERSUS PASSIVE IMMUNITY

If you contract a disease or receive a vaccine for it, you will eventually develop **active immunity.** But what if you are exposed to a serious disease and cannot wait for antibodies to form? In this instance, the danger is too great to allow time for your body to produce its own antibodies. Therefore, physicians may give you antibodies formed by another person or an animal, thus conferring **passive immunity.** The antibodies are found in certain proteins in the donor's blood, collectively called **gamma globulin.** Gamma globulin is used for passive immunization against infectious hepatitis and other diseases for which an effective vaccine for humans has not yet been devised.

In general, active immunity is long-term and in

some cases lifelong. Passive immunity lasts only a few weeks or months. Babies have passive immunity at birth: Antibodies that pass through the placental membrane become part of the immune system of the fetus. Within six weeks after birth the passive immunity begins to weaken, and the baby needs to begin the vaccination sequence that starts the development of active immunity.

The differences between the types of immunity are summarized in Figure 10.4.

◻—————————————————————

WHAT YOU CAN DO TO HELP GUARD YOUR OWN IMMUNITY—AND OTHER PEOPLE'S, TOO

Thanks to vaccines, we have greatly limited the pool of people who may be carrying certain infectious diseases and thus the total number of those microorganisms that exist in the United States. Effective and safe vaccines are now available for most viral diseases. Some need to be taken only once; others need only be followed by boosters to keep the level of antibodies in the bloodstream high enough to confer immunity. Today's American children are avoiding many of the diseases their parents experienced as a "normal" part of childhood: Rubella (German measles), varicella (chicken pox), and whooping cough are much less common today than ever before, and measles, some experts think, will probably be eradicated from the United States by the end of 1983.[24] More serious diseases such as polio, diphtheria, and tetanus have also dropped to almost insignificant levels.[25]

But some Americans have been lulled into complacency about these infectious diseases. They are not as well informed about them as they should be, nor are they as careful as they should be to keep up with the necessary immunizations. And this may mean trouble for all of us. Though it's not necessary for everyone in the population to be immune in order to prevent a disease from spreading, scientists don't know how far below 100 percent immunity we can go in our population without having new outbreaks of these diseases.[26] So it's important for all of us to keep our own vaccinations up to date and to urge others to do the same. Check back to see when you last had

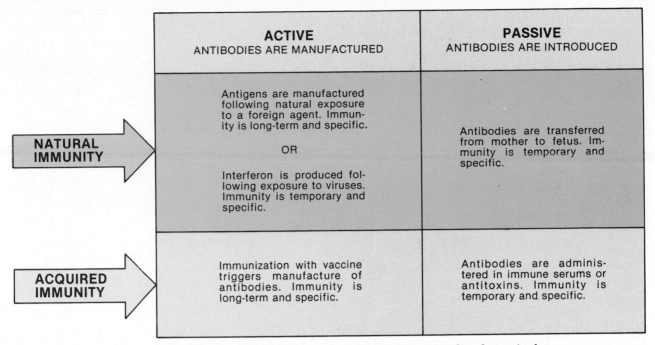

	ACTIVE ANTIBODIES ARE MANUFACTURED	**PASSIVE** ANTIBODIES ARE INTRODUCED
NATURAL IMMUNITY	Antigens are manufactured following natural exposure to a foreign agent. Immunity is long-term and specific. OR Interferon is produced following exposure to viruses. Immunity is temporary and specific.	Antibodies are transferred from mother to fetus. Immunity is temporary and specific.
ACQUIRED IMMUNITY	Immunization with vaccine triggers manufacture of antibodies. Immunity is long-term and specific.	Antibodies are administered in immune serums or antitoxins. Immunity is temporary and specific.

Figure 10.4   Types of immunity: active and passive, natural and acquired.

your "shots" and find out when you should go for any further shots or boosters (see Table 10.1).

TABLE 10.1 · Recommended Schedule for Active Immunization

Age	Vaccines
2 months	Diphtheria-tetanus-pertussis (DTP), oral polio vaccine
4 months	DTP, oral polio vaccine
6 months	Oral polio vaccine (recommended for infants in areas where polio is endemic)
15 months	Measles, rubella, mumps
18 months	DTP, oral polio booster
4 to 6 years (school entry)	DTP booster, oral polio booster
14 to 16 years	Combined tetanus and diphtheria toxoid, adult type (repeat every 10 years)

Source: American Academy of Pediatrics.

Interferon

Earlier we mentioned that promising research is being done on a substance that provides specific defense against viruses: **interferon.** Once one type of virus stimulates the body to make interferon, this same interferon can help protect the body against certain other types of viruses.

When a cell is attacked by a virus, that cell starts to produce interferon. It's too late for the interferon to protect the original cell against the virus; the original cell is destroyed. But the interferon moves out to other cells around the original cell, interacting with their cell membranes in such a way as to block viral invasion. Only certain viruses are highly effective as interferon triggers. Recently, however, scientists have discovered that certain bacteria—and certain synthetic chemicals as well—can stimulate interferon production.

Though interferon has been studied for twenty-five years, there is still much that scientists don't know about it. It was hoped that interferon would prove to be a "miracle drug" for cancer, but results to date have been disappointing. Researchers are now testing it against chronic hepatitis and some herpes virus infections of the eye and other parts of the body. Interferon does show some promise in reducing the severity of chicken pox in children who already have cancer. And in 1981–1982 English scientists used a nasal spray of pure interferon to try to protect a group of experimental subjects against an ordinary cold virus. The result was "virtually complete protection." The catch, of course, is that interferon would have to be used frequently in huge doses to prevent colds in the general population—an impossibly expensive approach.[27]

SEXUALLY TRANSMITTED DISEASES (STDs)

Now that so many of our bacterial diseases have been conquered or tamed by antibiotics, it is ironic that one of our most common types of infectious disease is one that is predominantly bacterial in origin. These are the **sexually transmitted diseases,** or **STDs**—and they are *not* totally responsive to antibiotics. STDs are infectious diseases that are almost always transmitted during sexual intercourse, homosexual relations, or other sexual activity.[28] Syphilis, gonorrhea, and herpes simplex virus Type 2 are by far the most prevalent STDs, but there are other types, including chancroid, granuloma inguinale, lymphogranuloma venereum, trichomoniasis (protozoa), and moniliasis (fungus). Many STDs have very serious consequences, and individuals usually *cannot* develop immunity to them. Nor does having one STD prevent the individual from catching another at the same time.

In the late 1950s, after a decade of being kept under reasonable control through antibiotics, these diseases began to increase dramatically, and today they are widespread. In most communities, gonorrhea cases alone outnumber all other reportable infectious diseases combined. Since 1973, the reported cases have leveled off at about 1 million per year. Recent trends seem to show that reported cases are decreasing slightly through time (990,864 cases in 1981), but many cases continue to go unreported.[29] One in every fifty teenagers will contract gonorrhea. At least half of all reported cases in the United States occur among those under age twenty-four, and particularly among those in their late teens.

◼─────────────────────────

WHAT YOU CAN DO: GENERAL PRECAUTIONS AGAINST STDs

Clearly, there are only two ways to minimize your own chances of contracting an STD: you can ei-

ther avoid all sexual activity with partners, or somehow make sure you never have sexual relations with anyone who has the remotest chance of being infected. The second alternative is perhaps most possible for those who are married. Those who are not married need to know some basic precautions—just to be on the safe side.

▶ Women on the Pill should be especially careful: The Pill makes the vagina less acid and hence less well protected against STDs.
▶ If you are thinking of having sexual relations with a person who might be infected, it's wise to bear in mind that disease can be transmitted in several ways —not only through genital contact, but also through kissing or through contact with broken skin or pores.
▶ It does help to have the man use a condom and for both partners to wash their genitals carefully. And women *may* run less risk of gonorrhea in particular if they use vaginal spermicides. But beyond that, the general rule should probably be this: Try to limit your sexual activity to partners you can trust and talk to honestly.
▶ Concern for others is part of health responsibility, too. If you go to a health professional for treatment of a suspected STD, you will probably be asked to name people you have had sexual contact with. Despite the embarrassment or hostility that this may create for you or your sexual partners, remember that you may ultimately be doing a number of people a very important favor by cooperating with health workers.
▶ Even if you yourself don't have a STD, you may know other people who think they may have and are reluctant or afraid to go for treatment. Perhaps they don't know how dangerous STDs can be, or they don't know what the symptoms are, or they don't know how to talk to health workers about such personal matters. You can help by passing along the facts and offering a certain amount of realistic reassurance —by pointing out that many cases of STD can be easily cured *if* they are recognized and treated early enough. Even herpes, which is still incurable, can be coped with.

─────────────────────────◼

The point is obvious: *Everyone* should know the basics about STDs. Let's look at some of the major ones, starting with gonorrhea and then moving on to syphilis, herpes, and others.

Gonorrhea

Gonorrhea is caused by gonococcal bacteria. It usually starts in the lower urinary and genital areas in both men and women. If it's not treated, it can spread upward in the genital tract and cause sterility. It can also enter the bloodstream and

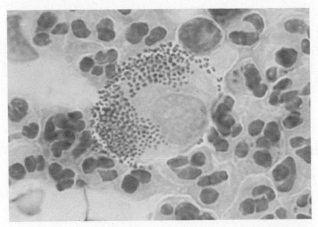

This is the pathogen that causes gonorrhea, surrounded by white blood cells. (© Holly Williamson/Taurus Photos)

cause severe arthritis and endocarditis (an inflammation of the heart). Thus it's potentially very serious. Happily, however, it's easily treated if it's caught early, through antibiotics such as penicillin.

If gonorrhea in a woman continues untreated, the symptoms may diminish. But the disease will continue unabated: The whole pelvis may eventually become inflamed. (This syndrome is known as pelvic inflammatory disease, or PID.) Even after this inflammation dies down, chronic difficulties may continue, including extensive damage to the reproductive tract.[30]

If a man does not receive prompt treatment, the infection spreads to the prostate gland and testicles. Here it can cause sufficient damage to produce sterility. In time, the urethra can become narrowed, making it difficult for a man to urinate. If the infection is severe, men can also suffer arthritis as well as heart damage.

HOW CAN I TELL IF I HAVE GONORRHEA?

▶ If you're a woman: You may not suspect you have gonorrhea at first. The early symptoms are frequently not pronounced, and most women with gonorrhea never develop any early symptoms. A few days after exposure, you may notice a mild burning sensation in the genital region and perhaps a vaginal discharge. (Occasionally the individual develops severe pain in just one joint.) Later, after the disease spreads from the vagina up through the uterus and into the Fallopian tubes and ovaries, you may have

pain and fever. These may be severe, or they may be so mild that you think they're due to a stomach upset.

▶ Sometimes a woman does not suspect she has gonorrhea until a man reports that he has contracted the infection from her. If you suspect you've been exposed to gonorrhea or if you have a vaginal discharge of any sort, you should see a physician promptly. The physician will be able to examine the vaginal discharge microscopically and confirm the diagnosis.

▶ If you're a man: The early symptoms of gonorrhea are more evident in men, although some men who have the disease have no early symptoms. About three to eight days after exposure, men notice a sharp, burning pain during urination. At about the same time, pus begins oozing from the penis, which causes many men to seek treatment.

NONGONOCOCCAL URETHRITIS: A SIMILAR, THOUGH MILDER, DISEASE

Nongonococcal urethritis (NGU) has symptoms similar to those of gonorrhea, though they are usually milder. The term *urethritis* simply means "an infection of the urethra." (The urethra is the canal leading out from the bladder, through which urine passes.)

Many organisms can cause urethral infection; a specific bacterial cause of NGU is usually difficult to identify. The treatment for this disorder is similar to that for gonorrhea, however. Though the means of transmission is generally thought to be sexual, many people have developed this disease even after having had no sexual contact in the relatively recent past.

Syphilis

Syphilis, caused by a spiral-shaped bacterium (a spirochete) known as *Treponema pallidum,* is another extremely dangerous disease. It can go on for years, moving through a number of stages. Fortunately, it can be cured with antibiotics in the first two stages or even in the latent phase.

PRIMARY SYPHILIS

Let's see what happens as syphilis begins.

WHAT TO LOOK FOR IN PRIMARY SYPHILIS

▶ The disease begins when one of the spirochetes enters a tiny break in the skin, usually in the warm, moist mucous membranes of the genital tract, rectum, or mouth. But there is usually no sign of the disease for ten to twenty-eight days. Then, you *may* discover a moist, painless open lump or swelling, about the size of a dime or smaller, somewhere in the visible portions of the genitals, anus, or mouth. This is known as a *chancre* (pronounced "shank-er").

▶ But this chancre can also develop out of sight, deep in the recesses of the vagina, the rectum, or the male urethra. So don't wait until you see a chancre. If you even faintly suspect that you may have been exposed to syphilis, see a physician at once.

▶ And be very careful not to let anyone else come into contact with the chancre: It is dangerously infective.

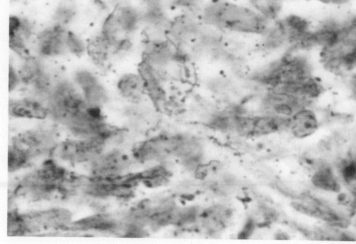

This is the pathogen that causes syphilis. (© Martin M. Rotker/Taurus Photos)

SECONDARY SYPHILIS

Even without treatment, the chancre will disappear within several weeks. Unfortunately, this may give the infected person a false sense of security. Meanwhile, however, the infection has entered the blood, and the spirochetes are being carried to all parts of the body. The secondary stage has begun.

WHAT TO LOOK FOR IN SECONDARY SYPHILIS

Secondary-stage symptoms appear from a few weeks to as long as a year after the appearance of the chancre.

▶ What are the symptoms and signs of secondary syphilis? They include: a skin rash, small flat sores in regions where the skin is moist, whitish patches on the mucous membranes in the mouth and throat, and spotty temporary baldness. There are also symptoms such as general discomfort and uneasiness, low-grade fever, headache, and swollen glands.

▶ Since these symptoms are easily mistaken for those of other diseases, it is important to consult a physician if any of them appear, particularly if you have been exposed to syphilis. Secondary syphilis, which lasts from three to six months, can always be diagnosed by blood tests.

▶ During the secondary stage, the disease is more contagious than at any other phase of its development. All the sores are filled with spirochetes, and any contact with them—even without sexual intercourse—can transmit the disease.

THE LATENCY PHASE

After the second stage of syphilis, all signs and symptoms of the disease disappear. The disease enters a latency phase, but it is not gone. Spirochetes are invading various organs, including the heart and the brain. This phase of the disease sometimes lasts only a few months, but it can last for twenty years or longer. In this stage, the infected individual appears disease-free and is usually not infectious, with an important exception— a pregnant woman can pass the infection to her unborn child. Although there are no symptoms, a blood test during this stage will reveal syphilis.

TERTIARY SYPHILIS: THE INCURABLE PHASE

The tertiary stage of syphilis generally begins ten to twenty years after the beginning of the latent phase, but it occasionally occurs much earlier. In tertiary syphilis, about one-fourth of all untreated patients become incapacitated.[31] Many develop serious cardiovascular disease. Some die of severe heart damage or rupture of the aorta. Others have slowly progressive brain or spinal-cord damage, which eventually leads to blindness, insanity, or crippling.

CONGENITAL SYPHILIS

Congenital syphilis occurs when a pregnant woman transmits the disease to her unborn child. Early in pregnancy, the infection may kill the fetus, produce various malformations, or result in an obviously diseased baby. A fetus infected late in pregnancy may seem healthy at birth, only to develop tertiary syphilis later. Treatment of the infected pregnant woman within the first four months of pregnancy halts the spread of the disease in the unborn child.

Herpes Simplex Virus Type 2

Until a few years ago, the herpes simplex Type 2 virus (HSV–2) was a rare condition. It was considered only a minor STD threat compared with syphilis and gonorrhea. Today, this highly contagious and often painful disease is epidemic throughout the country. Between 300,000 and 1 million new cases occur each year, according to the Centers for Disease Control. There is no cure for herpes at this time, but much active research is under way.[32]

Herpes virus Type 1 is the organism that causes the well-known fever blisters or "cold sores." This condition is only loosely related to the Type 2 virus. The blisterlike sores of the Type 2 virus might be described as fever blisters of the genital area; thus the disease is also known as *genital herpes.* Herpes Type 2 is usually spread by sexual contact, but the virus can be transmitted by any direct physical contact with herpes blisters. Lesions appear about six days after sexual contact with an infected person and may be spread over the genitals, buttocks, and thighs. Other symptoms include difficult urination, swelling of the legs, watery eyes, fatigue, and a general feeling of illness. The symptoms usually respond well to treatment, but the disease does not: The virus remains in the body indefinitely.

Symptoms recur periodically, often activated by sexual intercourse. Exposure to the sun, lack of sleep, infections, or physical or emotional stress can also bring them on. In some women the symptoms tend to reappear just before their menstrual periods. The disease can be spread any time during the recurrence. Occasionally symptoms are too mild to be noticeable, and a sexual partner may be infected without knowing it.

THE DANGERS OF HERPES

Pregnant women with genital herpes are likely to suffer even further misfortune: Their miscarriage rate is more than three times that of the general population.[33] When miscarriage does not occur, the birth process may expose the infant to the virus, causing death or irreversible brain damage. As a preventive measure, the baby may be delivered by Caesarean section (see Chapter 8). If the child is delivered vaginally, there is about a 50 percent chance that the newborn will contract the disease. Herpes is fatal for more than half of all infants who contract it.[34]

And if this weren't enough, several years of research indicate a strong relationship between herpes Type 2 and cancer of the cervix and prostate. Women with HSV–2 are more likely to develop cancer of the cervix than are other women.[35] Presumably, the virus penetrates the cervical cells, disrupting normal metabolism and setting off the typical uncontrolled growth of cancer. Women with genital herpes should have Pap smears annually (or more often) to check for early signs of cervical cancer.

HERPES' PSYCHOLOGICAL IMPACT

The physical symptoms of herpes can be painful, but many victims find the emotional impact of the disease even more distressing. Herpes sufferers often feel isolated, angry, and ashamed. The ailment can ruin relationships and make social lives difficult. In fact, sufferers' feelings of frustration and unhappiness about the disease are so characteristic that some psychologists refer to a "herpes syndrome" (see box). Moreover, the disease is so prevalent—experts estimate that between 5 million and 20 million Americans have herpes—and so widely feared that it may be changing basic patterns of sexual behavior. People are no longer certain that sexual encounters are physically safe, nor can they be sure of hiding infidelities from spouse or lover.

The problem is complicated by the medical profession's difficulties with the disease. The symptoms vary extraordinarily from person to

WHAT CAN BE DONE: Coping with Herpes

Why does herpes cause such serious emotional problems? It is not life-threatening, the symptoms grow progressively less annoying after the first bout, and half of those who contract it have no symptoms at all. To understand why so many people find it so difficult to manage, consider how it might affect a victim.

A TYPICAL CASE

Suppose that Kate is a college sophomore who is not seriously involved with anyone. It's not that no one is interested in her. Rather, she has been in relationships that didn't work out, and now she doesn't commit her emotions lightly. At a party she meets Paul, whom she remembers having seen in her psychology classes. They enjoy talking and spend the rest of the party together. Later that week, they go to a movie. Soon they're spending much of their free time together, and several weeks later they have sex.

A week later, Kate notices painful blisters on her thighs and genitals. At first, she is unconcerned. She has had bladder infections, and she supposes that this may be some variation of that ailment. Nevertheless, the next time she sees Paul, she asks him as casually as she can whether he has ever had a venereal disease. He denies it and she believes him. But when the blisters persist for a few days, she decides to go to the university health service. There, a doctor takes a culture. A week later, the doctor informs her that she has herpes. She learns that she almost certainly contracted the disease when she had sex with Paul.

When she returns to the dorm, she calls Paul and tells him she has to talk to him right away. When he arrives, she gives him the news and angrily asks him what he has to say for himself. Flustered, he denies that he has herpes; he goes so far as to accuse *her* of giving it to *him*. Kate was angry before, but this infuriates her. They have a brief but very nasty argument and then Paul stalks off. She's disgusted and upset. "That's the end of that," she says to herself.

Over the next few weeks, however, she slowly realizes the implications of what has

happened to her. The disease, of course, has not ended with the relationship—she has the disease, it's incurable, and she may give it to anyone she's intimate with. She tries to stop thinking about it, but that makes her feel devious, as if she's hiding something. She's ashamed to tell her friends, even her roommate. Her self-esteem plummets. "Why would anyone want to be involved with me now?" she asks herself. She worries: What would her parents say? Will it be safe for her to have children? Will she be alone for the rest of her life?

For a few months, she avoids men. Although she knows it's unreasonable, she finds that she distrusts all men. But when the new semester begins, she is assigned to a project in art class with a junior, Brian, and they are instantly attracted to each other. He's interesting and sympathetic, and it's soon clear that they are very fond of each other. Ordinarily, they would become lovers, but Kate is faced with a difficult choice. She can either tell Brian that she has herpes and risk losing him, or she can plunge into the relationship and try to avoid sex during the periods when the disease is most contagious, hoping that if he finds out he will care enough about her to stay with her.

If you were in Kate's position, what would you do? What would you want her to do if you were Brian?

Victims of herpes may feel that they have only two options—spread the disease or resign themselves to lives of celibacy and loneliness. In fact, there is a third option. Though at first life can seem very bleak indeed, people can and do learn to "manage" the disease and prevent it from disrupting their lives. It makes the already difficult task of sustaining a good relationship even tougher, but eventually most people make the adjustment.

HOW CAN I AVOID GETTING HERPES?

Other than giving up sex altogether, how can people avoid getting the disease? Several suggestions can be made.

▶ Herpes is a cyclical disease—the virus retreats periodically to the base of the spine. During these periods, the risk of transmitting it to a partner is low. So, if you're thinking of having sex with a person who has herpes, it is wise to wait till the "inactive" phase.

► It may also be helpful, if you don't know your partner well, for men to use condoms and for women to use a spermicide.

► One STD specialist recommends examining a prospective partner with the lights on: "If there are sores or discharge, it's time to put your clothes back on and find another partner."* (As you can imagine, following this advice does not contribute to a romantic atmosphere.)

► Perhaps the best recommendation is that people establish a trusting relationship before they have sex with each other.

HOW CAN A PERSON WHO HAS HERPES DEAL WITH THE SITUATION?

Those who have contracted the disease must deal with both the psychological upset and the physical symptoms. These two aspects of the disease are even more closely related than you might guess.

► One poorly understood peculiarity of herpes is that it can be influenced by emotional stress. Just as the physical symptoms can cause psychological distress, an emotional upset can lead to an outbreak of symptoms. For this reason, it is important that patients realize that the ailment can be lived with. As a leading herpes expert says, "One of the best things you can do for patients with genital herpes is tell them to stop worrying about it."† The ailment's susceptibility to emotions may explain why placebos so often prove effective against the disease. Researchers frequently find that a completely inert substance given to patients in control groups clears up blisters and prevents recurrences.

► Many sufferers find it easier to accept the disease after they join a discussion group. Groups are sponsored by the Herpes Resource Center at fifty locations around the country. These groups give victims a chance to talk over their problems in a sympathetic environment and provide emotional support for one another. Those who have herpes syndrome have many complaints in common. Like Kate, most are extremely angry at the person who gave them the disease. One study found that herpes sufferers experience symptoms resembling those often felt by victims of chronic diseases such

as multiple sclerosis. The first reactions are shock and denial, followed by loneliness, anger, fear, self-imposed isolation, depression, and a sense of being trapped. Herpes victims who attend such groups may find that talking over their problems cuts down the sense of isolation that is one of the worst aspects of the disease.

WHAT'S THE BEST THING TO TELL A NEW PARTNER?

One question often discussed is what to tell a prospective partner. Most Herpes Resource Center staff members recommend that sex partners be told, but there is no consensus on the best way.

► One psychotherapist suggests that prospective partners be told "as far away from the bedroom as possible." This therapist also warns against a dramatic presentation, such as saying in a quavering voice, "I have an incurable disease."†

► Those who choose *not* to tell sometimes regret it later. The disease may recur after years of dormancy, leaving the afflicted person with a lot of explaining to do to his or her current partner.

CAN MEDICATION HELP?

Although the disease is as yet incurable, recent medical advances do hold some promise. Some advice is just common sense—keep the affected area clean and dry and don't scratch. Other approaches have been developed in the laboratory. An ointment called *acyclovir,* marketed under the name Zovirax, is the first antiviral drug that has proved to be effective against genital herpes. It is not a cure, however—it merely shortens the contagious period by a day or two. Another promising treatment uses a laser beam to "vaporize" infected cells; others use *gossypol* (a cottonseed oil extract) or interferon. Vaccines are being developed, but it may be years before they are available to the public.

Such research does offer hope to the disease's victims. For now, however, the disease cannot be eliminated, and victims must learn to adjust to it.

Sources: *John Leo, "The New Scarlet Letter," *Time*, August 2, 1982, pp. 62–66; †Daniel Laskin, "The Herpes Syndrome," *The New York Times Sunday Magazine*, February 21, 1982, pp. 94–108; Matt Young, "Herpes: The VD of the '80s," *Newsweek*, April 12, 1982, pp. 75–76.

person. Some have no symptoms, others have excruciating pain almost constantly. For this reason and others, the ailment is hard to diagnose. It's not unusual for a person to visit several doctors before finding one who can recognize the disease and explain its implications. The only nationwide group that offers authoritative, up-to-date information on the ailment is the Herpes Resource Center, based in Palo Alto, California.

Other Common Sexually Transmitted Diseases

TRICHOMONIASIS

This disease is caused by a protozoan parasite, *Trichomonas vaginalis,* more commonly known as "trich." The organism produces a profuse white bubbly discharge with a characteristic odor and a general reddening of the vulva. This irritation can result in a secondary bacterial infection, in which case the discharge becomes greenish-yellow. As the name implies, trich normally affects only women, although men frequently act as carriers, and a few men may suffer mild irritation of the urethra.

Diagnosis is easily made by microscopic examination of vaginal secretions (usually the parasite will also appear in a urine specimen as well). Treatment is with a drug called Metronidazole. To be most effective, male sexual partners should also be treated to prevent any reinfection.

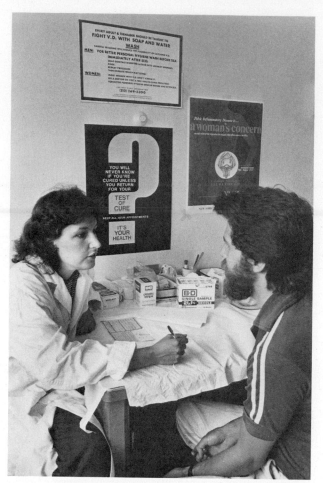

Health clinics offer counseling about STDs free or at low cost, on a confidential basis. (© Hazel Hankin 1981)

Trichomoniasis disease is not transmitted solely by sexual means: it can be contracted, for instance, from underwear or washcloths—so it's a good idea to be sure these are always fresh and clean.

MONILIASIS

Moniliasis, also known as candidiasis or thrush, is a yeast infection of the vagina. Most commonly it occurs from altered conditions of the vaginal lining, as in pregnancy or during antibiotic therapy. There has been a recent upsurge of the disorder among Pill users.[36]

Moniliasis is easily recognized by an almost intolerable itching around the entire vulva. The ac-

companying discharge is white, granular, and lumpy, with a yeasty odor. Treatment is somewhat difficult, since individual susceptibility plays a role in the infection: Users of the Pill usually require regular and frequent treatment by a physician. Moniliasis can also occur in the male genitals and result in a couple's passing the disease back and forth. The disease may also occur in the mouth or anus and on the skin.

A sore mouth, with white patches on the tongue and cheeks, indicates a need for prompt medical attention. It may mean the individual has moniliasis.

Rarer Sexually Transmitted Diseases

Besides syphilis, gonorrhea, and genital herpes, which unfortunately are common in the general population, there are a number of rarer STDs. Although they were once quite unusual in the United States, they have been reported more frequently in recent years.[37]

Chancroid involves a syphilislike, but usually painful, genital sore in men (in women it usually produces no symptoms). This sore can be distinguished from the chancre of syphilis by laboratory tests. In lymphogranuloma venereum, a small genital sore is followed in a few weeks by painful swelling of the lymph glands. Granuloma inguinale produces large, reddened, raw-looking (but usually painless) patches on the genitals. Fortunately, all three of these disorders respond to therapy with antibiotic drugs.

MAKING HEALTH DECISIONS

Sexually Transmitted Diseases: Your Attitudes and the Decisions You Make

Sexually transmitted diseases (STDs) occupy a unique place among diseases in our society. They are among the most common of all infectious diseases, yet we view them in a very different way from other infectious diseases. Our embarrassment and shame about STDs makes them very difficult to deal with, from a personal as well as a public health perspective.

If you are sexually active, then you are at some risk of contracting STDs. Not surprisingly, STDs are relatively rare among married couples. They are most commonly found among unmarried and sexually active people. STDs are common and effective treatment is readily available, yet many people do not take measures to prevent infection and they fail to seek prompt treatment when necessary. It is very important indeed to understand what lies behind these decisions.

What do *you* think about STDs? The items listed below are designed to focus your thoughts about STDs and thus promote thoughtful decision making. Check the response you choose. But note: There is no one correct answer to any of these questions—what's important is what *you* believe.

1. Which of the following do you think is the major cause of the high rate of STDs in our society?

   ☐ A breakdown in moral values

   ☐ Lack of education about sexuality and STDs

   ☐ Changing sexual values in our society

   ☐ Other_____

2. I believe the main reason people contract STDs is that:

   ☐ They are promiscuous

   ☐ They are not careful about choosing sexual partners

   ☐ They do not know enough about STDs

   ☐ Other_____

3. Look back at your responses to questions 1 and 2. How would you characterize your feelings abouts STDs? Are you afraid? unconcerned? ambivalent? other?_____

   _____

   _____

4. Would you decline a *highly desirable* opportunity for sex if you thought you *might* catch an STD? Would your decision be the same if you thought you could give the disease to your sexual partner? _____

   _____

   _____

5. What steps can you take to help ensure that you do not allow an STD to go undetected (if you are sexually active)? _____

   _____

SUMMARY

1. Of the billions of microbes in the human body, most are harmless, some are beneficial, and only a limited number cause disease. Endogenous microbes live in the human host and are normally harmless. Exogenous microbes live outside the body. Infection is an attack on the body by microbes. Disease occurs when microbes overwhelm the host or when they release toxins.

2. The six main types of infectious agents, or pathogens, are: bacteria, viruses, rickettsiae, fungi, protozoa, and worms.

3. Bacteria are single-celled organisms, most of which are not harmful. Bacteria that may be harmful include *E. coli*, streptococci, and staphylococci. Bacterial toxins can be dangerous as well.

4. Viruses are the simplest form of life and reproduce to cause infectious diseases like the common cold, influenza, hepatitis, and infectious mononucleosis.

5. Infections spread either by direct physical contact or by intermediaries (vectors) like insects, air, and drinking water.

6. The body's first line of defense against infectious disease includes the skin, mucosae, secretions, cilia and other hairs, and certain reflexes such as coughing. The second line of defense in the blood and tissues is the inflammatory response. Immunity is the body's third line of defense.

7. Immunity may be either natural or acquired through vaccination. The mechanism of immunity depends on the lymphocyte, a kind of white blood cell that is important for antibody production. Antibodies are proteins that can render certain invaders harmless. The invading microbes that stimulate the B lymphocytes to produce antibodies are called antigens. T lymphocytes fight infection in many ways. The body also manufactures interferon to protect itself against certain viruses and bacteria.

8. Sexually transmitted diseases have reached epidemic proportions since the 1950s, the result of changing lifestyles, greater mobility, drug use, increased use of the Pill and IUDs, complacency about the dangers involved, better diagnoses, and reluctance to seek treatment.

9. Gonorrhea, a potentially serious illness, is almost always transmitted by sexual intercourse. The early symptoms may be more noticeable in men than in women. Penicillin is the usual treatment. Nongonococcal urethritis is a similar but milder disease.

10. Syphilis develops in stages, following infection during sexual activity. During the primary, secondary, and latent stages, syphilis can be treated by antibiotics.

11. Herpes simplex Type 2, or genital herpes, is an STD that has become epidemic in recent years. It is not yet curable, although its symptoms respond well to treatment. Herpes is chronic and has inactive and active phases. Many people who get herpes develop a psychological "herpes syndrome." Medical professionals suggest that people can adjust to the disease and recommend that they tell sexual partners about the problem, avoid sex during active phases, avoid stress, and take medication.

GLOSSARY

abscess   A pus-filled cavity formed in the body as a result of destruction of local tissue in the inflammatory response.

active immunity   Long-lasting resistance to an infectious disease acquired through the body's production of antibodies as a result of either having the disease or being vaccinated against it. Compare **passive immunity.**

animal parasite   An organism that lives in or on the body of another animal (the **host**), obtaining food from it and in the process weakening it and causing disease.

antibiotics   A group of drugs that destroy or inhibit the growth of disease-causing bacteria.

antibodies   Chemical substances produced in response to an invading microorganism (the **antigen**) that can inactivate the microorganism.

antigen   An invading microorganism that stimulates the body to produce chemical substances (antibodies) that can inactivate the microorganism.

bacteria (singular: **bacterium**) Single-celled, plantlike microorganisms.

endogenous microorganisms Microscopic organisms that normally live within the human body, usually causing it no harm and often contributing to its welfare, but sometimes causing disease.

exogenous microorganisms Microscopic organisms that are not normally residents of the human body, many of which can cause disease if they enter the body.

fungi (singular: **fungus**) Many-celled, plantlike organisms that lack chlorophyll and must therefore obtain food from organic material—in some cases, from humans.

gamma globulin Certain blood proteins that contain antibodies.

host The human or animal in or on which an animal parasite lives.

immunity A group of mechanisms that help protect the body against specific diseases.

incubation period The time between first exposure to a virus or other disease-causing organism and the appearance of symptoms.

infection The invasion of the body by disease-causing organisms and the reaction of the body to their presence.

inflammatory response (inflammation) A general defense mechanism in the blood and tissues aimed at warding off any irritant or foreign body.

interferon A substance produced by the body to help protect it against viruses.

lymphocytes White blood cells that fight infection.

parasitic worms Many-celled animals such as pinworms, tapeworms, and flukes that live in human hosts, causing illness.

passive immunity Short-term resistance to infectious disease acquired through the administration of antibodies formed by another person or an animal. Compare **active immunity.**

pathogen An organism, such as a bacterium or virus, that can be an agent of infectious disease.

phagocytes White blood cells that protect the body from infection by engulfing and digesting invading microorganisms, toxins, and other foreign substances.

protozoa (singular: **protozoon**) Single-celled parasitic animals, some of which produce illness in human and animal hosts.

pus A sticky, yellow-white substance that fills an abscess as a result of the inflammatory response; it consists of fluid in which active and dead white blood cells are suspended.

rickettsiae Infectious organisms that grow in the intestinal tracts of insects and insectlike creatures and may be transmitted to humans through insect bites.

sexually transmitted diseases (STDs) Infectious diseases that are almost always transmitted during sexual intercourse, homosexual relations, or other sexual activity.

toxins Poisonous substances, such as those produced by disease-causing organisms.

toxoids Modified toxins, which are no longer poisonous, used to induce the production of antibodies that will inactivate specific microbial disease-producing toxins.

vaccine Killed or weakened viruses that are taken orally or by injection to stimulate the body to produce antibodies that give immunity to the specific disease caused by the virus.

vector A carrier of an infectious agent; insects, ticks, and rats are vectors of some human infectious diseases.

virus A microorganism that can reproduce only in living cells of a person or animal.

NOTES

1. C. Dobell, *Anton van Leeuwenhoek and His "Little Animals"* (New York: Harcourt, Brace & Co., 1932), p. 243.

2. K. N. Shands et al., "Toxic Shock Syndrome in Menstruating Women," *New England Journal of Medicine* 303, no. 25 (1980): 1436; Centers for Disease Control, "Toxic Shock Syndrome, U.S., 1970–1982," *Morbidity and Mortality Weekly Report* 31, no. 16 (April 30, 1982).

3. Ibid.

4. Centers for Disease Control, cited in "TB Is Found Still a Danger," *New York Times*, January 18, 1983.

5. Lawrence K. Altman, "Infections Still a Big Threat," *New York Times*, July 20, 1982, p. C2.

6. Harold M. Schmeck, Jr., "Flu Update: New Advances Promise Aid in Prevention," *New York Times*, September 28, 1982.

7. W. Paul Glezen, cited in ibid.

8. R. G. Douglas and R. F. Betts, "Influenza Virus," in G. L. Mandell, R. G. Douglas, and J. E. Bennett, eds.,

Principles and Practice of Infectious Disease (New York: Wiley, 1979).

9. Schmeck, "Flu Update."

10. *Public Health Reports* 96, no. 5 (1981): 478.

11. C. C. Boyd and H. Sheldon, *An Introduction to the Study of Disease,* 7th ed. (Philadelphia: Lea and Febiger, 1977), p. 304.

12. A. S. Evans, J. C. Niederman, and R. W. McCollum, "Seroepidemiologic Studies of Infectious Mononucleosis with EB Virus," *New England Journal of Medicine* 297 (1968): 1121.

13. Ibid.

14. A. S. Benenson, ed., *Control of Communicable Diseases in Man,* 12th ed. (Washington, D. C.: American Public Health Association, 1975).

15. K. L. Jones, L. W. Shainberg, and C. O. Byer, *Communicable and Noncommunicable Diseases* (San Francisco: Canfield Press, 1970).

16. I. L. Weissman, L. E. Hood, and W. B. Wood, *Essential Concepts in Immunology* (Menlo Park, Calif.: Benjamin/Cummings, 1978).

17. Lawrence K. Altman, "Transplants Are Surging as Survival Rates Improve," *New York Times,* October 5, 1982.

18. Weissman, Hood, and Wood, *Essential Concepts in Immunology.*

19. Ibid.

20. Ibid.

21. B. H. Park and R. H. Good, *Principles of Modern Immunology: Basic and Clinical* (Philadelphia: Lea and Febiger, 1974).

22. Ibid.

23. Jean Seligmann et al., "The AIDS Epidemic: The Search for a Cure," *Newsweek,* April 18, 1983, pp. 74–79.

24. Lawrence K. Altman, "End of Measles in U.S. Expected by 1983," *New York Times,* October 19, 1982, p. C1.

25. Centers for Disease Control, *Morbidity and Mortality Weekly Report* 30 (January 1, 1982): 50–51.

26. J. S. Mausner and A. K. Bahn, *Epidemiology: An Introductory Text* (Philadelphia: Saunders, 1974).

27. Harold M. Schmeck, Jr., "Interferon Makes Inroads Against Some Infections, Including Colds," *New York Times,* June 1, 1982.

28. C. E. Campbell and R. J. Herten, "VD to STD: Redefining Venereal Disease," *American Journal of Nursing* 81, no. 9 (September 1981): 1629–1635.

29. U.S. Public Health Service, *Annual Summary 1981, Morbidity and Mortality Weekly Report* 30, no. 54 (October 1982).

30. C. I. Fogel and N. F. Woods, *Health Care of Women: A Nursing Perspective* (St. Louis: Mosby, 1981).

31. Boyd and Sheldon, *An Introduction to the Study of Disease.*

32. L. B. Meeks and P. Heit, *Human Sexuality: Making Responsible Decisions* (Philadelphia: Saunders, 1982).

33. Campbell and Herten, "VD to STD."

34. Meeks and Heit, *Human Sexuality.*

35. A. J. Nahmias, W. E. Josey, and J. M. Oleske, "Epidemiology of Cervical Cancer," in A. S. Evans, ed., *Viral Infections of Man—Epidemiological Control* (New York: Plenum Press, 1975).

36. R. A. Hatcher, G. K. Stewart, F. Stewart, F. Guest, P. Stratton, and A. H. Wright, *Contraceptive Technology 1978–1979,* 9th ed. (New York: Irvington, 1979).

37. Campbell and Herten, "VD to STD"; H. H. Neumann, "Those 'Newer' Sexually Transmitted Diseases," *Connecticut Medicine* 49, no. 9 (September 1981): 612.

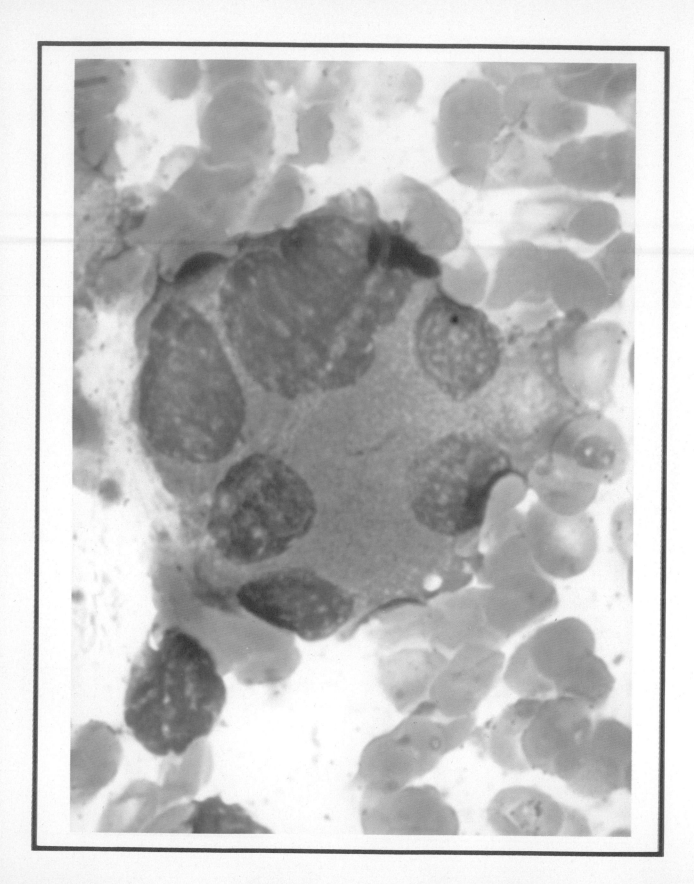

CHAPTER 11

Cancer

T he Big C," they called it in the old days. More often, people couldn't bring themselves to say even that. Asked what was wrong with someone, they answered simply, "Bad news" or "It's not good," or gave you a look that said it was better not to ask. Then you knew what it was—the most threatening disease of all, cancer.

Many people still resist saying the word, but times have changed and we now know that cancer is no longer synonymous with a death sentence. Thanks to medical research, greater public knowledge, and more open human communication and understanding, we are better able to deal with the fear—and the battle, too.

Cancer Today

The incidence of cancer has risen dramatically in recent decades, primarily due to cigarette smoking, and cancer is probably our most dreaded disease today. As a cause of death in the United States, cancer has climbed from less than 6 percent of all deaths in 1900 to over 20 percent today, based on recent statistics.[1] It is already the leading killer of women aged thirty to fifty-four.[2] And as a killer of the overall population, it is second only to heart disease, accounting for close to 430,000 deaths per year.[3] This figure has risen annually since 1949, and if present trends continue, cancer may well overtake heart disease as the number one cause of death.

Why has cancer recently been showing up more frequently in the mortality statistics? There are three major reasons. First, today's new techniques permit earlier, more accurate diagnosis than in the past, when many patients who had other disorders died without even knowing they also had cancer. Second, since the risk of cancer grows with age, our increasing life spans automatically increase the prevalence of cancer. And third, our changing lifestyles have increased our exposure to certain causative factors—such as the tobacco in cigarettes.

Can We Fight Cancer More Effectively Today?

Although there is still much to be learned about cancer, our knowledge of the disease has grown steadily in recent years. We have a better understanding of the disease and are finding ways to cope with it. Early recognition of the signs of cancer, prompt diagnosis, and aggressive treatment by the appropriate means have made cancer less deadly.

Even more important is the fact that some kinds of cancer are in part caused by preventable factors—for example, 25 to 30 percent of all cancer deaths are related to cigarette smoking, and most skin cancer is caused by excessive exposure to the sun.[4] Where such risk factors have been established, we can attempt to reduce the odds of developing those particular forms of disease.

WHAT IS CANCER?

Cancer is many things: it's a dangerous and sometimes fatal physical condition, and it's a psychological and social problem, too. First, let's look at the physical side of cancer.

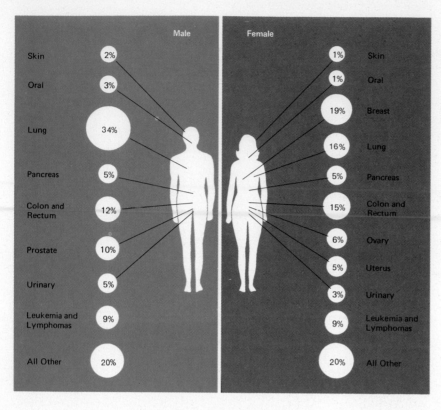

Figure 11.1   Percentage of cancer deaths by sex and site.

Source: American Cancer Society, *1982 Cancer Facts and Figures,* p. 12.

The Physical Aspects of Cancer: Know Your Terms

Cancer is a condition of abnormal cellular growth. It starts when one or a few cells undergo certain changes that make them no longer able to perform their intended functions in the body. Then, these altered (mutant) cells begin to reproduce very rapidly. If they go on reproducing unchecked, the patient will die.

TUMORS

To understand the peculiar nature of cancer, it is necessary to know how the physician (usually a pathologist) distinguishes cancerous tissues from other kinds of tissue. First of all, what is a **tissue?** This term refers to a collection of specialized cells in the body. Muscle tissue is composed of cells that are specialized to fulfill the function of muscles, nerve tissue is made up of cells specialized to fulfill the function of nerves, and so on.

The tissues in our bodies are constantly changing: Some cells are dying, and new cells are developing to replace them. Most of the cells in our bodies are constantly reproducing. Normally an individual cell divides to produce two new cells through an orderly and controlled process known as **mitosis.**

Sometimes, the controls that govern cell reproduction in our bodies somehow break down, and the reproductive process goes out of control. Cells within a tissue that normally cooperate with each other in performing a useful function no longer do so. They grow to an abnormal size and shape and begin to multiply independently, often rapidly, forming a swelling or mass known as a **tumor.** Such a group of cells, growing in this uncontrolled fashion, is called a **neoplasm** (a term that basically means "new growth").

When this happens, does it mean the individual has cancer? Not necessarily; he or she may have a **benign tumor**—a tumor that grows relatively slowly, in a growth pattern that keeps it localized. Benign tumors usually do not recur once they are removed. The fact that they are benign, however, does not mean they do no damage. They can cause pressure and subsequent harm to sur-

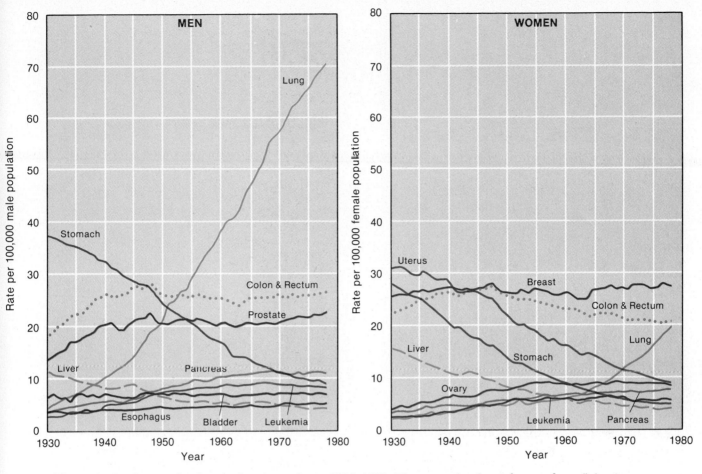

Figure 11.2 Cancer death rates by site and sex, 1930–1978. These graphs show the number of deaths per 100,000 men and women associated with certain types of cancer in the United States between 1930 and 1978. Most alarming is the dramatic increase in lung cancer deaths among both men and women.

Source: National Center for Health Statistics and the U.S. Bureau of the Census, in *CA—A Cancer Journal for Clinicians* 32, no. 1 (January–February 1982).

rounding structures, and they can rob normal tissues of their blood supply. A benign tumor can have serious consequences in a vital organ such as the brain. Benign tumors are usually curable by surgical removal.

The individual *does* have cancer, however, if the tumor turns out to be **malignant** (a *malignant neoplasm*). The cells that form malignant tumors are of a special type: They grow in abnormal ways and may invade other healthy tissues. Cancerous cells may break away and enter the lymphatic channels and the blood vessels. Either or both systems can then carry the cancerous cells to other parts of the body, where they may settle and form new tumors.

METASTASES

The new, or secondary, tumors that can form when cancerous cells break away from the original malignant tumor are called **metastases,** and the process by which they spread is called **metastatic growth.** Such new growths may develop a considerable distance from the original site, and each metastasis may be capable of seeding more new sites. In this way cancer can spread widely throughout the body.

KINDS OF CANCER

Malignant tumors are classified according to the tissues or organs from which they arise and their

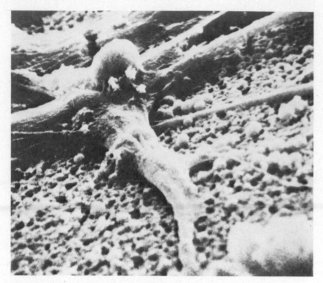

Metastasis: A cancer cell (magnified 3,000 times) spreads into normal cells. (© Omikron/Photo Researchers, Inc.)

appearance under the microscope. There are more than a hundred different forms of cancer; about thirty of them are fairly common.[5]

Carcinomas are cancers that arise from **epithelium**—the cells forming the skin, the glands, and the membranes that line the respiratory, urinary, and gastrointestinal tracts. **Sarcomas** are cancers that arise from supporting or connective tissues, such as bones, cartilage, and the membranes covering muscles and fat. These terms are often modified to indicate more specifically the type or location of the disease. In cancer of the breast, for example, cancers derived from cells lining the milk ducts are called **adenocarcinomas,** meaning that they are composed of glandular *(adeno-)* epithelial cells.

Further subdivisions identify cancers of lymphatic cells as **lymphomas,** cancers of blood-forming cells as **leukemias,** cancers of pigment-carrying cells of the skin as **melanomas,** and so on.

There are also cancers whose cellular structure is so abnormal that they no longer resemble the cells from which they originated, and no identification is possible. Such cancers are termed **anaplastic.**

HOW DOES CANCER KILL?

As cancer cells invade the body organs and begin to spread, they act as disruptive elements in the organ or organ system. As the cancer spreads, the disruption becomes more severe and the functioning of the organ becomes progressively reduced.

- If the cancer is in the stomach, digestion will become impeded, and the patient will lose weight and progress toward starvation.
- When the cancer involves the blood or the blood-forming organs (bone), the patient may become more susceptible to infection, may tire easily, or may suffer **hemorrhage** (profuse bleeding).
- When the cancer is in the liver, toxins and other harmful substances that would otherwise have been removed by the liver circulate through the blood.

When such disruptions become severe, death results because the affected organs cannot function properly. The body suffers starvation, infection, poisoning, and other similar problems, and all body systems decline.

The Psychological Impact of Cancer

> Miss B. felt very dizzy and unsteady. Leaving the doctor's office, she saw a sign, "Every three minutes someone dies of cancer," and burst into uncontrollable hysterical laughter. On reaching home, she sat bolt upright in her living room with the lights on throughout the entire night, quivering with fear.[6]

Patients almost always describe the initial impact of the news as feeling like a heavy blow on the head. They are stunned. From then on, reactions vary from patient to patient.

THE PSYCHIC PAIN OF CANCER

Everyone has experienced an emotional hurt, but cancer patients must be seen as people under a special and severe form of emotional stress. They are under the threat of a disabling illness or loss of a body part or mutilation or death. Their usual methods of coping with the world and striving for fulfillment no longer work. Their emotional needs and defenses are knocked off balance. Anxious about whether they will be able to go on meeting the ordinary demands of life, they often lose self-esteem, becoming vulnerable to feelings of condemnation or isolation from others.

A cancer patient's psychological problems may be particularly severe if the threatened event—loss of a body part, or perhaps a period of being bedridden—is likely to interrupt valued life activities and disturb the patient's body image. The expectation, moreover, may be as psychologically painful as the event itself. The patient may feel under attack on all fronts.[7]

DEPRESSION

Many cancer patients have to deal with depression. Those accustomed to being very active may feel it especially on days when they are unable to move about. Some develop excessive concern about their bodies. They say, "I treat my body like a soft-boiled egg, liable to break its shell at any moment," or "I have lost confidence in my body."[8] This attitude may lead to economic loss if it lowers the patient's productivity at work—and the financial loss may increase problems at home.

Other patients believe they have somehow brought the disease on themselves by some forbidden activity. The guilt and rage that accompany such beliefs can be very harmful to their emotional health.[9]

WHAT CAUSES CANCER, AND WHAT PREVENTIVE STEPS CAN WE TAKE?

The American Cancer Society estimates that approximately one-third of cancer deaths could be avoided with existing methods of treatment—if diagnosis and treatment were undertaken earlier.[10] Why do so many people with curable cancer have to die? The problem seems in part to be one of ignorance and fear. Cure depends on early diagnosis and treatment, but earlier treatment is possible only when people (1) know about the risk factors, (2) are aware of the danger signs of cancer, (3) have periodic health examinations, and (4) do not allow fear to keep them from seeking medical diagnosis. This is one situation where it is extremely dangerous to believe that "what you don't know can't hurt you."

The Role of Multiple Causes

As we've mentioned, the term *cancer* actually describes a group of more than a hundred different diseases. It's unlikely that such a wide variety of diseases could arise from a single cause. Furthermore, we know that some forms of cancer appear to result from the interaction of a specific *combination* of factors, such as cigarette smoking and exposure to asbestos (taken together). So, what we will discuss is not causes, but risk *factors*—any of which may affect an individual's chance of developing cancer. Obviously, our primary interest is in how we can help cut down these factors.

HEREDITY AND ENVIRONMENT

As in any disease, the chances of developing cancer depend on both the environment and the individual's genetic constitution. Let's look at a clear example of this genetic and environmental interplay: Many skin cancers are caused by exposure to sunlight, especially ultraviolet light. Persons with fair complexions are more likely to develop skin cancer after excessive exposure to sunlight than are persons with heavy pigmentation.[11]

Human beings of all races, colors, and environmental habits have been known to develop cancer of one type or another. There are, however, some intriguing differences in the cancers that occur among different human populations. The Japanese have very low rates of malignant melanoma and breast cancer, for example, but a very high rate of stomach cancer. Black people living in Uganda, Nigeria, and South Africa have low rates of cancers of the larynx, lung, stomach, colon, rectum, and brain, but are at a high risk of developing a certain type of liver cancer.[12] While we know that certain factors play a causative role in these cases, many questions remain. How important are the genetic factors and how important are the environmental ones? This is an important area for continuing research—and a difficult one, since it is often almost impossible to separate genetic patterns from environmental patterns. In fact, recent studies indicate that personal habits such as smoking, alcohol use, diet, and sexual behaviors may be much more important than environmental exposure (see Figure 11.3)—but this is still a very much debated question.[13]

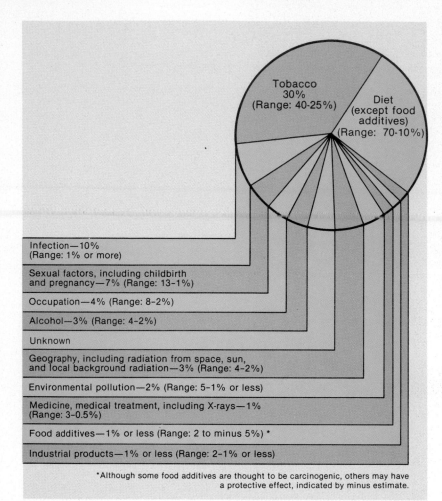

Figure 11.3   The relative import-ance of the major environmental factors linked to cancer. According to these estimates, work-related exposures to carcinogens account for only 4 percent of cancer deaths, and pollution in the air, water, food, and earth accounts for even less. As the chart shows, however, the range of uncertainty for all these estimates is very large —an indication of how much we still have to learn about cancer. And even if, for example, work-related exposures lead to only 4 percent of all cancer deaths in this country, that represents 16,000 unnecessary deaths each year. We cannot afford to be any more complacent about environmental cancer risks than about personal factors such as smoking.

Source: Estimates by Richard Doll and Richard Peto, reported in Philip M. Boffey, "Cancer Experts Lean Toward Steady Vigilance, but Less Alarm, on Envi-ronment," *New York Times,* March 2, 1982.

Tobacco
30%
(Range: 40-25%)

Diet
(except food
additives)
(Range: 70-10%)

Infection—10%
(Range: 1% or more)

Sexual factors, including childbirth
and pregnancy—7% (Range: 13-1%)

Occupation—4% (Range: 8-2%)

Alcohol—3% (Range: 4-2%)

Unknown

Geography, including radiation from space, sun,
and local background radiation—3% (Range: 4-2%)

Environmental pollution—2% (Range: 5-1% or less)

Medicine, medical treatment, including X-rays—1%
(Range: 3-0.5%)

Food additives—1% or less (Range: 2 to minus 5%) *

Industrial products—1% or less (Range: 2-1% or less)

*Although some food additives are thought to be carcinogenic, others may have
a protective effect, indicated by minus estimate.

CAN HEREDITY BE A RISK FACTOR IN ITSELF?

It is known that a few rare types of cancer are definitely hereditary—one example is cancer of the retina.

But, more important, there is evidence that families tend to inherit a predisposition toward particular types of cancer—and here's where the greater risk lies for most of us. Take, for example, breast cancer. One study found that relatives of patients who had contracted breast cancer before the age of forty were *nine times* as likely to develop the disease as the control group. In addition, a woman whose mother and sister have breast cancer has about a 50 percent chance of developing the disease herself.[14] Heredity is also a factor in cancer of the stomach, large intestine, uterus, or prostate.[15]

WHAT YOU CAN DO IF THERE IS CANCER IN YOUR FAMILY

This family tendency toward specific forms of cancer is only that—a tendency. You cannot change your heritage, but knowing about it should prompt you to do three things.

1. Eliminate as nearly as possible all other associated risks.
2. Familiarize yourself with your family's medical history.
3. Be especially attentive to the need for regular checkups.

Don't be an "ostrich" about it: you *can* help improve your chances.

Cutting Down Your Risk Factors: Lifestyle-Related and Other Controllable Causes

DIET

Preliminary evidence from a number of studies suggests that a high-calorie, fat-rich diet that is low in fiber may increase the risk of developing cancer of the breast, prostate, colon, and uterus.[16] An interesting example occurs in the Japanese cancer patterns mentioned earlier. Japanese who immigrate to the United States and adopt American dietary habits and cooking methods gradually tend to assume cancer patterns similar to those of native-born Americans. Specifically, the incidence of stomach cancer declines, while that of breast and colon cancers climbs.[17] This relationship between heredity and environment is not well understood, and more research is needed.

Scientists are also studying a possible relationship between breast cancer and dietary fat.[18] Postmenopausal women who are overweight may be at increased risk of breast cancer.[19]

HOW TO CHANGE YOUR DIET TO LOWER YOUR CANCER RISK

In 1982 a panel of the National Academy of Sciences concluded a study of nutritional factors that may be involved in causing cancer. The scientists who produced this 600-page study, called "Diet, Nutrition and Cancer," spent two years reviewing all the published research on the subject to date. The study suggested that certain adjustments in the average American diet would help lower the risk of cancer.[20]

▶ The most prominent of the study's recommendations was that Americans eat at least 25 percent less fat. This would mean eating less meat and less of such high-fat dairy products as butter, cheese, and ice cream, and cutting down the amount of cooking fats and oils we use.
▶ The study also recommended that salt-cured and smoked foods be eaten infrequently or not at all. This would mean, for most Americans, less bacon, ham, smoked sausage, and smoked fish.
▶ The study also recommended that we eat more fruits and vegetables rich in vitamin C (citrus fruits, tomatoes, peppers) and more vegetables in the cab-

bage family (cabbage, broccoli, cauliflower, kale, and brussels sprouts). There seems to be some evidence that these vegetables contain natural cancer-inhibiting substances.

Fortunately, the recommendations of this study coincide with the principles of good nutrition and with the recommendations of those who urge us to eat less fat to reduce our risk of heart disease. Once again, eating less fat and more fruits and vegetables would be a healthful switch for most Americans.

TOBACCO AND ALCOHOL

CIGARETTE SMOKING Currently more Americans (nearly 100,000) die annually of lung cancer than die in automobile accidents, and cigarette smoking has been overwhelmingly implicated as the cause of most lung malignancies.[21] Both the tar and the smoke from tobacco contain specific **carcinogenic** (cancer-producing) chemicals. Lung cancer is the most common cause of cancer death among American males age thirty-five and over. The risk appears to be greatest among men who have smoked cigarettes for twenty or more years.[22]

How is smoking related to lung cancer? The evidence indicates that inhaling carcinogenic irritants over a period of time triggers the cancerous potential in susceptible lung-tissue cells. Inhaled smoke paralyzes the bronchial cilia, interfering with their natural cleansing mechanism. The carcinogenic dusts, gases, and tars linger in the lungs, irritating them and causing precancerous changes, which can eventually trigger the cancer mechanism.

Nor is lung cancer the only danger. Cigarette smoking is unquestionably one cause of bladder cancer; this disease occurs two to three times as often among smokers as nonsmokers.[23] Apparently the body attempts to excrete the tobacco carcinogens by way of the urinary tract, irritating the bladder as it does so. Still other forms of cancer associated with cigarette smoking include oral cancers and cancers of the larynx, esophagus, and pancreas, and possibly the kidney.[24]

ALCOHOL Chronic, excessive alcohol consumption, a major social and health problem in itself (see Chapter 5), also seems to increase the risk of cancer in the mouth, throat, larynx, and esophagus when combined with the effects of tobacco smoking and poor nutrition.[25]

WHAT YOU CAN DO TO MINIMIZE CANCER RISKS FROM SMOKING AND ALCOHOL

► Give up tobacco. (See Chapter 6 for ways to kick the habit.) It is estimated that if everyone gave up smoking, 80 percent of lung cancers could be eliminated.[26]
► Keep your alcohol consumption moderate. If you smoke, avoid alcohol entirely. It enhances the carcinogenic effects of tobacco.

RADIATION

We are all exposed to various kinds of radiation in some degree, including sunlight and other forms. Can this radiation contribute to our risk of cancer? Here are the latest findings:

ULTRAVIOLET RADIATION Excessive exposure to the sun's ultraviolet rays can easily trigger skin cancers, particularly among fair-skinned individuals.

IONIZING RADIATION Exposure to radiation—from X-rays, radium, and atomic-bomb explosions, among other forms of ionizing radiation—indisputably increases the occurrence of leukemia (cancer of the blood) as well as cancers of the thyroid, skin, and bone. Opinions about avoiding such exposure differ, some scientists insisting that just one rad (a standard X-ray dose) ages the involved cells by one year.[27] (See Chapter 17 for a further discussion of the risks of radiation and nuclear energy.)

WHAT YOU CAN DO TO MINIMIZE RADIATION RISKS

► Don't broil yourself in the sun. Use a good sun*screen* (not sun*tan*) lotion.
► Expose yourself gradually to the sun, avoiding the hours between 11 A.M. and 3 P.M.
► Wear protective clothing even on cloudy days. This is doubly important if you are fair-skinned.

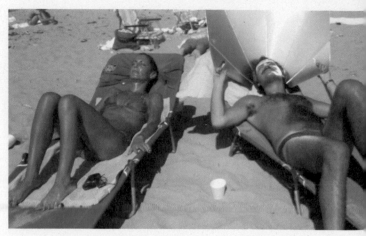

It is a mistake to think of a good tan as a sign of good health. Using a reflector to focus the sun's rays on the body only increases the risk of skin cancer. (© Barbara Alper)

► Avoid unnecessary X-rays. If you do need an X-ray, see that proper precautions are taken.
► Such exposure is especially dangerous to children and the developing fetus, so if you are pregnant do not submit to an X-ray except in an emergency.

These warnings do not mean that X-rays should never be used diagnostically, but they do mean that X-rays should be used with discretion and that exposure rates should be kept as low as is practicable.[28]

SEXUAL ACTIVITY AND CHILDBIRTH

Cancer of the cervix is known to be associated with such factors as poor sexual hygiene, sexual intercourse at an early age, and multiple sexual partners.[29] Women who have been infected with herpes virus Type 2 are also at risk: The precise cause-and-effect mechanism is still speculative, but a definite relationship has been established.[30]

Because of these relationships, good genital hygiene is particularly important, especially for women and uncircumcised males. Women who are sexually active should also be sure to have pelvic exams and Pap smears on a regular basis.

Childlessness and birth of a first child after age

30 also somewhat increase the risk of developing breast cancer.[31]

———————————————————— ◙

DRUGS

Certain drugs have come under scientific scrutiny as being possibly carcinogenic. Following are some highlights:

ESTROGEN Medicinal use of the hormone estrogen is associated with cancers of the breast, uterus, and testes in mice and other rodents. Studies of women who have used high doses of estrogen to relieve some common symptoms of menopause now indicate that there is an increased risk of cancer of the uterus associated with the medication. Apparently, the key problem here is misuse of the drug. Short-term use of *low* doses of estrogen does not seem to increase the risk of uterine cancer.[32]

BIRTH CONTROL PILLS Researchers still do not know if there is a relationship between oral contraceptives and cancer of the cervix, nor have they found clear-cut evidence of an increased or decreased risk of breast cancer among women who use oral contraceptives. Research among women who use the Pill is still going on. To date, cancer of the endometrium (the lining of the uterus) is the only malignancy that has been clearly linked to oral contraception, and this may be limited to one type—perhaps even a single brand, Oracon.[33]

DES In 1971 a very small but still unusual number of cases of a rare form of vaginal cancer was reported among women aged fourteen to twenty-two whose mothers had taken DES (diethylstilbestrol) to prevent miscarriage. Recent research has shown that DES is associated with many kinds of cancer. The women exposed to DES before they were born are now just entering the age range when cancers of the cervix and breast begin to appear, and it will be a number of years before they reach the usual age for cancers of the endometrium and ovary. Males whose mothers took DES may also be at risk. It is estimated that between four and six million Americans (mothers, daughters, sons) have been exposed to DES during pregnancy.[34]

DRUGS USED IN ORGAN TRANSPLANTS Certain drugs used during organ transplants to suppress the immune response and thus lessen chances of the body's rejecting the new organ have now been implicated as increasing the risk of cancer. Results of one study of over 16,000 kidney transplant patients showed that one type of lymphatic cancer developed at thirty-five times the normal rate.[35] Presumably, however, this increased risk is due to suppression of the immune defense system rather than to any carcinogenic properties of the drugs themselves.

ENVIRONMENTAL FACTORS: CHEMICALS, POLLUTANTS, AND WORKPLACE HAZARDS

As you'll discover when you read Chapter 17, experts disagree over the role of environmental factors, such as chemicals and pollutants, in the causation of cancer. Here we'll note some key findings—and some major areas of debate.

CHEMICALS Animal studies have suggested that many chemicals have cancer-causing properties: When high doses of the chemicals are injected or fed to animals, the animals tend to develop cancer. But it's not clear how closely these carcinogenic chemicals are connected with cancer in humans, because the conditions under which humans are exposed to them vary so widely. *Suspected* as potential contributors to human cancer are nitrites (used in curing ham, bacon, frankfurters, salami, and other processed meats), saccharin, hair dyes, and certain pesticides.

Consider these facts, however: Cancer of the stomach, which you would think might be most closely related to chemicals added to foods, has actually been *decreasing* in the United States in the past twenty-five years. During this period, the only form of cancer that has continued to rise is cancer of the lung—highly associated with cigarette smoking. Further, countries such as Poland and Czechoslovakia, which do not use our methods of food production or preservation, have overall cancer rates similar to or higher than those of the United States. So, connections between cancer and food additives and preservatives remain doubtful at this point.[36]

How to Help Lower Your Risk of Breast and Uterine Cancer

Breast cancer is the leading cause of death from cancer in North American women between the ages of 35 and 54. The American Cancer Society estimates that the American woman has a one in eleven chance of having breast cancer during her lifetime. Risks are increased by nutritional habits (particularly in high consumption of fats), environmental factors, and the delay of first pregnancy after the age of thirty.* You can do something about lowering at least some of these risks. In addition, you should know your family history of breast cancer and be sure your doctor has this very relevant information.

DETECTING BREAST CANCER

Methods of detecting breast cancer fall into two main groups. In the first group are methods that are still in the developmental stage. They have not yet established a good enough track record to be widely accepted. They are *thermography, ultrasound, diaphanography, computed tomographic mammography,* and *XERG mammography system (Xonics)*. The second group consists of three readily available methods of detection that have proven their worth. These are regular *examinations* by a medical expert, *breast self-examination (BSE),* and *mammography*.

What You Can Do

▶ Have a checkup every year: It is very important to have a thorough annual examination, lasting at least fifteen minutes, by a physician, nurse or paraprofessional.
▶ Learn to do breast self-examination: Your gynecologist or other specially trained person should teach you how to do a meticulous self-examination. (See Figure 11.4.) The importance of this cannot be stressed too strongly. Many of the cancers women find by BSE are at an earlier stage than those found accidentally or in routine physical examinations. One study estimated that breast cancer mortality might be reduced 18.8 percent by BSE, and 24.4 percent by routine annual physical breast examination by doctors and other trained personnel. The technique of mammography is credited as the only available method that will find breast cancer even earlier.†

DETECTING AND PREVENTING CERVICAL AND ENDOMETRIAL CANCER

For both cervical and endometrial cancer, it is possible to identify the high-risk patient, detect changes at an early stage, and begin appropriate therapy to prevent a more serious problem. The majority of these cancers, if discovered early, when they are still localized, can be cured by surgery and radiotherapy.

▶ Cervical cancer: Who is at high risk? Cervical cancer is found more often in women of low socioeconomic status, women who became sexually active at an early age, women who married at an early age, prostitutes, and others who have sex with many partners, particularly with men who are uncircumcised and practice poor hygiene.
▶ Endometrial cancer: Who is at high risk? Patients who are considered high risk for endometrial cancer are those who are obese, diabetic, or arteriosclerotic with dysfunctional bleeding. About 5 percent of cases occur in women under age forty.**

What You Can Do

▶ Find out whether you are at high risk (see the high-risk categories we have just mentioned).
▶ If you are, have a talk with your gynecologist about this problem.
▶ Regardless of whether you are at high risk for any of these kinds of cancer, be sure to have pelvic examinations and Pap smears regularly.
   Women whose mothers took DES have a greater risk of vaginal cancer than those not exposed and should start having regular pelvic examinations and Pap smears at the time of their first menstrual period. If you are not part of that group, you should start at age twenty (or earlier if you have already had intercourse) and should continue at yearly intervals. The Pap smear is a quick and painless screening device. If positive or suspicious cells are reported, your doctor can start a systematic approach to making a diagnosis.

Sources: *A. B. Miller, "Breast Cancer," *Cancer* 47 (1981): 1109–1113; †T. Carlile, "Breast Cancer Detection," *Cancer* 47 (1981): 1164–1169; **Hugh R. K. Barber, "Uterine Cancer (Prevention)," *Cancer* 47 (1981): 1126–1132.

How to Help Lower Your Risk of Testicular Cancer

Testicular cancer is a common type of cancer among white American males between the ages of twenty and thirty-four. And though this type of cancer accounts for only 1 percent of all cancers in men of all ages, there is an increasing incidence in young adults. Males with undescended testicles are at high risk, and for this reason the condition should be corrected in early childhood. Testicular cancers of germ cell origin account for at least 95 percent of malignant neoplasms of the testes of adult men.

What is causing the rise in testicular cancer? Several possibilities are being explored: Two million sons were born to women who took DES during their pregnancies between 1940 and 1960. Although studies have yet to prove any clear risk factor to a marked degree, scientists are concerned, and the research is continuing. Could oral contraceptives be responsible for some part of the increase? These pills were not commonly prescribed until after 1960, so scientists cannot complete their studies until more males born to women on the Pill reach maturity. Scientists also believe that environmental factors may lie behind the increase, and they are investigating the possible influence of medical care and nutrition of parents before and during pregnancy and of children from birth to puberty. Parental work histories are also being looked into.

What You Can Do

Self-examination can help you detect testicular cancer early. The American Cancer Society recommends the following testicle self-examination:

1. Perform the examination after a warm bath or shower, when the skin of the scrotum is most relaxed. (The scrotum is the pouch in which the testicles normally lie.)
2. Cup each testicle in the palm of one hand and examine it by feeling it with the fingers of the other hand. The normal testicle is smooth, egg-shaped, and somewhat firm to the touch.
3. At the rear of each testicle is a tube called the epididymis, which carries sperm away from the testicle. This is a normal part of your body; its presence does not indicate cancer.
4. If there is any change in shape or texture of the testicles—or any lumps, especially hard ones—consult a doctor immediately.

Repeat this examination every six or eight weeks. It is important that you know what your own testicles normally feel like so that you will recognize any changes.

Source: D. Schottenfield, "The Epidemiology of Cancer," *Cancer* 47 (1981): 1095–1108.

POLLUTION It has been well established that lung cancer rates are higher in urban areas, even after correction is made for smoking.[37] The role of water contaminants has also been extensively debated. Yet the studies aimed at resolving the question of risk from environmental pollution are mostly inconclusive.

WORKPLACE (OCCUPATIONAL) CANCER HAZARDS Here we are on somewhat more solid ground. High-dose, long-term exposure to various workplace chemicals have been shown to increase the risk of certain forms of cancer. These chemicals include asbestos (insulating and fireproofing), vinyl chloride (plastics), chromates (paint), benzene (rubber), and benzidene (dyes). Today occupation-related cancers account for a sizable percentage of cancer deaths in the United States. Asbestos workers are a prime example: Not only

do asbestos workers show an increased incidence of mesothelioma (a rare cancer that attacks the lining of the chest or abdominal cavity), but *asbestos workers who smoke* have a higher incidence of lung cancer than other smokers—in fact, about 60 times higher.[38]

WHAT YOU CAN DO ABOUT CANCER-CAUSING CHEMICALS, POLLUTION, AND OTHER ENVIRONMENTAL CARCINOGENS

It is neither practical nor desirable to eliminate from our lives every item that is thought to be linked to cancer. Since much of the evidence concerning these problems is still tentative, the best approach is to stay informed. If you think you may

Figure 11.4   How to Examine Your Breasts

1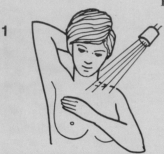

Examine your breasts during bath or shower; hands glide easier over wet skin. Fingers flat, move gently over every part of each breast. Use right hand to examine left breast, left hand for right breast. Check for any lump, hard knot, or thickening.

2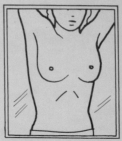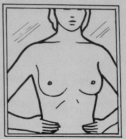

Stand before a mirror and inspect your breasts, first with arms at your sides, then with arms raised high overhead. Look for any changes in the shape of each breast, a swelling, dimpling of the skin, or changes in the nipple.

Then rest your palms on your hips and press down firmly to flex your chest muscles. Left and right breast will not exactly match; few women's breasts do.

3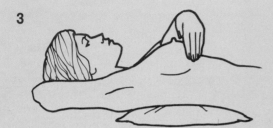

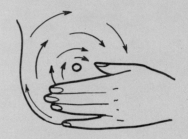

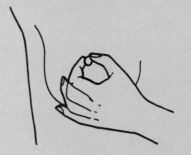

Lie down on a bed and put a pillow or folded towel under your right shoulder. Place your right hand behind your head; this distributes breast tissue more evenly on the chest. With left hand, fingers flat, press gently in small circular motions around an imaginary clock face. Begin at outermost top of your right breast for 12 o'clock, then move to 1 o'clock, and so on around the circle back to 12. A ridge of firm tissue in the lower curve of each breast is normal. Then move in an inch, toward the nipple, and keep circling to examine every part of your breast, including the nipple. This requires at least three more circles. Repeat this procedure on your left breast with a pillow under your left shoulder and your left hand behind your head.

Finally, squeeze the nipple of each breast gently between thumb and index finger. Any discharge, clear or bloody, should be reported to a doctor immediately.

Most breast cancers are discovered by women themselves. Every woman should examine her breasts every month. The best time to do so is about a week after the end of your menstrual period, when the breasts are usually not tender or swollen. If you do find a lump, discharge, or dimple, see a doctor as soon as possible. Most lumps or changes do not mean cancer, but only a doctor can make the diagnosis.

Source: American Cancer Society. Used by permission.

be exposed to industrial chemicals at work, find out the dangers associated with those chemicals and handle any that are known to be carcinogenic with extreme care.

THE DETECTION AND TREATMENT OF CANCER

Early detection and treatment give the cancer patient the best chance for complete recovery. The longer the time that elapses, the greater chance the cancer has of spreading locally—or of metastasizing to other sites in the body where it may compress, obstruct, or destroy vital organs. In this battle, you can't afford to lose any time.

If you want a dramatic example of the value of early detection, take a look at the cure rates for various forms of cancer. A dramatic example is the contrast between skin cancer and lung cancer. Skin cancers are easily seen, and they frequently receive early attention; in addition, they are readily accessible to treatment. Except for melanoma, a cancer of the pigment-carrying cells in the skin that is particularly resistant to treatment, the cure rate for skin cancers (taken as a whole) is more than 97 percent.[39]

For lung cancer, however, the cure rate is less than 10 percent. This disease is *not* immediately apparent; in fact, it frequently does not produce obvious symptoms until it has gotten out of control. Lung cancers have to be treated surgically; often one lobe of a lung or an entire lung must be removed. In some cases, the tumor at surgery appears to be confined to the lung. But only 15 to 20 percent of these patients will survive five years and be considered "cured"—a discouraging figure, since lung cancer is now so common.[40]

KNOW THE SEVEN WARNING SIGNS

Cancer often produces noticeable changes in our bodies, and we can often detect the changes through simple, painless self-examination. The American Cancer Society emphasizes seven warning signals of cancer. Know them and remember them.

1. A change in bowel or bladder habits
2. A sore that does not heal
3. Any unusual bleeding or discharge
4. A thickening or lump in the breast or elsewhere
5. Indigestion or difficulty in swallowing
6. Any obvious change in a wart or mole
7. A nagging cough or hoarseness.[41]

Don't be too nervous about these symptoms. *None of them automatically means that you have cancer.* They are only warning signals. But don't be too casual about these symptoms, either. A "maybe it will go away" attitude is just plain foolish if a signal lasts beyond two weeks. In such a case, see your physician promptly.

How Often Do You Need a Checkup?

The greatest hope for the cancer victim is in early diagnosis and prompt treatment. That is why it is so very important to be alert to the signals and have regular checkups. The American Cancer Society recommends a cancer-related checkup every three years for people between the ages of twenty and forty. The checkup should include testing for thyroid, oral, skin, and lymphatic cancers; cancers of the reproductive and digestive tracts; and, for women, breast cancer.

DELAY AND DENIAL

A recent study looked at 563 patients who had cancer to see how long they had put off getting help. They had delayed as long as patients had in similar studies made thirty and fifty years earlier! We now know so much more about the prevention, causes, and cures than we did half a century ago—and yet people are still afraid to deal with the disease. According to the study, "delay in seeking medical help appeared to be a conscious and deliberate act, rather than a failure to perceive the neoplasm or to comprehend the consequences."[42]

Why do people delay when they suspect they may have cancer? For many people, the problem is fear. Anticipating what we *think* will happen in treatment can produce so much anxiety that we delay going to see a doctor. In this study, fear and denial of the disease were evident: 8 percent a-

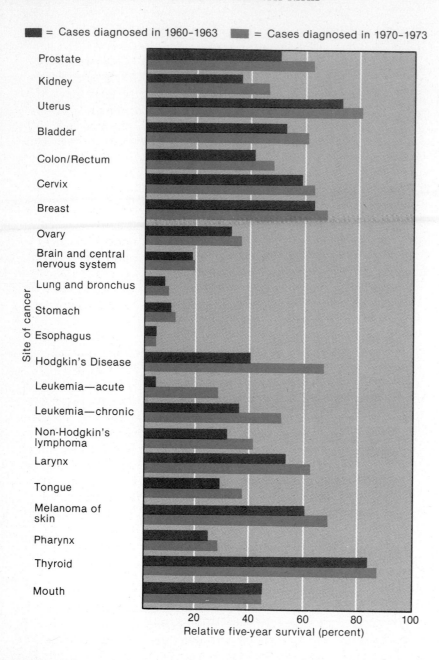

■ = Cases diagnosed in 1960-1963   ▬ = Cases diagnosed in 1970-1973

Site of cancer:
Prostate
Kidney
Uterus
Bladder
Colon/Rectum
Cervix
Breast
Ovary
Brain and central nervous system
Lung and bronchus
Stomach
Esophagus
Hodgkin's Disease
Leukemia—acute
Leukemia—chronic
Non-Hodgkin's lymphoma
Larynx
Tongue
Melanoma of skin
Pharynx
Thyroid
Mouth

20   40   60   80   100
Relative five-year survival (percent)

Figure 11.5 The gradually improving cure rates for many types of cancer provide grounds for hope. A cancer patient is considered "cured" if he or she survives for five years after the original diagnosis. As this chart shows, the survival rates for cancer patients diagnosed in 1970–1973 tend to be significantly higher than for those diagnosed ten years earlier. These figures are for whites; black patients have 5 to 10 percent lower survival rates, on the average, probably because they often get inadequate treatment.

Source: Adapted from Biometry Branch, National Cancer Institute, in American Cancer Society, *1982 Cancer Facts and Figures*, p. 7.

voided medical help until they couldn't function independently. And 33 percent of the group sought help only when their persistent pain became too hard to live with.

What Does Cancer Treatment Involve?

One of the reasons some people are afraid to face the possibility of having cancer is that they are afraid of what will happen during treatment. Will

it be painful? Will it disable them or make it hard for them to carry out their everyday activities? Today, there are many treatment options, and the physician can choose one that is best for a particular patient and disease. Some of these treatment approaches may actually cure cancer. If a total cure is not possible, treatment can help make the symptoms of the disease less severe.

TYPES OF TREATMENT

Following are some major treatment approaches and key facts you should know about them.

SURGERY: PROS AND CONS Because of improved diagnostic equipment and laser instruments, surgery is now more precise than ever before, and it has proven successful against some cancers—especially tumors involving the lung, colon, stomach, bowel, liver, and skin. Yet since surgery involves removing or disrupting entire organs of the body, it can mean more physical problems for the patient—sometimes with profound psychological effects.

Today, many cancer specialists examine other treatment options before recommending surgery. With breast cancer, for example, mastectomy-type surgery (removal of breast tissue and perhaps surrounding tissue) is no longer automatically recommended. Before physicians opt for it, they study the particular patient's hormonal picture, and determine if (or to what extent) the cancer has spread into the lymph nodes in the armpit. They may then decide that chemotherapy is the better treatment approach for a particular patient.[43]

◨—————————————————

A second opinion should always be sought before making a decision about *any* surgery.

—————————————————◨

RADIATION Radiation therapy uses energy in very high, concentrated doses to destroy cancer cells. It is now used as one of the primary treatments for cancers of the cervix, head, neck, larynx, prostate, and skin, among others.

The crucial thing to remember about radiation is this: It must be handled by a specialist who will tailor the therapy to the particular patient. No two cancers are alike, and no two people respond to radiation therapy in the same way.

CHEMOTHERAPY Chemotherapy is a course of treatment using chemicals that destroy cancerous cells. In recent years chemotherapy has become one of our biggest weapons against cancer. Today, for example, it is possible to *cure*, via chemotherapy, fourteen types of cancer that would have been considered all but incurable only a few decades ago.[44]

Recently there has been a trend toward using combinations of anticancer drugs, rather than just a single drug, for many types of cancer. Evidently, the cells in a tumor sometimes develop differ-ences, and not all of them will react to a given drug in the same way. Hence a combination of drugs has a better chance of destroying the growth.[45] But unfortunately there is still no drug or combination of drugs that can kill cancer cells selectively—that is, without harming normal cells and causing some side effects. Although they vary considerably, side effects generally include nausea, vomiting, and hair loss.

QUACKERY

Some cancer patients do not go to physicians and hospitals where they can be treated. They go instead to quacks and spend millions of dollars annually for ineffective drugs, diets, and other controversial forms of treatment. Among the publicized treatments that lack scientific support are laetrile, krebiozen, nucleic acid diets, vegetarian diets, and a variety of mechanical devices.

Laetrile, also known as "vitamin B_{17}" or "aprikern," is one of the most notorious quack cancer treatments. There is no such vitamin as B_{17}; this fact alone should make one suspicious right from the start! The substance is an extract of apricot pits. Repeated studies at reputable cancer and medical research institutes have failed to disclose any evidence whatever that laetrile will either cure or prevent any form of cancer. Nevertheless, advocates of laetrile and other quack treatments often claim success and offer testimonials of "cured" patients. What they do *not* say is that the "cure" they attribute to their treatment may very likely be the result of a naturally occurring improvement (remission) or a standard medical treatment such as chemotherapy.

Cancer quacks prosper not only because people are ignorant but also because they are afraid or desperate. Victims who fear they have incurable cancer, or who have had those fears confirmed by medical means, will often grasp at any straw. The greatest tragedy of cancer quackery is that the victim who might be cured often delays a trip to the doctor and instead relies on useless drugs and treatments. When he or she does finally seek appropriate treatment, it may be too late to curb the disease.

ACTIVE DECISION MAKING ABOUT TREATMENT

We owe it to ourselves to counter our fears of cancer by sensible information gathering. As with all health issues, the key is to go to a reputable source. The National Cancer Institute in Washington, D.C., cancer centers at major universities, and your local chapter of the American Cancer Society—all these are good sources for information on the value of various cancer treatments. Armed with reliable information, we are best able to make informed decisions about treatment. And again, we emphasize: Cancer treatment is one of today's fastest-growing medical areas. Through the recent developments in this field, we now have much more ammunition in our battle against cancer than many people realize.

LIVING WITH CANCER

"I'm living with cancer, not dying from it!" Jane Pike of Boston became, in her own words, a "cancer militant" when she herself was stricken. She decided to spread the word that cancer can be talked about—in fact, her message was, "Please talk." She founded a group called Omega aimed at making it possible for cancer patients and their relatives to get together and do just that.[46] There are many other such groups around the country, where members can share their feelings—whether happy or sad—and go on living productive lives as long as they possibly can.

Throughout this chapter we have spoken about the emotional and psychological impact of cancer. Depending on the nature of the disease and the family and friends involved, the effect of cancer may be catastrophic—or it may be an experience that, while never pleasant, can be dealt with and can even strengthen the people involved.

What to Tell the Patient— and When

How much—and when—a patient should be told is a big decision. More and more doctors are encouraging a candid approach with most patients—but it's a tough question. Undoubtedly, there are some patients who are simply unable to deal with the knowledge that they have cancer. Confronted with the truth, they are in danger of becoming so

depressed—perhaps even suicidal—that whatever time they have to live is lost. On the other hand, a patient who is not told the seriousness of his or her condition may not take the basic precaution of having periodic checkups after being successfully treated.

Other patients may need to be told the truth little by little. Still others, though, would much prefer to know the truth so that they can have "quality time" and structure their lives accordingly.

There is no black-and-white answer to the question of how much a cancer patient should know. We *can* say for certain, however, that those concerned must do all they can to prevent the patient from giving up all hope. There isn't a cancer specialist in the world who can't tell you of patients diagnosed as terminally ill with only months to live at most, who are still living years and years later.

Young Adults with Cancer

Denial is a frequent coping mechanism of young adults with cancer, and this denial may be extremely aggressive. They may be full of energy and certain they will "beat" the disease. In reality, there's nothing wrong with this pattern of denial. It can become a problem only if it interferes with treatment or encourages patients to become too active against medical advice. As a rule, teenagers are encouraged to continue as many activities as possible.

Young adults also tend to cope with cancer through overcompensation (trying to outdo everyone), intellectualizations, and anger. These are all normal responses. If you know a young adult who has cancer, try to accept these reactions, difficult as it may be to do so.[47]

It's often hard for young cancer patients to talk about their situation. Many adolescents have problems communicating with adults, and particularly their parents. Caregivers are working to help parents and their youngsters get over the hurdle of talking about cancer by encouraging open discussion of the disease and treatment. Many centers have peer-group sessions so that young people can share what they are going through with others their own age.

CONTINUING THE FIGHT

The days when cancer was mentioned in hushed tones—if at all—are past. We now know a great deal about the disease, and we are finding out more with each passing day. Survival rates climb as research continues and we learn more. Scientists, physicians, health educators, the media, and cancer patients themselves are teaching us and helping dispel fears.

Today, accurate and current information is available. You don't have to be a specialist to understand material from the American Cancer Society and other reputable sources. You need to know all you can about the dangers of radiation, pollution, toxic waste, and possible work hazards, so keep up to date and learn what is happening around you. Learn to discriminate between sensationalism and usable material, and keep yourself informed about prevention, treatment and cures. The war on cancer needs to be fought with brains, funding, responsive industry and government, a little help from our friends . . . and hope.

MAKING HEALTH DECISIONS

Assess Your Cancer Risk

Cancer is a group of diseases that are "caused," as far as we now know, by a number of factors. Only rarely are cancers directly associated with exposure to one factor. You should know what factors in your life may affect your risk of cancer. The following questions are intended to focus your attention on some of the factors associated with an increased risk of cancer. When you have answered all the questions, add up your total score to assess *your* susceptibility to cancer.

SMOKING AND TOBACCO USE

1. How much do you smoke?
   (0)_____ Not at all
   (1)_____ Less than one pack a day
   (2)_____ One to two packs a day
   (3)_____ More than two packs a day

2. How much do you use "smokeless" tobacco?
   (0)_____ Not at all
   (1)_____ Chew or dip occasionally
   (2)_____ Chew or dip regularly

3. How long have you used tobacco?
   (0)_____ I have never used tobacco.
   (1)_____ I gave up tobacco within the past year.
   (2)_____ I use tobacco now and have done so for the past two years.

   (3)_____ I use tobacco now and have done so for more than two years.
   (4)_____ I use tobacco now and have done so for more than five years.

DIET

4. How much fat does your diet contain?
   (0)_____ My diet contains less than 25 percent fat.
   (1)_____ My diet contains between 25 and 50 percent fat.
   (2)_____ My diet contains more than 50 percent fat.

5. How much fiber (raw fruit or whole grains, for example) does your diet contain?
   (0)_____ My diet includes fiber at least once every day.
   (1)_____ My diet includes fiber 3 to 5 times per week.
   (2)_____ My diet includes fiber 1 to 3 times per week.
   (3)_____ My diet seldom or never includes fiber.

(*Note:* For more information on dietary fats and fiber, see Chapter 13.)

PERSONAL RESPONSIBILITY FOR SELF-EXAMINATION

6. How often do you examine yourself?

Females: (0)_____I examine my breasts every month.

(1)_____I do not examine my breasts regularly.

Males: (0)_____I examine my testicles regularly.

(1)_____I do not examine my testicles regularly.

ENVIRONMENT

7. Where do you live and work?

(0)_____no (1)_____yes Is a report on air pollution a regular part of the weather forecast where you live?

(0)_____no (1)_____yes Is your community a site for treatment or disposal of toxic wastes?

(0)_____no (1)_____yes Does your work put you outside in the sun for most of the day?

(0)_____no (1)_____yes Do you handle hazardous chemicals at work?

(0)_____no (1)_____yes Does your work expose you to asbestos fibers?

(0)_____no (1)_____yes Does your work expose you to molten plastic?

HEREDITY

8. Have any of your blood relatives had cancer?

(0)_____ No relatives have ever had cancer.

(1)_____ One relative developed cancer after age fifty.

(2)_____ One relative of my sex developed cancer after age fifty.

(3)_____ Two or more relatives developed cancer before age fifty.

(4)_____ Two or more relatives of my sex developed cancer before age fifty.

Now add up your scores. If your total score is over 20, then your cancer risk is very high. If your score is between 10 and 20, then your risk is moderate. A score of less than 10 indicates relatively slight risk. You should realize, of course, that individual differences also play a major role in the development of cancer. A high score does not mean that you will get cancer; a low score does not mean that you are protected.

QUESTIONS

1. Of the five sections included in the assessment, which seem to contribute most to the risk of cancer indicated by your total score? _____

_____

_____

_____

2. What changes in your behavior are needed for you to reduce your total score?_____

_____

_____

3. Are there any risk factors that are really out of your control? _____

_____

SUMMARY

1. Cancer deaths have increased each year since 1949. The increase stems from more accurate diagnoses, people's greater longevity, and lifestyle trends. Knowledge about and treatments for cancer have also increased. Early diagnosis, prevention (as by not smoking cigarettes), and a wide range of treatments are major weapons in the war against cancer.

2. Cancer is a condition of abnormal cellular growth. A tumor is a swelling or mass that forms when cells that normally function usefully together begin to multiply independently, taking nourishment from surrounding, normal cells. Only malignant tumors, those that spread their damage to other parts of the body, are considered cancers. The process by which a malignancy spreads is called metastatic growth.

3. Cancer takes more than 100 different forms. Malignant tumors are classified by the types of cells from which they arise or by the site of the primary tumor.

4. Cancer kills by disrupting the normal functioning of organs or organ systems.

5. The psychological effects of cancer may include anxiety, depression, and enormous stress.

6. As with most other diseases, the onset of certain cancers appears to be associated with the interaction of hereditary, environmental, and psychological factors.

7. Cultural differences and family patterns in the incidence of certain cancers point to hereditary and environmental factors. It is often hard to separate the effects of these two sorts of causes.

8. Factors that people can control—such as diet, sexual behavior, drug and tobacco use, exposure to chemicals, radiation, and pollution—all affect the incidence of cancer.

9. People who stay alert to detecting cancer lower their risk. Therefore, know the seven warning signs of cancer. Regularly examine your genitals (and breasts, if you are female). Have regular checkups, Pap smears, and pelvic examinations. Do not smoke cigarettes or drink alcohol excessively. Avoid fats and high-cholesterol foods. Avoid unnecessary X-rays, exposure to the sun, environmental carcinogens, and drugs. Good personal hygiene also helps to prevent cancer.

10. The three forms of cancer treatment that most physicians rely on are radiation therapy, chemotherapy, and surgery. They may be used singly or in combination.

11. Cancer patients need help from relatives and friends in living with the disease. Young adults are especially likely to deny their illness or overcompensate for it.

GLOSSARY

adenocarcinomas Cancers arising from glandular epithelial cells, such as the cells lining the milk duct in the breast.

anaplastic Referring to cancers whose cellular structure is so abnormal that they no longer resemble the cells from which they originated, and no identification is possible.

benign tumor A tumor that grows relatively slowly and remains localized.

cancer A condition of abnormal cell growth.

carcinogenic Cancer-producing.

carcinomas Cancers that arise from epithelium.

chemotherapy A course of treatment using chemicals that destroy cancerous cells.

epithelium The cells forming the skin, the glands, and the membranes that line the respiratory, urinary, and gastrointestinal tracts.

hemorrhage Profuse bleeding.

leukemias Cancers arising from blood-forming cells.

lymphomas Cancers arising from lymphatic cells.

malignant tumor A tumor whose cells grow in abnormal ways and may break away and spread to other parts of the body.

melanomas Cancers of pigment-carrying cells of the skin.

metastases Secondary tumors that form when cancerous cells break away from the original malignant tumor and transfer to a new location in the body.

metastatic growth   The process by which cancerous cells break away from the original malignant tumor and transfer to a new location in the body.

mitosis   The orderly division of a cell into two new cells.

neoplasm   A group of cells growing in an uncontrolled fashion to form a tumor.

radiation therapy   The use of very high, concentrated doses of radiation to destroy cancer cells.

sarcomas   Cancers that arise from supporting or connective tissues, such as bones, cartilage, and the membranes covering muscles and fat.

tissue   A collection of cells in the body that are specialized to perform certain functions.

tumor   A swelling or mass formed by a group of cells within a tissue that grow to an abnormal size and shape and begin to multiply in an uncontrolled fashion.

NOTES

1. E. Silverberg, "Cancer Statistics 1982," *Ca—A Cancer Journal for Clinicians* 32, no. 1 (January–February 1982): 15.

2. E. Silverberg, "Cancer Statistics 1983," *Ca—A Cancer Journal for Clinicians* 33, no. 1 (January–February 1983): 9–25.

3. American Cancer Society, *1982 Cancer Facts and Figures* (New York, 1982).

4. *Harvard Medical School Health Letter* 7, no. 6 (April 1982): 2.

5. G. R. Newell, W. B. Boutwell, D. L. Morris, B. C. Tilley, and E. S. Branyon, "Epidemiology of Cancer," in V. T. De Vita, S. Hellman, and S. A. Rosenberg, eds., *Cancer: Principles and Practices of Oncology* (Philadelphia: Lippincott, 1982), pp. 3–32.

6. Harley C. Shands, Jacob E. Finesinger, Stanley Cobb, and Ruth D. Abrams, "Psychological Mechanisms in Patients with Cancer," *Cancer* 4, no. 6 (November 1951): 1159–1170.

7. Arthur M. Sutherland, "Psychological Impact of Cancer and Its Therapy," *CA—A Cancer Journal for Clinicians* 31, no. 30 (May–June 1981): 159–171.

8. Ibid.

9. Ibid.

10. American Cancer Society, *1982 Cancer Facts and Figures.*

11. American Cancer Society, *1982 Cancer Facts and Figures*, p. 17.

12. D. Schottenfield, "The Epidemiology of Cancer," *Cancer* 47 (1981): 1095–1108.

13. Philip M. Boffey, "Cancer Experts Lean Toward Steady Vigilance, but Less Alarm, on Environment," *New York Times*, March 2, 1982.

14. C. Bain, F. E. Speizer, B. Rosner, C. Belanger, and C. H. Hennekens, "Family History of Breast Cancer as a Risk Indicator for the Disease," *American Journal of Epidemiology* 111, no. 3 (1980): 301.

15. A. C. Upton, "Principles of Cancer Biology: Etiology and Prevention of Cancer," in De Vita, Hellman, and Rosenberg, eds., *Cancer,* pp. 33–58.

16. G. Saxon, "Diet and Cancer," *American Journal of Epidemiology* 112, no. 2 (1980): 247.

17 Schottenfield, "The Epidemiology of Cancer."

18. A. B. Miller, "Breast Cancer," *Cancer* 47 (1981): 1109–1113.

19. Saxon, "Diet and Cancer."

20. National Academy of Sciences, "Diet, Nutrition, and Cancer."

21. American Cancer Society, *1982 Cancer Facts and Figures.*

22. Ibid.; E. Silverberg and J. A. Lubera, "A Review of American Cancer Society Estimates of Cancer Cases and Deaths," *CA—A Cancer Journal for Clinicians* 33, no. 1 (January–February 1983): 2–9.

23. R. Doll and R. Peto, *Causes of Cancer,* (New York: Oxford University Press, 1981, pp. 1220–1223.

24. Ibid., pp. 1220–1224.

25. J. C. Rosenberg, J. G. Schwade, and V. Vaitkevicius, "Cancer of the Esophagus," in De Vita, Hellman, and Rosenberg, eds., *Cancer,* pp. 500–533.

26. American Cancer Society, *1982 Cancer Facts and Figures.*

27. Jon D. Boice, "Cancer Following Medical Irradiation," *Cancer* 47 (1981): 1081–1090.

28. Ibid.

29. Hugh R. K. Barber, "Uterine Cancer (Prevention)," *Cancer* 47 (1981): 1126–1132.

30. Ibid.

31. Doll and Peto, *The Causes of Cancer*, p. 1237.

32. Robert Hoover and Joseph F. Fraumeni, "Drug-Induced Cancer," *Cancer* 47 (1981): 1071–1080.

33. Ibid.

34. Ibid.

35. R. Hoover, "Effects of Drugs—Immunosuppression," in H. H. Hyatt, J. D. Watson, and J. A. Winsten, eds., *Origins of Human Cancer* (Cold Spring Harbor, N.Y.: Cold Spring Harbor Laboratory, 1977), pp. 369–379.

36. Schottenfield, "Epidemiology of Cancer."

37. Norton Nelson, "Cancer Prevention: Environmental, Industrial, and Occupational Factors," *Cancer* 47 (1981): 1065–1070.

38. Ibid.; American Cancer Society, *1982 Cancer Facts and Figures.*

39. American Cancer Society, *1982 Cancer Facts and Figures.*

40. Ibid.

41. Ibid.

42. Thomas P. Hackett, N. H. Cassem, and John W. Raker, "Patient Delay in Cancer," *New England Journal of Medicine* 28, no. 1 (July 5, 1973): 14–20..

43. Paul P. Carbone, "Options in Breast Cancer Therapy," *Hospital Practice* 16, no. 2 (February 1981): 53–61.

44. American Cancer Society, *1982 Cancer Facts and Figures.*

45. *Harvard Medical School Health Letter* 6, no. 6 (April 1982).

46. *A Time to Die*, CBS-TV, July 10, 1982.

47. National Institute of Health, U.S. Public Health Service, *Coping with Cancer*, September 1980 (NIH Publication No. 80-2080).

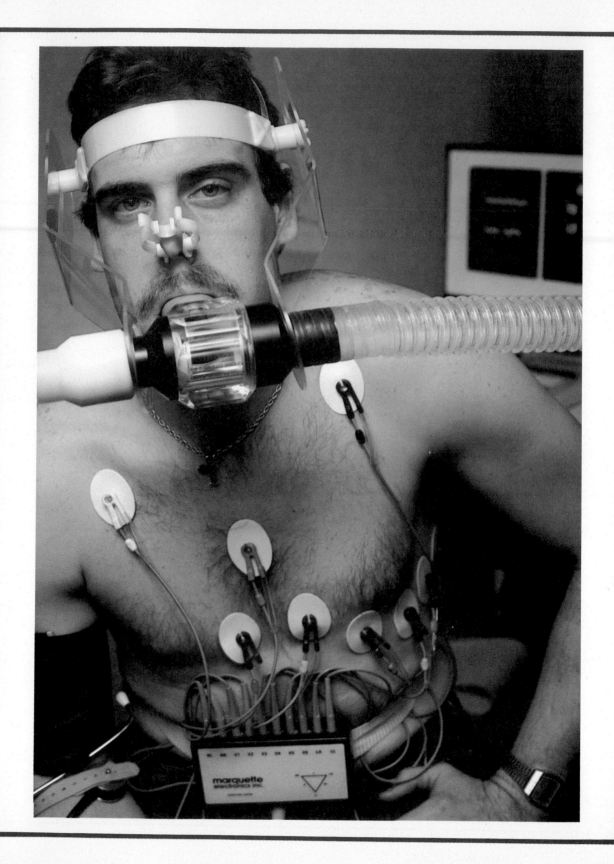

CHAPTER 12

Cardiovascular Diseases

It is one of the ironies of our society that people who rarely forget to fasten their seat belts, who scrupulously eliminate all known carcinogens from their diet, and who install sophisticated burglar alarm systems, may nevertheless take few precautions against cardiovascular disease (CVD), a class of highly *preventable* disorders that pose a severe threat to life, health, and well-being.

According to the 1983 edition of *Heart Facts,* a booklet published by the American Heart Association, diseases of the heart *(cardio)* and blood vessels *(vascular)* claim more American lives than all other causes of death combined. Cancer, which is far more widely feared, takes 400,000 lives in this country each year; but more than 1 million men, women, and children succumb to CVD annually.[1] A stealthy killer that develops slowly and without noticeable symptoms over a number of years, CVD takes many forms, including high blood pressure, coronary artery disease (disease of the arteries supplying the heart muscle), stroke, abnormal heart rhythms, and rheumatic heart disease. About 25,000 babies are born every year with heart defects, and a staggering total of 42.3 million Americans have some form of CVD.[2] In all, heart and blood vessel disorders cost the nation $60 billion annually in medical expenses, lost wages, curtailed production, and lost labor.[3]

Although CVD usually manifests itself during middle age, the seeds of the disorder seem to be sown decades earlier. In a now-famous study, army pathologists examined the hearts of 300 American soldiers who were killed in combat in Korea. These young men (their average age was twenty-two) were apparently in good health when they were killed, and none were known to be suffering from heart disease at the time of death. Yet in more than 75 percent of the men, the coronary atherosclerotic process (a process in which coronary arteries are narrowed) had already begun.[4] As the study shows, CVD *can* begin—"silently"—while people are still in their late teens and twenties. *But*—and this is the crucial point—we can help guard against it if we live in a healthy way. Many potential CVD victims lead sedentary lives, choose foods rich in salt and fats, are overweight, smoke cigarettes, and handle stress poorly. *If* we cut down on these risk factors, we can lower our chances of developing CVD.

Recently, for reasons that are not yet known, there has been a downward trend in CVD-related fatalities in the general population: The actual number of CVD deaths has been declining since the early 1970s.[5] Eighteen years after the Korean War study, for example, soldiers killed in Vietnam were the subjects of a similar study, and the results were not as alarming: Only 45 percent of the soldiers' hearts had narrowed arteries indicative of coronary atherosclerosis.[6] But this does not mean we can relax our guard against CVD; a sizable percentage of the population is still at risk. It continues to be important for us to know what causes CVD and what steps we can take to help prevent it. First, we need to know a few basic facts about the heart and circulatory system.

HOW THE HEART AND CIRCULATORY SYSTEM WORK

The major function of the **heart** is to pump blood into the lungs to pick up oxygen, and then to pump that blood throughout the body to supply the tissues with fresh, oxygen-rich blood (see Fig-

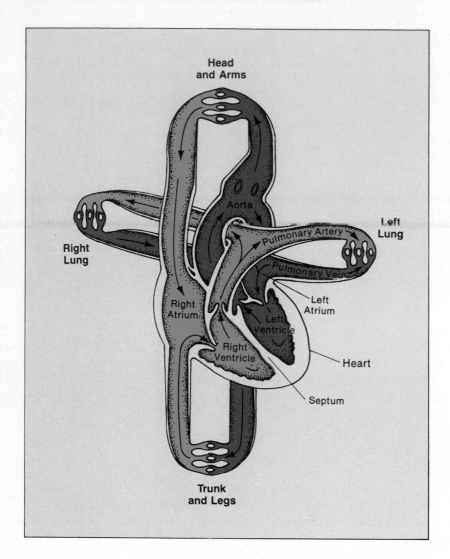

Head
and Arms

Aorta

Right
Lung

Left
Lung

Pulmonary Artery

Pulmonary Veins

Right
Atrium

Left
Atrium

Left
Ventricle

Right
Ventricle

Heart

Septum

Trunk
and Legs

Figure 12.1 The circulatory
system. This diagram shows how
the blood circulates, going to the
lungs to be cleansed of carbon
dioxide and to pick up oxygen
(blue area), being pumped through
the heart to the rest of the body
(red area), circulating back to the
lungs, and so on. The heart beats
about 100,000 times each day,
circulating the average person's
nine pints of blood 1,900 times.
Source: American Heart Association, *Heart Facts,* 1983, p. 5.

ure 12.1). This pumping process is carried out via
a continuous series of contractions and relaxations
not unlike the action of a bulb: Squeeze it and fluid
is squirted out; relax and fluid is sucked in, over
and over again. As you will see, your heart is somewhat like a system of four interconnected bulbs.[7]

Unlike other organ systems, such as the kidneys, that can shut down for a time without permanent harm to the body, the heart must work
nonstop. The only time it rests is during the split
second between beats. Each cell of the body needs
a constant supply of oxygen—the fuel that keeps
us alive—and because this oxygen is quickly used
up, it must be constantly replenished. Oxygen
starvation causes destruction of body parts—most
importantly the brain, the body's master control.
Brain death, which results if the brain is deprived

of oxygen, causes every other part of the body to
stop working within a few minutes.[8]

A Look at the Heart

The heart is a tough, four-chambered, muscular
organ the size of an adult's fist and weighing less
than one pound. It beats about 100,000 times per
day, pumping about one-half cup of blood with
each beat. Divided down the center by a solid
sheet of muscle, the *septum,* the heart consists of
four distinct chambers. Its thick muscular wall (the
myocardium) is surrounded by a tough protective
sac (the *pericardium*), and lined by a thin membrane (the *endocardium*). The top chambers, one
on each side of the septum, are termed the *atria*

TEST YOUR AWARENESS

Cardiovascular Disease: How Much Do You Know?

Sometimes, the more people fear an illness, the more misconceptions they develop about it. Not surprisingly, there are many myths about cardiovascular disease, America's number-one killer. How much do you know about CVD? Take this little quiz and see: You'll find out about CVD in this chapter.

True	False	
_____	_____	1. People with red faces and bulging eyes have high blood pressure.
_____	_____	2. People with quick tempers usually have high blood pressure.

True	False	
_____	_____	3. Heart attacks are definitely caused by a high-pressure, stressed life-style.
_____	_____	4. If you need surgery after a heart attack, you are really a "goner."
_____	_____	5. The best way to prevent heart disease is to "choose healthy grandparents."

ANSWERS

1 & 2. *False.* It is almost impossible to predict blood pressure from a person's appearance or temperament. Many people with dangerously high blood pressure appear cool and serene.

3. *False.* Heart attack is *associated* with a highly stressed lifestyle, primarily because such a lifestyle includes other risk factors for heart disease—but the stress in itself is not a direct cause of heart disease.

4. *False.* Surgery for heart disease is becoming increasingly common. In many cases heart disease is not discovered until a heart attack occurs.

5. *True.* This statement may sound silly, but it is a well-established concept that heredity plays a large part in the development of heart disease. If you have an inherited tendency toward heart disease, you are very likely to develop at least some aspect of the disease.

(singular: *atrium*). The lower chambers, one on each side of the septum, are called the *ventricles.* As the heart beats, the left atrium and ventricle work to form one pump, while the right atrium and ventricle form another.

Deoxygenated blood enters the right heart pump (right atrium) via large veins known as the *inferior* and *superior venae cavae;* then it starts on its journey to the lungs, passing through the right ventricle and the *pulmonary* (lung) artery before entering the lung. In the lung are millions of tiny air sacs (*alveoli*) at the ends of the branches of the respiratory tree. There, the blood is cleaned of waste gas (carbon dioxide) and saturated with a fresh supply of oxygen. Thus revitalized, the blood is pushed from the lungs into the heart's left atrium, then through the left ventricle and finally out of the heart through the **aorta** (the main vessel of the circulatory system), which is about as big around as a garden hose. From the aorta branch off the many arteries that carry blood bearing oxygen and other nutrients to all organs and tissues of the body.[9]

This constant refreshing process is made possible by the heart's natural *pacemaker,* an electrical impulse center located in the upper right chamber of the heart. The electrical impulse center regulates the heartbeat by stimulating the muscles of the heart to contract in a coordinated fashion. Valves separate the heart's four chambers, opening and closing to regulate the flow of blood through the heart and out into the body. The valves ensure that the blood always passes through the heart in the proper direction. Damage to any of the heart valves can result in backward movement of the blood within the heart, causing reduced efficiency and even failure of the whole system.

The Circulatory System

Approximately ten to fifteen seconds are required for blood to make a complete circuit of the cardiovascular system. Oxygenated blood leaving the heart via the aorta travels through a complex network of **arteries,** which divide and subdivide into smaller and smaller tubes until they terminate as tiny **capillaries.** These minute vessels connect with **veins,** which carry the blood back to the heart. The large arteries—the *subclavian* and *brachial* arteries of the shoulder and arm, the *carotid* arteries that carry blood to the head, the *iliac* and *femoral* arteries of the abdomen and lower extremities, the *pulmonary* arteries of the lungs, and the *coronary* arteries that nourish the heart itself—have three walls, an elastic outer layer that can be expanded and contracted, a middle layer of muscular tissue that does the expanding and contracting, and a smooth inner lining. Capillaries, the connecting links between the smallest arteries (**arterioles**) and the smallest veins (**venules**), have thin walls through which nutrients and oxygen pass from the blood into the tissues, and waste matter and carbon dioxide pass from the tissues into the bloodstream. Deoxygenated blood is returned via the veins to the lungs, where it absorbs a fresh supply of oxygen and then enters the heart for a return journey through the body.

Blood Pressure

Blood pressure is the force exerted by the blood on the walls of the arteries. When the powerful left ventricle contracts to pump blood throughout the body, the arteries receive more blood than can be instantly moved through the tiny arterioles and capillaries. Therefore, there is always a great deal of inner pressure in the arteries. Like liquid being poured into a funnel, blood pools up in an artery before entering the smaller areas of the circulatory network; healthy arteries are elastic and expand to accommodate the load.

Blood pressure is measured at two points during the beating of the heart: (1) when the left ventricle is actually pumping blood, and (2) when the left ventricle is relaxing and filling up with blood for the next pumping cycle. The heart beat phase, or **systolic** phase, causes the pressure to rise, while the resting phase, or **diastolic** phase, brings the

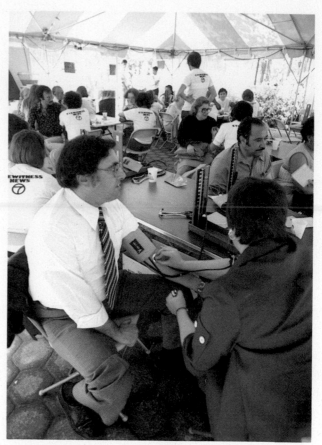

Everyone should have his or her blood pressure checked regularly. Many public agencies—and private companies, such as television stations—offer such checks to the public free of charge. (©Martin Adler Levick/Black Star)

pressure down. Much as air pressure in auto tires is measured in pounds per square inch, blood pressure is measured in millimeters of mercury. It is measured by means of an inflatable cuff, called a **sphygmomanometer,** that is wrapped around the upper arm.

KNOW THE NORMAL BLOOD PRESSURE RANGES

Blood pressure is extremely variable. What is "normal" is not clear. Young adults in good health may have a systolic, or contracting phase, pressure of between 100 and 140 millimeters of mercury; older adults may have a systolic pressure of from

120 to 180. Diastolic, or resting phase, pressure is usually below 95 millimeters of mercury in a healthy individual of any age. Thus, a good average blood pressure for a college student might be 120/80. Generally speaking, a continued diastolic blood pressure reading of over 95 is considered abnormal for people of any age. Elevated systolic blood pressure readings are usually of less concern, and in fact may increase with age as the blood vessels become less elastic.[19] It is normal for a person's blood pressure readings to vary from time to time. They may decrease when the individual is resting and increase during excitement, anger, or strenuous physical activity, when the heart pumps more vigorously.

The Coronary Arteries

The heart itself is a muscle, and like all other parts of the body it must have a blood supply to deliver

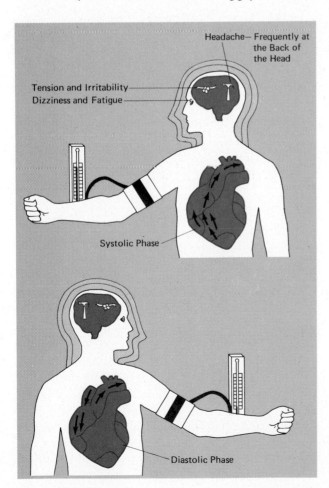

Headache— Frequently at the Back of the Head

Tension and Irritability
Dizziness and Fatigue

Systolic Phase

Diastolic Phase

oxygen and remove wastes. Surprisingly, very little of the thousand of gallons of blood circulating through the heart each day actually feeds the heart directly from within the heart chamber. Instead, the heart is nourished through the coronary arteries, two small blood vessels that arise from the aorta and encircle the heart, supplying blood to the heart muscle through numerous branches. Approximately one-eighth of an inch in diameter (about the width of a drinking straw), these arteries are critical: If they become blocked, a portion of the heart's cells die. This is what happens when a person suffers a heart attack.

HEART ATTACK

Essentially, a **heart attack** is the death of a portion of the heart muscle due to lack of oxygen. Heart attacks, which claim 570,000 lives in the United States each year, are usually a complication of **coronary atherosclerosis**—fatty thickening of the walls of the coronary arteries.

All that is needed to produce a heart attack is for a small blood clot to form in one of the narrowed coronary arteries, blocking the blood supply to a portion of the heart. Thus deprived of nourishment, the heart muscle that is fed by the affected artery dies. This event is called a **myocardial infarction** (death of a section of the heart muscle). Physicians also use the term **coronary thrombosis** (referring to a blood clot in a coronary artery). Another way the event can occur is via the formation of a **coronary embolism**: a piece of clotted material breaks away from the artery and floats down the bloodstream, lodging in—and damming up—a narrowed coronary artery (*embolus* is the Greek word for "wedge-shaped stopper"). Myocardial infarction—heart attack—follows.

Figure 12.2 High blood pressure. The heart exerts its greatest pressure when pumping in a fresh supply of blood (systolic phase, *top*) and the least pressure when pausing between beats to fill with blood (diastolic phase, *bottom*). The blood pressure is the measurement of pressure on the arterial wall at the extreme points of the systolic and diastolic phases. High blood pressure usually causes no symptoms until complications occur.

HEART ATTACK: What Happens, What to Do

Heart attack can strike anyone. When it occurs, there is no time for delay. Most heart attack victims survive if they recognize what is happening to them and get help quickly.

WHAT ARE THE SIGNALS?

Signals of heart attack vary, but these are the usual warnings:

1. The victim may feel uncomfortable pressure, fullness, squeezing, or pain in the center of the chest for more than two minutes.
2. Pain may spread to the shoulders, neck, or arms.
3. Severe pain, dizziness, fainting, sweating, nausea, or shortness of breath may also occur.
4. These signals are not continually present. Sometimes they subside, then return.

WHAT SHOULD YOU DO?

1. Heart-attack victims commonly deny their symptoms and delay getting help. That's the first thing to do—GET HELP. Phone a rescue squad, police, fire department, or whoever handles such emergencies in your community. DO YOU KNOW WHOM TO CALL? FIND OUT!
2. If you can get to the hospital faster than you can call for help, go immediately. The victim may find it more comfortable to be transported in a sitting or semireclining position.
3. If you discover someone who has collapsed, you have a chance to save that person if you can perform CPR (cardiopulmonary resuscitation). CPR training personnel will teach you the proper procedures to use to deliver immediate tempo-

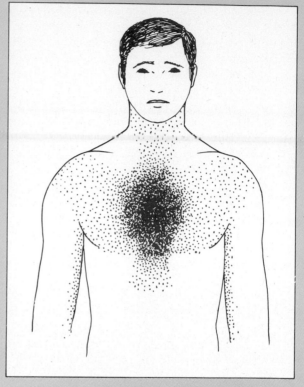

The characteristic intensity and location of pain during a heart attack.

rary aid to the victim. This aid may sustain the victim until medical help arrives.
4. Get trained in CPR. Your local American Heart Association can tell you where CPR is taught in your area.

Whether a heart-attack victim lives or dies depends in part on where the blockage occurs. If the flow of blood through one of the main arteries is blocked, large portions of the heart muscle may die, irreparably damaging the heart's pumping mechanism. Usually, however, only a small arterial branch is affected, and other areas of the heart are able to compensate for the loss.

A heart attack not only damages the muscle physically; it may also cause the heart's delicate electrical system to go out of control. When this happens, the heart beats in an abnormal rhythm (an **arrhythmia**). In one arrhythmia known as **fibrillation,** parts of the heart—the atria, the ventricles, or both—may beat irregularly at an extremely fast rate—hundreds of times a minute—and in an uncoordinated way. When this happens, the heart is incapable of pumping blood; unless

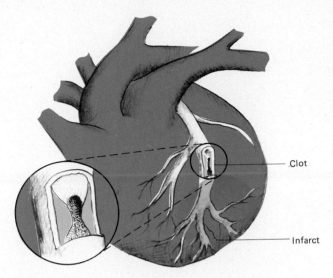

.Clot

Infarct

Figure 12.3   Coronary thrombosis. When a clot suddenly forms or migrates to a part of the heart muscle, the central area deprived of blood may die. The dead tissue is called a myocardial infarction or infarct.

TABLE 12.1 · Warning Signs of Heart Attack and Stroke

Heart Attack	*Stroke*
Prolonged, oppressive pain or unusual discomfort in *center* of chest	Sudden, temporary weakness or numbness of face, arm, or leg
Pain may radiate to shoulder, arm, neck, or jaw	Temporary loss of speech, or trouble in speaking or understanding speech
Sweating may accompany pain or discomfort	Temporary dimness or loss of vision, particularly in one eye
Nausea, vomiting, and shortness of breath may also occur	An episode of double vision
	Unexplained dizziness or unsteadiness
	Change in personality, mental ability, or pattern of headaches

Source: From Daniel M. Wilner et al., *Introduction to Public Health* (New York: Macmillan, 1978), p. 397.

the fibrillation can be stopped and normal circulation restored, the patient will die. CPR (cardiopulmonary resuscitation) should begin immediately.

Any heart-attack victim should be taken to a hospital as soon as possible, so that ventricular fibrillation can be immediately recognized and treated with special medicines and equipment.

What does it feel like to have a heart attack? Occasionally, heart attacks occur quietly and painlessly and are not discovered until months or even years later in the course of a routine electrocardiogram or during an autopsy (a medical examination of the body after death). Such "silent" heart attacks are just as damaging to the heart muscle as an overtly painful heart attack, and they are extremely dangerous because the victim rarely seeks medical attention or takes steps to ward off further episodes.

In most heart attacks, however, the victim knows something is wrong. Feeling one or more of the warning signs listed in Table 12.1, he or she may initially think the sensations are caused by indigestion or "heartburn." Ultimately, feelings of tightness, squeezing, or pain in the middle of the chest intensify (victims report feeling as though "an elephant were sitting on my chest" or "someone hit me in the chest with a sledgehammer").[12] The pain may radiate down the left arm, or to the neck, shoulders, and jaw. The victim becomes pale, sweats profusely, grows short of breath, and may vomit. It is not uncommon for victims to experience feelings of terror or a sense of impending doom. One cardiologist said, "It is like nothing the patient has ever known before, a feeling that something cataclysmic is happening."[13]

How Does Atherosclerosis Develop?

In **atherosclerosis,** fatty deposits circulating in the blood accumulate in one or more areas of the **intima,** the lining of the arteries. These deposits form mushy masses called **plaque,** which stick to the intima and cause the once-smooth arterial walls to become rough and thickened. Diseased arteries resemble sediment-clogged water pipes: The blood flow is sometimes reduced to a trickle instead of a healthy gush.

How atherosclerosis develops. (a) This diagram identifies the structures shown in the two photographs below it. (b) Photographic cross section of a normal artery, with its smooth inner lining, or intima. (c) An atherosclerotic artery. Over the years, the intima has become irregular and attracted fibrin, a blood protein important in coagulation. This fibrin matrix collects fat particles and other debris, thus producing plaque. Later in this degenerative condition, calcium is deposited and the plaque hardens. (Julius Weber; reprinted by permission from D. M. Wilner, R. P. Walkney, and E. J. O'Neill, *Introduction to Public Health*, 7th ed., © Macmillan Publishing Co., Inc.)

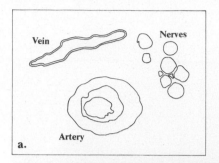

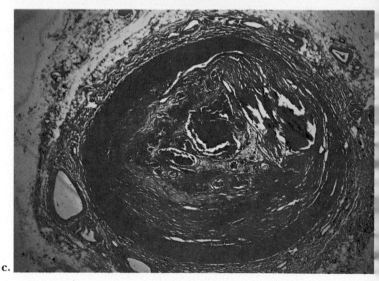

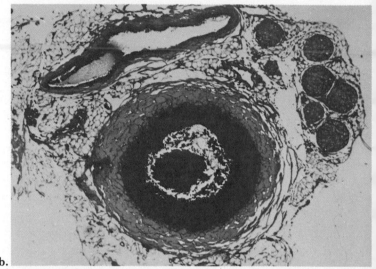

ANGINA: A SYMPTOM OF ATHEROSCLEROSIS

The reduced blood flow to the heart produced by atherosclerosis may not be noticeable when the heart is beating routinely and under little stress. But when extra demands are made on the heart muscle—for example, when a person sprints or shovels snow—the blood flow through the partially blocked coronary arteries becomes insufficient and the individual may experience **angina pectoris,** which is a tightness, pressure, and intense pain in the chest. Because it is a symptom of oxygen deprivation to the heart muscle, angina is one of the most important indicators of coronary heart disease.

Angina can be a stable medical condition in some persons. In other people, it can become more frequent and more severe; if the angina is unrelieved, a heart attack may ensue. Usually, the pain is relieved after a few minutes of rest but returns with more exertion. Taking a nitroglycerin tablet—which dilates (expands) the vessels, increasing the blood flow—gives prompt relief to anginal pain. Other drugs have been used with considerable success, and certain surgical techniques are helpful in more severe cases.

WHAT'S THE DIFFERENCE BETWEEN ATHEROSCLEROSIS AND ARTERIOSCLEROSIS?

You may have heard about arteriosclerosis—a disease that sounds a lot like atherosclerosis. **Arteriosclerosis** is a condition in which blood vessels become thick and hard and lose their elasticity. It is caused by calcium deposits—whereas atherosclerosis, as we have noted, technically refers to a *fatty* thickening of arterial walls (not a thickening caused by calcium). Just to make things more confusing, people sometimes use the term *arteriosclerosis* in a general sense to refer to any sort of "hardening of the arteries"—including atherosclerosis.

Recovering from a Heart Attack

After a heart attack, the patient must rest for a while to reduce the work load on the heart and allow it to heal. During the healing process, scar tissue will form around the area where the heart muscle has died. This scar tissue cannot contract, but if the scar is small, the heart may continue to function well and the patient may recover. Today, physicians are advising a shorter period of bed rest than they did in past decades. They stress starting a planned program of exercise under medical supervision as soon as the patient is well enough. Exercise can aid the process by which the heart develops **collateral circulation**—a system of smaller blood vessels that provide alternative routes for blood when a main artery is blocked.

People recovering from heart attacks experience many different emotions. Many are very frightened—and understandably so. They may have the idea that it will be dangerous to put any strain whatsoever on their heart: They may be afraid to exercise at all, even to get out of a chair and walk across the room. Their families are also affected by the experience. Spouses may try to encourage victims to avoid exercise, including sexual activity, and thus may reinforce any doubts the individual already has about his or her heart. The patient's fear of a recurrence of the heart attack symptoms, or even of sudden death, may interfere with rehabilitation.

The first step in cardiac rehabilitation, then, is to reassure patients that a careful, step-by-step exercise program is not likely to hurt them. Through rehabilitation, patients can be restored to a relatively high level of functioning and many can eventually return to normal life. Their chances for long-term recovery are better, of course, if they also make lifestyle changes, reducing some of the risk factors we will discuss later in this chapter.

OTHER CARDIOVASCULAR PROBLEMS

Heart attacks are, of course, one of the most dramatic manifestations of cardiovascular disease— but there are other problems of the heart and circulatory system that you should know about (see Figure 12.4).

Some Important Heart Problems

Among the heart problems you may hear about— either in connection with heart attack or in other

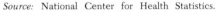

Figure 12.4 Heart attack is the most common cardiovascular disease, but it is not the only serious problem of the heart and circulatory system. This chart shows the estimated percentage and number of deaths from various types of CVD.
Source: National Center for Health Statistics.

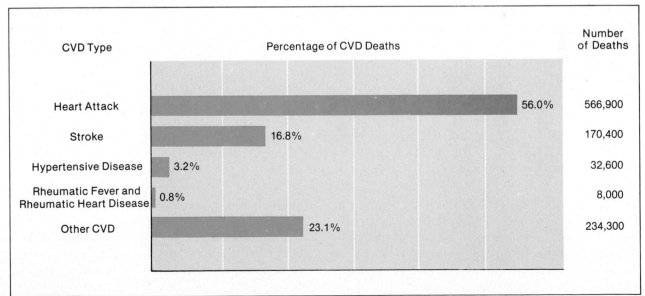

CVD Type	Percentage of CVD Deaths	Number of Deaths
Heart Attack	56.0%	566,900
Stroke	16.8%	170,400
Hypertensive Disease	3.2%	32,600
Rheumatic Fever and Rheumatic Heart Disease	0.8%	8,000
Other CVD	23.1%	234,300

contexts—are cardiac arrest and heart block. You may also hear about congestive heart failure, congenital heart disease, and rheumatic fever. We'll survey these below.

CARDIAC ARREST

Any time an individual's heart stops beating, he or she is said to be suffering **cardiac arrest.** The heart may stop because of heart attack or for many other reasons—drowning, electrocution, or strangulation, for example.

When cardiac arrest occurs, immediate action is necessary or the patient may die; the brain can survive without damage for only about four minutes after circulation is stopped.

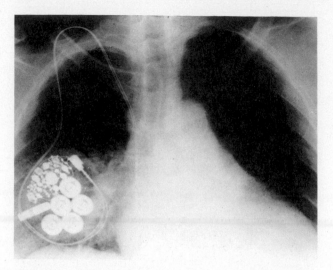

This X-ray shows an artificial pacemaker positioned in the chest. The pacemaker has proven to be highly successful in patients whose cardiac electrical system no longer delivers electrical impulses strong enough or regular enough to maintain the rhythmic contractions of the heart.

HEART BLOCK

Sometimes a heart-attack victim who seems to be recovering will experience a sudden slowing or stopping of the heartbeat. (This phenomenon may also occur for reasons other than heart attack, but in this setting it usually affects patients in their sixties or older, and is due to an aging process.) **Heart block** results from a failure of the electrical connection between the atria and the ventricles: Impulses do not reach the main pumping chamber often enough. Normal heart rate can be restored medically, with an electronic pacemaker. In most cases, the heart can then repair itself within a few days, and the natural rhythm returns. When this does not happen, an artificial pacemaker can be implanted and can take over the job indefinitely as long as the batteries are changed periodically.

CONGESTIVE HEART FAILURE

In **congestive heart failure,** the heart cannot pump enough blood and the result is a congestion, or backing up, of blood in the lungs. Fluid also oozes through the thin capillary walls in various parts of the body and collects in the tissues such as the lungs and skin, causing shortness of breath and **edema** (swelling).

Almost every known type of heart disease may produce congestive heart failure. Sometimes it can be aggravated by high blood pressure, which forces the heart to work harder to deliver sufficient blood to the body's organs and tissues. It can also be caused by heart attack, defective heart valves, a damaged section of heart muscle, or weakening of the entire heart by disease or toxins.

CONGENITAL HEART DISEASE

About eight infants out of every 1,000 are born with **congenital heart disease**—inborn defects of the heart.[14] Congenital heart disease varies in severity; it can affect any structure of the circulatory system—the pumping chambers, the valves that separate these chambers and force the blood to flow in one direction, or the blood vessels leading from the heart to the lungs and other parts of the body.

RHEUMATIC HEART DISEASE

Rheumatic fever is an inflammatory disease of connective tissues; as we noted in Chapter 10, it may occasionally follow a streptococcal infection, usually of the throat (strep throat). Although prompt treatment with antibiotics can prevent serious heart complications, approximately one-third of all rheumatic fever victims are left with heart damage, particularly of the valves.[15]

Rheumatic fever usually strikes children between the ages of five and fifteen, although it also occurs in older people. The ailment affects many parts of the body, but damage to the heart from scarring of heart muscle and valves is its greatest danger. Depending on the extent of the scarring, rheumatic heart disease will interfere with the normal functioning of the heart. An attack of rheumatic fever does not necessarily mean that one is left with a damaged heart. The disease tends to recur, however, and with each episode the chance of permanent damage increases.

Early detection and treatment of streptococcal infections of the throat, usually with penicillin, can effectively guard against rheumatic fever; it is therefore urgent that anyone with a persistent sore throat or earache seek medical attention.

Stroke: When CVD Affects the Brain

A **stroke,** also known as a **cerebrovascular accident (CVA)** or a **cerebrovascular occlusion,** is a sudden loss of brain function resulting from interference with the blood supply to one part of the brain. The word *stroke* is particularly apt: Victims compare it to being struck on the head with a blunt instrument.[16] Strokes usually result from degenerative cardiovascular disease; stroke is the third leading cause of death in the United States.[17] Three types of strokes are shown in Figure 12.5.

In many strokes, as in many heart attacks, the underlying cardiovascular disease begins to develop long before the critical event occurs. A stroke may "incubate" for thirty or forty years before symptoms become evident.

Some strokes are so mild, causing only temporary dizziness or slight weakness or numbness, that they are often ignored; these are called **transient ischemic attacks,** or TIAs. Other strokes are so severe that they kill within minutes by destroying the part of the brain that regulates heart and

lung functions. What makes stroke so devastating is that nearby cells, no longer fed by the blocked or ruptured artery, are deprived of oxygen and begin to die. Because the areas of the body controlled by these nerve centers can no longer function normally, a stroke victim may suffer partial paralysis and other crippling afflictions.

CAN STROKE BE PREVENTED?

By far the best way to reduce the mortality rate from strokes is to prevent their occurrence. Prompt treatment of causative conditions—such as hypertension or atherosclerotic disease in the carotid arteries in the neck which lead to the brain —may decrease the risk of a stroke.

TRANSIENT ISCHEMIC ATTACKS

Ominously, when a stroke, even a transient one, has occurred, the chances of a second stroke are increased. This is one reason it's a good idea to be alert to possible transient ischemic attack. Such an attack may last anywhere from a few minutes to twenty-four hours. It serves as a warning signal for possible impending stroke.

Symptoms that indicate TIA include any unexplained numbness, tingling, unusual weakness, or paralysis of any part of the body; difficulty in swallowing, speaking, phrasing sentences, or thinking clearly; sudden dizziness, fainting, altered vision, or severe headaches. Any such symptoms indicate a need for immediate medical testing.

REHABILITATION AFTER A STROKE

The patient's condition soon after a stroke can be very discouraging. Many stroke victims suffer loss of memory—especially short-term memory—and many exhibit general confusion. They become tired easily, and their ability to concentrate may also be impaired. Sudden and extreme mood fluctuations or inappropriate emotional reactions are fairly common.

Many stroke victims are left with some permanent physical impairment. Yet in many cases there

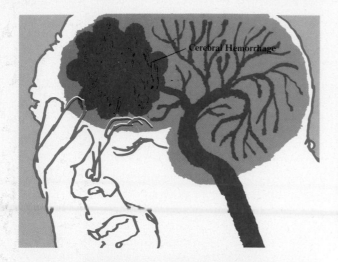

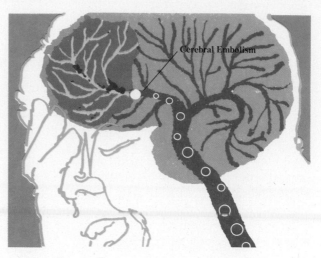

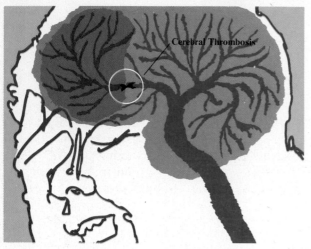

Figure 12.5   Three types of strokes. *(Top left)* Cerebral hemorrhage, in which blood flow to the brain is impaired due to rupture of a diseased cerebral blood vessel. *(Top right)* Cerebral embolism, in which a mass of abnormal material clogs a blood vessel. *(Bottom left)* Cerebral thrombosis, in which a blood clot forms in a cerebral blood vessel. In all cases, oxygen transport to parts of the brain is impaired, resulting in the death of some brain tissue. (Tom Lewis)

is hope for at least a partial recovery. Though brain cells do not regenerate (unlike most other body tissues), one area of the brain can learn to take over the functions of another after brain damage has occurred. With appropriate therapy, it is often possible for a stroke victim to relearn basic self-care skills—and sometimes other skills as well. Often, the degree of recovery is remarkable, as in the case of Patricia Neal, who went on to win an Academy Award—a slight limp the only evidence of the stroke that almost killed her!

Recovery from a severe stroke, however, is a slow, painstaking process. It requires enormous effort, patience, and strength on the part of the CVA victim and those around him or her. The most dramatic improvements occur in the first three to six months. Subsequent progress is extremely slow, often causing everyone involved to

become frustrated, resentful, and discouraged. Physiotherapists and others who help in the rehabilitation of stroke victims stress the importance of encouraging patients to do as much as possible for themselves, of helping them regain confidence in their abilities, and of preventing them from becoming too dependent on well-meaning friends and relatives.[18]

THE RISK FACTORS IN CARDIOVASCULAR DISEASES

Scientists have not been able to identify "causes" of most heart ailments. But there is an impressive accumulation of research material and statistical data pointing to certain physical conditions and

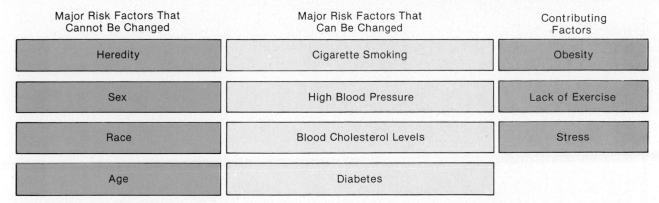

Major Risk Factors That Cannot Be Changed	Major Risk Factors That Can Be Changed	Contributing Factors
Heredity	Cigarette Smoking	Obesity
Sex	High Blood Pressure	Lack of Exercise
Race	Blood Cholesterol Levels	Stress
Age	Diabetes	

Figure 12.6 **The risk factors in cardiovascular disease—those that can be changed and those that cannot—are summarized here, along with factors that contribute to CVD and can also be controlled.**
Source: American Heart Association, *Heart Facts,* 1983, p. 13.

lifestyles in the development of heart attack and stroke. Some of these are beyond our control, but some are governed primarily by individual choices. Both types of factors are summarized graphically in Figure 12.6.

CVD Risk Factors You Cannot Control

Some risk factors—age, gender, race, and heredity —are built into our physical and genetic makeup:[19]

- The risk of heart attack increases with advancing years.
- Heart attack is more common among men than among premenopausal women.
- Whites in the United States suffer heart attack with greater frequency than blacks or Asiatics.
- Heredity plays an important part in heart disease, particularly that which occurs in the early years: People with blood relatives who have had CVD are at greater risk of developing CVD.

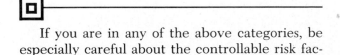

If you are in any of the above categories, be especially careful about the controllable risk factors discussed below.

CVD Risk Factors You Can Control

HIGH BLOOD PRESSURE

Often dubbed "the silent killer" because it rarely causes any noticeable symptoms, **hypertension,** or **high blood pressure,** affects close to 35 million people in the United States. And in both men and women, the higher the blood pressure, the greater the risk of coronary artery disease. One study showed that those with systolic pressure above 180 were seven times as likely to have coronary disease as those with systolic pressure below 120.[20] Persons with high blood pressure have a ten times higher risk of stroke than individuals with unelevated pressure.[21] Because hypertension forces the heart to work harder, the condition is a leading cause of congestive heart failure. In addition, unrelieved high blood pressure causes blood vessels to lose their elasticity and forces fatty materials onto the arterial walls, thus speeding the development of atherosclerosis.

A WIDESPREAD PROBLEM While hypertension is rarely found in persons under twenty years of age, systolic blood pressure (maximum pressure in the artery) tends to increase with advancing years. By age fifty, approximately one-half of the population has high blood pressure in some form, although many are unaware of it. Until the age of about fifty to fifty-five, men are far more likely than women to have high blood pressure. Nonwhites are two to five times more likely to be affected than are whites.[22]

HOW IS HYPERTENSION TREATED?   There is no cure for hypertension, but most cases can be controlled with medication and adjustments in the diet. A number of effective drugs are available: diuretics, which reduce the volume of blood and thereby lower blood pressure; tranquilizers, which calm the central nervous system; and the newly developed *beta blockers*, drugs that impede nerve impulses that tend to affect the width of small blood vessels. Hypertensive individuals are also warned to restrict salt intake, because salt causes retention of fluids, increasing blood volume and putting additional strain on blood vessels. Weight control, moderate exercise, and relaxation techniques such as meditation and biofeedback may also be helpful.

THE ISSUE OF AWARENESS   Since hypertension is dangerous, it is vitally important to treat even slightly elevated blood-pressure levels. Because there are no symptoms, many who have the condition may be unaware of it. As a result, many are receiving no treatment for it.[23]

Everyone should have blood pressure checks at regular intervals. If your blood pressure is not within normal ranges for your age, see a physician without delay *and follow his or her instructions.*

LOW BLOOD PRESSURE   If your blood pressure is below normal, should you be concerned? Probably not. Low blood pressure is generally a problem only in certain medical emergencies, such as hemorrhage and shock, and among the elderly.

CIGARETTE SMOKING AND HEART DISEASE

Cigarette smoking is as hard on the heart and circulatory system as it is on the lungs. It speeds up the heart rate, raises blood pressure, and constricts blood vessels, making persons who smoke one pack of cigarettes a day twice as likely to have heart attacks as nonsmokers.[24] Tobacco users also

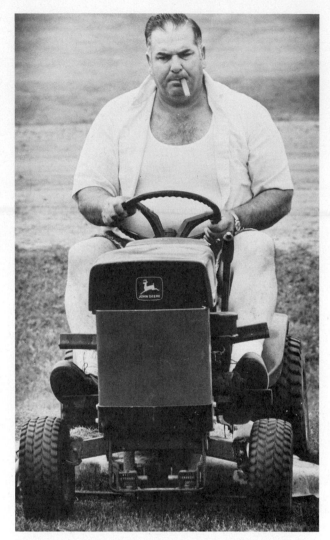

Smoking, overweight, and lack of physical activity are three risk factors in cardiovascular disease that the individual can change. (©Michael C. Hayman/Stock, Boston)

greatly increase their chances of developing atherosclerosis.

In recent years, an international series of medical reports confirmed a deadly, synergistic relationship between oral contraceptive use and cigarette smoking: The Pill acts in some not-yet-understood way to greatly increase the adverse effects of cigarette smoking.

Women who smoke moderately or heavily *and* use the Pill run significantly higher risk of heart attack than do nonsmoking Pill users, or smoking non-Pill users.[25]

The preventive value of *not* smoking has been clearly demonstrated. Three years after a smoker has given up cigarettes, his or her risk of having a heart attack drops back to that of a nonsmoker. (The role of smoking in heart disease is also discussed in Chapter 6.)

DIET AND HEART DISEASE

We have become accustomed to the irony that the foods we may like best—chocolate, hot dogs, French fries—are not necessarily good for us. Indeed, many specialists regard diet as the single most important factor in atherosclerosis, especially because one of the major constituents of atherosclerotic fatty deposits is cholesterol. Whether cholesterol actually *causes* narrowing and hardening of the arteries is questionable, but it may be an accomplice to the crime.

IS DIETARY CHOLESTEROL BAD FOR THE HEART? During the past few years, much has been written about the ill effects on the cardiovascular system of dietary cholesterol and saturated fats (fats from which the body synthesizes its own cholesterol). But careful analyses of these studies have revealed little, if any, correlation.[26] While disease of the coronary arteries occurs more frequently among individuals with high cholesterol levels, there is no indication that the elevated levels are due to *dietary* intake. In addition, some individuals with extraordinarily high cholesterol levels never show any signs of coronary heart disease.

THE ROLE OF HDL AND LDL More recent studies indicate a relationship between heart disease and **lipoproteins**—substances containing both fat and protein that transport fat molecules, including cholesterol. The heaviest of these is known as **high-density lipoprotein, or HDL. Low-density lipoprotein (LDL)** is lighter because it contains less protein. LDL is the medium by which most cholesterol is transported through the body. Greater concentrations of HDL than LDL appear to offer protection from heart disease, although

the reasons are not yet clearly understood. Apparently HDL is able to "lure" cholesterol away from arterial walls, carrying it to the liver (the only organ that can degrade it), where it is metabolized and destroyed.

SHOULD YOU CHANGE YOUR DIET TO BOOST YOUR HDL?

The significance for the healthy individual of the above findings about HDL is still unclear. Until further investigation suggests otherwise, there is probably no need for the average person to avoid moderate amounts of either fats or cholesterol. The key to good nutrition is a balanced, varied diet, which minimizes the possibility of excesses and maximizes the inclusion of all essential nutrients.

DIABETES

Diabetes cannot be cured, but it can be controlled to reduce the risk of complications, including heart disease. Once diabetes is detected, the physician can help the patient keep it in check by prescribing changes in eating habits, weight-control and exercise programs, and medication if necessary.

EXERCISE

The physical fitness craze that began in the 1960s and blossomed into a full-fledged industry in the 1970s and 1980s had as its genesis the widespread belief that exercise prolongs life. The value of exercise in preventing coronary disease has not been conclusively shown. Yet people who are physically active seem to be less prone to heart attacks and to tolerate them better than those who lead sedentary lives.

The *type* of physical activity undertaken is important. Certain forms of strenuous exercise, such as running, cycling, and swimming, lead to the development of extensive collateral circulation (growth of additional coronary blood vessels). Then, if a coronary artery is blocked, it can be immediately bypassed and circulation continued

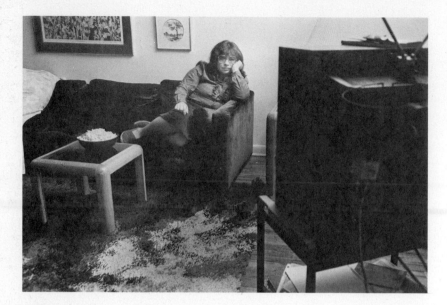

A person is never too young to examine his or her lifestyle, eliminating factors—such as poor diet and lack of exercise—that increase the risk of cardiovascular disease. (© Harvey Wang)

by way of the additional collateral arteries. Death and disability from heart attack are averted under these circumstances.

STRESS

As we noted in Chapter 2, there is no actual proof that stress in itself helps to cause heart disease. It has been suggested that "Type A" people, who live a competitive, aggressive, impatient, fast-paced lifestyle, constantly under pressure, may be more prone to heart attacks, but not all researchers agree with this concept. In any case, it is highly unlikely that stress will prove to be as important a factor as smoking, diet, or hypertension.

OBESITY

There is little indication that obesity itself causes heart disease. More likely, it is the *relationship* among obesity, hypertension, blood fat levels, and possibly diabetes that significantly contributes to increased risk of heart disease and atherosclerosis.

Multiplying the Risks

One of the most troublesome aspects of the coronary culprits is the way they tend to reinforce one another. People often eat more or smoke more when they are under stress. Overweight people tend to shun exercise. Working separately, the risk factors represent a considerable threat; in combination, they are even more deadly.

For example, a person with normal blood pressure and blood fat levels who neither smokes nor has diabetes has a one in twenty—or 5 percent—chance of having a heart attack prior to age sixty-five. If one risk factor is present, the chance of heart attack doubles (rises to 10 percent); with two risk factors, the chance becomes one in two, or 50 percent.[27] Take a fairly common combination, obesity plus smoking. Obesity puts a strain on the cardiovascular system as a whole; for every pound that is gained, the body must circulate new blood supplies to nourish that tissue, and thus obese persons are putting much more stress on their hearts than leaner people. If the obese person also smokes cigarettes, the risk is compounded: smoking acts to lessen the adaptability of the cardiovascular system as a whole. Consequently, a system that is already stressed by obesity is stressed synergistically much more than it would be by either of these two factors acting alone.[28]

The Framingham study—a controlled research project involving a large, representative sample of adult men and women who were examined every other year over a fourteen-year period—supported the theory that high blood pressure, elevated blood fats, and cigarette smoking are all associated with increased risk of heart disease. It also found that people who exercised regularly were more likely to survive a heart attack.[29]

If any *one* of the controllable CVD risk factors is applicable in your case—uncontrolled hypertension, cigarette smoking, an extremely rich and fatty diet, lack of exercise, extreme stress, or obesity—be especially careful about the *other* risk factors.

Issues in Behavioral Change

We know that many heart-disease victims share certain behavioral characteristics. Does this mean that if we alter selected aspects of our behavior, we can reduce our chances of getting heart disease? Actually, yes—but it isn't easy. Many of the behaviors associated with heart disease cannot be changed overnight. Furthermore, behavioral changes are usually connected: Those who change one aspect of their behavior may find they have more difficulty with other aspects of their behavior. The smoker who quits, for example, may then have to struggle to avoid gaining weight.

Take another example: a hard-driving, aggressive, successful salesman who is trying to change his way of dealing with life to reduce stress. He may find his employer is disappointed with his new personality—the company really liked the go-getter and is not so happy with the more relaxed person who is emerging. The problem here is that even when behavioral changes are strongly indicated in order to reduce the risk of heart disease, these changes may require changes in the very essence of an individual's existence. To the physician, the changes needed are a matter of survival in a physical sense. But to patients, the changes may represent a threat to their essential definition of themselves. It may be unrealistic to expect a hard-driving salesman to stop smoking, reduce dietary fat, begin an exercise program, and cut down on alcohol. Even asking him to reduce stress—the stress he equates with his success—may be asking far too much, from his point of view.

Each individual must decide what kinds of changes he or she can "live with"—in the psychological sense as well as the physical sense. People at every age should devote some thought to where they stand with regard to CVD risk factors, then make some plans for modifying those factors that are under their control. But when they decide to change their lifestyles, they should aim for changes that harmonize with their personalities.

MAKING HEALTH DECISIONS

Heart Disease Risks: Where Do You Stand?

How likely are you to develop heart disease? This activity can give you a fairly clear idea of your chances—though not, of course, a guarantee.

MEN

Everyone starts with a score of 10 points. Complete all four items, adding or subtracting points as instructed to arrive at your final score.

Starting Score   10

1. Weight

Locate your weight category in the table for men on the next page.

If you are in weight category

A, subtract 2
B, subtract 1
C, add 1
D, add 2
     Equals   _____

2. Systolic Blood Pressure

Use the "first" or "higher" number from your most recent blood pressure measurement. If you do not know your blood pressure, estimate it by using the letter for your weight category. If your blood pressure is

A 119 or less, subtract 1
B between 120 and 139, add 0
C between 140 and 159, add 0
D 160 or greater, add 1
     Equals   _____

WEIGHT TABLES

Look for your height (without shoes) in the far left column and then read across to find the category into which your weight (in indoor clothing) would fall. Because both blood pressure and blood cholesterol are related to weight, an estimate of these risk factors for each weight category is printed at the bottom of the table.

MEN

Your Height	Weight Category (Lbs.)			
	A	B	C	D
5'1"	up to 123	124–148	149–173	174 +
5'2"	up to 126	127–152	153–178	179 +
5'3"	up to 129	130–156	157–182	183 +
5'4"	up to 132	133–160	161–186	187 +
5'5"	up to 135	136–163	164–190	191 +
5'6"	up to 139	140–168	169–196	197 +
5'7"	up to 144	145–174	175–203	204 +
5'8"	up to 148	149–179	180–209	210 +
5'9"	up to 152	153–184	185–214	215 +
5'10"	up to 157	158–190	191–221	222 +
5'11"	up to 161	162–194	195–227	228 +
6'0"	up to 165	166–199	200–232	233 +
6'1"	up to 170	171–205	206–239	240 +
6'2"	up to 175	176–211	212–246	247 +
6'3"	up to 180	181–217	218–253	254 +
6'4"	up to 185	186–223	224–260	261 +
6'5"	up to 190	191–229	230–267	268 +
6'6"	up to 195	196–235	236–274	275 +

Estimate of Systolic Blood Pressure

119 or less	120 to 139	140 to 159	160 or more

Estimate of Blood Cholesterol

199 or less	200 to 224	225 to 249	250 or more

WOMEN

Your Height	Weight Category (Lbs.)			
	A	B	C	D
4'8"	up to 101	102–122	123–143	144 +
4'9"	up to 103	104–125	126–146	147 +
4'10"	up to 106	107–128	129–150	151 +
4'11"	up to 109	110–132	133–154	155 +
5'0"	up to 112	113–136	137–158	159 +
5'1"	up to 115	116–139	140–162	163 +
5'2"	up to 119	120–144	145–168	169 +
5'3"	up to 122	123–148	149–172	173 +
5'4"	up to 127	128–154	155–179	180 +
5'5"	up to 131	132–158	159–185	186 +
5'6"	up to 135	136–163	164–190	191 +
5'7"	up to 139	140–168	169–196	197 +
5'8"	up to 143	144–173	174–202	203 +
5'9"	up to 147	148–178	179–207	208 +
5'10"	up to 151	152–182	183–213	214 +
5'11"	up to 155	156–187	188–218	219 +
6'0"	up to 159	160–191	192–224	225 +
6'1"	up to 163	164–196	197–229	230 +

Estimate of Systolic Blood Pressure

119 or less	120 to 139	140 to 159	160 or more

Estimate of Blood Cholesterol

199 or less	200 to 224	225 to 249	250 or more

3. Blood Cholesterol Level

Use the number from your most recent blood cholesterol test. If you do not know your blood cholesterol, estimate it by using the letter for your weight category. If your blood cholesterol is

A 199 or less, subtract 2
B between 200 and 224, subtract 1
C between 225 and 249, and 0
D 250 or higher, add 1
      Equals   _____

4. Cigarette Smoking

If you

do not smoke, subtract 1
smoke less than a pack a day or smoke a pipe, add 0
smoke a pack a day, add 1
smoke more than a pack a day, add 2
      Final score equals   _____

WOMEN

Everyone starts with a score of 10 points. Complete all five items, adding or subtracting points as instructed to arrive at your final score.

Starting Score   10

1. Weight

Locate your weight category in the table for women, above. If you are in weight category

A, subtract 2
B, subtract 1
C, add 1
D, add 2
      Equals   _____

2. Systolic Blood Pressure

Use the "first" or "higher" number from your most recent blood pressure measurement. If you do not know your blood pressure, estimate it by using the letter for your weight category. If your blood pressure is

A 119 or less, subtract 2
B between 120 and 139, subtract 1
C between 140 and 159, add 0
D 160 or greater, add 1
   Equals   ____

3. Blood Cholesterol Level

Use the number from your most recent blood choles-terol test. If you do not know your blood cholesterol, estimate it by using the letter for your weight category. If your blood cholesterol is

A 199 or less, subtract 1
B between 200 and 224, and 0
C between 225 and 249, and 0
D 250 or higher, add 1

4. Cigarette Smoking

If you

   do not smoke, subtract 1
   smoke less than a pack a day, add 0
   smoke a pack a day, add 1
   smoke more than a pack a day, add 2
      Equals   ____

5. Estrogen Use

Birth control pills and hormone drugs contain estrogen. A few examples are: Premarin, Ogan, Menstranol, Prov-era, Evex, Menest, Estinyl, Meurium. Have you ever taken estrogen for five or more years in a row? Are you age 35 years or older and now taking estrogen?

   No to both questions, add 0
   Yes to one or both questions, add 1
      Final score equals   ____

WHAT YOUR SCORE MEANS

0–4 You have one of the lowest risks of heart disease for your sex.

5–9 You have a low to moderate risk of heart dis-ease for your sex, but there is some room for improvement.

10–14 You have a moderate to high risk of heart dis-ease for your sex, with considerable room for improvement on some factors.

15–19 You have a high risk of developing heart dis-ease for your sex, with a great deal of room for improvement on all factors.

20 and over You have a very high risk of developing heart disease for your sex and should take immediate action on all risk factors.

HOW TO REDUCE YOUR RISK

- Try to quit smoking permanently. There are many programs available.
- Have your blood pressure checked regularly, prefer-ably every twelve months after age 40. If your blood pressure is high, see your physician. Remember, blood pressure medicine is effective only if taken regularly.
- Consider your daily exercise (or lack of it). A half hour of brisk walking, swimming, or other enjoyable activ-ity should not be difficult to fit into your day.
- Give some serious thought to your diet. If you are overweight, or eat a lot of foods high in saturated fat or cholesterol (whole milk, cheese, eggs, butter, fatty foods, fried foods), then changes should be made in your diet. Look for the *American Heart Association Cookbook* at your local bookstore.
- Visit or write your local Heart Association for further information and copies of free pamphlets on many related subjects, including: reducing your risk of heart attack; controlling high blood pressure; eating to keep your heart healthy; how to stop smoking; exercising for good health.

SOME WORDS OF CAUTION

- If you have diabetes, gout, or a family history of heart disease, your real risk of developing heart disease will be greater than indicated by your score. If your score is high and you have one or more of these additional problems, you should give particular attention to re-ducing your risk.
- If you are a woman under 45 years or a man under 35 years of age, your score represents an upper limit on your real risk of developing heart disease. In this case your real risk is probably lower than indicated by your score.
- If you are a woman whose use of estrogen has con-tributed to a high score, you may want to consult your physician. Do not automatically discontinue your prescription.
- Using your weight category to estimate your systolic blood pressure or your blood cholesterol level makes your score less accurate. Your score will tend to *over-estimate* your risk if your actual values on these two important factors are average for someone of your height and weight. Your score will *underestimate* your risk if your actual blood pressure or cholesterol level is above average for someone of your height and weight.

SUMMARY

1. Cardiovascular disease (CVD) is a class of highly preventable disorders of the heart and blood vessels.

2. Although CVD usually becomes evident in middle age, its course actually begins years before.

3. For reasons not yet understood, the CVD death rate has been declining since the early 1970s. Many people are still at risk, however.

4. The heart works without ever stopping to pump blood to the lungs, where the blood picks up oxygen, needed by every cell of the body. The heart is a muscular organ that is divided into four chambers. Heartbeat is regulated by electrical impulses from one of these chambers. Valves open and close to regulate the flow of blood through the heart and body. Oxygen-rich blood leaving the heart travels through arteries. Deoxygenated blood returning to the heart travels through veins.

5. Blood pressure is the amount of force that blood exerts on the walls of the arteries. Healthy arteries are elastic and accommodate to shifts in blood volume. Systolic pressure is measured when the heart is pumping blood and diastolic pressure is measured when the heart is filling with blood for the next cycle.

6. A heart attack is the death of part of the heart muscle due to lack of oxygen. A fatty thickening of the walls of the coronary arteries, which supply the heart with oxygenated blood, is the disease called coronary atherosclerosis. Many heart attacks result from a blockage of these arteries. Heart attacks can damage the pumping ability and the rhythmic beating of the heart.

7. Most heart-attack victims survive if they recognize what is happening and get help immediately. A heart attack feels like pressure or pain in the center of the chest. Pain may spread to the shoulders, neck, or arms. Severe pain, dizziness, nausea, sweating, and shortness of breath may also occur, or may come and go.

8. Atherosclerosis is believed to be caused by cholesterol deposits. The relationship between dietary cholesterol and heart attacks is still not completely understood. Angina pectoris, intense chest pain, is an indicator of coronary heart disease.

9. People recovering from a heart attack need rest, but soon they are given programs of moderate exercise to build collateral circulation.

10. In addition to heart attacks, there are a number of other cardiovascular problems. Cardiac arrest is any heart stoppage. Heart block describes a sudden slowing or stopping of the heartbeat, usually in an elderly person recovering from a heart attack. Congestive heart failure can result from all forms of heart disease. Congenital heart disease is a general term for all inborn heart defects, which differ in severity. Rheumatic fever can damage the heart, especially the valves.

11. Stroke is a sudden loss of brain function that is the result of lack of oxygen in part of the brain. The best way to prevent strokes is to prevent the conditions, like high blood pressure or atherosclerosis, that can cause them. Transient ischemic attacks are warnings that a major stroke may be coming. A person recovering from a stroke may be able to relearn lost abilities by using other, undamaged parts of the brain.

12. The risk factors of CVD are correlates rather than absolute causes. They tend to reinforce one another. Some are not susceptible to control: advancing age, being a male, being white, or having a family history of CVD. Factors that one can control include: reducing one's blood pressure, not smoking cigarettes (and for women who smoke, not taking birth control pills), eating well, and exercising moderately and regularly. Stress and obesity may combine with other factors to put people at risk for CVD.

GLOSSARY

angina pectoris A tightness, pressure, and intense pain in the chest caused by insufficient blood flow through partially blocked coronary arteries.

aorta The main vessel of the circulatory system, carrying blood from the heart to the arteries.

arrhythmia An abnormal rhythm in the heartbeat.

arterioles The smallest arteries.

arteriosclerosis A condition in which the arteries become thick and hard and lose their elasticity; caused by calcium deposits.

artery A blood vessel that carries blood from the heart to the various parts of the body.

atherosclerosis A disease process in which fatty deposits circulating in the blood accumulate on the intima (the lining of the artery walls), forming plaque which causes the walls to become rough and thickened.

blood pressure The force exerted by the blood on the walls of the arteries. See **diastolic, systolic.**

capillaries Very small blood vessels that serve as links between arterioles and venules.

cardiac arrest Any stoppage of the heartbeat.

cerebrovascular accident (stroke, cerebrovascular occlusion) A sudden loss of brain function resulting from interference with the blood supply to one part of the brain.

collateral circulation A system of smaller blood vessels, which develop to provide alternative routes for blood when a main artery is blocked.

congenital heart disease Defects of the heart that are present at birth.

congestive heart failure A condition in which the heart cannot pump enough blood, resulting in a congestion of blood in the lungs.

coronary atherosclerosis A disease process characterized by fatty thickening of the intima (the lining) of the coronary arteries.

coronary embolism A blockage of a coronary artery that occurs when a piece of clotted material breaks away from the artery wall and dams up a narrowed coronary artery.

coronary thrombosis A blood clot in a coronary artery.

diastolic Referring to blood pressure inside the arteries when the left ventricle of the heart is relaxed and filling with blood between beats. Compare **systolic.**

edema Swelling caused by fluid collecting in the tissues.

fibrillation An arrhythmia in which the ventricles of the heart beat irregularly at an extremely fast rate.

heart A four-chambered, muscular organ that continuously pumps blood throughout the circulatory system.

heart attack The death of a portion of the heart muscle due to lack of oxygen.

heart block A sudden slowing or stopping of the heartbeat, caused by a failure of the electrical connection between the atria and ventricles of the heart.

hypertension (high blood pressure) An elevation of blood pressure above the normal range, which increases the risk of cardiovascular disease.

intima The lining of the arteries.

lipoproteins Substances containing both fat and protein that transport fat molecules through the body. **Low-density lipoprotein (LDL)** contains little protein and is the major medium of cholesterol transport. **High-density lipoprotein (HDL)** is heavier, and higher concentrations of it in the body seem to offer some protection from heart disease.

myocardial infarction Death of a section of the heart muscle caused by a reduction in the supply of blood to that area.

plaque Fatty deposits that stick to the lining of the artery walls, causing them to become rough and thickened.

rheumatic fever Inflammatory disease of connective tissue throughout the body; can cause scarring of heart muscle and valves.

sphygmomanometer Instrument used to measure blood pressure.

stroke See **cerebrovascular accident.**

systolic Referring to blood pressure inside the arteries when the left ventricle of the heart is contracting at each beat. Compare **diastolic.**

transient ischemic attack (TIA) A very mild stroke, causing temporary dizziness or slight weakness or numbness.

vein Blood vessel that carries blood from the body back to the heart.

venules The smallest veins.

NOTES

1. American Heart Association, *Heart Facts*, 1983, p. 1.

2. Ibid., pp. 18, 3.

3. Ibid., p. 2.

4. W. F. Enos, R. H. Holmes, and J. Beyer, "Coronary Disease Among United States Soldiers Killed in Action in Korea," *Journal of the American Medical Association* 152, no. 12 (1953): 1090.

5. American Heart Association, *Risk Factors and Coronary Disease: A Statement for Physicians* (Dallas: American Heart Association, 1980).

6. J. J. McNamara, M. A. Molot, J. F. Stremple, and R. T. Cutting, "Coronary Artery Disease in Combat Casualties in Vietnam," *Journal of the American Medical Association* 216, no. 7 (1971): 1185.

7. Stanley L. Englebardt, *How to Avoid Your Heart Attack* (New York: Readers' Digest Press, 1974), p. 40.

8. Ibid., pp. 38–40.

9. L. M. Elston, *It's Your Body: An Explanatory Text in Basic Regional Anatomy with Functional and Clinical Considerations* (New York: McGraw-Hill, 1975), pp. 485–486.

10. W. Boyd and H. Sheldon, *An Introduction to the Study of Disease*, 7th ed. (Philadelphia: Lea and Febiger, 1977), pp. 228–234.

11. American Heart Association, *Heart Facts*, 1983, p. 2.

12. Irving M. Levitas, *You Can Beat the Odds on a Heart Attack* (Indianapolis: Bobbs-Merrill, 1975), p. 5.

13. *Time*, June 1, 1981, p. 56.

14. American Heart Association, *Heart Facts*, 1983.

15. Boyd and Sheldon, *Introduction to the Study of Disease.*

16. *Psychology Today*, June 1977, p. 122.

17. American Heart Association, *Heart Facts*, 1983.

18. R. S. Fowler and W. E. Fordyce, *Stroke: Why Do They Behave That Way?* (Dallas: American Heart Association, n.d.); *Self-Care for the Hemiplegic* (Minneapolis: Sister Kenny Institute, 1977).

19. The following information on *non*controllable risk factors is derived from *Heart Facts*, 1983, p. 13.

20. William C. Roberts, "The Hypertensive Diseases," in J. H. Laragh, ed., *Topics in Hypertension* (New York: Dun-Donelly, 1980).

21. E. D. Fries, "Age, Race, Sex and Other Indices of Risk in Hypertension," in J. H. Laragh, ed., *Hypertension Manual* (New York, Dun-Donelly, 1974); American Heart Association, *Fact Sheet on Heart Attack, Stroke, and Risk Factors*, 1982.

22. Ibid.

23. American Heart Association, *Heart Facts*, 1983, p. 2.

24. U. S. Public Health Service, *Cardiovascular Primer for the Workplace*, National Institutes of Health Pub. No. 81-2210, January 1981, p. 7.

25. L. Rosenberg et al., "Oral Contraceptive Use in Relation to Non-Fatal Myocardial Infarction," *American Journal of Epidemiology* 111, no. 1 (1980): 59; D. E. Krueger et al., "Fatal Myocardial Infarction and the Role of Oral Contraceptives," *American Journal of Epidemiology* 111, no. 6 (1980): 655.

26. T. Gordon et al., "High Density Lipoprotein as a Protective Factor Against Coronary Heart Disease," *American Journal of Medicine* 62 (1977): 707.

27. Ibid.; U. S. Public Health Service, *Cardiovascular Primer for the Workplace.*

28. W. Winkelstein and M. Maimot, "Primary Prevention of Ischemic Heart Disease: Evaluation of Community Intervention," in L. Breslow, J. E. Fielding, and L. B. Lave, eds., *Annual Review of Public Health*, vol. 2 (Palo Alto, Calif.: Annual Reviews, Inc., 1981), pp. 253–273.

29. T. R. Dawber, *The Framingham Study: The Epidemiology of Atherosclerotic Disease* (Cambridge, Mass.: Harvard University Press, 1980).

PART FIVE

Promoting Well-Being: Lifestyle Decisions

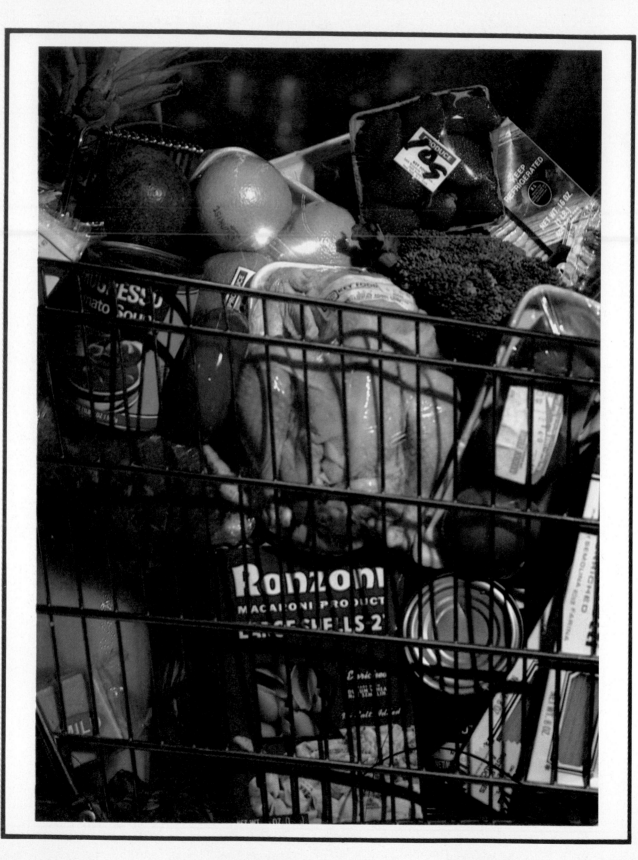

CHAPTER 13

Diet and Nutrition

An item on the television news connects the use of saccharin with cancer. A diet book that recommends eating large amounts of pineapple becomes a best-seller. A suburban supermarket begins to offer alfalfa sprouts and cakes of tofu to its customers.

As these examples suggest, Americans are now more interested in food and nutrition than they ever have been. We are concerned about whether certain foods may be hazardous to our health, and, quick to notice our concern, manufacturers have begun to label everything "natural," from tomato juice to potato chips. As a nation, we seem to be obsessed with keeping our weight down, and we are more likely than ever to choose "diet" soft drinks—and even "dietetic" chocolates and chewing gum. Our changing tastes in food have led some of us to sample new foods—yogurt, for example. Others of us seem to have so little time to cook and eat that we subsist on doughnuts, pizza, Big Macs, fries, and Cokes—a diet that has never before been eaten regularly by large numbers of people. Whatever we eat, we are probably wondering whether we're eating the right thing. Increasingly, we are concerned about nutrition.

food you take in ultimately feeds all the cells of the body as it makes material for bones, skin, hair, muscles, hormones, and enzymes and provides the fuel for efficient operation. Too little food or too much—or worse, too much low-nutrient food —tends to lead to poor health. We now have evidence that poor nutrition may be linked to many serious diseases—among them heart disease, stroke, and some types of cancer.[1]

Although most people are aware of the connection between good nutrition and good health, in recent years so many conflicting claims have been published about particular foods that the public has been left in confusion. Should you use saccharin in your coffee, on the theory that too much sugar is bad for you? But some studies have connected saccharin with cancer.[2] And what *about* that cup of coffee? Isn't caffeine a hazard?

You can avoid some of this confusion by studying what food is composed of and how it acts in the body. Good nutrition, as you will see, is not simply a matter of avoiding any one harmful food or filling up on any supposedly good food. We know that several types of food work together to produce good health.

What Is Nutrition?

Nutrition is the science of food, its use within the body, and its relationship to good health. It includes the study of the major food components—protein, carbohydrates, fat, vitamins, minerals, and water—and the more than fifty specific nutrients of which they are composed.

Nutrition is vital to the good health of all people of all ages. When you eat, you are doing much more than simply filling an empty stomach. The

THE FOUR BASIC COMPONENTS OF FOOD

All foods are composed of chemical compounds. During the process of digestion, our bodies break these complex compounds down into simpler ones, and then reassemble them into other kinds of chemicals that can be directly used by the body. There are four basic groups of chemicals in the foods we eat: (1) protein, (2) carbohydrates, (3) fat,

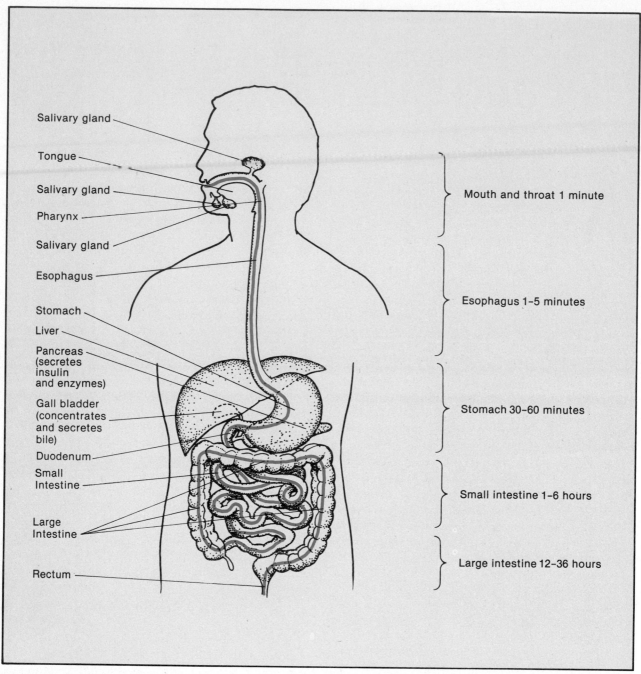

Figure 13.1 The human digestive system. After food is partially broken down by being chewed and mixed with saliva in the mouth, it is swallowed and enters the stomach, whose acids break it down further. As the food passes through the duodenum, secretions from the pancreas are added. Bile from the gall bladder is added in the small intestine. Digestive proteins and carbohydrates travel from the small intestine through the liver and into the bloodstream. Digestive fats move from the large intestine through the lymph system, which drains into the bloodstream via the heart. The large intestine reabsorbs excess water; the solid wastes that remain are collected in the rectum and excreted through the anus. The time that food spends in each part of the gastrointestinal tract is highly variable; the intervals shown here are averages.

and (4) vitamins and minerals. (Vitamins and minerals are often categorized together in this context.)

Protein

Protein, found in meat, eggs, dairy products, and some other foods, is essential for growth and repair of the body. The body uses protein to build muscle, hair, teeth, nails, bones, nerve cells, hemoglobin, and enzymes. There are also special proteins, known as nucleic acids, in the nuclei of all the cells in your body. The job of these nucleic acids—which include RNA, or ribonucleic acid, and DNA, or deoxyribonucleic acid—is to transmit hereditary characteristics.

OBTAINING THE PROTEIN BUILDING BLOCKS YOU NEED

Protein is made up of twenty-two different amino acids, the "building blocks" of the body. Of these twenty-two, eight are called essential amino acids, because the body cannot manufacture them. You must obtain them directly in your food. The body can make the other fourteen amino acids.

All eight essential amino acids must be present in your body at the same time in order for the body to form protein. Since free amino acids cannot be stored in the body, this means that you must consume the eight essential acids at approximately the same time—preferably at the same meal—for your body to use them.

HOW TO GET THE PROTEIN YOU NEED

▶ One way is to include foods of animal origin (meat, eggs, dairy products) in your daily diet. The protein in these foods is known as **complete protein:** It contains all eight of the essential amino acids.
▶ You can also get your protein from plant foods. However, protein of plant origin (in vegetables and grains) is almost invariably **incomplete protein.** That is, it lacks one or more essential amino acids. You can combine plant proteins, either with each other in specific combinations or with animal protein, to form complete protein. Familiar examples include cereal and milk, macaroni and cheese, rice and beans, a peanut butter sandwich on whole wheat bread.

HOW MUCH PROTEIN DO YOU NEED EACH DAY?

Clearly, it is vital to consume adequate amounts of protein each day. Most Americans, however, take in far more than is needed: Most young men need about 56 grams and most young women need about 45 grams, but our average daily consumption is about 100 grams.[3] One quick way to get a rough estimate of your protein need is to divide your weight in pounds by 3. Thus, if you weigh 150 pounds and divide this by 3, your approximate daily protein need is 50 grams. That's roughly the amount of protein found in two servings, each 2 to 3 ounces, of lean cooked meat, poultry, or fish. The body converts any excess protein to **glucose,** a type of sugar, which is then either burned as energy or stored as fat—a very expensive source of calories for such usage.

Getting too little protein can be dangerous. Low-protein fad diets (to be discussed in Chapter 14) can only have undesirable results. The dieter can become seriously ill (though this is rare). But even minor protein deficiencies over a period of time will cause fatigue and irritability, and they will reduce the body's production of antibodies, so that the individual becomes more susceptible to infection and recovers more slowly from disease. Wounds and burns heal more slowly. And continued protein deficiency may eventually lead to anemia and liver disorders.

Carbohydrates

Carbohydrates, found in spaghetti, bread, cereal, rice, potatoes, doughnuts, candy, most fruits and vegetables, and other foods, are our source of ready energy: They contribute approximately 50 percent of the body's energy needs and are its most economical energy source. They include two major types: **sugars** and **starches.** (Cellulose is also a carbohydrate, but since it is a nonnutrient, it will not be considered here.)

Carbohydrates are less complex compounds than proteins, and they can be burned (*oxidized*) in the body much more efficiently than either proteins or fats. They are broken down in digestion into chemicals known as **simple sugars,** which are then further converted by the liver into glucose. Some of this glucose goes right into the blood-

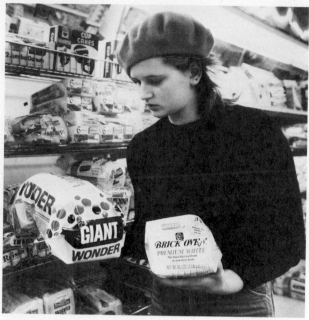

Carbohydrates—found in such foods as bread, spaghetti, and rice—are essential nutrients and should not be omitted from the diet, even of people who are trying to lose weight. These foods should not be thought of as necessarily fattening. Whole-grain, enriched, and fortified breads are especially recommended. © Ray Solomon/Monkmeyer Press Photo)

stream and is directly used by all the cells in the body for energy. Some glucose remains stored in the liver and muscles as a substance called **glycogen**, ready for immediate release into the bloodstream should blood glucose levels fall too low. Excess glucose—that which is neither burned as energy nor stored as glycogen—is converted to substances known as fatty acids, such as **triglycerides**, which are then stored in fat tissue.

In addition to fulfilling our energy requirements, our bodies also need carbohydrates to utilize fat efficiently. If an individual consumes less than 125 milligrams of carbohydrate per day, the body will not be able to burn fat from fat stores completely.

HOW MUCH CARBOHYDRATE DO YOU NEED EACH DAY?

Most nutritionists believe that a minimum of 50 to 100 grams of carbohydrates per day—four servings of bread, cereal, noodles, or rice—is necessary for optimal energy levels.[4] For this reason, low-carbohydrate fad diets are ill-advised. Your energy level will be lowered and you will feel weak, light-headed, and fatigued—not conditions that keep you operating at peak performance.

We all experience a condition of temporary low blood sugar, or **hypoglycemia**, from time to time when our blood sugar drops—when we are very hungry, for example. It's important to note that this temporary drop is not the same as the *disease* known as hypoglycemia, which is an extremely rare condition caused by malfunctioning of the pancreas.

TOO MUCH SUGAR CAN BE HARMFUL

Ordinary table sugars themselves—such as white sugar, brown sugar, and honey—are not necessary in the diet. In recent years, sugar has been suggested as the culprit in a variety of diseases and health disorders, including obesity, hypoglycemia, diabetes, heart disease, and tooth decay. The relationship between sugar consumption and a given disorder is not always simple or direct: For example, the consumption of sugar does not in itself cause obesity; what makes a person fat is consuming more calories than the body can use.

HOW IS SUGAR RELATED TO DIABETES?

Many of us know that the level of sugar in the bloodstream is somehow related to the disease known as *diabetes mellitus* (or "sugar diabetes"). Beyond that, our understanding of this condition may be hazy—and that's not surprising, since medical researchers are still debating about the disease.

There are two major types of diabetes, both characterized by abnormal processing of carbohydrates. In *juvenile-onset diabetes*, the body somehow fails to produce enough of a substance known as **insulin**, which helps the cells of the body take sugar (in the form of glucose) from the bloodstream and use it. In *adult-onset diabetes*, the body manufactures insulin, but somehow it cannot use this insulin properly.

Relatively high levels of sugar in the bloodstream, then, are the result, not the cause, of these problems with insulin—the body is not able to remove this sugar from the bloodstream and use it at the same rate a normal person's body would.

But there is a further difficulty. Diabetes has very dangerous complications, including degeneration of the large and small blood vessels and high blood pressure. Some scientists think that relatively high levels of sugar in the bloodstream may help bring on these complications.[5] And that's why some physicians teach their patients to monitor their blood sugar levels carefully and take steps to prevent wide swings in the level. Other physicians, however, don't agree that the high blood sugar levels are the cause of the complications; they think some other relationship may be involved.[6]

Fat

Fat has gotten a bad reputation recently—yet fat in the diet is essential to good health. Besides serving as an additional energy source, **fats**—also known as **lipids**—give flavor and juiciness to many of the foods we eat. Fats also insulate the body; cushion vital organs, protecting them from injury; serve as carriers for the four fat-soluble vitamins (A, D, E, and K); and contribute to hormone synthesis and the blood clotting mechanism. Unused fats, like extra carbohydrates, are stored as "fat tissue" and drawn on by the body when they are needed for energy. Stored fats are the greatest nutritional reservoir in the body.

TYPES OF FATS

Fatty acids are the building blocks of fats. They are made up of carbon, hydrogen, and small amounts of oxygen. The terms "saturated" and "unsaturated" are used to describe the hydrogen component of fats. **Saturated fats**, found in meats, butter, coconut oil, and palm oil, have all the hydrogen atoms they are capable of holding. A saturated fat is usually solid at room temperature. An **unsaturated fat** is capable of holding more hydrogen atoms than it does. *Polyunsaturated fats* (such as corn, soya, sunflower, and cottonseed oil) and *monounsaturated fats* (such as olive oil) are two classes of unsaturated fats. Polyunsaturated fats tend to lower blood cholesterol; monounsaturated fats do, too, but to a lesser degree. Unsaturated fats are usually liquid at room temperature. They can be changed to solids by **hydrogenation**, which involves bubbling hydrogen gas through the liquid oil. Margarine is processed in this manner. As we'll

see a little further on in our discussion, some experts think people who eat high proportions of saturated fats may have a higher risk of cardiovascular disease.

CHOLESTEROL

Cholesterol is a fatlike substance that has great physiological importance. It is one of the nonessential nutrients—that is, it is found in all foods from animal sources, and our bodies can also manufacture it.

Scientists have found that there is a relationship between high levels of cholesterol *in the blood* and increased risk of heart disease.[7] As we noted in Chapter 12, cholesterol is a major component of the **plaque** that can build up on the walls of blood vessels, including the vessels that supply the heart muscle, so that the blood vessels become narrowed and may eventually close off completely.

What is not precisely understood, however, is how much cholesterol *in the diet* (consumed in eggs and meat, for example) raises the level of *blood* cholesterol, and whether reducing dietary cholesterol significantly reduces the risk of heart disease.[8] It is not as if the cholesterol in our breakfast eggs and bacon immediately migrates to our arteries and begins to clog them up. Other factors in our diet or body metabolism, including exercise, may affect how much of the cholesterol we eat ultimately becomes part of our bodies and subjects us to increased risk of heart disease.

THE ROLE OF FIBER   Scientists believe that dietary fiber may also affect blood cholesterol levels directly.[9] As we shall see later in this chapter, the plant fiber present in fruits, vegetables, and grains is an important part of the human diet. Possibly, dietary fiber acts to lower blood cholesterol levels by reducing the amount of time that cholesterol-containing foods remain in the digestive tract.[10]

OTHER FACTORS   It is also thought that persons who are physically fit, who do not smoke, and who are not obese carry their blood cholesterol in a form that is less dangerous to the body.[11] In any case, we must realize that cholesterol and fats are not the only villains in heart disease; heredity, high blood pressure, and stress also play a role.

WHAT AMOUNT OF FAT DO YOU NEED EACH DAY?

Most people consume much more fat than they need. Between 40 and 50 percent of their daily calories come from fat.[12] They would be far better off if they kept their fat intake down to about 30 percent or less of their daily calories.

WHAT YOU CAN DO TO REDUCE YOUR BLOOD CHOLESTEROL LEVEL

We now know that saturated fats such as butter tend to raise blood cholesterol levels by serving as the starting material from which cholesterol can be synthesized in the body. Polyunsaturated fats such as corn oil, however, tend to lower blood cholesterol. Such knowledge makes it possible to reduce the amounts of fats and cholesterol you take into your body by adjusting your choice of foods.

▶ Use leaner cuts of meat; trim off all visible fat.
▶ Eat chicken and fish more frequently and beef, lamb, and pork—which are high in fat—less often.
▶ Drink skim milk instead of whole milk.
▶ Eat more vegetables and fruits and fewer fatty foods such as french fries and ice cream.
▶ Switch from butter to margarine.

It is especially important to choose foods that are low in cholesterol and fats if you know you are at increased risk of heart disease because, for example, you have relatives with heart disorders.

Vitamins

Vitamins, along with minerals, are often referred to as "micronutrients," because they are required in only trace amounts. Yet they are indispensable in triggering vital bodily functions. Vitamins do not form new compounds in the body, as proteins, carbohydrates, and fats do. Rather, they help other chemical reactions to take place: For example, vitamin D is necessary for calcium to become part of the bone structure. Tables 13.1 and 13.2 show the specific functions of each vitamin, its food sources, and the effects of deficiency and excess.

HOW MUCH OF EACH VITAMIN DO YOU NEED EACH DAY?

Most people get all the essential nutrients they need, including vitamins, if they eat a varied diet. A few people run the risk of not taking in necessary vitamins: This category includes some people who are on restricted diets (extremely low-calorie diets, for example), and some people with particular health problems (alcoholism, chronic diarrhea). But there is no evidence that most Americans need to take vitamin supplements routinely, nor that their use prevents disease or promotes health. We spend more than $1.2 billion a year on vitamin supplements, and the amount grows by about 10 percent each year.[13] For those who have not been diagnosed as suffering from a vitamin deficiency, this money would be far better spent in purchasing nutrients in the form of food.

THE DANGER OF VITAMIN OVERDOSE

Vitamins are subdivided into two major groups; the **water-soluble vitamins,** C and the B complex, and the **fat-soluble vitamins,** A, D, E, and K. The danger of excess consumption of the fat-soluble vitamins has long been known. These cannot be excreted, but rather are stored (as the name implies) in the fatty tissues, where they may build to toxic levels. More recently, evidence has begun to accumulate that vitamin C in doses above 2 to 4 grams may cause kidney problems and may increase the body's need for vitamin C in pregnant women.

For these reasons, a word should be said about the dangers of overdosing with vitamin supplements. Vitamin supplements can be of great help to persons who suffer from a deficiency of a particular vitamin or vitamins. But although vitamins are necessary to health, taking *more* of them is not necessarily better for you. Consumed in large doses, vitamins are properly considered drugs, not nutrients, and overdoses of the fat-soluble vitamins can cause illness or even death.[14]

HOW MUCH VITAMIN C DO YOU NEED?   The controversy over vitamin C has lingered since publication in 1970 of Linus Pauling's book *Vitamin C, the Common Cold, and the Flu.* In this book Pauling presented his theory that vitamin C would both prevent and cure common colds.[15] After an initial flurry of interest and a great deal of profes-

TABLE 13.1 · Water-Soluble Vitamins

Vitamin	Physiological Role	Food Source	Effects of Deficiency DISEASE	SYMPTOMS
C (ascorbic acid)	Collagen formation and maintenance; protects against infection	Citrus fruits, tomatoes, cabbage, broccoli, potatoes, peppers	Scurvy	Rough, scaly skin; anemia; gum eruptions; pain in extremities; retarded healing
B₁ (thiamin)	Changes glucose into energy or fat; helps prevent nervous irritability; necessary for good appetite	Whole-grain or enriched cereals, liver, yeast, nuts, legumes, wheat germ	Beriberi	Numbness in toes and feet, tingling of legs; muscular weakness; cardiac abnormalities
B₂ (riboflavin)	Transports hydrogen; is essential in the metabolism of carbohydrates, fats, and proteins; helps keep skin in healthy condition	Liver, green leafy vegetables, milk, cheese, eggs, fish, whole-grain or enriched cereals	Ariboflavinosis	Cracking of the mouth corners; sore skin; bloodshot eyes; sensitivity to light
Niacin	Hydrogen transport; important to maintenance of all body tissues; energy production	Yeast, liver, wheat germ, kidneys, eggs, fish; can be synthesized from the essential amino acid tryptophan	Pellagra	Diarrhea; skin rash; mental disorders
B₆ (pyridoxine)	Essential to amino-acid and carbohydrate metabolism	Yeast, wheat bran and germ, liver, kidneys, meat, whole grains, fish, vegetables	—	Greasy scaliness around eyes, nose, and mouth; mental depression
Pantothenic acid	Functions in the breakdown and synthesis of carbohydrates, fats, and proteins; necessary for synthesis of some of the adrenal hormones	Liver, kidneys, milk, yeast, wheat germ, whole-grain cereals and breads, green vegetables	—	Enlargement of adrenal glands; personality changes; low blood sugar; nausea; headaches; muscle cramps
Folacin (folic acid)	Necessary for the production of RNA and DNA and normal red blood cells	Liver, nuts, green vegetables, orange juice	—	Anemia yielding immature red blood cells; smooth, red tongue; diarrhea
B₁₂ (cyanocobalamin)	Necessary for production of red blood cells and normal growth	Meat, liver, eggs, milk	Pernicious anemia	Drop in number of red blood cells; irritability; drowsiness and depression
Biotin	Important in carbohydrate metabolism and fatty-acid synthesis; probably essential for biosynthesis of folic acid	Same as other B vitamins	—	Scaliness of skin; pain in muscles; sensitivity to light; can lead to eczema
Choline	Synthesis of protein and hormones of adrenal gland; important in maintenance of normal nerve-impulse transmission	Brains, liver, yeast, wheat germ, egg yolk	—	None observed and identified

TABLE 13.2 · Fat-Soluble Vitamins

Vitamin	Physiological Role	Food Source	Effects of Deficiency	Effects of Excess
A	Maintenance of epi-thelial tissue; strengthens tooth enamel and favors utilization of calcium and phosphorus in bone formation	Milk and other dairy products, green vegetables, carrots, animal liver; carotene in vegetables is converted to vitamin A in the body	Night blindness; growth decrease; eye secretions cease	Swelling of feet and ankles; weight loss; lassitude; eye hemorrhages
D	Promotes absorption and utilization of calcium and phosphorus; essential for normal bone and tooth development	Fish oils, beef, butter, eggs, milk; produced in the skin upon exposure to ultraviolet rays in sunlight	Rickets: a softening of the bones causing bow legs or other bone deformities	Thirst, nausea, vomiting; loss of weight; calcium deposits in kidney or heart
E	May relate to oxidation and longevity; may be a protection against red blood cell destruction	Widely distributed in foods: yellow vegetables, vegetable oils, and wheat germ	Increased red cell destruction	—
K	Shortens blood-clotting time	Spinach, eggs, liver, cabbage, tomatoes; produced by intestinal bacteria	Poor blood clotting (hemorrhage)	Jaundice in infants

sional criticism, dozens of attempts were made to either confirm or deny these claims. To date, results are still inconclusive. What is of great concern, as mentioned earlier, are the possible side effects of the massive doses recommended by Pauling. Even though vitamin C is water-soluble —so that excess amounts would ordinarily be excreted in the urine—the amounts involved here are too large to be excreted very quickly. A buildup may occur, resulting in diarrhea, kidney or bladder stones, or gout.

Minerals

Minerals are inorganic elements that we need in trace amounts daily to help form tissues and various chemical substances in the body. They assist in nerve transmission and muscle contraction and help regulate fluid levels and the acid/base balance of the body.

Minerals are needed in the diet in different amounts. Iron, zinc, selenium, copper, cobalt, and manganese, all of which are "trace minerals," are needed in only tiny amounts (a few micrograms) daily. The body needs much larger quantities of the major minerals such as calcium, phosphorus, potassium, and magnesium. Since minerals are absorbed, used, and excreted by the body, they must be continuously replaced.

Minerals are contained in almost everything we eat, and most people can obtain sufficient quantities of the essential minerals by eating a variety of foods, particularly fruits and vegetables. Table 13.3 provides a summary of the functions and sources of some of the most important minerals. Here we'll discuss in detail only two major minerals: iron and salt.

IRON

Iron is one of the body's most important nutrients, essential for hemoglobin production in the red blood cells, yet it is also the most frequently deficient nutrient in the diet. Only about 10 percent of the average person's iron intake is actually used,

TABLE 13.3 · Minerals*

Mineral	Primary Functions	Food Source
Calcium (Ca)	Building material of bones and teeth; regulation of body functions: heart muscle contraction, blood clotting	Dairy products, leafy vegetables, apricots
Phosphorus (P)	Combines with calcium to give rigidity to bones and teeth; essential in cell metabolism; serves as a buffer to maintain proper acid-base balance of blood	Peas, beans, milk, liver, meat, cottage cheese, broccoli, whole grains
Iron (Fe)	Component of the red blood cell's oxygen and carbon dioxide transport system; enzyme constituent necessary for cellular respiration	Liver, meat, shellfish, lentils, peanuts, parsley, dried fruits, eggs
Iodine (I)	Essential component of the thyroid hormone, thyroxin, which controls the rate of cell oxidation	Iodized salt, seafood
Sodium (Na)	Regulates the fluid and acid-base balance in the body	Table salt, dried apricots, beans, beets, brown sugar, raisins, spinach, yeast
Chlorine (Cl)	Associated with sodium and its functions; a component of the gastric juice hydrochloric acid; the chloride ion also functions in the starch-splitting system of saliva	Same as sodium
Potassium (K)	Component of the system that controls the acid-base and liquid balances; is probably an important enzyme activator in the use of amino acids	Readily available in most foods
Magnesium (Mg)	Enzyme activator related to carbohydrate metabolism	Readily available in most foods
Sulfur (S)	Component of the hormone insulin and the sulfur amino acids; builds hair, nails, skin	Nuts, dried fruits, barley and oatmeal, beans, cheese, eggs, lentils, brown sugar
Manganese (Mn)	Enzyme activator for systems related to carbohydrate, protein, and fat metabolism	Wheat germ, nuts, bran, green leafy vegetables, cereal grains, meat
Copper (Cu)	The function of copper has not been fully resolved although it is known to function in the synthesis of the red blood cell and the oxidation system of the body	Kidney, liver, beans, Brazil nuts, wholemeal flour, lentils, parsley
Zinc (Z)	The function is unknown although it is a component of many enzyme systems and is an essential component of the pancreatic hormone insulin	Shellfish, meat, milk, eggs
Cobalt (Co)	A component of the vitamin B_{12} molecule	Vitamin B_{12}
Fluorine (F)	Essential to normal tooth and bone development and maintenance; excesses are undesirable	Drinking water in some areas

*Several trace minerals—chromium, selenium, nickel, molybdenum, vanadium, and tin—are now known to be required in very small amounts by experimental animals. Their distribution in food varies considerably, depending in part on the composition of the soil in which plants are raised.

because iron cannot be absorbed in the small intestine. Iron-deficiency anemia is thus a fairly widespread health problem in the United States, particularly among women of child-bearing age, who regularly lose considerable amounts of iron through the menstrual process. A woman's iron requirement is almost twice that of a man's, and this is the one nutrient that frequently requires supplementation. Such supplements, however, should be recommended only by a physician.

Both men and women should attempt to include some iron-rich foods in their diet every day —liver, meat, shellfish, dried beans, and dried fruits.

SALT (SODIUM CHLORIDE)

Common table salt (sodium chloride) is a necessary part of the human diet, but if it is consumed to excess, it can cause problems. Numerous studies have demonstrated that too much salt can interfere with growth and raise blood pressure, and there is a known association between salt and congestive heart failure, and certain types of kidney diseases.

Furthermore, salt may be habit-forming: Human beings develop a "taste" for it. Some

Adolescents, whose bodies are still growing and whose activity levels are usually high, have special nutritional needs. Yet many teenagers eat poorly balanced diets, which are likely to be deficient in minerals and vitamins, especially iron, calcium, and vitamins A and C. (© Mimi Forsyth/Monkmeyer Press Photo)

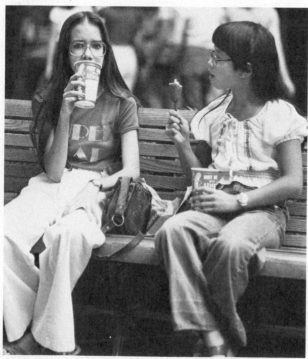

scientists believe that an excessive appetite for sodium develops largely because of the large amounts of salt in the diet during childhood and early adulthood. Today, many doctors and nutritionists recommend reduced use of salt from infancy in order to prevent the salt habit from developing. Manufacturers of baby food now add to their products only the barest minimum (if any) for accentuating natural flavors.

Recently, concern has focused on the relationship of excess salt in the diet to high blood pressure, or hypertension. Sodium intake is only one of many factors related to high blood pressure. Others include genetic predisposition, obesity, and stress. One view is that certain people inherit a susceptibility to high blood pressure, and too much sodium can trigger the disease. In many hypertensive patients, a low-sodium diet reduces blood pressure, and doctors often advise such patients to eliminate as much sodium as possible from their diets. Since a person may be susceptible without knowing it, some nutritionists and public-health authorities have urged that we all attempt to curb our salt habit.[16] Other investigators, however, have recently argued that general recommendations to cut back on sodium are inappropriate because the majority of Americans are not at risk of developing hypertension.[17]

For most of us, reducing salt intake is no easy matter, even if we throw out the salt shaker. There is some sodium in almost every processed food sold in our supermarkets, from peanuts, pickles, bacon, and potato chips to canned tuna, candy bars, and instant pudding. According to some estimates, American adults consume approximately twenty times the daily amount of salt they need— per person, as much as fifteen pounds of salt per year.[18]

OTHER KEY FOOD COMPONENTS

Water

Water in itself has no nutritional value. Yet it is perhaps the most important of all food components! Why? A major reason is that water is the medium both for transporting nutrients to the cells of the body and for removing cellular waste products. In addition, water acts as a medium for digestion, is the body's temperature regulator, serves to cushion vital organs, and lubricates the joints. Finally, water and some of the chemicals it carries are responsible for bodily structure: The cells in our bodies contain fluid, and there is fluid around the cells too. As much as 80 percent of the body weight may be water, although the average is closer to 60 percent.

HOW MUCH WATER DO YOU NEED EACH DAY?

While the body can survive for long periods without food, it can exist for only a few days without water. An average of two to two-and-a-half liters of water (slightly more than two quarts) per day is the recommended daily intake. Of course, not all of this need be consumed as plain water; other liquids serve as well. Generally speaking, only about 50 percent of the body's water requirement comes directly from liquids; another 25 to 50 percent is from food, and the rest is an end product of metabolism.

The actual amount of water our bodies require each day depends on our environment, our physical activity, the season of the year, and the type of food we eat.

Fiber

Fiber, also known as "roughage" or "bulk," is another nonnutritive substance that is necessary in the human diet. Fiber consists of indigestible carbohydrates, largely the cellulose that is part of the fruits, vegetables, and grains we eat. (Common examples of fiber are fruit skins and wheat bran.) Today, scientists are calling attention to the importance of fiber in the diet—largely because modern American diets may be deficient in it. Our diets nowadays consist predominantly of processed foods. In them, most fiber has been either milled or peeled away (white bread, white rice, french fries, instant potatoes), and so many traditional sources of fiber have disappeared from the diet.

Fiber is necessary in the digestive process. In the large intestine (the colon), it serves to bind other waste products with large amounts of water, forming an easily passed, soft, large stool. Ade-

quate amounts of fiber in the diet result in stools that are increased in both volume and frequency. This, in turn, helps to prevent diverticulitis, a physiological problem in which the large intestinal wall weakens and balloons out. The presence of fiber also provides a medium for the growth of certain bacteria that help the body synthesize nutrients such as vitamin K.

WHAT YOU CAN DO TO GET THE FIBER YOU NEED

Some recent studies have suggested that increased fiber in the diet will result in lowered risk of colon cancer.[19] But until further research offers more definite proof of the effects of high-fiber diets on the body, most nutritionists recommend that you simply consume moderate amounts of fiber as part of a balanced diet. This should include whole-grain breads and cereals and ample servings of salads, fresh fruits, and vegetables. Bran or other such supplements are unnecessary in most circumstances, unless you have ongoing bowel problems—in which case you should check with your physician.

Calories

Calories are not nutrients either; a calorie is just a unit of measurement, like a foot or an inch. Calorie listings indicate the potential energy value of foods or food components. Protein and carbohydrate each contain 4 calories per gram; fat contains 9 calories per gram. (Thus, you would consume more than twice as many calories in a teaspoon of butter as in a teaspoon of sugar.) Vitamins, minerals, and water contain no calories; neither does fiber, since it is indigestible to human beings.

Energy expenditure—the amount of energy your body needs in order to carry out an activity or bodily process—is also expressed in calories. For example, an average-sized apple contains about 100 calories. A twenty-minute walk will burn up just about as many calories. (However, it will take one to one-and-a-half hours to "walk off" a wedge of apple pie.)

How many calories do you need per day? This depends on your physical activity and other factors. This subject will be covered more thoroughly in Chapter 14.

YOU NEED A BALANCED DIET

Since foods vary so much in their combinations of both nutrients and calories, how can you achieve a "balanced" diet each day? There are complicated ways to perform all the necessary calculations, but few people have the time or interest to do this. The simplest way to plan adequate nutrition on a daily basis is to use the "Basic Four" food groups.

The Basic Four

The Basic Four provide most of the Recommended Dietary Allowances (RDAs) established by the National Academy of Sciences/National Research Council (see Table 13.4).[20] The RDAs, which are reviewed for possible revision every five years, are estimates of the optimal quantity of each nutrient required—the *most* a person would be likely to need. Thus, if the food you eat supplies all the recommended allowances, you can be assured of meeting all your daily nutritional needs. It should be noted that refined sugar, fats, and oils are not included in the Basic Four, since they provide mainly calories (but not nutrients such as proteins, carbohydrates, vitamins, and minerals) and are rarely lacking in the American diet.

Briefly, the four groups are:

MEAT GROUP

This group includes meats, poultry, fish, eggs, and legumes such as dried beans, peas, and nuts—all good sources of protein. In addition, these foods supply iron and B vitamins such as thiamine, riboflavin, niacin, B_6, and B_{12}.

MILK AND MILK PRODUCTS

These foods supply more calcium per serving than any other. Indeed, it is difficult to meet your daily calcium requirement if you don't eat milk or cheese. Foods from this group are also valuable sources of protein, many of the B vitamins (especially riboflavin), vitamin A (if the milk is whole milk), and vitamin D if it has been added to the milk, as it should be.

FRUITS AND VEGETABLES

Foods in this group supply 100 percent of the vitamin C requirement, 60 percent of vitamin A, many other vitamins and minerals, and much of the body's fiber requirement.

BREADS AND CEREALS (WHOLE-GRAIN OR ENRICHED)

Foods from this group (including macaroni, sphaghetti, noodles, rice, and similar products) are valuable sources of carbohydrates, thiamine, riboflavin, niacin, and iron. In fact, it is difficult to obtain enough thiamine and iron (particularly for females) if this group is excluded from the diet.

Nutrition Labeling

If you want to find out what nutrients from the Basic Four are in a processed or packaged food, one thing you can do is read the label. Since 1973, nutrition labeling has been required for any food that has been enriched with additional nutrients or that makes a specific nutritional claim.[21] **Enrichment** refers to either the restoring of specific nutrients that have been lost in processing or the addition of nutrients that were not originally present in a food.

Food labels must show the following:

▶ Serving size
▶ Number of servings per container
▶ Per-serving amount of calories, protein, carbohydrates, and fat, as well as the percentage of U.S. Recommended Daily Allowances per serving for certain essential nutrients—protein, vitamins A and D, thiamine, riboflavin, niacin, calcium, and iron.
▶ An asterisk (*) placed next to the name of an essential nutrient if the quantity of that nutrient in one serving of the food is below 2 percent of the RDA.

Labeling regulations have provided the consumer with valuable information. None of this information is helpful, however, if it is not used. Reading labels is a good habit.

ACTIVITY: EXPLORING HEALTH

NUTRITION: The Decisions You Make

It has become increasingly clear that our eating habits can play a very powerful role in improving or reducing the quality of our lives and our health. The area of nutrition offers perhaps more opportunities for improving our health than any other area of our lives. Just think about it! You probably eat three meals a day, plus snacks, seven days a week, fifty-two weeks a year. In one year alone, this offers more than a thousand opportunities for you to do something positive for yourself.

So how do you go about choosing your diet and adopting good dietary habits—whether you happen to be a junk-food junkie or you just want to improve in this area? Let's see what your eating habits are right now.

PART I: HOW YOU EAT

The activity that follows is designed to assess your eating habits.

Eating Habits (Place a check next to all that apply.)

1. Which meals do you eat daily?
   _____ breakfast
   _____ lunch
   _____ dinner
   _____ snacks

2. How much salt do you use?
   _____ I do not use salt.
   _____ I add little salt.
   _____ I add moderate salt.
   _____ I add lots of salt to most things.

3. Which of the foods listed below do you eat often?
   _____ french fries
   _____ cake/cookies/pie
   _____ potato chips/pretzels
   _____ candy/chocolate bars

4. Which beverages do you drink each day, and how much?
   _____ soft drinks _____
   _____ fruit or vegetable juices _____
   _____ water _____
   _____ beer/wine _____
   _____ other alcoholic beverages _____
   _____ coffee/tea _____

5. How many calories do you think you take in daily?
   _____ probably too many
   _____ probably too few
   _____ the proper amount

6. Which of the foods listed below do you eat daily?
   _____ salads (vegetable or fruit)
   _____ fresh fruits
   _____ cooked vegetables
   _____ raw vegetables

7. Which do you eat the most of?
   _____ fresh vegetables
   _____ canned vegetables
   _____ frozen vegetables

8. What mainly governs your eating habits?
   _____ what is convenient to me
   _____ what tastes good to me
   _____ a combination of what tastes good and what is nutritious

Review the items you've checked. Are your eating habits like those of most Americans—too high in salt, sugar, fat, and calories and too low in fresh fruits and vegetables? Do you usually skip breakfast? Maybe you'd like to improve your eating habits. If so, you'll want to do the activity at the end of this chapter.

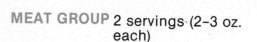

Figure 13.2   Guide to Good Eating: A Recommended Daily Plan

Humans need about 50 nutrients, including water, daily for optimum health. There are 10 "leader" nutrients: protein, carbohydrate, fat, vitamin A, vitamin C, thiamin, (B₁), riboflavin (B₂), niacin, calcium, and iron. If you include proper amounts of these 10 nutrients in your daily diet—and especially if you vary your choice of foods within each food group—you are likely to obtain sufficient amounts of the other 40 nutrients. This chart shows at a glance the kinds of foods found in each of the four basic food groups; the recommended number of daily servings of foods from each group; and the "leader" nutrients that each group supplies.

Source: Adapted from National Dairy Council data.

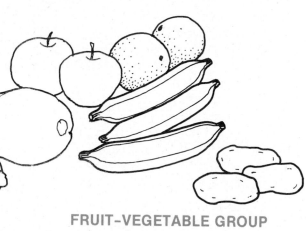

MEAT GROUP 2 servings (2–3 oz. each)

Protein
Niacin
Iron
Thiamin (B₁)

Sample serving: two eggs or one 2–3 oz. hamburger. Dry beans and peas, soy extenders and nuts combined with animal protein (meat, fish, poultry, eggs, milk, cheese) or grain protein (rice, spaghetti, etc.) can be substituted for a serving of meat.

FRUIT–VEGETABLE GROUP 4 servings

Vitamin A
Vitamin C

Each week, three or four servings from this group should consist of dark-green, leafy, or orange vegetables and fruits for vitamin A. Citrus fruit (oranges, lemons, grapefruit, etc.) is recommended daily for vitamin C.

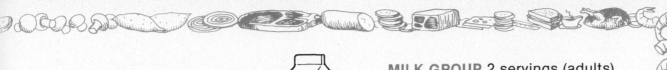

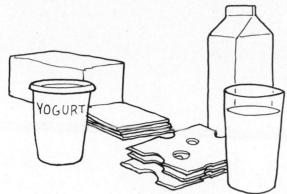

MILK GROUP
**2 servings (adults)
4 servings
   (teenagers)
3 servings
   (children)**

Calcium
Riboflavin
(B₂)
Protein

Sample serving: one 8-oz. glass of milk; 1½ oz. of cheese; 1 cup of yogurt. Foods made from milk, such as cheese, yogurt, and pudding, contribute some of the nutrients supplied by a serving of milk.

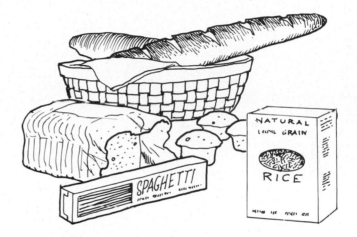

BREAD-CEREAL GROUP
4 servings (1 slice of bread, or equivalent)

Carbohydrates
Thiamin (B₁)
Iron
Niacin

Whole-grain, fortified, or enriched grain products are especially recommended.

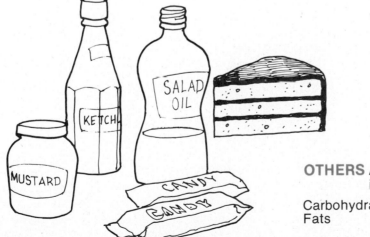

OTHERS
Amounts determined by individual caloric needs

Carbohydrates
Fats

Fatty or sweet snacks and condiments complement but do not replace foods from the four basic groups.

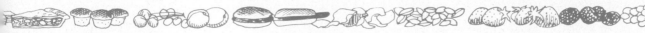

TABLE 13.4 · Recommended Daily Dietary Allowances for Healthy Adults

	Males		Females	
Nutrient	AGE 23–50	AGE 51+	AGE 23–50[b]	AGE 51+[a]
Energy (kcal)	2,700	2,400	2,000	1,800
Protein (gm)	56	56	44	44
Vitamin A (RE)	1,000	1,000	800	800
Vitamin D (μg)	5	5	5	5
Vitamin E (mgαTE)	10	10	8	8
Vitamin C (mg)	60	60	60	60
Folacin (μg)	400	400	400	400
Niacin (mg NE)	18	16	13	13
Riboflavin (mg)	1.6	1.4	1.2	1.2
Thiamin (mg)	1.4	1.2	1.0	1.0
Vitamin B₆ (mg)	2.2	2.2	2.0	2.0
Calcium (mg)	800	800	800	800
Phosphorus (mg)	800	800	800	800
Iodine (μg)	150	150	150	150
Iron (mg)	10	10	18	10
Magnesium (mg)	350	350	300	300
Zinc (mg)	15	15	15	15
Vitamin K (μg)[c]	70–140	70–140	70–140	70–140
Biotin (μg)[c]	100–200	100–200	100–200	100–200
Pantothenic acid (mg)[c]	4–7	4–7	4–7	4–7
Copper (mg)[c d]	2.0–3.0	2.0–3.0	2.0–3.0	2.0–3.0
Manganese (mg)[c d]	2.5–5.0	2.5–5.0	2.5–5.0	2.5–5.0
Fluorine (mg)[c d]	1.5–4.0	1.5–4.0	1.5–4.0	1.5–4.0
Chromium (mg)[c d]	0.05–0.2	0.05–0.2	0.05–0.2	0.05–0.2
Selenium (mg)[c d]	0.05–0.2	0.05–0.2	0.05–0.2	0.05–0.2
Molybdenum (mg)[c d]	0.15–0.5	0.15–0.5	0.15–0.5	0.15–0.5
Sodium (mg)[c]	1,100–3,300	1,100–3,300	1,100–3,300	1,100–3,300
Potassium (mg)[c]	1,875–5,625	1,875–5,625	1,875–5,625	1,875–5,625
Chlorine (mg)[c]	1,700–5,100	1,700–5,100	1,700–5,100	1,700–5,100

[a]For age 76 and above, the energy RDA for men is 2,050 kilocalories and for women 1,600 kilocalories.

[b]Nonpregnant, nonlactating.

[c]Estimated safe and adequate daily dietary intakes of additional selected vitamins and minerals. Because there is less information on which to base allowances, these figures are provided in the form of ranges of recommended intakes.

[d]Trace elements. Since the toxic levels for many trace elements may be only several times usual intakes, the upper levels for the trace elements given in this table should not be habitually exceeded.

Source: Food and Nutrition Board, National Research Council, *Recommended Dietary Allowances,* 9th ed. (Washington, D.C.: National Academy of Sciences, 1979).

Are Food Additives Safe?

If you do take the time to read the labels on the processed foods you buy, you're bound to notice that they usually list some additives and preservatives. Virtually all processed foods contain one or more of these chemical substances, most of which are synthetically produced.

The law requires manufacturers to test for the safety of food additives, and the Food and Drug Administration (FDA) must approve their use in food. No chemical that is found to be a health hazard may be added to food. But in spite of these regulations, both independent and government studies indicate that some food additives now in use are not as safe as was formerly believed. For example, the safety of nitrites (added to bacon and other smoked meats to preserve freshness and enhance color) is now being investigated. Some additives that were once widely used—such as Carbon Black and Red Dye No. 2—are now banned.[22]

Does Eating "Organic" Foods Help?

When you see the label "organic" on a food such as a bunch of carrots, this *implies* (though it does not really prove) that the food was grown in a specific way: While it was growing, it was not subjected to pesticides, chemical fertilizers, and so on. Instead, the soil was (supposedly) fertilized by such natural substances as manure. Proponents of "organically" grown food believe that it is more healthful than food grown with chemical fertilizers—that is, that it contains more vitamins and minerals.

In reality, however, there is no scientifically documented difference between the nutrient content of organically grown and inorganically grown crops. Plants can only absorb nutrients from the soil in an inorganic form. *All* fertilizers, including natural ones such as manure, have to be broken down into their chemical constituents before the plant can use them.

With regard to the pesticide issue: *Consumer Reports* reported that tests made by various agencies over the years have found little difference between the level of pesticide residue found on "organic" produce in health-food stores and that of similar "nonorganic" produce found in supermarkets.[23]

Runners engage in last-minute "carbohydrate loading" the night before the New York Marathon. (© Gayle Jann)

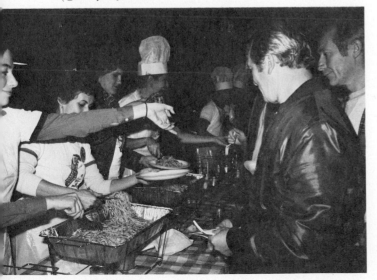

SPECIAL NUTRITIONAL NEEDS

Nutrition and Athletics

Football players who once found enormous hunks of steak on their training tables may today find plates of spaghetti instead. As nutritional knowledge has advanced, it has become clear that if strenuous exercise creates special nutritional needs, the most important need is for more energy, and carbohydrates are the body's best energy source. Athletes do need protein but not in significantly greater proportion than most other people. In general, athletes, like the rest of us, are best off eating a well-balanced Basic Four diet and consuming enough calories and water to replace those that are spent in strenuous activity and perspiration.

One special diet developed in recent years seeks to make the most of carbohydrates as energy foods. In this diet the athlete eats a low-carbohydrate diet for a period of time before an athletic competition and then switches to a very high carbohydrate diet a day or two immediately before the event. This procedure, called "carbohydrate loading," does indeed seem to increase the athlete's energy level, particularly in sports that call for prolonged endurance, such as long-distance running. However, carbohydrate loading may also cause the body to retain more water than usual, which can hamper athletic performance. And worse, some people who have tried carbohydrate loading have experienced cardiac abnormalities and chest pain: This occurs in people who have fasted first, then consumed a high-protein diet prior to the carbohydrate-loading phase. For this reason, it is best not to attempt the procedure of carbohydrate loading without medical supervision.[24]

Vegetarians

Vegetarian diets have long been followed by millions of people acting out of religious convictions: in the East, by some Hindus and Buddhists; in our own society, by Seventh-Day Adventists and other groups. Only recently, however, has vegetarianism become common among Americans.

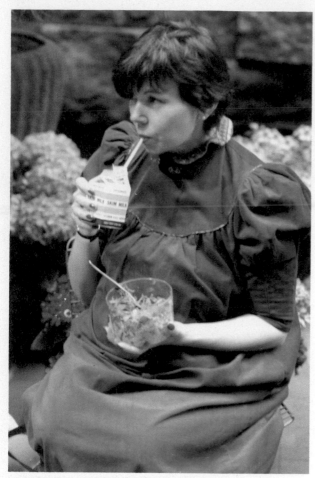

Contrary to once-popular opinion, a woman does not need to "eat for two" when she is pregnant. According to the National Academy of Sciences, a 5-foot, 5-inch woman weighing 130 pounds needs approximately 2,100 calories per day when she is not pregnant or is one to two months pregnant; 2,400 calories when she is three or more months pregnant; and 2,600 to 2,800 while she is breast-feeding. Total weight gain should be from 22 to 27 pounds, most of it during the fifth to ninth month of pregnancy. (© Leonard Speier 1983)

There are several kinds of vegetarians. The two most common are ovolacto vegetarians and vegans. Ovolacto vegetarians eat eggs (ovo-) and dairy products (lacto-) as well as plant foods. Vegans eat plant foods only—no eggs, cheese, or milk.

Although either diet can be quite adequate for health—with the reservations expressed below—it is far easier to obtain the necessary nutrients from the ovolacto diet than from the vegan. As we saw earlier, proteins from eggs and dairy products are complete, and it is a simple matter to substitute an egg or cheese dish for a meat dish. Proteins from plant sources, however, are usually incomplete (that is, they do not contain all the amino acids that the body needs). Therefore the vegan must plan meals that combine incomplete proteins so as to form complete ones. Typically, this means a combination of grains and legumes: rice and beans, bread and peanut butter, corn muffins and pea soup, for example. By selecting foods carefully, the vegan can consume adequate complete protein.

The real problem in the vegan diet is the lack of vitamin B_{12}, which is most often found in animal foods. The vegan *must* consume a source of B_{12} or suffer a deficiency. The non-meat source may be a special form of yeast, soybean milk, or a B_{12} supplement.[25] Besides B_{12}, iron may be a problem for the vegan, since its richest sources are animal foods. The vegan should make a special effort to eat plant foods high in iron (beans, spinach, prunes, tofu) and iron-enriched foods or should take an iron supplement.

DIETARY DEFICIENCIES

In the United States, most nutritional disorders are primarily a result of dietary excesses of several kinds. The American diet is characterized by excesses. On average, we take in too many calories, we eat too much fat, protein, salt, and sugar, and we drink too much alcohol.

Deficiency disorders, less common, are primarily related to low intake of trace minerals. Some people in our society simply do not have enough good food to eat, despite decades of social programs aimed at eradicating hunger. Although public assistance and food stamps have aided many needy people, they have not yet reached every distressed household. It can only be hoped that future social policy will attempt to help these people, in particular children, who cannot provide for their own nutritional needs.

A fairly high percentage of people in our society do not go hungry. Many of us may go without nourishing food, though, as our lives become more hurried. We often skip breakfast and snatch lunch from a fast-food stand. At home, we may substitute low-nutrient, high-calorie snack food or processed food for conventional meals. Fast-food outlets do a huge business selling us hamburgers, french fries, pizza, fried chicken, and soft drinks each year. One-fourth of the $20 billion Americans spend on eating out is spent on fast foods, and it is estimated that by the end of the 1980s, half of all expenditures for food will go to fast-food chains.[26] We may be paying a nutritional price as well. The typical fast-food meal is high in calories, fat, and salt, and low in fiber, iron, vitamin A, and several other trace nutrients.[27]

A similar problem is the widespread acceptance of processed and fabricated foods. Once again, these are often high in fat, calories, and salt (and often sugar as well). Many have been stripped of important nutrients in processing. Even "enriched" foods may have deficits. Although white bread, for example, may be enriched with a number of nutrients that were removed when the flour was milled, it still is not as nutritious as a whole-wheat loaf. The whole-wheat kernel may contain trace nutrients not restored to the loaf by "enrichment." And of course, the "enrichment" does not return the fiber that was present in the natural whole-wheat kernel.

Neither fast foods nor processed foods are threats to our health if we consume them in moderation, but we should not rely on them as a steady diet.

Those who eat fast foods or processed foods frequently should make sure that their other meals include whole grains and a variety of fresh fruits and vegetables.

Unacceptably large numbers of Americans still suffer from "silent undernutrition," in spite of food stamps and other programs. Dietary deficiencies, especially lack of protein, are particularly harmful to growing children. (© Michael O'Brien/Archive Pictures)

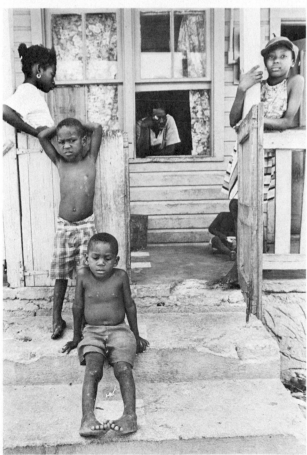

HEALTHY NUTRITION

The selection of an adequate, balanced diet is a fundamental requirement of lifelong good health. As we can see from our analysis of the excesses of the average American diet, many of us are not eating as well as we might. In 1977 a government body—the Senate Select Committee on Nutrition and Human Needs—completed an intensive study of the American diet by issuing *Dietary Goals for the United States.*[28] These guidelines were designed to reduce current nutritional knowledge to a few basic principles that the public could follow as they made dietary choices (see Table 13.5). Of course, any attempt to issue rules, especially in a field with as many conflicting claims as nutrition, was bound to stir up controversy. But although various groups and individuals have disputed one or more of the guidelines, they remain a generally reliable guide to healthful diet, given American eating habits. A similar government study, sponsored by the U.S. Departments of Agriculture and Health and Human Services, issued quite similar dietary guidelines in 1979, adding a recommendation that alcohol, if consumed at all, be taken in moderation—not more than one or two drinks a day.[29]

TABLE 13.5 · Dietary Guidelines for Americans

1. To avoid overweight, consume only as much energy (calories) as is expended; if overweight, decrease energy intake and increase energy expenditure.
2. Increase the consumption of complex carbohydrates and "naturally occurring" sugars from about 28 percent to about 48 percent of energy intake.
3. Reduce the consumption of refined and other processed sugars by about 45 percent to account for about 10 percent of total energy intake.
4. Reduce overall fat consumption from approximately 40 percent to about 30 percent of energy intake.
5. Reduce saturated fat consumption to account for about 10 percent of total energy intake and balance that with polyunsaturated and monounsaturated fats, which should account for about 10 percent of energy intake each.
6. Reduce cholesterol consumption to about 300 mg per day.
7. Limit the intake of sodium by reducing the intake of salt (sodium chloride) to about 5 g per day (2 g sodium).

Source: U.S. Senate, Select Committee on Nutrition and Human Needs, *Dietary Goals for the United States,* 2nd ed. (Washington, D.C.: U.S. Government Printing Office, 1977).

Following the dietary guidelines will not guarantee good health. Even the healthiest diet will not keep some people from developing heart disease, cancer, or other disorders. The dietary guidelines are also only part of the story: Their recommendations must always be used in conjunction with the RDAs and with a knowledge of individual differences. Nevertheless, there is no doubt that reducing the amount of fat, sugar, salt, and total calories in the American diet is a healthy step. For the individual this probably means forming new eating habits. Although it may be difficult to learn to choose a salad plate instead of a hamburger and fries, or an apple or orange instead of a piece of chocolate cake, good nutrition is a worthwhile goal. In the end, such choices should pay off in better health.

MAKING HEALTH DECISIONS

Making Decisions About Your Diet

If you're going to change your behavior, you'll need three things. First, you'll need *knowledge* about nutritionally sound eating practices. This chapter has given you the basics; the books listed in the Recommended Readings for this chapter can supply more detailed information. Second, you'll need *skills:* you'll need to be able to choose and combine the right foods for good nutrition. But most of all, you'll need to *believe* that nutrition is tremendously important for your health.

Let's see what you believe about nutrition. Then, we'll look at the factors in your environment that may affect whether you will be able to change your nutrition pattern.

SA = strongly agree, A = agree, U = undecided, D = disagree, SD = strongly disagree

Do You Believe That:	SA	A	U	D	SD
1. diet contributes to diseases such as heart disease, cancer, diabetes, and obesity?	____	____	____	____	____
2. diet can affect your energy levels?	____	____	____	____	____
3. diet can enhance or detract from your overall health status?	____	____	____	____	____

Do You Believe That:	SA	A	U	D	SD
4. improving your diet will benefit your health and that you'll feel better?	_____	_____	_____	_____	_____
5. changing your diet will reduce your chance of developing heart disease, cancer, etc.?	_____	_____	_____	_____	_____
6. changing your diet is compatible with your lifestyle?	_____	_____	_____	_____	_____
7. changing your diet is compatible with what your friends and peers believe to be good?	_____	_____	_____	_____	_____
8. changing your diet is compatible with whatever deeply rooted cultural patterns of eating you may have?	_____	_____	_____	_____	_____

Interpretation: SA = 5, A = 4, U = 3, D = 2, SD = 1. Compute your score. Add all the numbers you've checked.

A score of 30–40 means that you have a great chance for success in changing your eating habits. You believe that nutrition plays a key role in health. Your values and beliefs support a change.

A score of 20–29 means that while you do hold some attitudes and values that will support dietary habit changes, you're probably not highly motivated to make the changes.

A score of 5–19 may mean either that your knowledge of nutrition is poor or that you do not see yourself as particularly vulnerable to the diet-related diseases. The likelihood of your attempting to change eating habits, much less succeeding at them, is remote.

WILL YOU BE ABLE TO CHANGE YOUR BEHAVIOR?

When you try to improve eating habits, you are in fact changing a behavior. The chance for successful behavior changes depends on *enabling* and *reinforcing factors.* Let's look at these.

	YES	NO	UNSURE
1. Are you in a situation where you can make choices regarding food purchase and preparation?	_____	_____	_____
2. Do you have the ability to pay for nutritious foods?	_____	_____	_____
3. Are you willing to devote the necessary time preparing nutritious meals, and/or eating nutritious meals in restaurants or at home rather than fast-food?	_____	_____	_____
4. Will your family and friends support and approve your changed food choices?	_____	_____	_____
5. Is there another person—a friend or family member—who would also like to change his or her eating habits? (This should be someone who would like to work with you on good nutrition.)	_____	_____	_____
6. Do you have the cooking and food preparation skills to make nutritious meals?	_____	_____	_____

Interpretation:

If you checked yes five or six times you are well on your way to permanent changes in your eating habits. The outlook is especially good if you checked item 4. Supportive feedback from other people is an essential ingredient to behavior change.

If you checked yes three or four times you can successfully change your eating habits, but you'd probably be wise to incorporate some personal rewards for achieving your dietary habit goals. (For example, if you go for 2 weeks without drinking a Coke, reward yourself with a new blouse or shirt.) Also, it's possible to change your answer from no to yes on some of the questions by developing skills or through other changes.

If you checked one or two yeses, it is unlikely you have the factors you would need to change your eating habits and to maintain them once you've changed them.

MAKING YOUR PLAN

Will you change your dietary habits? How? What do you do first? People most frequently make nutritional changes in the following sequence:

1. First, try to eliminate caffeine, nicotine, and alcohol.
2. Next, see if you can reduce your consumption of red meat.
3. Then try to increase your intake of fresh produce (and fiber).
4. Last, reduce refined carbohydrates (ice cream, pastries, soft drinks).

But there's no hard-and-fast rule. Some people start with step 4, some with step 3—they start eating more salads because salads taste good. So approach your changes in whatever way seems best for you.

SUMMARY

1. Nutrition is the science of food, its use within the body, and its relationship to good health. Nutrition includes the study of the major food components and the nutrients they are made of.

2. Food fuels all the cells of the body. Both too much and too little food contribute to poor health.

3. All foods are made of chemical compounds. The process of digestion breaks down these compounds into simpler forms that are reassembled into chemicals that the body can use directly.

4. The four basic groups of chemicals in foods are proteins, carbohydrates, fat, and vitamins and minerals.

5. Protein is essential for body growth and repair. Special proteins called nucleic acids transmit hereditary characteristics. Meat, eggs, and dairy products contain complete proteins. Plant proteins are usually incomplete. To make complete proteins, plant foods can be combined with one another or with animal proteins.

6. Carbohydrates include sugars and starches. They contribute about 50 percent of the body's energy needs and are the most economical energy source. Carbohydrates are needed for fat metabolism. Sugar is associated with obesity, tooth decay, diabetes, and other disorders.

7. Fats provide energy, give flavor to foods, and insulate and cushion the body. Stored fats are the greatest nutritional reservoir in the body. Depending on its hydrogen component, a fat may be either saturated or unsaturated. Saturated fats tend to raise the level of cholesterol in the blood, which increases the risk of heart disease.

8. Vitamins are necessary for triggering body functions and are needed in only trace amounts. Minerals are inorganic elements that help form tissues and various chemical substances in the body. Many people consume too little iron and too much sodium for good health.

9. Water has no nutritional value but is nevertheless one of the most important components of the diet because it is essential for digestion, transportation of wastes, and bodily structure. Fiber, an-

other nonnutritive substance, is also necessary for digestion.

10. A calorie is not a nutrient, but a unit of measurement of the energy value of food.

11. The simplest way to plan a balanced diet is to select enough foods every day from each of the Basic Four food groups: the meat group, which includes poultry, fish, eggs, and legumes as well as red meats; milk and milk products; fruit and vegetables; and breads and cereals (whole-grain and enriched).

12. The label on processed or packaged food must conform to certain regulations. The label shows what percentage of daily nutrition requirements are in each serving of the product.

13. Additives and preservatives are often added to processed foods. Fairly strict laws regulate the food industry, but some scientists question the safety of many additives and preservatives currently in use.

14. Research has shown that organically grown fruits and vegetables have no more nutrients and no less pesticide residue than other produce.

15. Among those with special nutritional needs are athletes, who must be careful to get the right amounts of calories, water, and carbohydrates; and vegetarians, who must plan their diets to ensure adequate intake of complete proteins and vitamin B_{12}.

16. Chronic nutritional diseases may be associated either with dietary deficiencies (poverty-related undernutrition, reliance on fast foods and processed convenience foods) or with dietary excesses (too much fat, sugar, salt, and alcohol). An adequate, balanced diet is essential to good health and contributes to the prevention of diseases, including cancer.

GLOSSARY

carbohydrates   One of the four basic components of food, found in the form of sugars and starches in bread, potatoes, most fruits and vegetables, and other foods. Carbohydrates are the body's source of ready energy.

cholesterol   A fatlike substance that is found in all foods from animal sources and is also manufactured by the human body.

complete protein   Protein that includes all eight of the essential amino acids.

diabetes mellitus   A chronic illness characterized by abnormal processing of carbohydrates as a result of the body's inability to produce enough insulin (**juvenile-onset diabetes**) or to use insulin properly (**adult-onset diabetes**).

enrichment   The restoring to food of specific nutrients that were lost in processing or the addition of nutrients that were not originally present in a food.

fats (lipids)   One of the four basic components of food, found in oils, meats, and other foods. Fats are essential as a source of energy, for insulation and protection of the body, and for many body processes (such as hormone synthesis and blood clotting).

fat-soluble vitamins   One of the two major types of vitamins, consisting of vitamins A, D, E, and K. Excess consumption of these vitamins is dangerous because surplus amounts cannot be excreted, but rather are stored in fatty tissue, where they may build to toxic levels. Compare **water-soluble vitamins.**

glucose   A type of sugar.

glycogen   The form in which glucose is stored in the liver and muscles; it is released into the bloodstream when blood sugar levels fall too low.

hydrogenation   The process of changing a liquid fat to a solid by bubbling hydrogen gas through it.

hypoglycemia   Low blood sugar. Temporary low blood sugar is a normal condition; the disease hypoglycemia is a rare condition caused by malfunctioning of the pancreas.

incomplete protein   Protein that lacks one or more of the eight essential amino acids.

insulin   A substance produced by the body that enables it to take sugar (in the form of glucose) from the bloodstream and use it for energy.

minerals   With vitamins, one of the four basic components of food, consisting of inorganic elements that humans need in trace amounts daily to help form tissues and various chemical substances in the body.

nutrition   The science of food, its use within the body, and its relationship to good health.

plaque   Fatty deposits, made up largely of cholesterol, that can build up on the walls of blood vessels, narrowing them and eventually perhaps closing them completely.

protein   One of the four basic components of food, consisting of amino acids and found in meat, eggs, dairy products, and some other foods. Protein is necessary for growth and repair of the body.

saturated fat   A fat that has all the hydrogen atoms it is capable of holding; usually solid at room temperature.

simple sugars   Chemicals that are an intermediate step between carbohydrates and glucose.

starches   A group of chemicals that are one of the two major types of carbohydrates. See **sugars.**

sugars   A group of chemicals that are one of the two major types of carbohydrates. See **starches.**

triglycerides   One of a number of fatty acids into which excess glucose is converted and stored in the body's fat tissue.

unsaturated fat   A fat that is capable of holding more hydrogen atoms than it does; usually liquid at room temperature.

vitamins   With minerals, one of the four major components of food, needed in very small amounts but essential for triggering vital bodily functions.

water-soluble vitamins   One of the two major types of vitamins, consisting of vitamin C and the B-complex vitamins. Because these vitamins are soluble in water, any excess amount can be excreted. Compare **fat-soluble vitamins.**

NOTES

1. M. Winick, *Nutrition in Health and Disease* (New York: Wiley, 1980).

2. W. L. Pines and N. Glick, "The Saccharin Ban," *FDA Consumer* 11, no. 4 (1977): 10; "NAS (National Academy of Sciences) Warns Against Saccharin," *CNI Weekly Report,* November 9, 1978, p. 1; I. I. Kessler and J. P. Clark, "Saccharin, Cyclamate, and Human Bladder Cancer," *Journal of the American Medical Association* 240, no. 4 (1978): 349.

3. Food and Nutrition Board, National Research Council, *Recommended Dietary Allowances,* 9th ed. (Washington, D.C.: National Academy of Sciences, 1979).

4. Ibid.

5. T. S. Danowski, "Sugar and Disease," *American Pharmacy* 20, no. 1 (January 1980): 49–51.

6. See ibid.

7. W. M. Bortz, "The Pathogenesis of Hypercholesterolemia," *Annals of Internal Medicine* 80 (1974): 738.

8. Leon Abrams, "Anthropological Research Reveals Human Dietary Requirements for Optimum Health," *Journal of Applied Nutrition* 34, no. 1 (1982): 38–45.

9. Woodrow Monte, "Fiber: Its Nutritional Impact," *Journal of Applied Nutrition* 33, no. 1 (Spring 1981): 63–103.

10. Ibid.

11. A. S. Truswell, "Diet and Plasma Lipids: A Reappraisal," *American Journal of Clinical Nutrition* 31 (1978): 977.

12. U.S. Senate, Select Committee on Nutrition and Human Needs, *Dietary Goals for the United States,* 2nd ed., Committee Report, 1977 (Washington, D.C.: U.S. Government Printing Office, 1977).

13. H. Seneker, "Body-Building at Hoffman-LaRoche," *Forbes* 123, no. 3 (February 1979): 92–94.

14. Food and Nutrition Board, National Academy of Sciences–National Research Council Committee on Nutritional Misinformation, "Hazards of Overuse of Vitamin D," *Nutrition Reviews* 33 (1975): 61–62.

15. Linus Pauling, *Vitamin C and the Common Cold* (San Francisco: Freeman, 1970).

16. George A. Bray, "Dietary Guidelines: The Shape of Things to Come," *Journal of Nutrition Education* 12, no. 2, Supp. 1 (1980).

17. Louis Tobian, "Dietary Salt (Sodium) and Hypertension," *American Journal of Clinical Nutrition* 32, Supplement (December 1979): 2659–2662.

18. Patricia A. Kreutler, *Nutrition in Perspective* (Englewood Cliffs, N.J.: Prentice-Hall, 1980).

19. D. M. Hegsted, "Food and Fiber: Evidence from Experimental Animals," *Nutrition Reviews* 35 (1977): 45.

20. Food and Nutrition Board, *Recommended Dietary Allowances.*

21. Special Report, "The Nutritive Quality of Processed Foods: General Policies for Nutrient Additions," *Nutrition Reviews* 40, no. 3 (March 1982): 93–96.

22. E. M. Foster, "How Safe Are Our Foods?" *Nutrition Reviews* Supplement (January 1982): 30–34.

23. "It's Natural! It's Organic! Or Is It?" *Consumer Reports* 45, no. 7 (July 1980): 413.

24. P. O. Astrand and K. Rodahl, *Textbook of Work Physiology*, 2nd ed. (New York: McGraw-Hill, 1977).

25. "Position Paper on the Vegetarian Approach to Eating," *Journal of the American Dietetic Association* 77 (July 1980): 66.

26. *Nation's Restaurant News*, reported in Virginia De Moss, "The Good, the Bad, and the Edible," *Runner's World*, June 1980, p. 44.

27. Kreutler, *Nutrition in Perspective*, pp. 442–443.

28. U.S. Senate, Select Committee on Nutrition and Human Needs, *Dietary Goals for the United States*.

29. "Dietary Guidelines for Americans," *Nutrition Today* 15, no. 2 (March–April 1980): 14–18.

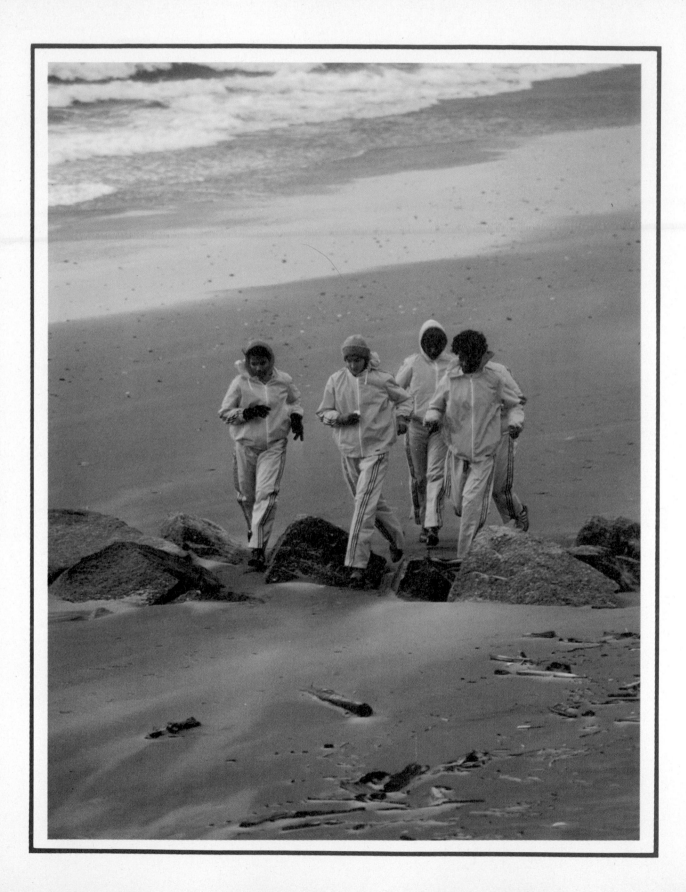

CHAPTER 14

Weight Management

Fat. Few of us want it, but millions of us have too much of it, and we'll do almost anything to get rid of it. We buy diet books and diet foods. We visit weight-loss centers and diet doctors. Every year, Americans spend $10 billion trying to take off fat.[1]

Why are we so obsessed with weight? In other times and in other cultures, a plump body was a social asset, a sign of prosperity and well-being. But today, thin is in. Style dictates that to be attractive, we must be slim. And there is another reason that compels many Americans to lose weight. It is now well known that serious overweight is linked with a number of potentially life-threatening health problems; in fact, being severely overweight is clearly associated with premature death.

The statistics on obesity and disease are fairly frightening. Some experts indicate that from 20 to 50 percent of adult Americans are overweight; according to the National Center for Health Statistics, both men and women in most age and height categories are heavier than they were in the 1960s.[2] And obesity is associated with at least twenty-six known medical conditions. These conditions could account collectively for 15 to 20 percent of the mortality rate in this country.[3]

One of the most crucial ways serious overweight can affect an individual's health is by increasing his or her risk of heart disease (discussed in Chapter 12). One expert has stated that on the average, for every 10 percent increase in weight, there is about a 30 percent increase in coronary heart disease.[4] In the Framingham study, a classic study of one group of people over a period of years, coronary mortality rates—especially rates of sudden death—were higher in obese people.[5]

Obesity itself does not directly cause heart disease. Rather, it works with other risk factors in setting up the preconditions for cardiovascular illness. Overweight people tend to have higher levels of blood fats and to exercise less—both of which are risk factors for heart disease.[6] They are also more susceptible to hypertension (high blood pressure).[7]

Even if a seriously overweight person is lucky enough not to develop heart trouble, he or she risks other health complications. Again, we're talking not so much about the direct effects of overweight as about the way it combines with other factors to create risk. If the overweight person develops hypertension, this in turn increases his or her chances of suffering a stroke or developing kidney disease. If he or she develops diabetes—as many seriously overweight people do—this increases the chances of suffering blindness, heart attack, stroke, or atherosclerosis. Diabetes, a disease in which the body fails to use sugar properly, is itself a major cause of death.

Health considerations and the bias of our culture both lead us to want to take off our extra pounds and keep them off. But controlling our weight is not always as simple as it sounds. First we have to determine the ideal weight for our own bodies—and this depends on our height, how muscular we are, and other individual characteristics. Next we have to understand *why* we are overweight. And then we have to look at what researchers have learned lately about the best and safest ways of taking off our excess poundage.

These are some of the topics we're going to take up in this chapter. We're also going to look at problems of *underweight,* and at the eating disorders anorexia nervosa and bulimia.

BODY COMPOSITION, OVERWEIGHT, AND OBESITY

In 1982 millions of American women helped to make actress Jane Fonda a best-selling author. *Jane Fonda's Workout Book* does not promise to transform the reader into a Fonda look-alike, but many women hope that following Ms. Fonda's advice will yield miracles.[8] At last, they think, they will look like an American model or actress—slim-hipped and long-legged. For many women, though, this look is simply not possible. Nor is it possible for the slenderly built man to have the physique of a weightlifter—or for the stocky man to be as lithe as Fred Astaire. People are made in an almost infinite variety of shapes and sizes; each has his or her own individual body composition.

Body Composition

Our bodies are made up of two kinds of tissue: lean, or nonfat, tissues—including muscle, bone, cartilage, connective tissue, skin, nerves, and the internal organs—and fat tissue. Our body composition is the relationship, or ratio, between lean and fat tissue in our body.

Let's look at both types of tissue in more detail.

FAT TISSUE

Everyone *must* have some fat tissue in order to stay alive. There are two kinds of fat tissue: essential fat and storage fat (also known as excess fat).

ESSENTIAL FAT Essential fat—usually about 3 percent of body weight for men and 12 percent for women—is used up and created anew constantly, day after day, in the course of the body's normal physiological functioning. It forms part of the chain of chemical reactions by which we store nutrients from our food and burn them up (metabolize them) to get energy.[9] Essential fat is stored in the bone marrow; in the spinal cord and the brain; and in organs such as the heart, lungs, liver, spleen, kidneys, and intestines.

STORAGE FAT Storage fat is deposited beneath the skin; layers of it also surround the various internal organs, to protect them from injury. Storage fat is sometimes called "excess fat," but that doesn't mean we don't need it. We all must have *some* "excess fat." Generally, men should have about 12 percent and women 15 percent of their body weight in excess fat.[10] (The higher percentage of fat in women is due to an additional layer of fat in female skin, plus fat deposits in the breasts, hips, thighs, and lower abdomen.)

HOW MUCH FAT IS HEALTHY? When we add up the two kinds of fat, "essential" fat and "storage" (or "excess") fat, we get the following: In adult men, no more than 16 to 19 percent of total body weight should be fat. In women, the proportion should not be higher than 22 to 25 percent.[11] Obviously, we'd be better off with less fat than this.

LEAN TISSUE: THE ROLE OF MUSCLE

So far, we've divided body tissue up into two categories, fat and lean. Now let's look more closely at that "lean" category. As we mentioned above, lean, or nonfat, tissue includes a number of different kinds of tissue—bone, cartilage, connective tissue, skin, nerves, internal organs, and *muscle.* Muscle is the crucial variable. If you have a lot of it, you're going to weigh more, even if you're not particularly fat. Shifts in the body's ratio of fat *and* muscle can cause our weight to vary from one week or month to the next. We can carry additional weight in the form of extra flab at the waistline or of well-toned muscle throughout the body.

When scientists look at body composition, they are interested in three variables: **mesomorphy,** or degree of muscularity; **ectomorphy,** or degree of "linearity" or "long-bonedness"; and **endomorphy,** or degree of fatness. Athletes usually have a relatively high proportion of muscle to other types of tissue. In scientific language, they are relatively *mesomorphic* (muscular). One athlete (perhaps a professional basketball player) may be quite long-boned as well; another athlete (perhaps a soccer player) may be relatively short-boned or stocky. But they both have quite a lot of muscle tissue relative to the amount of storage fat on their frames.

You yourself may be relatively long-boned or relatively stocky; this is part of your genetic heritage, and it can't be changed. Yet, by exercise, you *can* alter your overall body composition. If you begin to exercise regularly, the ratio of fat to lean tissue in your body will begin to change.[12] You will become less fat and more lean. Ironically, this may mean that your *total* weight stays the same—or possibly even increases—since lean muscle tissue weighs more than fat. But despite this, your vigorous exercise will have a positive effect on your body: Lean muscle tissue is what your body needs to function efficiently and to look its best.

ASSESSING BODY COMPOSITION

How can you determine the proportion of fat tissue in your body? One do-it-yourself method is the *mirror test*, which we all use from time to time: simply looking at yourself nude in a full-length mirror. "If you *look* fat," says nutritionist Jean Mayer, "you probably *are* fat." The mirror test is not objective, however; it is possible to make significant errors in judging one's own proportion of fat tissue.

A more objective do-it-yourself method is the *pinch test.* With your thumb and forefinger, grasp as much skin as you can at your waistline two to three inches to one side of the navel. If the skinfold is more than an inch thick, you are probably fat. Another fairly good method for men is the *abdominal circumference test.* If the circumference of your abdomen exceeds the circumference of your chest, you are probably obese.

Scientists have several more precise methods of assessing a person's actual proportion of lean and fat tissue. In the **densimetric method**, a person is weighed first in air and then weighed again while totally submerged in water, to find out his or her specific gravity, or overall density relative to water. Lean tissue is heavier than water, while fat tissue is lighter than water; thus, scientists can calculate, using appropriate formulas, the total amount of fat tissue in the body. This method, if used with careful attention to precise measurement, can be quite reliable.

Another fairly accurate method, more convenient than immersing the subject in a tank of water, involves taking **anthropometric measurements**. Using calipers (instruments rather like large tweezers), scientists measure the diameters of various parts of the body, such as the front of the

thigh, the shoulder blade, the abdomen, the back of the calf, and the triceps (bottom of the upper arm). From these data, they can compute the proportion of fat in the body, following an accepted formula. Again, the measurements must be extremely precise for this method to produce reliable results.

How Much Should You Weigh?

No two people are exactly alike. A 5-foot, 3-inch woman of delicate build, without a lot of muscle, should weigh about 110 pounds; a stockier, more muscular woman of that height, perhaps around 125 pounds. People also vary greatly in their activity level, their metabolism, and their cultural and religious background—so setting weight "standards" is risky.

As a point of departure, however, physicians often refer to a set of tables that are published by life-insurance companies, based on statistics on the average weights of men and women of different heights and body types. Though these tables indicate averages, they also imply that the given weights are *approximately* the ideal weights for health. In fact, they were devised as a way of identifying high-risk insurance customers: People who are seriously obese are known to die at a younger age, on the average, than people of normal weight.

Debate arose in 1983 when the Metropolitan Life Insurance Company issued revised tables that seemed to suggest that some Americans—shorter people, in particular—could safely carry slightly more weight than the company's statistics had indicated in the past (see Table 14.1). Some observers feared that the public would interpret the new tables as a "green light" to gain weight. But company spokesmen emphasized that it was still better to be lean than fat.

Generally, if your weight varies less than 10 percent—either more or less—from the weight the insurance-company tables recommend for your sex, height, and body frame, it is of no health significance. A weight 15 percent above that recommended in the table is usually considered **overweight;** 20 to 30 percent above the recom-

TABLE 14.1 · Ideal Weights for Men and Women, by Height and Size of Frame
(in indoor clothing and shoes; subtract 5 pounds for clothing and 1 inch for shoe heels)

	Men				Women		
HEIGHT	SMALL FRAME	MEDIUM FRAME	LARGE FRAME	HEIGHT	SMALL FRAME	MEDIUM FRAME	LARGE FRAME
5'2"	128–134	131–141	138–150	4'10"	102–111	109–121	118–131
5'3"	130–136	133–143	140–153	4'11"	103–113	111–123	120–134
5'4"	132–138	135–145	142–156	5'	104–115	113–126	122–137
5'5"	134–140	137–148	144–160	5'1"	106–118	115–129	125–140
5'6"	136–142	139–151	146–164	5'2"	108–121	118–132	128–143
5'7"	138–145	142–154	149–168	5'3"	111–124	121–135	131–147
5'8"	140–148	145–157	152–172	5'4"	114–127	124–138	134–151
5'9"	142–151	148–160	155–176	5'5"	117–130	127–141	137–155
5'10"	144–154	151–163	158–180	5'6"	120–133	130–144	140–159
5'11"	146–157	154–166	161–184	5'7"	123–136	133–147	143–163
6'	149–160	157–170	164–188	5'8"	126–139	136–150	146–167
6'1"	152–164	160–174	168–192	5'9"	129–142	139–153	149–170
6'2"	155–168	164–178	172–197	5'10"	132–145	142–156	152–173
6'3"	158–172	167–182	176–202	5'11"	135–148	145–159	155–176
6'4"	162–176	171–187	181–207	6'	138–151	148–162	158–179

Source: Metropolitan Life Insurance Company.

mended value may be considered **obesity;** and weight that is 30 percent or more above the recommended value almost always indicates obesity.[13] Among Americans, from 20 to 50 percent of adults are overweight; 10 percent of non-aged adults are moderately overweight; and 12 percent are severely obese.[14]

WHAT CAUSES OVERWEIGHT AND OBESITY?

Maintaining a constant weight involves a number of factors. One is fairly straightforward: the number of calories we take in relative to the number we burn for energy. If we take in only as many calories as we burn up, we don't get fatter. Most of us have behavior patterns that enable us to maintain this balance fairly automatically. If we are living a rather sedentary life, studying a lot or holding down an office job, we may not feel like eating large amounts of food. If we exercise a little more vigorously than usual, however, we may compensate by eating a little more—we may allow ourselves an extra plate of spaghetti or slice of cake.

Suppose we exceed that one extra plate of spaghetti, however, and start to eat much more than we need to maintain this balance. Where do the excess calories go? They get stored in our bodies in special cells known as *fat cells.* When we are lean, we carry many of these cells on our bodies in an "unfilled" or shrunken state. When we start eating a lot of extra desserts—without jogging a lot of extra miles to compensate—we start to store fat in our fat cells. For every excess 3,500 calories, the average person gains one pound of fat.[15] Result: a slight tendency to pudginess, which may become overweight or even true obesity if we don't start to control our eating behavior and exercise habits.

Scientists don't fully understand all the mechanisms that come into play as an individual starts to become overweight and that encourage the process to continue. Excess calorie intake, some researchers think, is only one of the conditions involved.[16] Let's take a look at some of the other factors.

Genetic Factors

We take for granted that hair and eye color, facial features, and height are inherited traits. No one is surprised when a 6-foot, 2-inch father has a taller than average son. Similarly, overweight parents tend to have overweight children: Evidence suggests that the genes we inherit influence our weight just as they influence our other physical traits. In one study, when both parents were of normal weight, only 9 percent of children were obese. When one parent was obese, however, 40 percent of the children were obese too. And when *both* parents were obese, the proportion of obese children rose to *80 percent.*[17] This study strongly suggests that genes play a significant role in determining weight.

Lack of Physical Activity

It's hard to tell whether obesity causes lack of exercise, or lack of exercise causes obesity, but the two patterns are often seen together. One study of twenty-eight obese and twenty-eight normal-weight girls showed that the obese girls actually ate *less* than the normal girls—but also exercised strikingly less. Motion-picture studies of obese and nonobese children on school playgrounds and adults in factories also showed that the obese exercised much less, both in amount and intensity.[18]

Why is exercise so important in this context? Obviously, exercise means that the individual is working hard and using up a lot of energy. But that's not the whole story. Interestingly enough, an individual's metabolic rate (the rate at which energy is used up) stays up even after the workout is over—for at least six hours after exercise. If you exercise daily, you can lose four or five pounds a year due to this effect alone—over and above the weight loss that will result from your expenditure of energy while exercising.[19]

Changes in Metabolic Rates with Age

How many people have parents who weigh what they did at age twenty-five? Most, probably, have gained a few pounds each year. "Between the ages of 28 and 42 years . . . the average adult tends to gain 1 to 5 pounds per year and averages 15 pounds overweight by middle age."[20]

Research studies help to explain why gaining weight in middle age is such a common problem. As you age, especially if you don't remain physically active, your metabolism (the rate at which

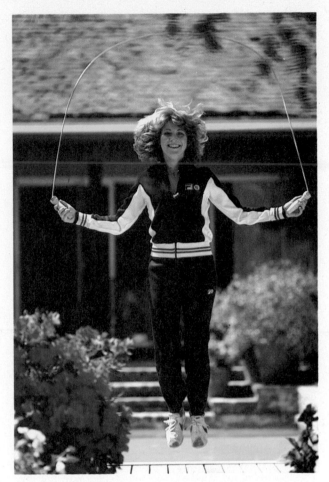

Regular exercise is essential to successful weight management. (©Douglas Kirkland/Contact/Woodfin Camp & Assoc.)

you burn up calories) may slow down. Thus, your body's energy level decreases: it may decrease 3 percent, on the average, from age twenty-two to thirty-five, and correspondingly into the middle and older years.[21]

People age at different rates, and their metabolisms may or may not change a great deal, depending on the person; but a decrease in caloric needs *is* common as people get older.

Unhealthy Eating Habits

"Have a cookie," says the parent to the crying child. "Eat your vegetables if you want dessert." Food can be a great comforter, a special treat.

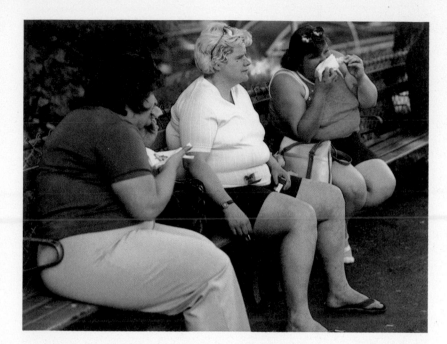

Unhealthy eating habits, often developed in childhood, are a major factor in overweight for many people.   (©Dan McCoy/Rainbow)

Such uses of food do not, by themselves, lead to weight problems. If they did, most of us would be seriously overweight. Many people eat something they especially like when they are feeling low. One double-fudge brownie eaten for consolation every now and then does not lead to obesity.

The trouble comes when eating takes over as the primary means of coping with tensions and frustrations. Some people do not stop at one brownie. They eat three or four. And obesity itself may become a defense. People who find close personal relationships threatening, for example, may use their obesity as a way of avoiding such intimate ties with other people. Extreme overweight may also lead to a very poor self-image. It is easy to see how the psychological aspects of obesity can lock a person into a cycle of overeating that is very difficult to break.

Families can have eating traditions that make it harder for family members to control their weight. Children raised by parents who eat double portions of high-calorie foods may be encouraged to eat more than they really need. Second helpings may flatter the cook, but they may also lead to a lifelong weight problem.

It is risky to generalize, though, about the social and psychological aspects of obesity. The explanation for one person's weight problem may have no bearing at all on another's.

Fat Cells: Are Obese People's Bodies Different?

One of the most hotly debated questions in the area of weight control is whether an obese person's body processes food in a way that is fundamentally different from the way a nonobese person's body does. One theory holds that many obese people have more fat cells in their body—two or even three times as many as people of normal weight—and thus more potential "storage space" for fat.[22] Once an obese person develops an overabundance of fat cells, this theory holds, these cells seem to be there for life. Even if the person loses a good deal of weight, he or she still has all those fat cells, carried on the body in an unfilled or shrunken state. The body may be ready to put weight right back on again in large amounts if the individual is not careful.

Scientists are not sure when most fat cells develop in an individual's life. This means that a person's *potential* capacity for getting fat as an adult may depend on what has happened during his or her early years. At this point, however, scientists don't know whether people can control what happens during those early years, or whether fat-cell development is simply part of the individual child's unchangeable genetic makeup. For example, can parents help cut down on the growth of fat cells in their child by feeding him or her less food? At this point there is no evidence to tell us the answer.

The Setpoint Theory

Have you ever had the experience of going on a diet, losing a few pounds in a week or two, then hitting a plateau at which your weight seems determined to stay no matter *how* little you eat? If so, you have a lot of company: This experience is common. A new theory has suggested an explanation for this phenomenon. It is known as the "setpoint theory," and its basic idea is that each of us has a given weight range known as the **setpoint** that is natural to our bodies.[23]

According to the setpoint theory, some of us tend to stay thin and others to stay fat regardless of what we eat. Those of us who have a high setpoint are going to have problems conforming to our culture's ideal of slenderness: Our bodies simply "want" us to be fat. The setpoint theorists argue that our bodies are able to change their metabolic rate to keep our weight at the setpoint. Our bodies react to a strict diet as if preparing for a prolonged famine—hoarding our fat reserves to keep us from starving to death. Suppose, for example, that a person who happens to have a high setpoint decides to try to lose weight by stringent dieting. The setpoint theorists hypothesize that this person's brain will "sense" what is happening via a feedback system that operates between the hypothalamus in the brain and fat cells throughout the body. The body will respond by slowing its metabolism—burning food more slowly—to keep weight stable.

If the setpoint theory is correct, dieting will not work as a weight-control strategy over the long run: No matter how hard you try, your body will defeat you. Yet, although there is some evidence for the setpoint theory, there are also many examples of people who have managed to sustain significant weight loss by working at it very carefully through weight-loss programs such as Weight Watchers. So perhaps the setpoint is not the only factor that determines weight in everyone. And even if the setpoint theory is ultimately confirmed, it doesn't mean that if you're fat you must stay that way. There *are* ways to lower your setpoint. The safest way is by increasing physical activity, which seems to raise the overall metabolic rate. Once again, exercise seems to be the key to permanent weight loss.[24]

UNDESIRABLE METHODS OF WEIGHT CONTROL

Millions of Americans are on unsupervised weight-loss programs—following this diet expert or that, eating lots of pineapple, grapefruit, or celery, or perhaps trying diet pills or even diet candies.

Fad diets are often promoted by books with catchy titles—*Diet Revolution, Quick Weight Loss, Live Longer Diet, The Beverly Hills Diet, The Dolly Parton Diet, The I Love New York Diet, The Zen Macrobiotic Diet, The Last Chance Diet*—that are ballyhooed by news stories, advertisements, magazine articles, and authors' appearances on television and radio talk shows. (Theodore Berland's book *Consumers' Guide: Rating the Diets* [New York: Signet, 1983] is a good resource for anyone who wants the facts on diets.)

These books offer every conceivable means of juggling food intake. Many fad diets are wildly unbalanced. They may be high in fat and low in carbohydrates, or high in protein (and fat) plus plenty of water, or low in protein and fat and high in carbohydrates.

One recent diet aid claimed to block the digestion of starch and the absorption of starch calories. If you swallowed enough "starch blocker" pills, the manufacturers claimed, you could eat all the pasta, potatoes, and bread you wanted. The starch blocker fad caught on quickly but was soon quelled by the Food and Drug Administration. Many of the pills' users complained that they developed stomach maladies, including vomiting and diarrhea.[25]

Many fad diets may work over the short term, but few if any produce long-term weight loss. Worse, they can be dangerous. Concern about this widespread dieting phenomenon has prompted the American College of Sports Medicine (ACSM) to issue a position paper titled "Proper and Improper Weight Loss Programs."[26] Noting that most popular diets entail a severe restriction of calorie intake, the ACSM has described in detail the adverse health results that are likely to be the

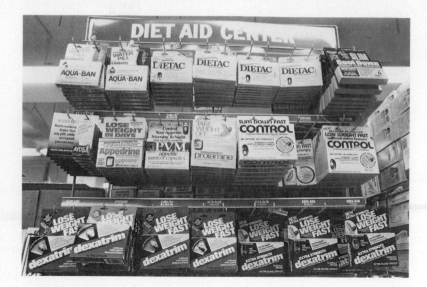

Appetite-depressing pills are among the ineffective approaches to permanent weight loss, and they can be risky. (© Hazel Hankin 1981)

consequences of such a regimen. If a person goes on one of these very-low-calorie diets, he or she may lose water, electrolytes, and minerals from the body; and he or she may suffer weakness, faintness, anemia, and a number of other possible medical problems. Ironically, reports the ACSM, putting the body through this stressful experience generally does *not* help the body shed fat. (Most of the "weight" lost in such a way consists of body fluids.) This means that all those suffering dieters trying to exist on 500 calories a day are taking the wrong approach.

So, avoid weight-reduction programs that employ techniques such as fasting, spot reducing, sweating, or a fad diet. These techniques are ineffective at best, and can be dangerous.

SUCCESSFUL WEIGHT CONTROL

If a strict diet will not banish fat, what will? The most successful weight reduction programs combine a *little* less eating and a *lot* more exercise. The ACSM paper is quite clear on this point:

A nutritionally sound diet resulting in mild caloric restriction coupled with an endurance exercise program along with behavioral modifica-

tion of existing eating habits is recommended for weight reduction. The rate of sustained weight loss should not exceed 1 kg (two pounds) per week. To maintain proper weight control and optimal body fat levels a lifetime commitment to proper eating habits and regular physical activity is required.[27]

This recommendation makes sense in the light of the findings we discussed earlier in this chapter regarding the possible causes of overweight.

True weight control is not achieved by going on a "diet" for a while and then going off it (and usually gaining the weight back). Instead, it means changing your whole way of life—permanently. You will need to make certain habits of living part of your own individual lifestyle. Usually, if you adopt these correct habit patterns, your body will find its ideal weight.

What are these habit patterns? Below, we'll describe some important ones that can result in "natural" weight management. The plan we'll outline avoids the rigors of dieting, and allows you to eat an abundance of nutritious foods, in harmony with your bodily needs. It is a physiologically and scientifically correct program for living. It involves two components: an exercise plan and an eating plan.

Planning Exercise for Weight Control

Over the long term, exercise is a useful—in fact, essential—tool in a weight-loss program. It has a

TABLE 14.2 · Number of Calories Burned in Various Physical Activities
(computed by multiplying the number of calories given here by your weight and by the number of minutes spent in performing the activity; an example is given in the right-hand columns for a 150-pound person)

Activities	Calories per Pound per Minute	Calories per 150 lbs, per Minute	Activities	Calories per Pound per Minute	Calories per 150 lbs, per Minute
Badminton	.039	6	Running:		
Bicycling			6 mph (10 min/ mile)	.079	12
Slow (5 mph)	.025	4	10 mph (6 min/ mile)	.1	15
Moderate (10 mph)	.05	8	12 mph (5 min/ mile)	.13	20
Fast (13 mph)	.072	11	Sailing	.02	3
Calisthenics (general)	.045	7	Skating:		
Canoeing:			Moderate	.036	5
2.5 mph	.023	3	Vigorous	.064	10
4.0 mph	.047	7	Skiing (snow):		
Dancing:			Downhill	.059	9
Slow	.029	4	Level (5 mph)	.078	12
Moderate	.045	7	Soccer	.063	10
Fast	.064	10	Stationary run		
Football (tag)	.04	6	(70–80 counts/ min)	.078	12
Golf	.029	4	Swimming (crawl):		
Handball	.063	10	20 yds/min	.032	5
Hiking	.042	6	50 yds/min	.071	11
Jogging, 4.5 mph (13:30 mile)	.063	10	Tennis:		
Judo, karate	.087	13	Moderate	.046	7
Mountain climbing	.086	13	Vigorous	.06	9
			Volleyball	.036	5
			Walking:		
			2 mph	.022	3
			4 mph	.039	6
			5 mph	.064	10
			Water skiing	.053	8

cumulative effect on the body's calorie expenditure. Even if you don't change your eating habits, beginning a program of regular physical exercise will start to shrink your body's fat tissues: You may be able to lose a pound of fat in seven to twelve exercise sessions (see Table 14.2).[28] If you also decrease your caloric intake—even modestly—you will, over time, experience a substantial weight loss. One expert has estimated that an exercise program consisting of a moderate jog of thirty minutes (or a brisk walk of sixty minutes) three times per week, plus a reduction of 100 calories a day in food consumed—say, by cutting out one buttered slice of bread or one glass of dry white wine a day—will produce a weight loss of twenty to thirty pounds in a year.[29] Plus, there are the benefits claimed by the setpoint theorists: Exer-

cise may encourage our brains to "program" our bodies for lower weight.

If you have any doubts about whether exercise is really important for a weight loss program, consider this: If you try to lose weight via diet alone, not only will you lose a lot of pounds by dehydration (water loss—very dangerous in large quantities!) but you may lose other types of lean tissue too. That means you could even lose some of your muscle mass. And that you don't want.

Perhaps you're thinking that there's a problem here: Isn't increasing my physical activity likely to make me eat much more? Studies have shown that exercise that lasts only a short time (such as one hour per day) does not seem to stimulate the appetite.[30] And one more question may have occurred to you: What if I gain back, in the shape of bigger muscles, the pounds I've lost in fat tissue? This *can* happen during the first six to eight weeks of an exercise program. But after that, you're not likely to add more pounds unless you embark on an ambitious weight-lifting program. Jogging, biking, and the like may enlarge your muscles somewhat, but these activities will still help you lose total weight eventually if you cut down on calories too.

All right, then, exactly how should you plan to exercise for weight control? Here's how.

EXERCISE FOR WEIGHT CONTROL: BASIC POINTS

1. The ACSM recommends a program of exercise at least three days a week—and preferably four or five days a week.
2. Each workout should be at least twenty minutes long.
3. The exercise should be of the type known as endurance training—continuous, rhythmic exercise such as walking, jogging, swimming, and bicycling (see Chapter 15).
4. Inactive people over the age of thirty-five should not begin any strenuous exercise program without a complete medical checkup that includes an exercise stress test (see Chapter 15).

Planning Your Diet for Weight Control

Now that you have set up your exercise plan, it's time to make a plan for eating. You need to decide how many pounds you want to lose, and how long you will take to lose them. You can then determine how many calories you should take in each day, what foods you should be eating (and what foods you should be avoiding), and how you're going to organize your daily meals.

YOUR WEIGHT-LOSS GOAL

The first step in planning your diet is to set a reasonable goal for the number of pounds you would like to lose—and the time frame in which you're going to do it. For example, you might decide you want to lose ten pounds over the next three months.

We would like to caution you here: *It is not wise to lose more than two pounds a week unless you are under a doctor's care.* If, for example, you are thirty pounds overweight, aim toward shedding that weight gradually, over the course of a year. Don't expect to lose it in just a few weeks.

YOUR DAILY CALORIE TARGET

Once you have set your weight-loss goal, the next step is to figure out about how many calories you should eat each day in order to achieve the goal. First, use the Calorie Calculator and Activity Level Guide (Figure 14.1) to determine the number of calories you *need* to take in daily to maintain your present weight. You are going to subtract a certain number of calories from this—let's say, 500 calories per day—in order to dip below your present weight.

Here's an example: An eighteen-year-old male student, who stands 5 feet, 9 inches tall, weighs 180 pounds, and has a part-time job in the library finds out by using the Calorie Calculator that he will need approximately 3,100 calories each day to remain at his present weight. Let's say his goal is to bring his weight down to 160 pounds by losing twenty pounds over a period of twenty weeks—that is, losing weight at the rate of one pound each week. (It has been found that when a person loses one to two pounds per week, the weight loss is more likely to be permanent.)[31] Since one pound of fat equals 3,500 calories, in order to lose one pound of fat in a week he needs to eat 3,500 fewer calories than he uses each week, or 500 fewer calories each day. The student therefore could achieve his goal by eating 2,600 calories a day (3,100 minus 500 calories).

Important note: in general, do not cut your total calorie intake below 1,200 calories a day. If you do so, it is almost impossible for you to take in enough food to supply yourself with the nutrients you need. (And a vitamin pill is only a supplement to a balanced diet, not a substitute for one.)

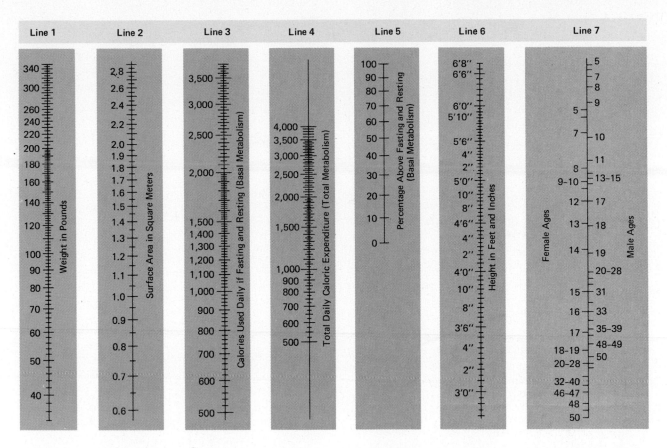

Line 1	Line 2	Line 3	Line 4	Line 5	Line 6	Line 7

Figure 14.1 The calorie calculator and activity-level guide. To determine the number of calories needed to maintain your present weight, follow these instructions:

1. Using a pin as a marker, locate your present weight on line 1.
2. Setting the edge of a ruler against the pin, swing the other end of the ruler to your height, located on line 6.
3. Remove the pin from line 1, and now place it at the point where the ruler crosses line 2.
4. Keeping the edge of the ruler firmly against the pin on line 2, swing its right-hand edge to your sex and age on line 7, using the age of your nearest birthday for the purpose.
5. Remove the pin, and place it where the ruler crosses line 3. This will give you the calories used daily (in twenty-four hours) if you are resting and fasting.
6. To the basal calories thus determined, add the percentage above fasting and resting for your usual type of daily activity, using the following guidelines:

- Add 40 percent if you are a nonworking student whose physical activity is limited to walking to and from classes.
- Add 50 percent if you are involved in physical activity (such as clerical or library work) that includes about two hours of walking or standing daily.
- Add 60 percent if you participate in limited physical exercise (such as disco dancing) or intramural sports of a moderate nature.
- Add 70 percent if your work involves heavy physical activity (such as construction work) or if you participate in a regular, daily exercise program (such as intercollegiate team sports).
- Add 80 to 100 percent if you are engaged in strenuous physical work or participate in intercollegiate sports that have a high rate of calorie expenditure (basketball, track, and the like).

7. Leaving the pin in line 3, swing the edge of the ruler to the right to the proper percentage on line 5. Where the ruler crosses line 4, you will find the number of calories necessary to maintain you at your present weight if you maintain your present activity level.

Source: Adapted from George A. Brey, *The Obese Patient* [Philadelphia: Saunders, 1976], p. 305.

FOODS TO CHOOSE AND FOODS TO AVOID

It's important to eat nutritious foods every day, even though you are trying to control your weight. Unless a doctor prescribes a special diet for you, each meal you eat should contain foods—in moderation—from each of the four basic food groups (see Chapter 13).

But you should probably cut down on certain types of foods. It has been estimated that 86 percent of the calories Americans eat come from meat, dairy products, fats and oils, flour and cereal products, and sugar and other sweeteners. Only 8.6 percent of our calories come from fruits and vegetables.[32] So, one simple step toward losing weight is to increase your consumption of fruits, nuts, grains, and vegetables while decreasing the amount of food you eat from the other food groups. Our young man might find that he normally eats many fried foods and rich snacks. Cutting out fried foods, rich desserts, sugary drinks and pastries, and the extra glass of wine or beer can make a big difference in calories.

Fats are a type of food to watch carefully. They are essential nutrients in every diet, but they are also the most concentrated source of calories in the food we eat. They contribute twice as many calories or more per portion as a serving of protein or carbohydrate does. Forty percent or more of the average American diet is composed of fat—and you don't need that much![33]

To get a clear picture of which foods you should continue eating and which foods you should cut down on or cut out altogether, take a look at your current eating patterns—the kinds of foods you are eating now. Begin by recording everything you eat for five consecutive days. Keeping a "food diary," like the one shown in the activity on pages 352–353, will tell you the types of foods you tend to eat habitually; then you can pinpoint the ones that should stay in your new eating plan and the ones that should be eliminated. Tips on modifying your eating behavior are given in the box on pages 354–355.

YOUR DAILY MEAL PLAN

If you're trying to control your weight, eating several modest-size meals per day may be more effective than eating just one large meal per day. The reason: Eating a large meal causes your body to secrete more insulin—the substance which, as we mentioned in Chapter 13, helps the body utilize blood glucose—and that means ultimately more fat storage, which you don't want.

MEAL TIPS: WHAT YOU CAN DO

▶ Eat a good breakfast every day, including a source of complete protein. This will keep your blood sugar up throughout the morning. You'll feel better, and you'll be less likely to gobble a huge lunch.
▶ Do not skip lunch.
▶ To help cut down fat storage, make the evening meal the lightest meal of the day.

IF YOU ARE UNDERWEIGHT

While millions of Americans are preoccupied with weighing too much, many others are concerned about being underweight and believe that they are "too skinny," "bony," or "shapeless." As with overweight, underweight usually results from a genetic predisposition plus eating and exercise habits. Some of the factors involved in underweight include undereating, compulsive hyperactivity, nervous tension that burns up calories, and lack of exercises to develop muscle mass and shape the body.

Correcting underweight also requires permanent changes in your eating and exercise habits. Like the person who wants to lose weight, you should start by estimating your daily calorie expenditure. This will help you see how many calories you need to add to your daily diet.

Then make a plan for boosting your daily calories. Programs of increased calorie intake and moderate exercise, plus control of stress, will usually result in weight gain. The increased calorie intake should generally be mostly carbohydrates such as corn, rice, and potatoes, because there is some evidence that high-protein and high-fat diets can be hazardous. It's also a good idea to eat frequent, small meals. Note, too, that while it is sometimes possible to build up certain areas of the body by selectively exercising certain muscles, it is not possible to add fat deliberately to desired locations, such as the breasts.

HOW TO GAIN WEIGHT SENSIBLY

To put on a pound of lean weight, you must consume about 2,500 additional calories. Of course, you should not try to do this all at once. Aim at consuming 1,000 to 1,500 calories more than your daily expenditures. You should exercise regularly so that the weight you gain won't be mostly fat.

EATING DISORDERS

In recent years, two extreme forms of eating disorders have gained increasing attention: anorexia nervosa and bulimia. These conditions are not yet fully understood, but let's take a brief look at what is known about them.

Anorexia Nervosa

At the extreme end of the weight-control spectrum is a disorder in which people severely limit the amount they eat, virtually starving themselves. This condition is called **anorexia** (loss of appetite) **nervosa** (nervous or psychogenic). It occurs almost exclusively among preadolescent and adolescent girls or young women, and it has been increasing in frequency in the past decade.[34]

Most anorexics are people who come from upper- or middle-class homes, and who may have seemed like model children before they developed the disorder. In the typical case, the young girl suddenly becomes obsessed with the idea that she is fat. She begins to diet, often following a fad diet. For some reason, even as she begins to lose weight seriously, she still feels fat and begins to starve herself. Eventually she begins to look like a skeleton, sometimes losing more than a third of her body weight. She may avoid food altogether, or she may seem to take a perverse pleasure in it —preparing gourmet meals for the rest of the family, for example, but eating nothing herself. Or she may occasionally gorge herself on a huge meal and then immediately make herself vomit it all. If her strange eating habits are questioned, she will typically deny that there is anything wrong with her behavior. Eventually, she may grow negative, passive, and apathetic. Left untreated, up to 10 percent of anorexics eventually die of starvation.[35]

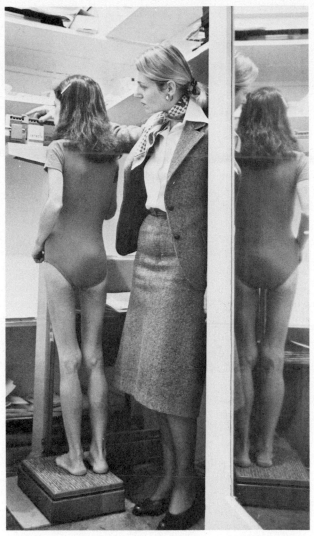

The incidence of anorexia nervosa, the "starving disease," is on the increase. (©Neal Boenzi/The New York Times)

Why should an apparently healthy, well-adjusted person decide to starve herself in such a bizarre and tragic way? Unfortunately, no one has yet been able to answer this question; the precise cause of anorexia nervosa remains a mystery. Occasionally, the disorder is seen in connection with mental illness, such as schizophrenia. Cases of this kind are known as *secondary anorexia nervosa*. *Primary anorexia nervosa*, in which the disorder does not seem to be produced by obvious mental illness, is a more puzzling problem. The consensus is that anorexia nervosa has a psychological cause, but researchers disagree over what this cause is.[36]

ACTIVITY: EXPLORING HEALTH

BEHAVIOR MODIFICATION: Keeping a Food Diary to Analyze Your Eating Habits

Before you can learn to control your own eating behavior, you may need to analyze your specific habits.

People have an amazingly wide range of patterns when it comes to eating: Some snack while they're talking on the phone; some reach for food whenever they're nervous or depressed; some avoid eating as much as possible (children sometimes avoid eating in order to manipulate their parents); some eat whenever they're feeling especially happy, while others console themselves with sweet treats.

The Food Diary, opposite, can help you chart your own eating patterns. Fill it out for a single day—today or yesterday—putting in as much detail as you can remember about when and where you ate, and what you were doing at the time. Then try filling in the diary for five consecutive days; and after that, one day a week for a month. You may find that simply having to fill out a diary makes you more aware of your eating habits, and makes you tend to change them—for the better.

ANALYZING YOUR EATING HABITS

The quality and amount of food you take into your body, and the atmosphere in which you eat, will do a great deal to determine the quality of the life that goes on in each cell of your body. As you review your Food Diary notations, ask yourself these questions:

1. Are you spending enough time at each meal to eat slowly and chew your food completely? Do you finish eating before most of the people around you or after them? Your body is best able to digest food and use its energy when you eat slowly and chew completely.
2. Do you separate eating from other activities? Do you pause and assume a calm and relaxed attitude before eating? Or is your pattern of eating hurried—grabbing food on the run or while doing other things like driving or reading? Eating in a calm, relaxed frame of mind aids digestion. Separating eating from other activities can make you more aware of how much food you can eat.
3. Do you eat only when you are hungry? Before eating, pause and ask yourself if you're hungry. If you are not, ask yourself why you are sitting down to eat at this time.
4. Do you eat only as much food as leaves you feeling pleasantly satisfied—as opposed to uncomfortably stuffed? For health and weight-control reasons, you should eat only the amount of food that is most comfortable for your body.
5. What kinds of feelings do you get from eating in general? From eating specific foods? Does food make you happy, sad, angry, disappointed, indifferent? Are there other emotions you associate with food?

Source: Adapted from M. Samuels and H. Bennett, *The Well Body Book* (New York: Random House, 1973).

FOOD DIARY

DAY OF WEEK_____

Time of Food Intake	*Minutes Spent Eating*	*Meal (M) or Snack (S)*	*Degree of Hunger (0=None, 3=Max.)*	*Other Activity While Eating*	*Location While Eating*	*Body Position While Eating*	*Eating With Whom*	*Feeling While Eating*	*Number of Calories in Meal/ Snack*

Adapted from James M. Ferguson, M.D., *Learning to Eat* (Palo Alto, Calif., Bull Publishing Co., 1975).

EATING CORRECTLY: How to Modify Your Eating Behavior

Think about the way you use food in your life. When do you overeat? When you are alone or with friends? When you're feeling good or when you're unhappy? In other words, what feelings and behaviors do you associate with eating? If you are overweight, changing some of your food-related behaviors may be the key to successful reducing.

In fact, the behavior-modification method described below is the most successful technique discovered to date for long-term weight control. This method is often used in weight-reducing groups led by professionals, but, to a certain extent, you can use it yourself.

STEP 1: MAKING A RECORD OF YOUR EATING BEHAVIOR

To become aware of your eating habits, *write them down.* Behavior therapists often recommend that you keep a detailed written diary of your eating behavior for several days or a week, writing down the following information about each meal or snack:

- ▶ The time you begin and finish the meal or snack
- ▶ The place where you eat it (if you eat at home, be sure to write down the room where you eat, such as bedroom or den—many people snack away from the dining room)
- ▶ Whether you are sitting, standing, or lying down when you eat
- ▶ Whether you are alone or with other people
- ▶ Any activity associated with the meal or snack, such as reading, watching television, or talking
- ▶ Your mood
- ▶ How hungry you were just before eating
- ▶ The foods you eat
- ▶ An estimate of the calories in the meal or snack

Therapists also recommend keeping a daily record of your activities, including a record of your exercise periods.

STEP 2: ANALYZING YOUR EATING PATTERNS

From these records, you should be able to identify the situations that prompt you to eat more than you should. Do you overeat when you catch a whiff or sight of some tempting but high-calorie goodie? Or when you are feeling bored or tense or lonely? Or do you eat too much when you are relaxed and socializing with friends? You may discover, for instance, that you are ingesting unneeded calories during a morning coffee-and-doughnut break with fellow workers on your job. Or you may be eating an excessively large breakfast while you watch a particular morning television show.

STEP 3: "REPROGRAMMING" YOURSELF

Once you have discovered the cues that prompt your overeating, you can consciously devise ways to

---

Some experts suggest that anorexics may have abnormal fears of their approaching womanhood. In losing so much weight, the girls lose their feminine curves, stop menstruating, and begin to look like little girls again.

Specialists in treating anorexia feel strongly that both psychological *and* medical treatment are imperative. Tube feeding and a high-calorie diet may be necessary at the start: Not only is the anorexic's weight dangerously low, it is also impossible for her to reason effectively when her thinking processes have been disrupted by chronic malnutrition. Treatment is not easy. Until the anorexic is able to establish a more realistic out-

look on her situation, therapy results in little more than cycles of remission and relapse.[37]

Bulimia

Bulimia, a pattern involving eating binges followed by vomiting purges, is considered a type of anorexia nervosa.[38] Typically, the bulimia sufferer is a woman in her early twenties, college-educated, single, and white. Like anorexics, bulimics "are usually perfectionists . . . but they tend to be older, of near-normal weight, with healthy, outgoing appearances."[39] Bulimia is not change your eating and activity habits by removing, avoiding, substituting, or ignoring these cues. While it is probably not feasible to reorganize your life so as to remove all such cues, you can usually avoid the most powerful ones. For instance, if you have developed the habit of having a drink and a snack while watching television before dinner, you might, for a week or two, take a walk instead or do exercises while watching the news—or move the TV set out of the kitchen or dining room.

Some people who are trying to improve their eating patterns make a point of never combining eating with any other pleasant or relaxing activity, such as reading or watching television or listening to music. Others make themselves follow a rule that they will eat only when seated at a table that is properly set with tablecloth or placemat, napkin, dishes, and silverware. This rule tends to cut down on snacking, since it is inconvenient to set the table just for a snack.

STEP 4: REWARDING YOURSELF

You should also devise some system for rewarding yourself for even small successes. People who do this often are more successful at losing weight than are those who reward themselves less frequently. One system is to give yourself a point each time you are able to change a problem behavior. When you have accumulated the predetermined number of points, treat yourself to something you want. Another system is to make a contract with yourself, setting goals and rewarding yourself when you meet these goals. Your primary reward, however, should be your satisfaction at being able to change your habits and improve your control of your weight.

THE IMPORTANCE OF MOTIVATION

The best and most important factor in any weight management program is a real desire to lose weight—whether to change the way you look or just to improve your health. Losing a lot of weight requires a total commitment to changing lifelong habits of eating and exercise, and this is not easy. In the end, what will encourage you to change your eating habits is your own inner motivation. Believe you can do it, be patient, and persevere.

One important caution: You should not judge your adequacy or inadequacy as a person by your success or failure at weight control. You should think well of yourself regardless of your weight. Weight control can simply be something you add to your life; it is not a measure of your worth.

A final point: Guard against giving in to negative thoughts such as "Exercise won't make any difference" or "If this method of weight reduction didn't work for Joe, it sure won't work for me." And don't let the people around you suggest such attitudes to you. Instead, urge your family members and other people who are important to you to reinforce the changes that you have made in your eating and exercise behaviors.

Source: Arnold Weiss, "Characteristics of Successful Weight Reducers: A Brief Review of Predictor Variables," *Addictive Behaviors* 2 (1977): 193–201.

just eating a lot, or "pigging out"; there is a distinct pattern to the bulimic's binges. The bulimic typically eats secretly, consuming an enormous amount of food at one sitting. The urge that drives such eating is clearly something beyond simple hunger. Commonly, a binge will follow one "slip" from a self-imposed diet: The bulimic will eat one favorite forbidden food—a brownie, a piece of pecan pie—and then feel compelled to consume virtually every bit of food in sight. Then comes the need to vomit or to take quantities of laxatives to make sure that the food doesn't stay in the body to produce weight gain.

What causes bulimia? As with anorexia, the condition is not fully understood. Psychiatrists who have studied bulimics agree that they have an abnormal fear of becoming fat. The onset of bulimia usually occurs during adolescence, when staying slim seems to be the one way to please overly critical parents. The binge-purge syndrome can over time be very harmful. Potassium depletion, urinary tract infections, kidney failure, weight loss, ulcers, and hernias are all possible side effects. Curing bulimia is difficult because the disease is still so poorly understood, but the number of treatment programs is growing.

MAKING HEALTH DECISIONS

Setting Up a Weight-Loss Plan

If you're interested in losing weight, you need to make a plan that will suit *you.* No two people are alike; you must find your own individual best method.

YOUR OVERALL APPROACH

First, you need to decide whether you are simply going to reduce the number of calories you take in each day, or reduce your caloric intake *and* increase your caloric expenditure via exercise. Some people find that if they don't exercise while they are trying to lose weight, they tend to feel nervous, cranky, tired, and hungry most of the time; their bodies remain flabby, and they go through long "plateau" periods during which they don't lose a single pound. Still, some people seriously dislike exercise—or are so busy right now that they don't have time for regular exercise sessions, but would like to start cutting down calories anyway. You *may* decide that just watching your calories is the method that will work best.

In contrast, many people who exercise regularly while trying to lose weight tend to feel more energetic and relaxed; they find that their appetite seems to be controlled, and that their muscles are toned up and their bodies look attractive even before the pounds actually start to drop off. Thus, the "exercise plus calorie-counting" approach *may* be right for you.

Mark your choice here:

_____I'm going to concentrate on lowering my daily caloric intake.

_____I'm going to cut down on calories *and* begin an exercise program.

Whichever one you choose, don't be discouraged. If you feel firmly committed to improving your weight, appearance, and health, you'll do what's best for *you.*

A SPECIFIC PLAN

Let's assume for the moment that you have decided that you are going to cut down calories *and* increase your daily exercise. Here's a handy method for establishing a sensible plan.

A. Estimate the number of calories that you are probably consuming to maintain your present weight.

(1) _____Your present weight

(2)× _____(Men multiply by 17; women multiply by 16)

(3)= _____Calories consumed per day

B. *By contrast,* calculate the calorie intake needed to maintain your *goal weight.*

(4) _____Your goal weight

(5)× _____(Men multiply by 17; women multiply by 16)

(6)= _____Calories needed per day

C. To lose weight, you must use up more calories than you consume.
   1. To do that you must eat less and exercise more.
   2. Right now, consider decreasing your calorie intake by 500 to 800 calories per day (but not below 1,200 calories or so, to ensure proper nutrition).

(7) 3. _____Present calories consumed per day (from line 3, above)

(8)− _____(Subtract 500–800 calories)

(9)= _____Daily calorie goal

D. Estimate the number of calories you will use by walking each day (all at one time).

(10) _____Your present weight

(11)× _____ Miles you plan to walk per day (It is suggested that you begin with 1.5 to 3.0 miles per day.)

(12)= _____

(13)× ___.75___

(14)= _____ Calories "burned" by walking each day

E. Now, make a *realistic* prediction of how long it will take you to lose enough weight to reach your individual weight goal.

(15) _____ Decrease in calories per day (from line 8)

(16)+ _____ Calories "burned" in exercise each day (from line 14)

(17)= _____ Total

F. Weight loss plan

(18) _____ Number of calories to give up and burn up daily (from line 17)

(19) _____ Number of days to lose 1 pound at that rate (see chart below)

(20) _____ Total number of pounds you want to lose

(21)× _____ Your number from line 19 (multiply that number by line 20).

(22) _____ Product (The number of days it will take for you to reach your desired weight)

INCREASE ACTIVITY AND CUT YOUR DAILY INTAKE OF CALORIES BY	DAYS IT TAKES TO LOSE ONE POUND
100	35
200	17.5
300	12
400	9
500	7
600	6
700	5
800	4.5
900	4
1000	3.5
1100	3.1
1200	3

G. Count ahead from today the total number of days that it will take to reach your goal weight. Record that success date below.

(23)_____

A PERSONAL WEIGHT MANAGEMENT CONTRACT

If you are committed to losing enough weight to achieve your goal weight, you may wish to complete the following personal contract.

I, _____, do hereby contract to begin a weight-control plan of restricting my calorie intake and increasing my activity by _____ calories daily (from line 17, above), beginning on the date of _____ _____ . I am fully aware that at this rate I will reach my desired weight in approximately _____ days (from line 22, above). I further realize that when I reach my desired weight on or before _____ (date from line 23, above) I must continue on a sensible eating and activity program for the rest of my life if I am to maintain my desired weight.

_____   _____
DATE   SIGNATURE

                             _____
                             WITNESS

Source: Adapted from "The Better Weigh," a weight-control program developed by Tempe Community Hospital (now Tempe St. Luke's Hospital), Tempe, Arizona; and based on ideas in Jack D. Osman and Bobbie J. Van Dolson, *Thin from Within* (Washington, D. C.: Review & Herald, 1981), p. 49.

SUMMARY

1. Serious overweight is associated, usually indirectly, with several forms of disease. Overweight increases the risk of incidence of heart disease, diabetes, and emotional problems. Estimates are that half of all adults in the United States are overweight. Both men and women in most height and weight categories are heavier than they were in the 1960s.

2. Genetic and environmental factors both contribute to one's body shape. All bodies are made of two kinds of tissue. One is lean tissue, including muscle, bone, cartilage, connective tissue, skin, nerves, and internal organs. The other is fat tissue, in the form of essential fat and storage fat.

3. The amount of muscle in one's body significantly affects how much one weighs. Regular exercise can change the ratio of fat to lean tissue in the body. Lean muscle tissue weighs more than fat tissue does, but lean muscle looks better and is healthier than too much fat.

4. Life insurance tables indicate approximately ideal weights for men and women of different heights and body types. A weight 15 percent above that recommended by such a table is considered overweight. A weight 20 to 30 percent above is considered obese.

5. Overweight begins when a person takes in more calories than his or her body burns in the form of energy. Factors that may contribute to overweight include genetic inheritance; lack of physical activity; a decrease in the metabolic rate as the individual gets older; unhealthy eating habits; the development of an overabundance of fat cells in the overweight person's body; and, according to setpoint theory, the body's effort to maintain its "natural" weight by adjusting its metabolic rate.

6. Severe, unhealthy weight-loss diets can cause the body to lose not just fat, but essential fluids, electrolytes, and minerals. The best diets combine a small, steady reduction of calories with a significant increase in exercise. Short periods of exercise do not increase the appetite.

7. For weight management, a person should exercise at least three times a week for 20 minutes each time. The exercise should be of the endurance type. People over thirty-five need a medical checkup before they begin a strenuous exercise program.

8. Permanent weight loss and weight control result from permanent changes in eating and exercise habits. A weight loss of more than two pounds a week is likely to be temporary. Eating fewer than 1,200 calories a day means missing some essential nutrients.

9. Underweight people must contend with the genetic and environmental factors that underlie their problem. To gain weight, they must change their eating and exercise habits. Increased calories, moderate exercise, and control of stress can usually produce the desired weight gain.

10. Anorexia nervosa, which is voluntary starvation, and bulimia, which is the alternating of food binges with purges, are eating disorders that can have severe, even fatal, effects. Their causes are not fully understood; it is known that both medical and psychological treatment are necessary.

GLOSSARY

anorexia nervosa   An eating disorder in which people severely limit the amount of food they eat, virtually starving themselves.

anthropometric measurements   Measurements taken, using calipers, of various parts of the body to calculate the proportion of fat in the body.

bulimia   A type of anorexia nervosa characterized by eating binges followed by purges.

densimetric method   Technique for assessing the proportion of lean and fat tissue in the body by weighing the person first in air, then again when submerged in water, to determine overall body density in relation to water.

ectomorphy   Degree of "linearity" or "long-bonedness" of a person's body build.

endomorphy   Degree of fatness of a person's body build.

essential fat   Fat that is necessary for the body's normal physiological functioning in the storage and usage of nutrients. Compare **storage fat.**

mesomorphy Degree of muscularity of a person's body build.

obese Weighing 20 percent or more above the recommendation in insurance-company tables.

overweight Weighing 15 percent or more above the recommendation in insurance-company tables.

setpoint The weight range that is natural to an individual's body, which, according to the "setpoint theory," the body strives to maintain by adjusting its metabolic rate.

storage fat Fat deposited under the skin and around the internal organs to protect them; although it is sometimes called *excess fat,* some storage fat is necessary to the body's well-being. Compare **essential fat.**

NOTES

1. George E. Schauf, "Is the Caloric Theory Valid?" *Nutrition Today,* January–February 1979, pp. 29–31.

2. Vital and Health Statistics: Data from the National Health Survey, Weight and Height Survey for Adults 18–74 Years: U.S. 1971–1974 (Series 11, No. 208, U. S. Department of Health and Human Services, September 1979); reprinted in *Statistical Abstracts of the United States, 1981.*

3. A. L. Stewart, R. H. Brook, and R. L. Kane, "Conceptualization and Measurement of Health Habits for Adults in the Health Insurance Study: Vol. II," *Overweight* (Santa Monica, Calif.: Rand Corporation, R-2374/2 HEW, July, 1980); Schauf, "Is the Caloric Theory Valid?"

4. Frantz W. Ashbey and William B. Kannel, "Relation of Weight Change to Changes in Atherogenic Traits," *Journal of Chronic Disease* 27 (1974): 103–114.

5. W. B. Kannel and T. Gordon, "Obesity and Cardiovascular Disease: The Framingham Study," in W. L. Burland, P. D. Samuel, and J. Yudkin, eds., *Obesity* (London: Churchill-Livingstone, 1974), pp. 24–51.

6. S. Matter et al., "Body Fat Content and Serum Lipid Levels," *Journal of the American Dietetic Association* 77 (1980): 149.

7. Norman M. Kaplan, "The Control of Hypertension: A Therapeutic Breakthrough," *American Scientist* 68, no. 5 (September–October 1980): 537–545.

8. Jane Fonda, *Jane Fonda's Workout Book* (New York: Simon & Schuster, 1981).

9. Frank Katch and William McArdle, *Nutrition, Weight Control, and Exercise* (Boston: Houghton Mifflin, 1977), p. 102.

10. Ibid.

11. M. L. Pollack, J. H. Wilmore, and Samuel Fox, *Health and Fitness Through Physical Activity* (New York: Wiley, 1978), p. 47.

12. David Clark, *Exercise Physiology* (Englewood Cliffs, N.J.: Prentice-Hall, 1979), p. 129.

13. C. Corbin et al., *Core Concepts in Physical Education,* 4th ed. (Dubuque, Iowa: William C. Brown, 1981), p. 60.

14. Anita L. Stewart and Robert H. Brook, "Effects of Being Overweight," *American Journal of Public Health* 73, no. 2 (February 1983): 171–177.

15. S. R. Williams, *Nutrition and Diet Therapy,* 4th ed. (St. Louis: Mosby, 1981), p. 538.

16. D. Jacobs, F. P. Heald, P. L. White, and W. J. McGanity, "Obesity 1. Prevention," *Journal of the American Medical Association* 186 (November 9, 1963): Supp. 27-40.

17. Jean Mayer, "Obesity: Physiological Considerations," *American Journal of Clinical Nutrition* 9 (September–October 1961): 530.

18. B. A. Bullen, R. B. Reed, and Jean Mayer, "Physical Activity of Obese and Nonobese Adolescent Girls Appraised by Motion Picture Sampling," *American Journal of Clinical Nutrition* 14 (April 1964): 211.

19. Herbert DeVries, *Physiology of Exercise* (Dubuque, Iowa: William C. Brown, 1980), p. 344.

20. Maria Simonson, "An Overview: Advances in Research and Treatment of Obesity," *National Livestock and Meat Board Reports* 53, no. 4 (March–April 1982): 2.

21. S. Le Vasseur, "Obesity Update '81," lecture presented at symposium, Johns Hopkins Medical Institute, March 1980; cited in ibid.

22. Katch and McArdle, *Nutrition, Weight Control, and Exercise.*

23. R. E. Keesey et al., "The Role of the Lateral Hypothalamus in Determining the Body Weight Set-Point," in D. Novin, W. Wyrwicka, and G. A. Brav, eds., *Hunger: Basic Mechanisms and Clinical Implications* (New York: Raven Press, 1976).

24. William Bennett and Joel Gurin, "Do Diets Really Work?" *Science 82,* March 1982, pp. 42–50.

25. "Drug Agency Sees Peril in Starch-Blocker Diet Aids," *New York Times,* July 2, 1982, p. 1A.

26. American College of Sports Medicine, "Position Statement on Proper and Improper Weight Loss Pro-

grams," *Medicine and Science in Sports and Exercise* 15, no. 1 (1983): ix–xiii.

27. Ibid.

28. Pollack, Wilmore, and Fox, *Health and Fitness,* p. 28.

29. Ibid.

30. David Clark, *Exercise Physiology,* p. 127.

31. R. B. Stuart and B. Davis, *Slim Chance in a Fat World* (Champaign, Ill.: Research Press, 1972).

32. "National Food Situation in the U.S.," *Nutrition Notes,* July 1971.

33. George A. Brey, ed., "Obesity in America," U.S. Public Health Service, DHHS Pub. No. 80-359, May 1980).

34. Jane E. Brody, "Anorexia Nervosa, an Ailment Rising Among Teen-Age Girls, Is Yielding to a New Therapy," *New York Times,* July 14, 1982, p. C6.

35. "Anorexia: The Starving-Disease Epidemic," *U.S. News and World Report,* August 30, 1982, pp. 47–48.

36. Sadrudin Bhanji, "Anorexia Nervosa: Physicians' and Psychiatrists' Opinions and Practice," *Journal of Psychosomatic Research* 23 (1979): 7–11.

37. "Anorexia: The Starving-Disease Epidemic."

38. Paul E. Garfinkel, Harvey Moldofsky, and David M. Garner, "The Heterogeneity of Anorexia Nervosa," *Archives of General Psychiatry* 37 (September 1980): 1036–1040.

39. "The Binge-Purge Syndrome," *Newsweek,* November 2, 1982, pp. 68–69.

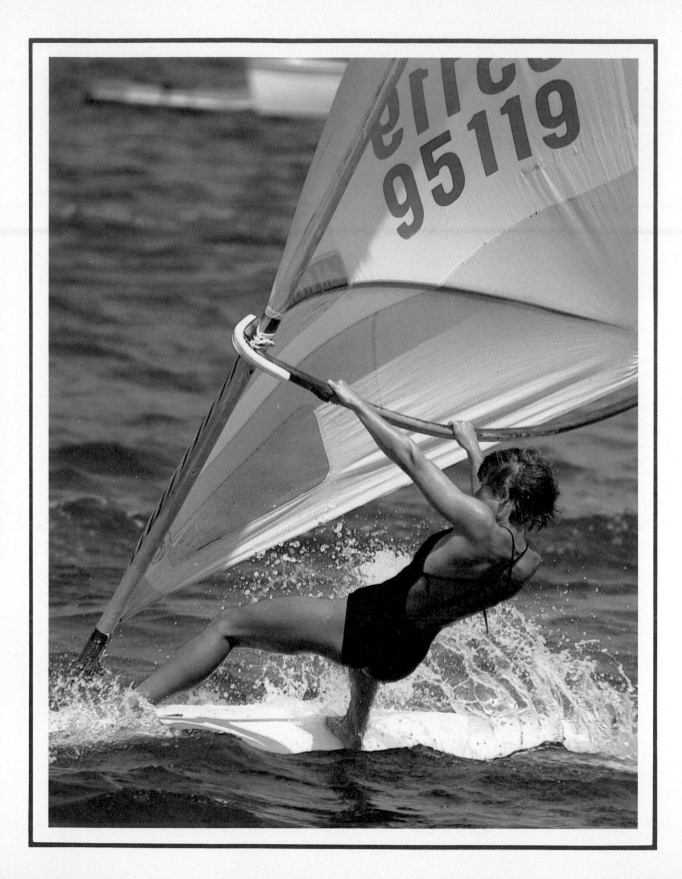

CHAPTER 15

Exercise and Physical Fitness

Millions of Americans have begun to walk, jog, bicycle, swim, and play tennis, with the goal of improving their physical fitness. Today it is considered fashionable, not eccentric, to be seen around town in warm-up suits or tennis togs; and a vast industry has sprung up to provide sports clothes, footwear, and other gear for all this new physical activity. Exercise and fitness are definitely "in." This phenomenon, which appears to be permanent and growing, may well be the most important health-promoting shift in the American lifestyle in this century.

Why are so many people devoting time and money to physical exercise today? Many may have begun to exercise in an effort to control their weight. But they have found additional benefits as well. Regular exercise not only helps them look and feel better physically but also brightens their entire outlook on life. They are more relaxed and have more energy, and they feel better about themselves. As we learn more about the body's need for physical exercise, it becomes apparent that we get a lot more from our jogs around the neighborhood and our workouts on the tennis court than a stronger heart and stronger muscles: We get an increased sense of inner power, tranquility, and self-esteem.

THE HEALTH BENEFITS OF EXERCISE

Our bodies were designed to be *used*—to be kept in fairly constant motion. Until recently in human history, the daily tasks of life required physical work: From the Stone Age up to our own century, most people spent their days in strenuous exertion—swinging a scythe in the fields, manipulating machinery in factories, or scrubbing floors and lugging tubs of wet laundry around at home. In modern life, however, few of our daily activities demand physical exertion. Most of our waking hours are spent sitting—at a desk, behind the wheel of a car, in front of a television set; even our toothbrushes and pencil sharpeners are motorized.

If we are to give our bodies the activities they need, we must make an effort to exercise. Otherwise, we may bring on, or make worse, a good many health problems. As we grow more sedentary, we may become obese, our muscles may become limp and soft, and our joints may begin to deteriorate. We may find that we tire easily and sleep poorly. We may be irritable and subject to a variety of minor ills—upset stomach, aches and pains.[1] These effects may not be detectable in people in their early twenties, but as people reach their late twenties or early thirties, the signs of lack of exercise may begin to show.

Exercise and Physical Well-Being

Recent studies have shown that exercise benefits the body because it stimulates all the body systems, especially the muscular, cardiovascular, and respiratory systems (see Table 15.1). The body of a person who exercises regularly seems to work at a higher level of efficiency—much like a car engine after a tune-up. Admittedly, fitness is not a cure-all: Even diseases that have been shown to

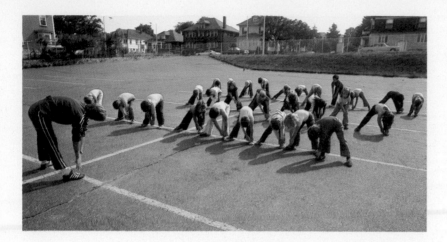

Ideally, the habit of regular exercise begins in childhood and continues throughout life. (©Erik Anderson/Stock, Boston)

occur less often in active people, such as heart disease, cannot be prevented by exercise alone. (Heart disease, like many other ailments, has no single cause. As we saw in Chapter 12, it is associated with a number of risk factors, among them obesity, stress, high blood pressure, and a family history of heart disease.[2]) Yet exercise is one important variable in the equation of overall health. For most of us, the beneficial effects of an active life—in keeping our weight down, in helping us feel and look better—will induce us to make use of our bicycle or running shoes.

Exercise and Psychological Well-Being

Those who walk, run, swim, or cycle regularly are familiar with the psychological and physical "glow" that often follows exercise. Exercise seems to discharge the tension that accumulates when we are under stress. After a strenuous workout, the body naturally relaxes, with beneficial effects on the body *and* the mind. Researchers are only beginning to understand how exertion affects the mind, but some research has shown that exercise

TABLE 15.1 • Physical Benefits of Regular Exercise

Heart	*Lungs*
Reduced resting heart rate	Increased functional capacity during exercise
Reduced heart rate for a standardized exercise session	Increased blood supply
Increased rate of heart rate recovery after a standardized exercise	Increased diffusion of respiratory gases
Increased blood volume pumped per heartbeat	Reduced nonfunctional volume of lung
Increased size of heart muscle	
Increased blood supply to heart muscle	*Neural, Endocrine, and Metabolic Function*
Increased strength of cardiac contraction	Increased glucose tolerance
	Reduced strain and nervous tension resulting from psychological stress
Blood Vessels and Blood Chemistry	Increased enzymatic function in muscle cells
Reduced resting systolic and diastolic arterial blood pressure, if originally elevated	Reduced body fat content
Reduced serum lipids or fats (that is, cholesterol, triglycerides)	Increased muscle mass
Increased blood supply to muscles	Increased functional capacity during exercise (oxygen uptake capacity)
Increased blood volume	
More efficient exchange of oxygen and carbon dioxide in muscles	

Source: Adapted from unpublished material prepared by W. L. Haskell and J. H. Wilmore for the Preventive Medicine Center, Palo Alto, California, as cited in Jack H. Wilmore, "Individualized Exercise Prescription," in Ezra Amsterdam, Jack H. Wilmore, and Anthony De Maria, eds., *Exercise in Cardiovascular Health and Disease* (New York: Yorke Medical Books, 1977), p. 271.

has a protective effect against any disease and especially heart disease. Since exercise has been shown to act as a tension reducer, there may be reason to believe that the stress of exercise may almost "immunize" the body against more destructive kinds of stress.[3]

Thaddeus Kostrubala, a psychiatrist and author of *The Joy of Running,* has recently discovered that endurance training—jogging at three-fourths of one's maximum capacity (as determined by a medical stress test) for one hour or more three times a week—produces psychological benefits such as relieving depression and anxiety.[4] Some long-distance runners have even reported feelings of euphoria—the "runner's high"—and a trancelike state after an hour or more of running.[5] This pleasurable response may be responsible for the almost religious zeal with which so many people are becoming committed to running. Another psychiatrist, William Glasser, has found that runners and other athletes who do endurance activities develop a "positive addiction."[6]

Admittedly, in a few people there is evidence of "negative addiction": When deprived of their daily exercise, they have reported what might be considered withdrawal symptoms—irritability, tension, restlessness, and anxiety.[7] Yet most people who begin a regular exercise program report that they sleep better, work more efficiently, have more energy, and feel more relaxed and self-confident. As an additional benefit, regular exercisers are often motivated to stop smoking and to eat more healthful diets, producing not only physiological benefits but also a rise in self-esteem.[8]

CONCEPTS IN FITNESS

When a fitness expert measures your overall level of fitness, he or she looks for four qualities:

1. Muscular **strength**—how much force can your muscles generate?
2. Muscular **endurance**—how many times can your muscles contract against a moderate force?
3. **Flexibility**—how freely can you stretch your muscles, bones, tendons, and ligaments?
4. **Cardiorespiratory endurance**—how well do your heart, lungs, and blood vessels function to enable you to mobilize your body's energy and sustain movement over a period of time?

All four of these elements are linked; a certain amount of strength is necessary, for example, to develop cardiorespiratory endurance. But it is possible for your body to exhibit one or more of these qualities without exhibiting all four. Some people can lift heavy barbells, for example, but cannot jog for more than ten minutes without getting "winded."[9]

If fitness experts were planning a training program for you, they would bear in mind the concept of **specificity:** The activity you select to build one of the above four elements of fitness must be specific to your goal. For example, if your goal is to develop strength in your biceps, you will need to do arm curls with barbells or some other biceps exercise in a flexed position. But if you want to develop or increase your cardiorespiratory endurance, you must select an activity that offers continuous, rhythmic exercise, such as jogging or swimming. Jogging won't help you develop flexibility or bicep strength, but it will improve the condition of your heart and lungs.

Fitness experts also work with the concept of **overload,** subjecting muscles to a greater than normal load to increase their size and strength. Systematic and progressive overloading can increase muscle strength, flexibility, and cardiorespiratory endurance. Once the muscles adapt to the overload, an additional increase in the load is necessary for further improvement.

For example, let's say you begin training with weights, doing arm curls at a forty-pound weight load. After you arrived at the point where you can do three sets of six repetitions easily at forty pounds, you would add five to ten pounds at your next session. Or perhaps you have taken up jogging; in that case, once you were able to run two miles in twenty minutes easily, you would increase the distance you're trying to cover by one-third to one-half of a mile if you wanted to continue improving your cardiorespiratory endurance.

Developing Muscular Strength

As we have noted, strength is the amount of force a muscle can generate. Your muscles develop strength when they are overloaded by being systematically and progressively subjected to a greater than normal load. Generally, you do not overload muscle groups heavily enough and regularly enough to improve muscle strength through such normal everyday activities as carrying bags of groceries or climbing stairs. Rather, you must engage in one of three scientifically developed methods: isokinetic, isotonic, or isometric training programs.

ISOKINETIC PROGRAMS

Isokinetic programs are a fairly new development in strength training. They rely on specialized apparatus, such as Nautilus and Universal gym equipment, that provides maximum resistance throughout a range of motion. The resistance is exactly equal to the force that the user applies. Today, many experts believe these programs work best for developing muscle strength: Properly used, equipment such as the Nautilus machines provides a highly effective way of building strength, giving the body the benefits of both isotonics and isometrics (which we'll discuss below). There is a problem with isokinetic training programs, however: They require special machinery that is normally available only at health clubs and gyms. Unfortunately, not everyone has access to such equipment.

ISOTONIC PROGRAMS

Another good way to develop muscle strength is through **isotonic** programs, such as weight training. Isotonic exercise involves muscle contractions: The muscle shortens, as when lifting a heavy object. By using weights properly, you can increase the strength and endurance of your muscles. Progressive resistance programs are another form of isotonic exercise. Such programs overload muscles through a complete range of motion. These increase flexibility as well as strength and endurance.

ISOMETRIC PROGRAMS

Least useful, experts now think, are **isometric** programs, in which the individual pushes or pulls against a fixed resistance or an immovable object. It was once believed that isometric programs might be superior to isokinetic programs. Today,

however, most experts agree that isometric programs have drawbacks: They seem to increase muscle strength over a narrower range of movement than isotonic exercises do.

WHERE TO FIND OUT MORE

Most people who want to develop muscle strength should do some weight training. A complete description of a typical beginner's weight-training program is beyond the scope of this chapter, but if you are interested, you should consider reading a book on the subject or consulting a qualified instructor. Note, too, that while weight training is not vigorous or sustained enough to produce cardiorespiratory fitness, it is a good supplement to a jogging or swimming program.

Developing Muscular Endurance

The term *muscular endurance* refers to the number of times a muscle can contract against a moderate force. Stated another way, it is the degree of prolonged and repetitive exertion of which you are capable. Many daily activities—washing windows, shoveling snow, using a hand saw, even vacuuming—require a certain degree of muscular endurance.

Properly designed weight-training programs build muscular endurance as well as strength. However, if your goal is to emphasize muscular endurance development over strength, note that you should do a relatively large number of repetitions ("reps") of each exercise, using a low to moderate load. If you are training for strength, however, you will need to do a relatively small number of "reps"—with a heavier load.

Developing Flexibility

As we have noted, flexibility is the condition of muscles, bones, tendons, and ligaments that permits full range of movement in a joint. A person may be flexible in some joints but not others. There may even be large differences in flexibility between the same joints on opposite sides of the body; many people, for instance, have a greater range of movement in one shoulder than the other. It's important to try to stay flexible: Immobilization or restricted movement of a limb or joint often leads to reduced flexibility and may give rise to postural or orthopedic problems.

How flexible are you? Try touching your toes with your feet placed together on the floor. If the muscles along the backs of your thighs feel tight, you should probably do some work in this area. You can maintain your flexibility if you do periodic bending and stretching exercises. Stretching is an especially important injury-preventive measure for those who do vigorous exercises, particularly runners. Stretching exercises such as the Achilles tendon stretcher, the hamstring stretcher, and the low-back stretcher (see Figure 15.1) warm up the muscles and make them better able to withstand the stress of strenuous exercises. Stretching exercises are also recommended after running. They ease the muscular tightness that may result from exertion.

One important point about flexibility exercises: To avoid injury, *do not* bounce or move jerkily from one position to another. (Forget what you may have done in a dance or calisthenics class long ago.) *Slowly* move to the stretched position and hold that position for 10 seconds.

Developing Cardiorespiratory Endurance

As we have noted, cardiorespiratory endurance is the quality that enables you to mobilize energy and sustain movement over an extended period of time. It requires your heart, lungs, and blood vessels to function efficiently. Since your life depends on the capacity of these organs to deliver nutrients and oxygen to your tissues and remove wastes, cardiorespiratory endurance is the most essential component of physical fitness. It is normally achieved through sustained exercise of the whole body—the kind of exercise you get from running, bicycling, swimming, cross-country skiing, and aerobic dancing. Exercise of this type uses the large muscles and puts the major joints through a wide range of motion.

An exercise program aimed at developing cardiorespiratory endurance must be tailored to the individual: Some people must start at a lower level and progress more slowly than others. Yet the basic principles of developing cardiorespiratory endurance are the same for everyone, and any person who regularly exercises vigorously enough will, in time, see improvements in endurance. Compared with an unfit person, the fit individual is leaner, is stronger for his or her body size, has better blood circulation, has more energy, and recovers more quickly after exercise.[10] Endurance conditioning also helps develop cardiovascular fitness, which some scientists believe may be a defense against heart and blood-vessel diseases (see Chapter 12).

Vigorous swimming—not just dog-paddling or playing in the pool—is an excellent aerobic exercise, helping to develop cardio-respiratory endurance. (©Harvey Stein)

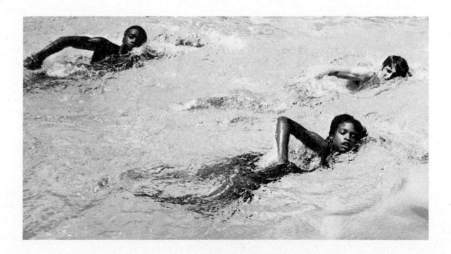

Achilles Tendon Stretcher

Stand an arm's length from the wall, knees straight, toes pointed inward slightly, heels flat on the floor. Rest your hands on the wall and bend your elbows slowly to let your body lean forward, keeping legs and body straight and heels on the floor. Push back to starting position. Repeat 3 to 5 times.

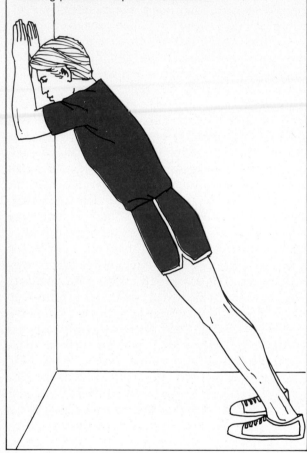

Hamstring Stretcher

Sit on the floor with knees extended and legs spread at a 45-degree angle. Bend forward slowly at the waist. Grasp one ankle with both hands and try to touch your head to your knee. Stop when you feel stretching pain in the back of the leg and hold for two or three seconds, then return to starting position. Alternate, repeating 3 to 5 times for each leg.

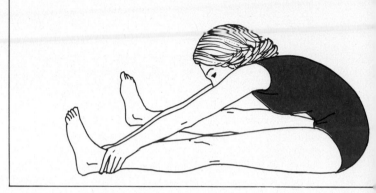

Figure 15.1   Stretching exercises like these are recommended for warming up the muscles before strenuous exercise and for easing them afterward.

Low-Back Stretcher

Lie on your back, knees straight. Grasp one leg just below the knee and pull the knee toward your chest, at the same time curling your head and shoulders toward the knee. Hold for three or four seconds, then return to starting position. Alternate, repeating 4 to 6 times for each leg.

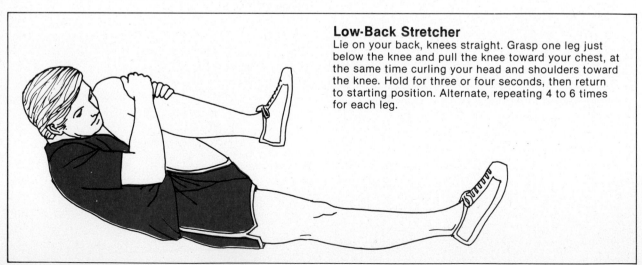

"AEROBICS"

"Aerobics," a major concept in cardiorespiratory endurance exercise, involves an approach developed by the physician Kenneth H. Cooper, who conducted major research projects in adult fitness for the United States Air Force. **Aerobic exercise** means "exercise with oxygen." To understand this concept, remember that as the body exercises, its oxygen needs increase. Aerobic exercise is sustained exercise at a level that allows the body to meet its oxygen needs continually. Some examples are vigorous walking, running, jumping rope, bicycling, swimming, and cross-country skiing. Exercise that causes the body's demand for oxygen to exceed the supply—producing "oxygen debt"—is termed **anaerobic.** An example of anaerobic exercise is sprinting 100 meters: The runner goes so fast that he or she can replace only part of the oxygen the body uses during the sprint itself and has to make up for the oxygen debt afterward.

During *anaerobic* exercise, energy-rich substances (adenosine triphosphate and creatine phosphate) stored in the muscle cells are broken down. Eventually, the supply of these substances starts to run low; the muscle grows tired and is unable to continue working. During *aerobic* exercise, in contrast, the body gets enough oxygen to continually replenish its supply of these substances. Cooper's studies and others have shown that continuous, rhythmic aerobic exercise of sufficient duration and intensity is the only effective way to promote cardiorespiratory fitness.[11]

THE EFFECTS OF CARDIORESPIRATORY ENDURANCE EXERCISE ON THE BODY

Exactly how does cardiorespiratory endurance exercise improve your physical health? First, it makes your heart, lungs, and blood vessels work hard. Your body responds by adapting; that is, it becomes able to accommodate future training demands with less or no stress. In time, the muscles involved develop a more extensive network of blood vessels, so that your blood has more available routes for oxygen transport. The body develops more red blood cells (which carry oxygen) and a greater volume of blood. Furthermore, is typically an increase in the amount of air the lungs can take in and breathe out at one time (the vital capacity) and an increase in the amount of air the lungs can take in over a period of time (the maxi-

mum breathing capacity). And the exchange of oxygen and carbon dioxide in the tiny chambers (alveoli) of the lungs becomes more efficient.[12]

EFFECTS ON THE HEART   With training, your heart becomes stronger and more efficient. Though the heart does not increase much in actual size, it pumps an increased amount of blood on each beat and is emptied more completely each time. Between beats, it can slow down and rest more: The normal adult resting pulse rate is around seventy beats per minute, and eighty to ninety beats is not unusual in sedentary individuals. In contrast, the physically fit adult usually has resting pulse rates of only fifty-five to sixty beats per minute. (The pulse may be even lower sometimes: In trained athletes, such as runners, it is not unusual to see rates of forty beats per minute.) Consequently, the heart makes thousands fewer beats per day, which reduces wear and tear on heart valves and blood vessels.

OTHER EFFECTS   Endurance exercise may also reduce some forms of hypertension (high blood pressure): It tends to relax the tiny arteries (arterioles) that work much like nozzles in controlling blood pressure. Further, experts believe that endurance exercise increases the ratio of high-density lipoprotein (HDL) to low-density lipoprotein (LDL) in the blood: Higher ratios of HDL to LDL are associated with a lower risk of heart disease.[13]

Last but not least, endurance exercise burns calories, thus contributing to weight control. Research shows that in typical adult conditioning programs—involving twenty-minute sessions three days a week—partially trained participants expending energy at about 400 calories per session can lose about seventeen pounds a year if their calorie intake remains constant.[14]

PLANNING FOR FITNESS

When it comes to exercise, Americans often seem to do either too much or too little. They will play football all Saturday afternoon and then get no exercise for the rest of the week. What is essential for lifetime fitness is regular vigorous exercise involving the whole body, in a program that's tailored to the individual.

What sort of exercise should you include in your fitness program? That depends on your specific needs. Exercise serves many purposes. The professional golfer might take up weight training to increase arm and upper-body strength so that she can put more speed into her golf swing and consequently gain distance. A middle-aged executive might perform a series of exercises specially designed to improve back flexibility in order to relieve chronic low-back pain. A college student who wants to improve his health and manage stress more effectively could begin a jogging program. Some people simply need a minimal, though scientifically based, exercise plan—one we might call a "fitness for health" plan.

A "fitness for health" plan suits the individual who has no interest in becoming a marathon runner or a world-class athlete. Often, such an individual may not even enjoy exercising, but wants the health benefits that can be derived from the program—cardiorespiratory endurance, muscular strength and endurance, flexibility, improved body composition (more muscle, less fat), relaxation, and improved emotional health. Men and women who are fit have greater ability to work and play and are less likely to injure joints or muscles through "overexertion."

Other people need a more ambitious plan—we might call it "fitness for its own sake" or "fitness for high-level performance." A "fitness for performance" plan is geared to the individual who wants to improve his or her skill in a specific sport or activity. A football player, for example, will follow a program of training with weights or other strength-training equipment; he will also engage in agility and cardiovascular activities to improve his speed, strength, and endurance on the field. A gymnast will train with weights to gain strength to improve her performance on the uneven bars and in floor exercises. Some of the performance-related benefits of exercise are the same as the health-related benefits—improvements in cardiorespiratory endurance, muscular strength and endurance, flexibility, and body composition. But a performance-oriented plan will also help develop agility, speed, and coordination and can help refine a specific athletic skill. We will not discuss the components of a "fitness for performance" exercise program here, but if you are interested, you may want to seek guidance from a qualified trainer or coach.

Your Exercise Plan

When you are designing a "fitness for health" plan, your primary emphasis should be on devel-

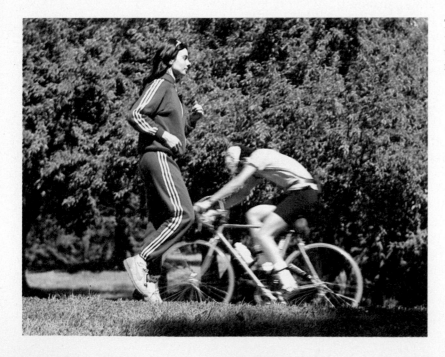

The individual can choose from a wide variety of exercise activities to match his or her interests, needs, and abilities. (©Ken Karp)

oping cardiorespiratory endurance. But you should also include activities that improve muscular strength, muscular endurance, and flexibility. A very basic and minimal "fitness for health" plan would include the following:

1. An activity that can improve your cardiorespiratory endurance (jogging, walking, cycling, swimming). You should engage in it at least three times a week for at least twenty minutes per session, at 75 percent of your maximum heart rate. (We will explain the concept of maximum heart rate later in this chapter.) If you choose walking or cycling, you will need to put in more than twenty minutes per session, say forty to sixty minutes, since these activities are not as demanding as jogging.
2. Bent-knee sit-ups and push-ups, at least three times a week.
3. Basic flexibility exercises for legs, back, and shoulders, at least three times a week.

If you don't have access to an exercise physiologist or other qualified physical educators who can help you design your fitness program, you can design your own program by following some fairly simple guidelines. And if you design your own program, or at least have some say in designing it, you will be more likely to keep up your efforts because you have chosen an activity you enjoy. For best results, you need a planned program that lets you see progress. A sample "fitness for health" exercise program is described in the box on page 371. The details of such a program are discussed below.

START WITH A MEDICAL OK

It is wise to obtain medical clearance for beginning a fitness program, especially if you are inactive, over thirty-five, or under thirty-five and have suspected or documented coronary artery disease or significant risk factors. A number of medical conditions can be aggravated by physical exertion, and the possibility of such conditions should be ruled out by a medical examination and an exercise stress test before the endurance program begins. It is also a good idea to set up a tentative plan for your fitness program and show it to a doctor who is familiar with your physical condition and medical history.

Some colleges and universities have set up "human performance laboratories" that are equipped to conduct exercise tolerance tests using a piece of equipment known as a treadmill. You might find out whether your campus has such a facility, staffed by an exercise physiologist who will give you the graded treadmill test.

FINDING YOUR CURRENT FITNESS LEVEL

The next step is to find your current fitness level. You can do this by means of a simple test. All you need is a running track or other measured surface.

Here's what to do: After five to ten minutes of warm-up exercises, start running along the track. Note your starting time on a watch with a second hand. Run as fast as you can for 2.0 miles (men) or 1.5 miles (women). (Pause and walk for a while if you get out of breath.) Then compare your time with the figures given in the "Cardiorespiratory Endurance" section of the self-assessment activity on pages 373–374. This will tell you the level at which you should *begin* your fitness training. Later, as your fitness improves, you can add to your pace or distance and increase the total time of your workouts.

CHOOSING YOUR ACTIVITY

For best results, you should plan your training around an exercise that involves vigorous, continuous whole-body movement. Possibilities include jogging, swimming, walking, hiking, skating, bicycling, rowing, cross-country skiing—even rope skipping, trampolining, and aerobic dance. The activity you choose should be one you enjoy: As one writer put it, "Not everyone wants to jog, not everyone can jog, and furthermore, not everyone *should* jog!"[15] Generally, if you enjoy something, you'll do it; if you don't, you won't.

Whatever the activity, it must be strenuous enough to tax your body. If it is too easy, it will not produce a conditioning effect. If you go out for bowling, golf, softball, or backyard badminton, you won't be expending enough continuous effort to build your cardiorespiratory endurance. Highly competitive sports are undesirable: Many are an-

A Sample "Fitness for Health" Exercise Program

It is easy to design a safe, effective, and enjoyable fitness program that is tailored to your needs. As an example of how an effective program might work, suppose that José Sanchez, twenty-year-old man in good health, decides to embark on a "fitness for health" program. First, he identifies his current fitness level by completing the 2.0-mile test (see the norms for 1.5- and 2.0-mile runs given in the self-assessment activity on pages 000–000.) He covers the 2.0 miles in 17:49 minutes, which puts him in the "fair" category. He sets his goal to reach the "good" category by the end of four months and the "excellent" category by one year.

Next, José selects an aerobic activity that he believes he will enjoy enough to make it a lifetime pursuit. He decides to begin with a jog-walk program and then to move on to a jogging program as his cardiorespiratory fitness improves.

José engages in his fitness program three days a week. In order to maintain flexibility and avoid stiffness, he precedes each jogging workout with ten minutes or so of bending and stretching all limbs and joints through their full range of motion. Since he has selected jogging, he focuses on the hamstring muscles at the backs of his legs. He also does push-ups and bent-knee sit-ups to develop muscular strength and endurance. Once the warm-up is complete, José begins his jog-walk conditioning. He begins with sixty seconds of jogging, followed by thirty seconds of brisk walking. He continues alternating sixty seconds of jogging with thirty seconds of brisk walking for a period of twenty minutes.

The key to an individualized program is to establish the work load you can safely handle, as measured by your targeted exercise heart rate. José computes his exercise heart rate to be 155 ($180 - 80 = 100 \times 0.75 = 75$; he adds 75 to his resting pulse, which is 80 beats per minute, and gets 155). The alternating sixty-thirty jog-walk program he is engaged in results in an exercise heart rate of 155 beats per minute, at least for the time being.

Over the first month of his program, José builds up to jogging for four minutes, alternating with a one-minute brisk walk, for three miles. During that month, he has constantly monitored his exercise heart rate; whenever he has found that it was below the target level of 155 beats per minute, he has gradually increased his work load. As a result, his physiological condition has improved: He has made progress on the road to fitness.

Over the next two months José gradually adds to his pace and distance until he is able to jog continuously for twenty to thirty minutes for a distance of two to four miles. He has improved in all the complex physiological procedures involved in his exercise activity. He feels more vigorous and alive, and he feels better about himself in general.

Following each exercise bout, José cools down properly: For five to ten minutes after his vigorous workout, he keeps moving and continues his activity, but at a lower level of intensity (he slows down and walks). He knows that if he doesn't cool down, he runs the risk of passing out: Blood will pool in his arms and legs, meaning that there will be insufficient blood for other organs of the body, including the brain.

---

aerobic and require quick bursts of energy and sudden movement. (This is why professional baseball and football players must also train by doing aerobic exercises such as running and vigorous calisthenics.) The highly competitive sports are also more likely to result in injury for the untrained person.

The potential for injury is another factor you will want to consider in selecting an aerobic activity. "Any aerobic activity, too vigorously undertaken by a novice, may present dangers."[16] According to the American College of Sports Medicine (ACSM), endurance activities that require running and jumping generally cause more debilitating injuries—especially to the feet, legs, and knees—than do non-weight-bearing activities such as cycling or swimming.[17] If you're a begin-ning exerciser, especially if you already have orthopedic problems, you should use caution in selecting an activity.

Other considerations are the intensity with which you will have to do the sport, and the length of time you will need per session, in order to produce a conditioning effect. Each time you exercise, you should aim for the same level of intensity (your "exercise heart rate"—a concept we discuss below). Jogging, for example, is a more intense activity than cycling, so if you are exercising with a bicycle, you must pedal twice as long and twice as fast as you would have to run if you were jogging to achieve the same level of conditioning. That is because a session of about forty minutes of cycling is required for an adequate workout (as opposed to a twenty-minute session of jogging).

ACTIVITY: EXPLORING HEALTH

How Fit Are You? A Self-Assessment

This activity is intended to help you evaluate your level of physical fitness. After completing this assessment, you'll have an insight into your strengths and weaknesses and a basis for setting your personal fitness goal. The tests in the assessment represent major areas of physical fitness—flexibility, strength, and endurance.

MUSCULAR STRENGTH AND ENDURANCE

There is a close relationship between your muscular strength and endurance and your overall physical fitness. This test will allow you to evaluate the level of your muscular strength and endurance.

Bent-knee sit-ups. Purpose: To assess the strength and endurance of your abdominal muscles. Directions: Lie down on your back and interlock your hands behind your neck. Draw your feet toward your buttocks until your knees are bent at about a 90 degree angle. Your feet should be flat on the floor. Have a partner hold your feet on the floor by grasping your ankles. A full sit-up is counted when you have curled your back and raised your trunk until it is perpendicular with the floor, and then returned to the starting position. Your hands must be interlocked for the sit-up to count. Do as many sit-ups as you can in two minutes if you are a male, or one minute if you are a female. Resting is permitted.

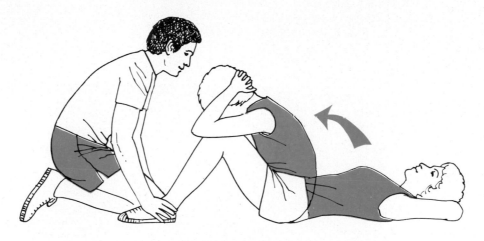

SCORING SIT-UPS

FITNESS CATEGORY	MEN		WOMEN	
	T-score	Raw Score	T-score	Raw Score
Super	80	91	80	45
	70	79	70	38
Good	60	67	60	31
Average	50	56	50	24
Fair	40	44	40	17
Poor	30	32	30	10
Very Poor	20		20	3

Your raw score is the number of sit-ups completed in the prescribed time to determine your muscular strength category. Compare your raw score with the corresponding T-score, which is a standardized score ranging from a high of 80 to a low of 20. Next, find the fitness category that corresponds to your T-score. You may not find a raw score on the chart that contains the exact number of sit-ups you completed, but this should give you a rough estimate of your abdominal strength and endurance.

FLEXIBILITY

Flexibility refers to the ability to use a muscle through its full range of motion. Sedentary living leads to a shortening of the muscles. This test will allow you to evaluate the flexibility of two major muscle groups.

Trunk flexion. Purpose: To assess the ability of your back muscles and back thigh muscles to stretch. Directions: Sit with your legs fully extended and the bottoms of your feet against a box projecting from the wall. Extend your arms and hands forward as far as you can. Hold for a count of three. Using a ruler, measure the distance that you can reach before or beyond the edge of the box. Distances before the edge are recorded in negative scores (−); distances beyond the edge are recorded in positive scores (+).

SCORING TRUNK FLEXION

	MEN	WOMEN
Normal range	−6 to +8 inches	−4 to +10 inches
Average	+1 inch	+2 inches
Desired range	+1 to +5 inches	+2 to +6 inches

CARDIORESPIRATORY ENDURANCE

To measure cardiorespiratory endurance and health, several tests have been devised which rely on vigorous, sustained physical movement. Here is one of them: the 1.5- or 2-mile run.

1.5- or 2-mile run. Below are five fitness classifications. To figure out which one you belong in, find the time it takes you to run a 1.5-mile distance (for women), or a 2-mile distance (for men).

SCORING 1.5- or 2-MILE RUN

FITNESS CATEGORY	1.5 MILES (WOMEN)	2 MILES (MEN)
Super	Faster than 11 min., 30 sec.	Faster than 12 min.
Excellent	11:30 to 12:59	12:00 to 13:59
Good	13:00 to 14:29	14:00 to 15:59
Fair	14:30 to 15:59	16:00 to 17:59
Poor	16:00 or slower	18:00 or slower

Source: Bud Getchell, *Physical Fitness: A Way of Life* (New York: Wiley, 1979).

Swimming for conditioning requires approximately a thirty-minute session if you swim vigorously. So, which sport you choose may depend in part on how much time you want to allot to each exercise session. Not everyone has time for a forty-minute cycling session three times a week.

HOW OFTEN SHOULD YOU EXERCISE?

Researchers have found that exercising at least three days a week provides the greatest cardiorespiratory benefits. Exercising two days a week or less is not adequate. And if more than two days pass between exercise sessions, "detraining" begins—you start to lose the good effects of earlier sessions. For this reason, the ACSM has recommended that people embarking on a training program exercise three to five days a week to achieve the greatest cardiorespiratory benefit.[18]

Will you progress faster if you exercise more than five days a week? The value of so intense a program for the nonathlete has not been documented.

HOW LONG SHOULD YOU EXERCISE IN EACH SESSION?

The ACSM recommends twenty- to sixty-minute sessions of continuous aerobic activity. As we have noted, the duration depends on the intensity of the activity. With higher-intensity activities such as moderate jogging or swimming, you can achieve a training effect in as short a time as twenty or thirty minutes. With activities of lower intensity, such as walking and bicycling, longer sessions are needed. (See Table 15.2.)

In general, nonathletic adults are advised to choose activities of low to moderate intensity and to work out longer. But any activity that uses large muscle groups and that can be maintained continuously may be chosen.

HOW INTENSELY SHOULD YOU EXERCISE DURING EACH SESSION?

The ACSM recommends that normal, healthy adults exercise at a rate known as the "target heart rate" or "exercise heart rate." Your pulse should not exceed the exercise heart rate during your session; you can determine the level of intensity you are reaching by checking your heart rate during exercise.

TABLE 15.2 · **Time, Pace, and Distance Needed per Session to Benefit from Various Aerobic Activities**

Activity	Pace	Time	Distance
Jogging	60–90 sec. over 220 yds.	20–30 min.	2–4 miles
Bicycling	30–60 sec. over 220 yds., 12–15 mph	40–60 min.	10–20 miles
Swimming	30–40 sec. for one 25-yd. length	30–40 min.	400–1600 yds.
Walking	Steady, brisk pace	45–60 min.	4 miles

HOW TO TAKE YOUR OWN PULSE

Place the tips of your fingers on the inside of your wrist or on the side of your neck. Feel the throbbing? Once you've located the pulse, count the number of beats per minute, using a watch with a second hand. Or count the number of beats in ten seconds and multiply by six.

The exercise heart rate should be somewhere between 60 and 90 percent of the difference between your resting heart rate and your "maximum heart rate" or "training rate" (a measure of physiological stress on the body). Most young people have a maximum heart rate of somewhere between 180 and 200 beats per minute. A typical resting pulse for a young person might be around 80 beats per minute; so the *difference* between a hypothetical young person's maximum heart rate and resting heart rate might be 200 − 80, or 120 beats per minute. Sixty percent of this difference would be .60 × 120, or 72. When we add this to the resting heart rate, we get 80 + 72, or 152 beats per minute; this is the *lowest* intensity at which this young person should exercise in order to gain benefits from his or her fitness program. Ninety percent of the difference would be .90 × 120, or 108. When we add this to the resting heart rate, we get 80 + 108, or 188 beats per minute; this is the *highest* intensity at which this young person should exercise in order to benefit.

Research has found that the best intensity for most people is 75 percent of the difference between resting heart rate and maximum heart rate. For this young person, 75 percent of the difference would be .75 × 120, or 90. So the best intensity at which to exercise would be 80 + 90, or 170 beats per minute. Then, as the individual gradually progresses, it may be possible to raise the exercise heart rate; many conditioned people can work out safely at a level of 85 percent of the difference between resting heart rate and maximum heart rate. Remember, whatever activity you do must be done at a level (usually a speed) that is sufficiently strenuous or demanding to produce the conditioning effect, systematically overloading your muscles and other body systems as we described earlier. Most fitness experts recommend that beginners start with a program that combines jogging and walking: With this type of activity, you can easily establish a safe, reasonable intensity level.

YOUR ORDER OF BUSINESS IN EACH SESSION

You should begin each session with about ten minutes of warm-up stretching exercises. This warm-up will help you avoid cramps, sprains, and other problems and injuries.

After your warm-up, do your chosen activity for no less than twenty and no more than sixty minutes. Then repeat your stretching exercises, or spend at least five minutes in continuous movement—walking around, for example, or swimming slowly. This cool-down period is important; it helps your body return to normal gradually. If you neglect the cool-down period, you may find yourself feeling faint.

GUARDING AGAINST INJURIES AND SORENESS

The last thing you want to do in a fitness program is to hurt yourself. The beginning of an exercise program is particularly hazardous, since your body is not used to the new demands you are placing on it. Start slowly. Don't try to make up for years of neglect in a single exercise session. *Al-*

ways warm up adequately with stretching exercises.

Sore muscles are a symptom of overexertion. Some soreness is almost inevitable when you start using muscles that have not been used recently. Again, the best way to minimize soreness is to start slowly, increase your effort gradually, and do stretching exercises that will gently work out any kinks that develop.

Soreness usually comes on gradually and—unless you've really overdone it—is fairly mild. Pain, which may be sudden and severe, is something else again.

Pain is always a signal to stop. Your body is telling you that something is wrong, and you should try to figure out what it is. If you have

A brief warmup before each exercise session is essential to avoid injury and soreness. (©Larry Lawfer/The Picture Cube)

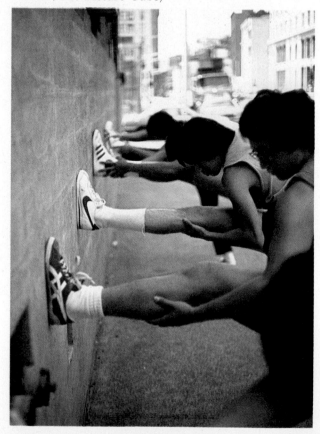

repeated problems with pain, especially in the chest, see your doctor.

Also, be sure to avoid getting exhausted. If you're very fatigued for an hour or more after your workout, your program is too demanding. Your exercise should leave you feeling relaxed and comfortable—not totally drained.

Equipment

First let us note: it is wise to be suspicious of fitness fads, which come and go with regularity. Not surprisingly, our consumer-oriented culture has developed a range of fitness gadgets and devices; these may be useful, but they are certainly not essential. Weights, springs, and other devices for increasing resistance help build strength beyond minimum levels, but they have little use in developing cardiorespiratory endurance. Exercise bicycles and minitrampolines do help develop cardiorespiratory endurance, but jogging is just as helpful—and it requires a relatively small financial outlay.

Depending on the activity you choose, you may need to buy a few pieces of equipment and special footwear and clothing. As you shop, remember to think of safety and comfort first, not stylishness: Exercise doesn't require a designer wardrobe.

For runners, the most obvious necessity is a good pair of shoes. To economize here is to invite blisters and other injuries to your feet, your legs, and possibly your back. Don't buy bargain-basement or discount-store tennis shoes to run in. Go to a good sporting-goods store and have yourself fitted by someone who has a good knowledge of footwear and of running. Make sure the shoes feel good on your feet; try on several pairs made by different manufacturers. As you will see when you look over the many kinds of shoes on display, other sports such as tennis, basketball, and hiking call for specially designed shoes as well.

Good running shoes should allow your toes plenty of movement; they should support your feet adequately and should have enough padding to protect your feet when they strike against pavement.

As for clothing, if you are a swimmer, all you need is a comfortable suit that fits without binding. For running and most other exercise, choose lightweight T-shirts, sweatshirts, shorts, or sweatpants. The fit should be loose, so you can move around comfortably, and the garment(s) should preferably be made of cotton (cotton "breathes" better than synthetic materials such as nylon, allowing perspiration to evaporate.) Rubberized suits, sometimes sold as weight-reduction devices, should be avoided: They can cause your body to overheat. For proper support during strenuous movement, men need an athletic supporter and women a comfortable bra. In cold weather, an extra sweatshirt or jacket, a hat, and gloves may be needed for comfort and prevention of frostbite.

When and Where to Exercise

Running on busy streets is dangerous. Cars may not see you, or the right-of-way may be so narrow that a driver cannot dodge you and an oncoming car as well. Worse, some drivers may be daydreaming or drunk and may not be on the alert for you. To avoid being hit, choose quiet streets or run on the sidewalk. Better yet, run in a park that has an even, grassy surface; this will minimize the likelihood of foot, leg, and back injuries, and will cut down on the amount of exhaust fumes you inhale. If you work out after dark, wear light-colored clothing or a reflective garment designed for running at night.

The time of day you choose to exercise depends on your schedule; no one particular time is best. Some people like to do their exercises early in the day; others find that jogging or biking at the end of the work or school day serves as a relaxing change of pace.

Very hot or very cold weather sometimes poses a problem. Humidity may reduce the body's normal ability to dispel heat; on an extremely humid day, body temperature may rise much more than normal, resulting in heat stroke. But you can exercise regardless of the weather if you use common

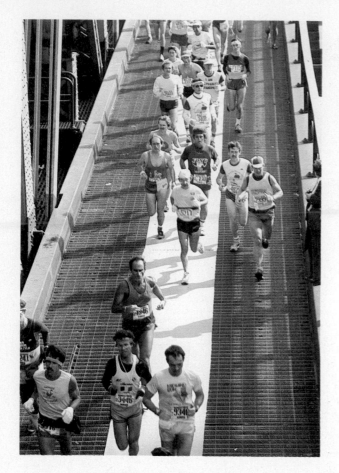

sense. When it is cold, you usually need do no more than protect yourself with extra clothing. If streets and sidewalks are icy, switch to an indoor track or gym, or do calisthenics or jump rope at home. In hot, humid weather, you may be able to keep up with your jogging or cycling by exercising very early in the morning, when it is coolest. Another alternative is swimming, which is especially pleasant in the heat.

One point to remember: Always drink lots of water to replace body fluids you have lost through sweating.

The thousands of people who participate in marathon races each year attest to the popularity of running as an exercise program. (©Birgit Pohl 1982)

MAKING HEALTH DECISIONS

Deciding for Physical Fitness

People who engage in exercise conditioning programs on a regular basis have reasons for doing so. And their goals for exercising regularly are different; they view the benefits of being in good shape differently. Some exercise simply to achieve a minimum level of fitness. Others exercise because it is fun: They enjoy exercise for its own sake, and seek higher levels of achievement. Other people choose *not* to engage in a reguular exercise or conditioning program. They too have their reasons. Some say it's boring; others say they get enough exercise in their daily work.

Exercise is actually the cheapest form of preventive medicine available. Some also find it the most enjoyable form; others don't. This activity is designed to help you explore the reasons why you do or do not regularly engage in a vigorous exercise program.

I. SOME PRELIMINARY QUESTIONS

1. Do you feel that you get enough exercise?

_____Yes   _____ No

2. Do you now exercise on a regular basis? (If your answer is no, answer questions a to d below and then skip to question 8.)

_____Yes   _____ No

Whether or not you are already engaging in an exercise program, if you answer yes to the following questions, insufficient exercise is beginning to show its effect on you.

a. Have you experienced an increase in body fat over the past few years? Having to wear a larger clothes size is one indication; so is the "pinch test" described in Chapter 14.

b. Do you have a loss of muscle tone? Muscle trembling or spasms following or during demanding exercise is one sign.

c. Has your breathing capacity lessened? Does walking briskly up a flight of stairs leave you panting?

d. Do normal day-to-day activities leave you fatigued at the end of the day?

3. How often do you exercise on a weekly basis?

_____ 1 time per week

_____ 2 times per week

_____ 3 times per week

_____ 4 times or more per week

4. When you do exercise, for how long a time (in minutes) do you exercise per session?

_____ 15 minutes

_____ 20–30 minutes

_____ 30–45 minutes

_____ 1 hour or longer

5. Which of the following exercises are you now doing?

_____ Walking   _____ Jogging

_____ Bicycling   _____ Calisthenics

_____ Swimming   _____ Weight training

Interpretation

If you are exercising only once a week, you should increase the frequency to three times a week. Research has shown that "detraining" occurs when more than forty-eight hours pass between exercise sessions.

If you are only exercising for fifteen minutes at each exercise session, you should gradually in-crease the duration of your exercise bouts to at least thirty minutes, and perhaps eventually up to sixty minutes, depending on the level of fitness you have established as your goal.

If you are only engaging in calisthenics or weight training, you should consider adding an aerobic activity such as swimming or jogging to your conditioning program. Calisthenics and weight training do little to improve your cardio-vascular fitness; aerobic activity is the most helpful form of adult exercise.

II. QUESTIONS ABOUT YOUR MOTIVATION

6. Do you enjoy exercising or the benefits you derive from exercising?

_____ Yes   _____ No

7. Of the following benefits, which do you enjoy the most, or which are most important to you? Rank the items in order of priority.

_____ Weight control

_____ Improved body appearance

_____ Tension release/stress management

_____ Cardiovascular health benefits

_____ Increased energy levels

_____ Enhanced capacity to enjoy life

_____ Better sleep

_____ A sense of power and improved self-worth

_____ Social contacts it makes available

_____ Sheer fun

_____ Success and achievement through competing against myself for self-improvement

8. If you are not engaging in a conditioning or exercise program, why don't you? Select the three most important reasons from the list below.

_____ I lack time.

_____ I lack money.

_____ I lack someone to exercise with.

_____Exercise is boring.

_____It hurts, and it's too demanding to get in shape.

_____I get enough exercise from my daily work to be in shape.

_____My past experience with exercise was bad (ridicule/embarrassment or punishment in P.E. classes)

_____Females only: It's unfeminine because it will result in bulging muscles.

_____I don't need it for weight control, stress management, or improved energy levels.

_____Exercise won't improve my health or capacity to enjoy life.

_____None of my friends are fitness freaks.

_____I just don't enjoy it.

_____I just can't seem to get in the habit of exercising regularly.

Interpretation

Lack of time: The time required for a basic conditioning program is only about one and a half to three hours per week—not a huge time investment by any standard. Besides, some people believe that if you don't take time for health now, you'll have to take time for sickness later!

Lack of money: Most conditioning programs don't require a big financial outlay. Jogging requires only a good pair of shoes, at a cost of about $40 to $50. Brisk walking is even less expensive. Swimming requires only that you own a swimsuit. You could begin a conditioning program that incorporates any of these activities for less than the cost of a pair of designer jeans!

None of my friends are fitness freaks: Keep your non-fitness-freak friends for socializing, and make some new friends who do like to exercise. Sign up for a physical conditioning class at your school or a local YMCA or YWCA—or join a cycling club. You'll meet some people who are turned on to fitness.

I get enough exercise in my daily work: Unless you are a postal worker who hand-carries and delivers mail from house to house each day on foot or by bicycle—or work at some similar job that gives you a comparable amount of exercise—it's very unlikely that your daily work provides you with sufficient activity for cardiovascular health and fitness.

It will result in bulging muscles: Exercise will not result in bulging muscles in women. This is a common misconception that has been refuted through scientific research. However, women who exercise will find themselves firming up and developing a lower ratio of fat to muscle. What could be more desirable than improved body composition?

III. MAKING YOUR DECISION

1. List your reasons for not starting a regular exercise program or for not continuing it. (Refer to question 8.)_____

_____

_____

_____

2. Now, identify three ways in which you can overcome these blocks to enjoying stimulating exercise and improved cardiovascular health.

_____

_____

_____

Here are some hints that may help you get started:

- Make a *firm* commitment that you will set aside one hour, three times a week for exercise for the next eight weeks.
- Make a schedule: Block in the hours you work, go to school, sleep, and eat. Include your commuting time. Now, plug in the three hours a week you'll devote to exercising. Find the time that's best for you: morning? midday? early evening? Stick to the time you set! It's an appointment you have with yourself.
- Persist. It may not be fun at all in the beginning; it may even hurt. But don't give up.
- Be patient. You won't notice results right away, but you will notice them if you give yourself a chance.

- Find a friend to exercise with you. While each person in the end must provide his or her own motivation to keep up a program, the companionship of others may motivate you to stay with it in the beginning.
- Reward yourself. After the first four weeks and then eight weeks are up, reinforce your commitment with a dinner out or a new pair of running shoes.

The Bottom Line

Do you now think you have resources and desire that will enable you to start and maintain an exercise program?

_____Yes   _____No

SUMMARY

1. Millions of Americans now exercise and try to keep fit. People have different reasons for exercising. Some want to control their weight. Others enjoy the increased sense of inner power, tranquility, and self-esteem that exercise brings.

2. The human body was designed to be used, but modern life has rendered many people sedentary. People must therefore make special efforts to exercise their bodies.

3. Exercise has physical benefits because it stimulates all of the body systems, especially the muscular, cardiovascular, and respiratory systems. Exercise also has psychological benefits.

4. A person's fitness level depends on four qualities: muscle strength; muscle endurance; flexibility; and cardiorespiratory endurance. These four qualities are interdependent.

5. Overload is the systematic and progressive loading of muscles. It can increase muscle strength, flexibility, and cardiorespiratory endurance.

6. To improve muscle strength, isokinetic exercises are best. They provide maximum resistance, equal to the force applied, throughout a range of

motion. Isotonic exercises involve contracting muscles through a complete range of motion. Isometric exercises are the least useful; they involve pushing or pulling against an immovable object through a relatively narrow range of motion.

7. Aerobic exercise can improve cardiorespiratory endurance. It involves sustained exercise in which the oxygen needs of the body are met continually. In contrast, anaerobic exercise exhausts the body's oxygen stores, creating an "oxygen debt" that must be made up for afterward.

8. A basic "fitness for health" exercise plan would include: a cardiorespiratory endurance exercise of some kind at least three times a week, for at least twenty minutes per session, at 75 percent of maximum heart rate; at least three sessions a week of bent-knee sit-ups and push-ups; and flexibility exercises at least three times a week.

9. In embarking on a "fitness for health" plan, a person should get medical clearance, determine his or her current fitness level, and choose a suitable activity. Research has shown that a minimum of three exercise sessions a week, each fifteen to sixty minutes long, preceded and followed by stretching and limbering exercises, are the most beneficial. A major investment in exercise equipment, footwear, and clothing is seldom necessary.

GLOSSARY

aerobic exercise Sustained exercise during which the body is able to meet its oxygen needs continually. Compare **anaerobic exercise.**
anaerobic exercise Exercise in which the body's demand for oxygen exceeds its supply, producing "oxygen debt." Compare **aerobic exercise.**

cardiorespiratory endurance The ability of the heart, lungs, and blood vessels to mobilize the body's energy and sustain movement over a period of time.
endurance The number of times the muscles can contract against a moderate force.
flexibility The freedom with which the body's muscles, bones, tendons, and ligaments are able to move.

isokinetic Referring to the strength training of muscles through the use of specialized apparatus that, throughout a complete range of motion, provides resistance that is exactly equal to the force the user applies.

isometric Referring to the strength training of muscles by pushing or pulling against a fixed resistance or an immovable object through a relatively narrow range of motion.

isotonic Referring to the strength training of muscles through exercises that involve muscle contractions throughout a complete range of motion.

overload Subjecting muscles to a greater-than-normal load to increase their size and strength.

specificity The concept whereby the activity chosen is specific to the individual's physical-fitness goal.

strength The amount of force the muscles can generate.

NOTES

1. Wilhelm Raab and Hans Kraus, *Hypokinetic Disease* (Springfield, Ill.: Charles C. Thomas, 1960).

2. Joseph A. Bonanno, "Coronary Risk Factor Modification by Chronic Physical Exercise," in Ezra Amsterdam, Jack H. Wilmore, and Anthony De Maria, eds., *Exercise in Cardiovascular Health and Disease* (New York: Yorke Medical Books, 1977), pp. 274–279.

3. J. T. Falonen, P. Puska, and J. Tuomiolehto, "Physical Activity and Risk of Myocardial Infarction, Cerebral Stroke, and Death," *American Journal of Epidemiology* 115 (1982): 526–537.

4. Thaddeus Kostrubala, *The Joy of Running* (Philadelphia: Lippincott, 1977), p. 115.

5. W. F. Ganong, *Review of Medical Physiology,* 10th ed. (Los Altos, Calif.: Lang Medical Publications, 1981), p. 74.

6. William Glasser, *Positive Addiction* (New York: Harper & Row, 1976).

7. Michael L. Sachs, "Compliance and Addiction to Exercise," in Robert C. Canta, ed., *The Exercising Adult* (Lexington, Mass.: Collamore Press, 1982), p. 23.

8. James Skinner, *Body Energy* (Mountain View, Calif.: Anderson World, 1981), p. 15.

9. For the discussion of concepts in this major section of our chapter, we are indebted to Bud Getchell, *Physical Fitness: A Way of Life* (New York: Wiley, 1979).

10. *Healthy People: The Surgeon General's Report on Health Promotion.* U.S. Department of Health and Human Services Pub. No. 79-55-071, 1979, pp. 133–135.

11. Kenneth H. Cooper, *Aerobics* (New York: Evans, 1968), and Cooper, *The New Aerobics* (New York: Evans, 1970).

12. Jack H. Wilmore, *Training for Sport and Activity: The Physiological Basis of the Conditioning Process,* 2nd ed. (Boston: Allyn & Bacon, 1982), p. 62.

13. Philip L. Hooper and R. Philip Eaton, "Exercise, High Density Lipoprotein and Coronary Artery Disease," in O. Appenzeller and R. Atkinson, eds., *Health Aspects of Endurance Training, Encyclopedia of Medicine and Sport,* Vol. 12 (Basel, Switzerland: S. Karger, 1978), pp. 72–81.

14. M. Pollack, J. H. Wilmore, and S. Fox, *Health and Fitness Through Physical Activity* (New York: Wiley, 1978).

15. "Is There Life After Jogging?" *Harvard Medical School Health Letter,* April 1982, p. 3.

16. Ibid., p. 4.

17. American College of Sports Medicine, "Position Statement on the Recommended Quantity and Quality of Exercise for Developing and Maintaining Fitness in Healthy Adults," *Medicine and Science in Sports and Exercise* 10, no. 3 (Fall 1978): vii–x.

18. Ibid.

PART SIX

Making Responsible Choices: Health and Societal Issues

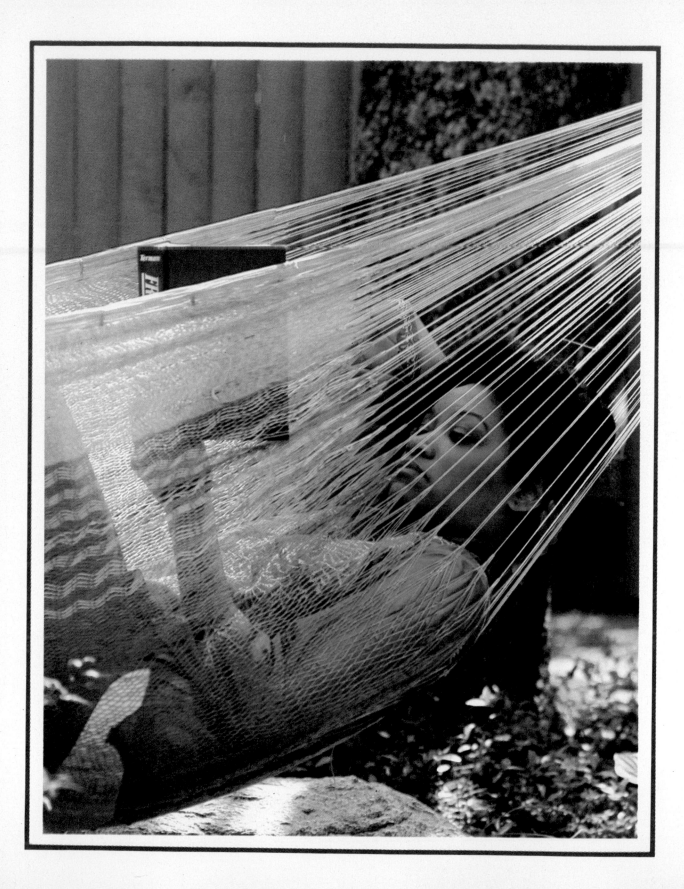

CHAPTER 16

Health Care and the Consumer

In pioneer days people often lived miles from the nearest doctor, and they had to learn how to deal with many medical problems themselves. But then in this century, as it became easier to get to a doctor, and as medicine became better able to treat disease, many people lost this self-reliance.

Today, a new trend is in evidence: a trend toward "self-care" and the "activated patient." More and more people want to stop receiving medical care passively: They want to be active participants in their own care and treatment.[1] Consumers have welcomed a flood of books and magazine articles on medical subjects. They are receiving more medical information, in more detail, than might have been available to the average turn-of-the-century family doctor. And as people have become more knowledgeable about health and medicine, they have begun to ask their doctors more questions and to demand more, and more informative, answers. Some medical practitioners have resisted these efforts. But many thoughtful physicians have come to realize that the patient who grasps basic health-care principles, and applies them intelligently, can be the doctor's most valuable asset.

BECOMING HEALTH-ACTIVATED: WHAT CAN YOU DO?

In many ways you are in a position to do a great deal more for your health, on a continuing basis, than your personal physician—or *any* physician.[2]

Learning to Judge Health-Care Problems

You can save substantial amounts of time and money if you can tell the difference between medical problems that require professional care and problems that can be treated at home. It has been estimated that as many as 70 percent of visits to the doctor are unnecessary.[3] Many common ailments run their course within a short period of time, no matter what anyone does about them. Furthermore, many are caused by viruses that cannot be killed by antibiotics or other drugs. (As we have noted in other chapters, antibiotics are effective primarily against bacterial diseases.) Physicians generally cannot cure these ailments. They can only tell you what you can do for yourself: You can rest, you can ease your symptoms with over-the-counter drugs, if necessary, and you can drink fluids as appropriate.

You should also know when you have an unusual or uncommon or truly alarming symptom and be able to act promptly to obtain appropriate professional treatment or advice. The goal of becoming health-activated is not to replace your physician. Rather, it is to know how to make the best use of medical advice, while assuming basic responsibility for your own overall health. Becoming health-activated really means taking the necessary steps to stay healthy and knowing how to manage minor illnesses so that they don't become major ones.[4]

To be health-activated, you need to interpret the messages your body sends you via symptoms and signs. **Symptoms** are sensations you experience (such as fatigue, a headache, chills, or a stuffy nose), which may or may not be apparent to an observer. **Signs** are observable indications, such as a rash, a fever, or a swollen ankle, that another person (such as a physician) can objectively verify. Often your body is sending you a perfectly logical message via signs and symptoms. If you have diarrhea and/or vomiting, for example, this sign generally means there is something your body wants to get rid of, such as a "bug" or some spoiled food. If you are unusually thirsty after a bout of diarrhea or vomiting, your body is warning you that its fluid supplies have been depleted.

What should you do in response to a sign or symptom? When the message your body is sending you is a familiar one, such as the stuffy nose and scratchy throat that come with the common cold, then you can proceed to self-treatment. When the message is one you're *not* familiar with, then it's time to take steps: Use your home health reference library, and perhaps then contact the appropriate health-care professional.

Learning to Treat Some Problems at Home

The second way you can equip yourself to take responsibility for your own health is to learn some basic skills for home treatment. In this chapter we'll teach you how to check some key body functions such as temperature, breathing rate, and blood pressure; and we'll take up the subject, introduced in Chapter 3, of over-the-counter medications. We'll also talk about how best to approach some common ailments.

HOME HEALTH CARE

To carry out home health care responsibly, you'll need a few basic techniques. You'll also need a few basic medications.

Know Your Normals

How do you know when you, or someone else, has a medical problem? First, you must be able to distinguish a problem situation from the norm—

not a statistical norm, but the norm for you. If you know your "baseline" or "normal" values, you will be able to recognize departures from the norm, so you will know when it is necessary to call a physician.

THREE BASIC MEASUREMENTS: TEMPERATURE, RESPIRATION, PULSE

Everyone should know how to take a temperature and measure respiration and pulse. It is also important to know how to examine the throat; this skill was discussed in Chapter 10.

 ———————————————

HOW TO MEASURE TEMPERATURE

Most people think 98.6° Fahrenheit (37° Celsius) is the universal "normal" human body temperature. But an individual's norm may vary within a degree or two on either side. Temperature may also vary during the day; in women, it varies slightly during the menstrual cycle.

In most cases, you should use a regular oral thermometer. For infants, and for anyone who is unconscious, you will need to use a rectal thermometer (which has a more rounded bulb). Fever will register rectally in thirty seconds, orally in one to two minutes. Extremely high temperature, especially in the very young or the elderly, should be treated as a medical emergency.

HOW TO MEASURE RESPIRATION

The normal range for respiration is twelve to nineteen breaths per minute. Here's how to measure respiration in yourself or another person: Count the number of breaths over three to five minutes, then divide the total number by the number of minutes that have elapsed. (Use a watch or clock with a second hand, so you're sure you are measuring an exact number of minutes.) Also, become familiar with the *sound* of the individual's normal respiration, so that in an illness affecting respiration you can observe not only whether respiration *rate* has changed, but also whether it is shallower (or deeper) than usual and whether there are any unusual noises associated with it. One final point about measuring respiration: Try not to let the person know you are calculating it.

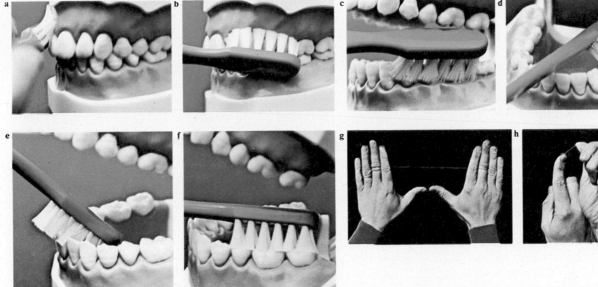

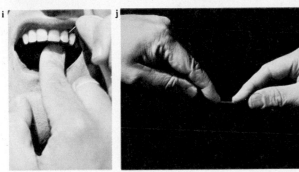

Home care of the teeth and gums is a crucial but often neglected aspect of self-care. These photographs demonstrate the Bass technique of oral hygiene. To clean the outside surfaces of all teeth and the inside surfaces of the back teeth, position the brush at the junction between the teeth and gums (a). Use short back-and-forth strokes. Do the outer surfaces first (b, c), and then do the inner surfaces (d, e) in the same manner. To clean the inner surface of the upper front teeth, hold the brush vertically, using several gentle back-and-forth strokes over gums and teeth. Brush back and forth on biting surfaces (f). After brushing, rinse the mouth vigorously to remove the loosened plaque from the teeth and mouth. The use of dental floss is encouraged for getting into the crevices between teeth. Wrap an 18-inch length of dental floss around the middle fingers to anchor it (g). Pass the floss over the left thumb and the forefinger of the right hand for cleaning the upper left teeth (h, i); reverse the hold for the upper right. Clean the bottom teeth by holding the floss between the forefingers of both hands (j).

HOW TO MEASURE PULSE (HEART RATE)

In a healthy, resting adult, the heart normally beats between 60 and 90 times a minute. Athletes may have rates of 40 to 60 a minute; young children, 90 to 120 (and even higher in infants).

You—or your "patient"—should be completely at rest, since the heart rate increases with physical exertion and with stress. With the "patient's" palm up, press your fingers down on the thumb side of the wrist until you feel the artery throbbing. Do not use your own thumb; it has a pulse of its own that will confuse your count. Using a watch with a second hand, count the number of beats you feel in fifteen seconds. Multiply this number by four to get the heart rate in beats per minute.

The pulse rate may be affected by age, physical exertion, stress, and, of course, heart disease. It may also be affected by other factors, including emotional state, pain, sex, and body size and build. Typically (there are certain exceptions), the pulse rate rises with fever.

BLOOD PRESSURE

As we saw in Chapter 12, the blood pressure is the rhythmic pressure of the blood as it is pumped through the arteries. Blood pressure is affected by a number of factors, including the strength and speed of the heartbeat, the total blood volume, and the condition of the arteries. It is measured by a device called a sphygmomanometer, which consists of a gauge attached to an inflatable cuff wrapped tightly around the upper arm.

WHAT IS NORMAL BLOOD PRESSURE? Blood pressure, like pulse rate, can vary considerably, both with age and among individuals. A reading of 120/80 is considered ideal in a healthy young adult. Pressures in children are normally lower; pressures generally edge upward as people age. An individual's blood pressure may vary with the time of day and the circumstances, and many factors may cause additional variations. Excitement, weight gain, kidney disease, hormonal malfunction, and other events may cause pressure to rise, while malnutrition, injury, extensive bleeding, and a number of illnesses can cause it to fall.

Unless your doctor recommends otherwise, you don't need your own blood pressure kit. It is a good idea, however, to note your usual blood pressure when it is taken by your physician at a regular checkup, so that you can report that norm to another physician who may treat you at some other time. If your physician does recommend that you or another member of your household check blood pressure regularly at home, follow that physician's advice as to the type of equipment to purchase.

The Home Pharmacy

There are many situations in which home treatment is perfectly appropriate, and it makes sense to have a few simple over-the-counter (OTC) medications on hand. Bear in mind, though, that special characteristics of the patient may mean you must exercise special caution: A minor mistake in self-treatment that would do no lasting damage to a generally healthy young adult could have serious consequences for a ninety-year-old suffering from chronic heart disease. You should always consult a physician before giving *any* medication to a very young child or an elderly person, or to anyone who is pregnant, is nursing a baby, or suffering from any serious chronic condition. And if the person is taking any other medication (prescription or not), you should consult either your physician or your neighborhood pharmacist regarding possible interactions between that medication and the one you are contemplating.

Which OTC drugs should you keep in your medicine cabinet? That depends somewhat on your circumstances. A healthy single person living near pharmacies usually needs to stock fewer home remedies than a large and active household in an isolated rural area. One recommendation for what your medicine cabinet should contain is given in Table 16.1.

The widespread availability of over-the counter medications makes it imperative to observe basic rules for safe storage and use in the home. The Food and Drug Administration recommends the following safety measures:

1. Date all over-the-counter drugs when you buy them.
2. Buy medicines and health supplies in realistic quantities—only enough for your immediate needs. Old drugs may deteriorate and become ineffective or even dangerous.
3. Store all drugs out of the reach of small children, under lock and key if necessary.
4. Read the label carefully and observe all warnings and cautions.
5. Do not give or take medicine from an unlabeled bottle. Transparent tape over the label will help protect it.
6. Do not give or take medicine in the dark. Be sure you can read the label clearly.
7. Pay attention when you measure drugs.
8. Do not take several drugs at the same time without consulting your doctor.
9. Weed out leftovers regularly from your home medicine chest, especially any prescription drugs used for a prior illness.
10. Flush discarded drugs down the toilet. Be sure that children or pets cannot reach the empty containers.

(©Martin M. Rotker, 1982/Taurus Photos)

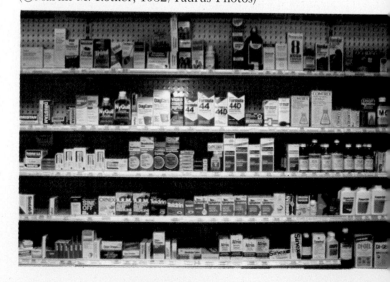

TABLE 16.1 · Recommendations for Stocking Your Medicine Cabinet

Name of Product	Reason for Use
ESSENTIAL PRODUCTS	
Aspirin	Fever, headache, minor pain
Antacid	Stomach upset
Adhesive tape and bandages	Minor wounds
Hydrogen peroxide, iodine	Cleansing minor wounds; antiseptic
Sodium bicarbonate (baking soda)	Soothing minor wounds, skin rashes, burns
Liquid acetaminophen	Pain and fever
Syrup of ipecac	To induce vomiting in case of poisoning
PRODUCTS FOR OCCASIONAL USE	
Antihistamines, nose drops and sprays	Allergies
Cold tablets, cough syrups	Colds and coughs
Milk of magnesia, bulk laxatives	Constipation
Sodium fluoride	To help prevent dental problems
Kaopectate, Parepectolin	Diarrhea
Eye drops and artificial tears	Eye irritations
Antifungal preparations	Fungus
Hemorrhoid preparations	Hemorrhoids
Hydrocortisone cream	Skin rashes
Elastic bandages	Sprains
Sunscreen agents	To prevent sunburn

Source: Donald Vickery and James Fries, *Take Care of Yourself: A Consumer's Guide to Medical Care,* rev. ed. (Menlo Park, Calif.: Addison-Wesley, 1981), pp. 61–62.

Remember, *all* drugs, including OTC drugs, have a potential for side effects. It therefore makes sense for you to own reference books that tell you a lot more about OTC drugs than you can find on their labels. Excellent sources of such information include Benowicz's *Non-Prescription Drugs and Their Side Effects,* Graedon's *The People's Pharmacy,* Zimmerman's *Essential Guide to Non-Prescription Drugs,* the *Handbook of Nonprescription Drugs,* and the *Physicians' Desk Reference for Nonprescription Drugs.* [5]

Which Problems Cannot Be Treated at Home?

Some health problems that can be treated at home are discussed in the accompanying box. But before you deal with any medical problem at home, the first question to ask is whether you should consult a physician. Sometimes home treatment is not effective; in these cases, a physician should be consulted.

WHEN TO SEE A PHYSICIAN

It's beyond the scope of this chapter to detail all those situations that demand professional rather than home treatment. Nevertheless, we can give some simple guidelines:

Emergencies. There are certain obvious emergency situations in which the patient should be seen by a physician immediately: massive bleeding that cannot be stopped, major burns, suspected broken bones, suspected poisoning. You should also get immediate medical help if the person:

▶ Is in severe pain
▶ Has cold sweats, particularly if combined with light-headedness or with chest or abdominal pain
▶ Is short of breath at rest (if not because of simple exertion)
▶ Is unconscious or in a stupor
▶ Is so disoriented that he or she cannot tell you what has happened, or does not know his or her name or whereabouts

How to Treat Some Common Health Problems at Home

UPSET STOMACH

The symptoms: Symptoms are variable, but diarrhea and a feeling of general malaise are typical; there may also be vomiting, low-grade fever, and abdominal discomfort.

The cause: The cause of upset stomach is frequently overeating or drinking too much, emotional stress, or one of a number of common viruses.

When to see a physician: See a physician immediately if there is evidence of internal bleeding (bloody or very dark-colored vomit or stools), or if abdominal pain is severe; these symptoms may indicate serious illness. You should also see a doctor promptly if you're unusually thirsty, if you're pregnant or possibly pregnant, if you're diabetic, or if there are also urinary symptoms (pain or unusual frequency of urination).

If the problem is due to a virus (this ailment is often called "intestinal flu," although it has no connection with influenza), it typically subsides within twenty-four to forty-eight hours. If the upset persists for more than seventy-two hours, it's time to consult your physician.

Home treatment: Home treatment for upset stomach is designed to put as little strain as possible on the gastrointestinal (GI) tract. Eat small amounts of bland food; take mostly fluids. As symptoms subside, add easily digested solid foods—soup, gelatin, soft-boiled eggs—and gradually increase your intake until you're back to normal.

Should you take OTC medications? Over-the-counter antidiarrheal medications such as Kaopectate or Pepto-Bismol may be helpful. Be sure to follow the directions on the label carefully.

ACID INDIGESTION

The symptoms: A feeling of stomach irritation or an acid taste in the esophagus ("heartburn"—but note that this ailment has nothing to do with the heart).

The cause: The stomach normally secretes hydrochloric acid. Acid indigestion, or hyperacidity, results when acid is overproduced—typically as a result of overeating or of eating while tense or anxious. The excess acid irritates the stomach lining.

When to see a physician: Chronic hyperacidity can cause peptic ulcers. If acid indigestion has occurred repeatedly or over a period of time—or if there are any additional symptoms, such as vomiting or extremely dark stools—medical consultation is advised. See a physician also if you have hyperacidity while you are taking any prescription medication or if you suffer from any chronic disorder, especially heart or kidney disease or hypertension.

Home treatment and use of OTCs: An occasional, isolated episode of acid indigestion can be treated with an over-the-counter antacid product. A liquid antacid is preferable to a tablet, gum, or an effervescent powder. Among the liquid products that contain one or two effective antacid ingredients are Delcid, Haley's M-O (this also contains mineral oil), and Phillips' Milk of Magnesia.

CONSTIPATION

The symptoms: Constipation is much rarer than advertising would have you believe! Despite what the ads say about the importance of once-a-day "regularity," healthy people may have a bowel movement anywhere from three times a day to three times a week; if you fall within this range, you are not constipated.

When to see a physician: True constipation is often a symptom of something serious, and chronic difficulty

Persistent Symptoms. It is recommended that you call a physician if you have been running a fever for more than a week, or if any other problem that you have been treating persists beyond a reasonable length of time.

New Findings. You should see a physician if you:

▶ Find an unexplained lump anywhere in your body
▶ Suspect you are pregnant
▶ Have any of the seven warning signs of cancer described in Chapter 11
▶ Have an unexplained weight loss or gain
▶ Cough up blood
▶ Find blood in your feces or urine

—that is, very infrequent or painful defecation—is a signal to see a physician.

Home treatment and use of OTCs: Do not automatically reach for a laxative. Try increasing the fiber in your diet. If this does not bring relief, remember that only brief, temporary episodes of constipation should be self-treated with a laxative. It is safe to do so *if* there are no other symptoms (if there are, *see a physician*) and *if* you can relate the problem to some recent circumstance such as a stressful situation, marked inactivity, or changes in your diet.

There are a number of kinds of laxatives. Probably the safest are the mild ones that work as bulk-formers by drawing water into fecal matter; such products may also contain a stool-softening agent. Among products of this type are Dialose, Hydrolose, Metamucil, Petro-Syllium, and Serutan. Don't use a laxative for more than one week without consulting your doctor.

COLDS AND FLU

When to see a physician: The first step is to distinguish these very widespread viral infections—which a physician cannot cure—from bacterial ones, which would respond to antibiotics. You should see your doctor if:

▶ The condition persists for more than two weeks.
▶ You run a fever for more than one week.
▶ There is pain in one or both ears.
▶ Throat soreness is the dominant symptom.
▶ A cough produces something other than what you would expect in an ordinary cold (for example, brownish sputum or puslike material).

Home treatment: For once, the TV commercials are right. The ideal treatment for flu (and for colds as well) consists of aspirin (or acetaminophen, if you don't tolerate aspirin well), rest, plenty of fluids—and a well-balanced diet.

Use of OTCS: Should you take over-the-counter drugs other than simple pain relievers? Many physicians point out that these "combination" OTCs may include many components you *don't* need, and few you

do. A single-ingredient product, to deal with a particular symptom, is probably wisest. If you have a cough, you might take an expectorant (during the day) or a cough suppressant (for night-time). During the early, runny-nose stage of a cold, you might take an antihistamine (it has a drying effect). For the stuffy stage you might use a decongestant spray (use it sparingly, to avoid the "rebound" effect that can make the situation worse).

A SPECIAL NOTE ON ASPIRIN

Aspirin is the drug of choice for pain, fever, and inflammation, since it is effective against all of them. Aspirin is not a cure for any underlying condition, but it is effective in relieving symptoms. Aspirin is also effective against rheumatoid arthritis and related conditions. But the dosages for these conditions are far higher, and the schedule of administration is different from that recommended for ordinary use; therefore, aspirin should not be employed in these disorders except under a physician's supervision.

There are a number of precautions of which you should be aware, even with this common household remedy:

1. Aspirin may interact with prescription medications. Anyone who is taking an anticoagulant, oral medication for diabetes, or drugs for gout should not use aspirin without checking with the prescribing physician. Aspirin can also aggravate a peptic ulcer.
2. Aspirin should not be combined with alcohol; the two substances can act synergistically to irritate the stomach.
3. Some evidence suggests a connection between aspirin and a rare but sometimes deadly children's disease known as Reyes' Syndrome. The American Academy of Pediatrics has advised physicians not to prescribe aspirin for children who have chicken pox or influenza; researchers believe children may be at risk if they are given aspirin under those conditions.

INTERACTING WITH HEALTH–CARE PROFESSIONALS: STEPS TOWARD HEALTH ACTIVATION

The human body can often heal itself. But sometimes the body needs assistance—when an infection threatens to overwhelm its defenses, when an organ threatens to fail, when a broken bone must be properly aligned if it is to heal properly. Modern medicine, through health-care professionals, can provide this assistance.

In this section, we will use the term *physician* when describing the health partnership, but you should know that the same principles apply when you are interacting with a nurse, a pharmacist, a dentist, or any other health-care professional.

Patient–Physician Communication

When you call or visit a physician, be prepared to explain why you are seeking medical assistance. Organize ahead of time the way you will describe your symptoms.

DESCRIBING YOUR PROBLEM

Without your accurate reporting, the physician knows only what can be determined by visual examination and by other objective diagnostic procedures such as X-rays, blood tests, and measurements of pulse, temperature, and blood pressure. If you do not report clearly and accurately, precious time may be wasted while a not-so-serious problem becomes critical.

Be explicit. Don't say "I feel terrible," or "I ache." Do say, for instance, "I have a temperature of 103°F and my throat is swollen," or "Johnny's pulse is such-and-such, and his eardrum looks red."

HOW TO PREPARE FOR A TALK WITH YOUR PHYSICIAN

Here are some of the questions only *you* can answer—questions you should ask yourself, and answer, *before* you call or visit your doctor:

▶ What is the chief symptom that has made you seek medical help?
▶ Are there *other* symptoms, *other* "something's-wrong" messages your body is sending or has sent you recently?
▶ Exactly where is each symptom?
▶ When did the symptom begin? If it comes and goes, how does it relate to time of day, meals, and so on?
▶ Can you relate the time of onset of the problem to any other event in your life? For example, your upset-stomach symptoms may have begun just a few hours after you dined on some food you now realize tasted odd. Have you been around a sick person? Have you returned from a trip within the past few weeks, especially one outside the United States? Have you recently acquired a pet, or purchased something new that's been in contact with your body? (Allergic reactions can involve animals, cosmetics, soaps, clothing fibers, and other substances.)
▶ What home remedies, if any, have you tried for the problem, and what was the result?
▶ Are you taking (or have you recently taken) any

other medication? If so, what is it, for what condition is it being taken, and what is the exact schedule and dosage? This is important for two reasons: First, your present problem may be a side effect of that drug; and second, certain drugs may alter the values in blood tests the physician may conduct as part of the diagnosis. Be sure to mention *all* drugs you are taking, whether recreational, prescription, or over-the-counter. You should also mention any allergies you may have. People who are allergic to eggs, for example, cannot safely receive certain inoculations.
▶ Do you know anyone, whether in your household or not, who has—or has recently had—a similar complaint? (An affirmative answer could mean something contagious *or* something—food poisoning, for instance—arising from a common environment.)

USING NOTES AND RECORDS

Depending on the complexity of the problem, you might even write out some notes for yourself and take them along to the doctor's office so that you won't forget any symptoms. You might also take along your home medical records, so you can refresh your memory and add new notations. (The accompanying activity explains how you can set up your medical record.) You should also have, on paper or in your mind, a list of questions that you want to ask the doctor, as well as paper and pencil for writing down the answers. Tell the physician —whether or not he or she asks you—if you are seeing another physician for another problem.

CLEAR COMMUNICATION

Before you leave the doctor's office, make sure you understand the diagnosis of your problem and what the treatment will be. Find out what to expect as the treatment progresses and what side effects to watch for. Ask whether you should return for another visit or report to the doctor by telephone—and, if so, how soon. And if the physician prescribes a drug, make sure you know how to take it. If you don't understand what your physician is saying, speak up and ask questions. If necessary, learn the basic medical vocabulary relevant to your particular problems, especially if you have a chronic condition that you and the doctor will be dealing with over a long period of time.

ACTIVITY: EXPLORING HEALTH

Setting Up Your Own Medical Record

Since ours is such a mobile society, keeping your own health history (and your family's) is very important. If you move and your medical records are forwarded by your last physician, some information may be missing. By maintaining your own health history (medical records), you can: keep an accurate record of your lifetime exposure to X-rays; answer tough questions such as when you had your last tetanus shot; and guard against loss of records. Here is a form to follow to set up your personal health history:

NAME _____   DATE OF BIRTH _____

1. IMMUNIZATION HISTORY
   Check off all "shots" you can remember having.

   DPT (diphtheria, whooping cough, tetanus)   _____

   Polio: Salk shots   _____
          Sabin drops or cubes   _____

   Measles   _____

   German measles (rubella)   _____

   Tetanus booster   _____

   TB skin test   Result_____   _____

   Chest X-ray   Result_____   _____

   Others:

   _____   _____

   _____   _____

   Note: Diphtheria and tetanus immunization is recommended every ten years for life, with a tetanus booster for any contaminated wound.

2. CHILDHOOD DISEASES
   Check off any diseases you can remember having had.

	DATE	PLACE	TIME
Whooping cough	____	____	____
Chickenpox	____	____	____
Measles	____	____	____
German measles (rubella)	____	____	____
Mumps	____	____	____

Other: **DATE**   **PLACE**   **TIME**

_____   _____   _____   _____

_____   _____   _____   _____

3. OTHER DISEASES
Check off any diseases which you have had diagnosed by a physician.

Mononucleosis   _____   _____   _____

Rheumatic fever   _____   _____   _____

Gonorrhea   _____   _____   _____

Syphilis   _____   _____   _____

Pneumonia   _____   _____   _____

Tuberculosis   _____   _____   _____

Hepatitis   _____   _____   _____

Other:

_____   _____   _____   _____

_____   _____   _____   _____

Allergies:

_____   _____   _____   _____

_____   _____   _____   _____

_____   _____   _____   _____

4. HOSPITALIZATION RECORD
Make a list of any times you have been hospitalized for treatment of a disease or for an operation.

HOSPITAL NAME AND ADDRESS	DATE	REASON
_____	_____	_____
_____	_____	_____
_____	_____	_____

5. FAMILY MEDICAL INFORMATION
Some diseases are familial; that is, they tend to show up generation after generation in the same family. Here are some diseases that are thought to be familial. Check those that apply to you:

_____ Allergies: asthma, hay fever, eczema   _____ Glaucoma

_____ Cancer   _____ Sickle-cell anemia

_____ Diabetes   _____ Migraine headache

_____ Heart diseases, stroke, high blood pressure   _____ Alcoholism

Physical Examinations

Physical examinations vary considerably in their complexity. Some involve extensive screening, lengthy questionnaires, multiple observations by physicians, laboratory tests of the blood and urine, and monitoring tests such as an electrocardiogram. Other physicals are simpler, involving only a few key tests and observations.

HOW OFTEN SHOULD YOU HAVE A CHECKUP?

Physicians and professional medical associations have long debated the question of periodic exams. Some physicians feel that extensive routine annual checkups aren't worth the time and expense for healthy adults. Other doctors do recommend annual physicals, and some employers require them.

The rule of thumb is that as we grow older, the regular checkup has greater potential for spotting adverse conditions. While you are young, you should have enough physicals to establish a baseline of what is normal for you: Between ages two and twenty, the American Medical Association recommends a checkup every year or two. Between ages twenty and thirty, routine annual checkups may not be worth the money, since they rarely reveal an illness that has not already shown itself via some symptom. If you are between twenty and thirty, it is probably better to wait until you have unusual symptoms—and when and if you do have unusual symptoms, to respond to them promptly by either phoning or visiting your physician. (Note, however, that it is wise for a woman of any age to have a general physical examination before becoming pregnant; see Chapter 8). At all ages, people who do have any abnormal symptoms or who are taking any medication (including birth-control pills) should have physicals more often.

WHAT TESTS MUST YOU HAVE PERIODICALLY?

There are specific items that *should* be checked regularly, particularly in high-risk people. The most essential of these items are the following:[6]

BLOOD PRESSURE Everyone—even healthy adults with no symptoms of heart disease or hyper-

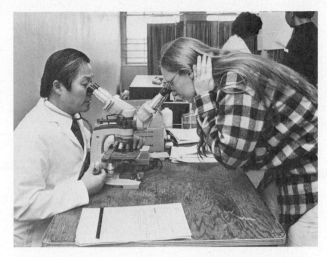

At a community health fair, this woman is looking at her own Pap smear, which the physician will examine for signs of cancer of the uterine cervix. (©Hazel Hankin)

tension—should have his or her blood pressure checked every year or so. Hypertension often does not reveal itself by any overt symptoms. It is dangerous—but it is treatable.

TB TEST You should have a skin test (called the Mantoux or PPD test) for tuberculosis every three to five years—unless you have been exposed to TB, in which case you should have it more often.

PAP TEST There is some difference of opinion about how often a "Pap" (or "Papanicolou") smear should be done to screen for cancer of the uterine cervix. The American College of Obstetricians and Gynecologists recommends that all women have it done annually. Other authorities recommend that it be done once between the ages of eighteen and twenty-four, then at five-year intervals until age seventy-five. Check with your physician for his or her recommendation. Cervical cancer is usually completely curable if caught early. During the same time visit, the physician will generally also check for breast cancer, as mentioned earlier in this chapter. (You should also perform a breast self-examination monthly; see Chapter 11 for details.)

MAMMOGRAPHY Mammography involves X-raying the breast to detect abnormalities, especially cancer. The American Cancer Society recommends that a procedure be done between the ages of thirty-five and forty to establish a baseline for the individual, and once a year thereafter.

GLAUCOMA TEST Glaucoma is a condition in which the pressure inside the eyeball increases; if not treated, it can lead to blindness. You should have your eyes checked for this disease every two years after the age of thirty-five.

MISCELLANEOUS Take your doctor's advice about whether you need to have your urine checked, and (for people over thirty) whether or not you need to be screened for bowel cancer. You should also have your eyes, ears, and teeth checked periodically.[7]

THE HEALTH-ACTIVATED CONSUMER

Just as you take responsibility for interacting effectively with your physician, so you should take responsibility for dealing sensibly with the health marketplace.

Let's say, first of all, that you are discussing a prescription with your physician. What is the drug likely to cost? This question is particularly important if you must take a drug over a long period of time.

Brand-Name Versus Generic Drugs

Sometimes you can save money if your doctor prescribes the drug by the generic name rather than brand name, and you should raise this question if your physician has prescribed a brand-name product. There are, however, two reasons why a brand-name prescription may be necessary in certain instances. First, the drug may be available only in the brand-name form. Second, the generic version of this particular medication may not be exactly equivalent to the brand-name version.

Purchasing Medications

Prices on generic drugs vary widely, and even brand-name drugs may be priced differently at different drugstores. In 1981, for example, a block association in New York City compared prices for half a dozen commonly prescribed drugs at pharmacies within a five-block radius. For 90 5-milligram tablets of the hypnosedative Valium, prices varied by 50 percent, ranging from $11.49 to $18; for 100 50-milligram tablets of generic hydrochlorothiazide (a medication for high blood pressure), the range was from $2.99 to $7.65—a difference of 150 percent.[8]

If you have some of the medication left after you have taken it as long as instructed, ask your physician or your pharmacist whether it can be kept for use on another occasion. If it can be kept, place clear tape over the label so that the information will not become smudged. (A medication that is not clearly labeled has no place in your medicine chest.)

Using Reference Resources

Two of the most valuable, periodically updated books on prescription drugs are the *Physicians' Desk Reference* and *AMA Drug Evaluations;* there are also two excellent subscription updates on drugs, *The Medical Letter* and *Physicians' Drug Alert.*[9] While these publications are not inexpensive, a group purchase or subscription may enable you to acquire them if you can't afford to do so on your own.

Avoiding Quacks

One of the factors that contribute to poor decisions about health is fear—of pain, of illness, or of death. Frequently this fear leads to a counterproductive reaction in which people delay seeing a doctor for their symptoms because they don't want their fears confirmed.

Quacks take advantage of such fears by advertising "cures" that they claim are both painless and fully guaranteed. The drugs and devices sold by these unscrupulous charlatans are sometimes harmful and, according to the Food and Drug Administration, occasionally lethal. Most are harmless but ineffective; when they "work," as they appear to sometimes, it is due to the user's emotional expectations, or to the fact that the problem would simply have abated by itself in any case, or to the coming-and-going nature of the condition.

HOW TO SPOT A QUACK

The best line of defense against quackery is to learn both about health generally and about how quacks work, since quackery often follows certain patterns. If the answers to the following questions tend to be yes—watch out.

1. Does the promoter of a product or service claim to be battling the medical profession, which is supposed to be trying to suppress the wonderful discovery? Does he or she maintain that surgery, X-ray, or medication prescribed by reputable physicians will do more harm than good?
2. Is the remedy sold from door to door by a self-styled "health adviser" or advertised in public lectures? Is it promoted in a sensational magazine, by a faith healer's group, or by a crusading organization of lay people?
3. Does the seller use scare tactics, predicting all sorts of harmful consequences if you do not use the product?
4. Is the product or service offered as a "secret remedy"?
5. Does the promoter show testimonials to demonstrate the wonders that the product or service has performed for others?
6. Is the product or service claimed to be good for a vast array of illnesses, or guaranteed to provide a quick cure?

"Guarantees in medicine," point out Donald Vickery and James Fries, "are almost a guarantee that the product or service is worthless. In medicine, a guarantee is not possible. . . . No worthwhile medical service is accompanied by a guarantee. . . . The offer itself strongly suggests a suspicious product."[10]

DEALING WITH HEALTH-CARE PRACTITIONERS

There's more to finding the health-care assistance you need than avoiding obvious quackery. You need to find the right person to help you—not only a reputable practitioner, but one with the skills appropriate to your problem. Below, we'll discuss independent practitioners—physicians and dentists—in detail.

Physicians and Dentists: Their Training and Qualifications

Physicians and dentists are the most highly trained workers in the health-care field. There are actually two types of physicians: the M.D., or medical doctor, and the D.O., or doctor of osteopathic medicine. Lengthy education is required to become a physician. After four years of college, the M.D.-to-be must spend four years in medical school, one year of internship in a hospital, and one or two years in residency. Only after all these years can the physician be licensed. Those who wish to specialize—in, say, gynecology or surgery—need additional residency training to qualify to take specialty board examinations.

Osteopaths, or D.O.s, who nowadays treat diseases in virtually the same way as M.D.s, must complete educational and training requirements similar to those of M.D.s. In fact, in some states, such as California and New York, M.D.s and D.O.s take the same licensure examination.

Dentists also undergo rigorous training. Most have already earned a bachelor's degree before they enter dental school. To get either the degree of D.D.S. (doctor of dental surgery) or the equivalent D.M.D. (doctor of medical dentistry), they usually must spend four more years in dental school; then they must pass both a written and a clinical examination to qualify for a state license.

MEDICAL SPECIALTIES

Whether he or she is an M.D. or a D.O., a physician may practice general medicine or may choose to enter any one of a number of specialties and subspecialties. Increasingly, the old-time general practitioner is being replaced by the new "family physician," a physician who specializes in comprehensive primary care for persons of all ages in a family and community context.

Depending on your age, sex, and the medical-practice patterns where you live, your basic primary-care physician will be a family physician, an internist (a specialist in internal medicine), or a pediatrician (who typically does not treat patients beyond the teen years).

ASSESSING A PHYSICIAN'S QUALIFICATIONS

Any physician licensed to practice may *call* himself or herself a specialist in a particular area—but that's no guarantee of expert, specialized care. If you want to know whether a physician is really a qualified specialist, find out whether he or she has received certification by the appropriate medical board. The boards, which are made up of distinguished experts, hold periodic examinations for qualifying physicians—physicians who have served a residency and have had a specified amount of experience. Physicians who have passed the examination receive certificates and are called *diplomates* in that specialty; they are sometimes referred to as "board-certified."

___

HOW DO YOU GO ABOUT FINDING A SUITABLE PHYSICIAN OR DENTIST?

There are a number of approaches you can take to finding a physician.

Ask your former physician. If you are moving to a new community, ask your present physician to recommend someone in the new area. If your physician is moving or retiring, he or she will generally be pleased to suggest a replacement.

Ask someone you know. Your friends, neighbors, relatives, or colleagues at school or work may be able to suggest physicians they find satisfactory —but keep in mind that your acquaintances may not necessarily be qualified to evaluate a physician's competence.

Ask the county medical society. County medical societies will usually give out the names of physicians willing to take new patients—but they will not evaluate them for you (and some of the most competent—and busiest—physicians remove their names from such lists).

Inquire at a hospital. You can also locate the nearest good hospital and find out the names of the physicians who practice there. Talk to nurses and young staff physicians (residents) to find names of the established physicians they most admire. Top physicians in private practice frequently contribute time to clinical teaching in teaching hospitals, or work at hospitals affiliated with medical schools.

Go to the library. Libraries have reference books in which you can check out a physician's educational background, training, and other credentials. The American Medical Association pub-

lishes a directory of physicians, organized by state, and the *Directory of Medical Specialists* lists physicians who are certified by the professional board of their specialty.

Finding a good dentist requires similar steps, and here, recommendations by friends, colleagues, and neighbors may be particularly valuable. You might also check the faculty of a university dental school—or ask your physician to suggest a dentist. A qualified dentist has either a D.D.S. or D.M.D. degree. There are also specialties in dentistry; most general dentists are capable of minor procedures in these specialty areas but will refer you to a specialist for more complex problems.

___

Why Must Physicians and Dentists Charge So Much?

Critics of the health care system have noted that in the twentieth century, medical care has moved from the home into the marketplace, where it has become a commodity. The medical profession, through its professional organization, the American Medical Association (AMA), has been able to control the supply of this commodity. It has restricted entry to the profession by getting state licensing laws passed and by limiting admissions to medical school. It has exerted influence over government regulation of medication. Through all these controls, critics say, the medical profession has been able to withstand outside pressures to lower its prices.

But there are also more practical reasons why the cost of a visit to a physician or dentist is often so high. Typically, these professionals run private offices and must pay all the overhead—rent, heat, light, office staff, laundry, phone bills, and so on— out of the receipts of their practice. Today, some physicians are moving away from this pattern. Some are forming group practices, some are becoming salaried employees of hospitals, some work in health maintenance organizations (to be discussed later), some work in public health centers or clinics. In these group settings, it is sometimes possible for physicians to charge patients less per visit than they would have to charge in a

Evaluating Your Medical and Dental Care

EVALUATING A PHYSICIAN

When you become ill, you quite naturally feel worried —and possibly helpless and fearful as well. These are not the ideal circumstances in which to initiate a partnership with a health-care professional! Such a relationship should be entered into when you are well.

The Preliminary Meeting

Once you have the names of two or three qualified physicians, it's a good idea to set up an appointment —*before* you get sick—to talk about establishing a partnership. (The physician may or may not charge for this appointment, but is entitled to do so.) That will give you a chance to assess the doctor and the doctor's office and to obtain some basic information.

Among the questions you should ask, if the answers aren't immediately apparent:

► Is the physician licensed and board-certified?
► Where would you be hospitalized, should it become necessary? (The physician should have admitting privileges at a good hospital nearby.)
► How available is this physician—say, in the middle of the night?
► Is there a "call hour" when you can phone to ask nonurgent questions? Does the physician have an efficient answering service?
► What are this physician's fees? (Generally, fees of doctors practicing in the same specialty in the same community are comparable. But one who is board-certified may charge a little more than one who is not, and a physician further certified in a subspecialty may charge still more.)

If, at the end of the preliminary visit, you're not sure that this physician is for you, simply explain that several were highly recommended and you plan to talk to all before coming to a decision; then go on to the next on your list.

After You Have Received Care from the Physician

The following tips can help you evaluate the care your doctor is providing.

► A good physician emphasizes preventive medicine. He or she should ask about your lifestyle—diet, exercise, smoking and drinking habits, occupational risks—and make suitable suggestions for improvements.
► A good physician takes a careful medical history from you and listens carefully to your complaints. He or she explains any proposed treatment to you in nontechnical language and is willing to answer your questions.
► A good physician takes enough time to do a thorough examination.
► A good physician keeps records on you, making notes of every office visit. He or she should always ask you about possible drug allergies; if you have any, this fact should appear prominently on your records.
► If a physician gives you a prescription, he or she should give you thorough directions as to how to take it.
► If surgery seems necessary, a good physician welcomes a second opinion.

EVALUATING A DENTIST

You should choose a dentist in much the same way as you choose a physician: Get the names of two or three dentists from friends and relatives, and have a preliminary visit with each. Once you have chosen a dentist, you can evaluate the dental care you receive on the basis of the following guidelines:

► *Checkups.* A good dentist will suggest that you come in at least once a year for a checkup and will probably recommend twice-yearly visits.
► *Fillings.* Fillings should stay in place for at least twelve years. If they fall out sooner, a new dentist may be warranted. If your dentist tells you that your caries are due to soft teeth, find another dentist.
► *Extractions.* If your dentist suggests pulling your teeth, find out why. You may want to get another opinion. No replacement does the job as well as your own.

Sources: R. Shipley and C. Plonsky, *Consumer Health: Protecting Your Health and Money* (New York: Harper & Row, 1980), pp. 145–146; H. Cornacchia and S. Barrett, *Consumer Health: A Guide to Intelligent Decisions* (St. Louis: Mosby, 1980), p. 268.

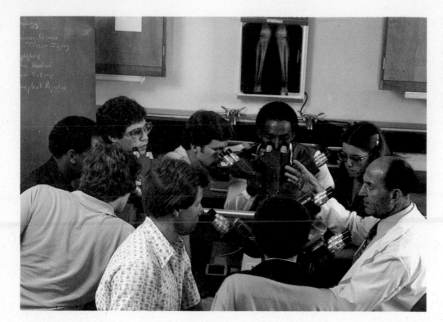

Most new physicians emerge from medical school owing thousands of dollars in education loans, and they must recover those costs from their patients—another reason physicians charge high fees. (© Charles Harbutt/Magnum)

private practice. But there may be drawbacks. In some such group arrangements, patients may not see the same physician every time, and they may have to wait longer to see a physician.

Can some of the physician's tasks be performed by nonphysicians? Today, there is a movement toward encouraging hospitals and doctors to allow nurses and other health-care professionals to take on more responsibility. The recognition that much routine medical care can be provided by someone with less extensive training than that of the physician has led to the acceptance of new health professionals known as physician's assistants and nurse practitioners. In certain circumstances you may be able to save some money by consulting one of these health professionals rather than a physician.

New Pressures on Physicians

Physicians often work under severe pressure. Some of the stresses they endure today have existed since the beginning of medicine: Life-and-death decisions must be made, and unending series of patients must be dealt with. Other problems are of more recent origin. In 1950 the typical G.P. saw an average of 91 patients a week. Today, such physicians are seeing an average of 171 patients a week, and more than a third are seeing in excess of 250 a week![11] Furthermore,

new discoveries are being made constantly, and even good doctors may have a hard time keeping abreast of all the latest developments in their field. After seeing forty or fifty patients a day, even the most devoted physician may find it difficult to spend hours reading journal articles.

WHAT MALPRACTICE SUITS MEAN TO ALL OF US

A wide range of injuries may give rise to malpractice suits, and cases of unremoved sponges, clips, and other surgical instruments are well publicized. Some malpractice suits are justified: A Senate subcommittee recently found that most malpractice suits result from actual injuries suffered during medical treatment or surgery, and the report concluded in part that "the majority have proved justifiable."[12]

It's important to state that some malpractice suits are undoubtedly brought by greedy patients and lawyers, trying to collect large sums from physicians who may have made unavoidable errors (or no errors at all). Lawyers would probably insist that people are better informed today about their medical rights and are more willing to sue doctors for sloppy or incompetent care. Physicians might argue that because no-fault insurance has eliminated many automobile liability cases, lawyers have turned to malpractice suits to make a living.

Juries tend to be very sympathetic to patients who bring malpractice suits. And judgments against physicians (who are usually well-to-do and heavily insured) are often for extraordinary sums of money: Settlements of more than $2.5 million have been awarded. As a result, physicians' malpractice insurance has become extremely expensive—in some parts of the country, $20,000 a year or more. This malpractice bill is largely paid by patients in the form of higher doctor bills. The malpractice threat has also led many physicians to practice "defensive medicine"—to be overly cautious in their diagnosis and treatment to avoid successful malpractice claims. This means that extra —and costly—laboratory tests and X-rays may be ordered. (Ironically, some of the tests are risky in themselves.) Like the cost of malpractice insurance, this cost is largely borne by the consumer. It has been estimated that the practice of defensive medicine increases U.S. medical costs by $3 billion to $5 billion a year.[13]

Alternative Approaches to Health Care

You may have heard about certain types of health practitioners whose approaches are very different from those of conventional American medicine.

ACUPUNCTURE

Acupuncture is a centuries-old Chinese medical treatment.

In acupuncture, fine needles are inserted into the body at different points along "meridians," lines through which (the theory holds) energy flows throughout the body. These needles are then moved in a circular fashion (by hand or by electrical current) to stimulate the energy flow. In treating disease, the goal of acupuncture is to restore the balance of the life forces, thereby restoring health. While the effectiveness of acupuncture in curing disease has not been documented, there have been reports of success in the United States in cases where acupuncture has been used to treat pain—as with headache, joint pain, and tooth extractions. But its acceptance and use as an anesthesic in the United States is unlikely, since it does not completely block pain and the patient remains conscious.

CHIROPRACTIC

Chiropractic is a healing system based on the theory that "subluxations," or misalignments of spinal vertebrae, interfere with proper functioning of the central nervous system and ultimately cause disease. Chiropractors treat patients by manipulation and adjustment to restore proper alignment of the spine. They receive a degree of Doctor of Chiropractic (D.C.) after four years of training at a chiropractic school. In order to practice, chiropractors must pass a state licensing examination. While chiropractic is generally considered to be useful in treating problems like stiffness or pain in the neck or back, its effectiveness in treating chronic or communicable diseases is open to controversy. The controversy over the effectiveness of chiropractic lies in two areas; its theory of disease causation and the scope and quality of chiropractic education. However, medical expenses for chiropractic are now reimbursed by Medicare and Medicaid in most states.[14]

OTHER ALTERNATIVE APPROACHES

You should exercise great caution in considering other alternative approaches to health care—especially *naturopathy*, which holds that diseases are the body's effort to purify itself (the textbook *Basic Naturopathy* states, "smallpox is certainly to be preferred to vaccination"), and *homeopathy*, which holds that diseases or symptoms can be cured via tiny doses of the very same substance that is causing the problem. Even the general name "holistic medicine," which is often used even in orthodox medical circles to describe efforts to help the "whole person," is also used by practitioners who are much less orthodox, sometimes useless, sometimes even dangerous. Among the nontraditional methods that you may hear about under this category are rolfing (realigning the body by vigorous manipulations), psychosynthesis, rejuvenation exercises, psychoelectronics, balancing body chemistry, and others. If a nontraditional practitioner advocates rest, balancing work with relaxation, "tuning in" to yourself, and getting plenty of exercise and fresh air, fine; these measures will certainly help you feel better. But you should not rely on them *instead* of seeing a physician if you have an actual medical problem.

HEALTH–CARE INSTITUTIONS: DEALING WITH HOSPITALS

Many hospitals have so many departments and offer so many services that it's understandable if we feel a bit overwhelmed by the prospect of choosing a good hospital. Yet you *can* deal effectively with hospitals and other health-care institutions if you know some basic rules.

CHOOSING A HOSPITAL: WHAT YOU SHOULD KNOW

▶ Although all hospitals must be licensed according to state law, only certain hospitals are accredited by the Joint Commission on Accreditation of Hospitals (JCAH). The JCAH is a professional group that sets minimum standards for hospital performance. Since the JCAH standards are considered a necessary minimum for adequate care, try to select a hospital that has JCAH accreditation.
▶ Good hospitals have few empty beds. (Those with many empty beds may pressure physicians to bring in patients or may extend patients' hospital stays.)
▶ Good hospitals offer good medical care. The best hospitals are often "teaching hospitals" affiliated with respected medical schools; they have full "house staffs" of interns and residents.
▶ Good hospitals have a range of services: X-ray laboratory, intensive-care unit, coronary-care unit, postoperative recovery room, emergency room, outpatient department, blood bank, and pathology laboratory.
▶ Good hospitals have physicians in a broad range of specialty areas (internists, surgeons, neurologists, psychiatrists, pediatricians, and so on); specialists and department heads are board-certified, as are all surgeons who practice there.
▶ Good hospitals regularly assess the quality of their own care. For example, a committee of physicians should regularly review the hospital's surgical cases to make sure that all surgery performed is necessary and appropriate.

Using Clinics for Outpatient or Ambulatory Care

It's helpful to be familiar with the various types of clinics. First, there are hospital clinics. If you have ever been taken to the hospital after injuring yourself or suddenly becoming ill, you are probably familiar with the hospital emergency room, which is set up to deal with accident victims and other emergency cases. Hospitals also have outpatient clinics, which provide follow-up services for those who have received hospital treatment, either as inpatients or as emergency-room patients.

Do *not* use a hospital emergency room for a routine medical problem that could more inexpensively and appropriately be handled by an office visit.

There are also public health department clinics, financed with city or county tax dollars. These clinics provide free care, or, in some cases, care on a sliding fee scale (based on ability to pay) to residents of particular geographical areas. They typically provide routine primary care, including immunization, health screenings, diagnosis and treatment for sexually transmitted diseases, and prenatal care. Some clinics may also offer drug rehabilitation and family-planning services.

Patients' Difficulties with Hospitals

Probably the most common complaint about the quality of medical care today concerns the dehumanization of treatment. Patients are sometimes annoyed by curtness on the part of an overworked nurse or a physician whose manner is a bit too brisk. Worse, there are instances when patients are not given adequate explanations of their condition, of the procedures being used to diagnose it, or of the risks involved in a certain course of treatment. Directions for taking drugs and information about their side effects may be inadequate as well.

A further problem is that of **iatrogenic** (doctor-caused) and **nosocomial** (hospital-caused) illnesses. Most common are infections passed on to the patient via hospital staff, dressings, injections and visitors. Studies by the federal Centers for Disease Control reveal that 5 percent of patients hospitalized in the United States contract nosocomial (hospital-acquired) infections.

Costs of Hospitalization

Even if you feel the staff in your hospital has treated you well, you may still be alarmed by your hospital bill. Since 1950 the cost of a one-day hospital stay has increased by 1,000 percent. Hospitalization accounts for the largest portion of health expenditures (more than 40 percent), and its costs are among the fastest rising—increasing three times as fast as the general cost of living (see Figure 16.1).

There are several good reasons why hospitals are so expensive. First, hospitals have many fixed costs: emergency rooms with expensive equipment that sits idle much of the time but must be ready twenty-four hours a day; operating rooms; salaries for administration, nurses, and supporting staff; heating, cooling, lighting, and custodial costs; and so on. Second, a hospital is a workshop for doctors, who need and expect up-to-date, sophisticated equipment.

However, hospital costs are probably a good deal higher than they need be. For one thing, some hospitals seem to be in an equipment "arms race": Though some equipment could be shared by several adjacent metropolitan hospitals, most hospitals want to have their own equipment. For another, many patients in hospitals today do not need to be there. It is believed that as many as 40 percent of the patients in hospitals could be adequately cared for in less expensive facilities, or on an outpatient basis, or even at home.[15]

A third key problem has been the traditional "fee-for-service" arrangement, whereby hospitals have obtained payments from the government for care of the elderly under the federal Medicare insurance program (discussed below). Until 1983, hospitals were allowed to bill the government for all the services they felt were necessary, naming the costs themselves. The 1983 Social Security Amendments Act promised to change this system. Henceforth, the government would *specify* how much it would pay of costs in 467 diagnosis-related categories, and would penalize hospitals whose costs exceeded these limits.

A major cost problem relates to surgery. Some critics have estimated that some 17 percent of operations performed annually, or 2.4 million operations each year, are not medically necessary. A professor of public health estimated that fully half of all heart surgery is unjustified; almost a quarter of all appendectomies are not necessary; and more than 90 percent of all tonsillectomies performed in the United States are technically unnecessary, yet 20 to 30 percent of all children still undergo the operation. Unnecessary operations have a high price tag—an estimated $4 billion and 11,900 deaths each year.[16]

Figure 16.1 Hospital care is the largest single component of health expenditures. It is also the fastest-growing cost, having increased since 1950 by a larger percentage than any other component.

Source: Health Care Financing Administration, U.S. Department of Health and Human Services, *Health Care Financing Review* (Washington, D.C.: U.S. Government Printing Office, 1982).

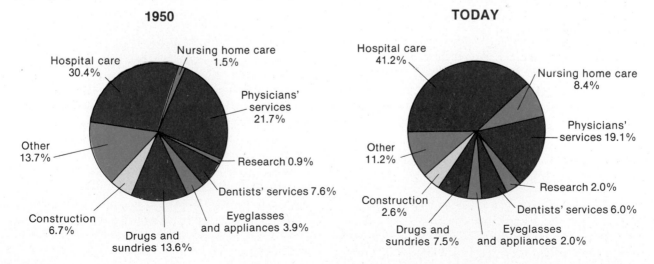

1950

Hospital care 30.4%
Nursing home care 1.5%
Physicians' services 21.7%
Other 13.7%
Research 0.9%
Construction 6.7%
Drugs and sundries 13.6%
Dentists' services 7.6%
Eyeglasses and appliances 3.9%

TODAY

Hospital care 41.2%
Nursing home care 8.4%
Physicians' services 19.1%
Other 11.2%
Research 2.0%
Construction 2.6%
Drugs and sundries 7.5%
Dentists' services 6.0%
Eyeglasses and appliances 2.0%

HEALTH INSURANCE

Most Americans do not have the financial resources to pay for extended medical care out of their own pockets. When our medical bills exceed a certain amount, we need help. This help is provided by insurance—for *some* people. Many people, however, either totally lack medical insurance or have inadequate coverage.

It's essential for everyone to have a basic knowledge of how health insurance works. Many people never look into the exact provisions of their policy until they have a problem—only to find that its coverage does not extend as far as they thought! Since there are more than 1,700 companies selling health insurance, and each company issues a number of different policies, insurance is complex. In this section, we will discuss the ABCs of health insurance to help you find your way through the tangle.

Private Plans: Which Ones Are Best?

Most private (prepaid/fee-for-service) health insurance is provided by one of two groups: (1) nonprofit corporations, the best known of which is Blue Cross-Blue Shield, or (2) profitmaking insurance companies. Both these categories offer insurance via two kinds of policies: group and individual.

Group policies account for the majority of all private insurance plans; most are offered by employers to groups of employees. Individual policies are bought by single persons, couples, or families, typically by those who do not have access to group plans.

You should try to get into a group plan if at all possible, because group plans offer the same basic coverage as individual plans, but are usually cheaper.

Kind of Policy

Before you buy into a plan, be sure to read the fine print to find out what kind of policy you are getting. This will determine how much of your medical expenses your insurance will cover.

Several kinds of coverage are available. **Basic health insurance** pays benefits for hospitalization and for medical and surgical expenses. This means that *part* of your hospital bill and *part* of your physician's and surgeon's fees—but *only* up to a given amount—will be paid by insurance. **Major medical insurance** is designed to protect you from the high medical expenses that will accumulate if you are seriously injured or ill for a long time. Typically, major medical coverage is bought in addition to basic medical for an extra fee. **Disability insurance** pays you benefits if you are unable to work because of accident or illness.

Don't think you're completely covered if you just have a "basic" health insurance policy! Try to get at least some major medical and disability coverage as well.

Public Plans: How Much Government Help Is Available?

If a person cannot afford private health insurance, he or she *may* still get some coverage by way of public plans. There are two types of public plans; they have the confusingly similar names "Medicare" and "Medicaid."

MEDICARE: FOR THOSE OVER SIXTY-FIVE

Medicare, a federal health insurance program designed to benefit people aged sixty-five or older, has two parts, A and B. Part A is a compulsory hospitalization insurance program that operates through the social security system. (Thus, everyone who reaches the age of sixty-five has some hospitalization coverage under Medicare.) Part B is a voluntary program, by which those sixty-five and older can receive additional medical insurance by making a monthly contribution to the program. Medicare coverage is limited, however: Parts A and B together pay only about 60 percent of the total health bill for persons sixty-five and older.

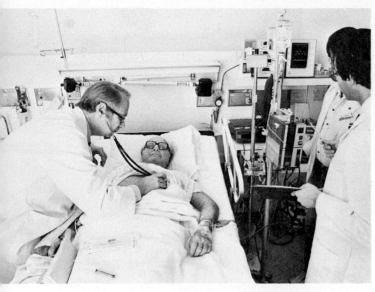

Medicare has put adequate health care within the reach of thousands of elderly Americans who could not have afforded it otherwise. (©Sepp Seitz, 1982/Woodfin Camp & Assoc.)

MEDICAID: FOR THOSE WHO CANNOT PAY FOR MEDICAL CARE

Medicaid is a federal-state health insurance program designed to assist people of any age who cannot pay for medical care. Those who can meet the standards of "medical indigence" are wholly or partly covered for hospital stays and other medical expenses. Medicaid has helped substantially in getting medical care to low-income people who had previously lacked access to the health-care system.

Health Maintenance Organizations (HMOs)

Some critics of traditional fee-for-service care believe it encourages physicians and hospitals to give you more care (such as tests) than you really need —and to charge for the extra care, of course. Partly in response to this problem, a new approach has developed: the **health maintenance organization,** or **HMO.** This is a type of prepaid group practice plan in which consumers pay a set fee every month and in return receive all their health care—whatever care they need—at little or no ad-

ditional cost. In an HMO, instead of going to a private or family physician, you choose a group of physicians, usually ten or more, specializing in various branches of medicine; these physicians all work for the HMO. As one writer has emphasized, HMOs are uniquely structured to encourage patients to "think preventive":

> The idea is to make services easily available, mostly under one roof, and to encourage you to come in soon enough to prevent a minor condition from becoming serious and costly. Since you pay in advance for guaranteed care, HMO proponents say, you won't put off visits at the expense of your health, and this kind of vigilance not only keeps you fitter but also results in lower costs for health care.[17]

HMOs have advantages over traditional health-care systems: Some studies have shown that patients under HMOs have less frequent hospitalization, shorter periods of hospitalization, and less surgery than those under the care of fee-for-service practitioners.[18] HMOs also stimulate competition: The hospitalization rate goes down when an HMO enters a community. HMOs have been quite successful in limiting their cost increases, largely because people are treated on an outpatient basis whenever feasible. Of course, HMOs are not a magical solution to health-care reform.

TAKING ACTION TO CONTROL HEALTH-CARE COSTS

Coping with high medical costs may seem to be too big a problem for any one person to tackle. Yet there are some steps that we, as individuals, can take to help keep our own medical costs down (see Figure 16.2).

WHAT YOU CAN DO TO CONTROL YOUR OWN COSTS

Here are some basic points you need to know if you want to try to keep down your own medical bills:[19]

1. *Practice prevention.* Make sure your lifestyle is healthy: don't smoke; try to stay at your optimum

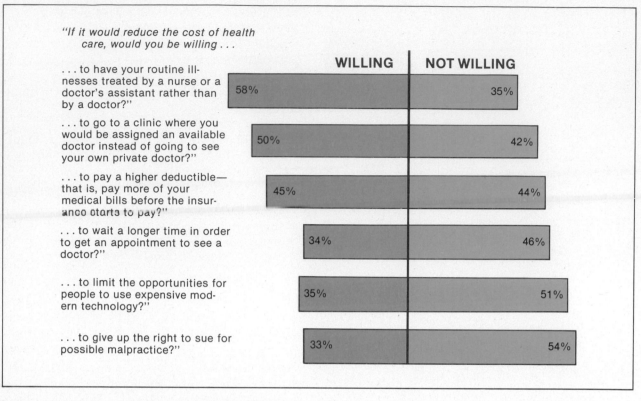

"If it would reduce the cost of health care, would you be willing . . .

	WILLING	NOT WILLING
. . . to have your routine illnesses treated by a nurse or a doctor's assistant rather than by a doctor?"	58%	35%
. . . to go to a clinic where you would be assigned an available doctor instead of going to see your own private doctor?"	50%	42%
. . . to pay a higher deductible—that is, pay more of your medical bills before the insurance starts to pay?"	45%	44%
. . . to wait a longer time in order to get an appointment to see a doctor?"	34%	46%
. . . to limit the opportunities for people to use expensive modern technology?"	35%	51%
. . . to give up the right to sue for possible malpractice?"	33%	54%

Figure 16.2   Each of us contributes to the high cost of health care. But what steps are we willing to take in order to cooperate in the effort to cut those costs? A recent survey revealed that a majority of Americans would indeed accept a number of changes in the nation's health-care system if that meant a reduction in their medical bills. For example, a sizable majority said that they would be willing to have their routine illnesses treated by a nurse or physician's assistant rather than by a physician. However, only one-third would be willing to wait longer for an appointment to see a doctor.

Source: Robert Reinhold, "Majority in Survey on Health Care Are Open to Changes to Cut Costs," *New York Times*, March 29, 1982, pp. A1, D11.

weight; don't drink too much; get regular exercise; keep your immunizations up to date; and wear your seatbelt when you're in a car.

2. *Know how to obtain some medical services free of charge.* Occasionally you can get needed information via a short, well-planned phone call to your doctor. You may be able to have certain tests done without cost by local diagnostic clinics; the clinic will inform your physician of the results. And you may be able to get free immunizations or other health services from the local health department.

3. *Try to have X-rays and other diagnostic procedures done before you enter the hospital.* By doing so, you can cut down your stay by two or three days, and your insurance carrier will probably pay for tests done on an outpatient basis.

4. *Try to choose a surgeon who has admitting privileges at a hospital with a single-day program for minor surgery.* You will be able to leave the hospital the same day you have the surgery performed.

5. *Get an itemized copy of your hospital bill.* Check it to make sure it doesn't list services you haven't actually received.

6. *Be reasonably skeptical.* Whenever your doctor recommends elective surgery, ask for details. And get a second opinion.

7. *Watch how you purchase drugs.* Shop around for prescription drugs. Don't waste money on vitamins and food supplements unless your doctor says you need them.

8. *Be sure you have enough health insurance.*

SUMMARY

1. Today, more and more people want to participate actively in their medical care and treatment. In turn, more and more physicians have come to believe that an informed patient is a better patient.

2. People can become "health-activated" by: learning to judge symptoms and signs in order to determine which medical problems they can safely treat on their own and which ones require professional attention; and learning basic skills for home treatment.

3. Responsible home health care includes a knowledge of baseline data for temperature, respiration, and pulse so that these can be compared to measurements taken when symptoms arise.

4. Home treatment with over-the-counter medications is often appropriate for otherwise healthy adults with self-limiting ailments such as colds, intestinal upsets, and minor infections. Home treatment of the very young or old, the chronically ill, and pregnant or nursing women is inadvisable.

5. A doctor should be consulted and self-treatment should not be attempted: in obvious emergencies (massive bleeding, broken bones, and so on); when symptoms persist beyond a reasonable length of time; and when new findings are made, such an unexplained lump or suspected pregnancy.

6. Good health care requires interaction between patients and health-care professionals. Health-care professionals need lay people to take responsibility for their own basic health, to report clearly and accurately what the professional cannot find out otherwise, and to respond intelligently to medical advice.

7. In communicating with a health-care professional, a person should report accurately: the chief symptom; other symptoms, if any; where each symptom is; when each symptom began; whether the symptoms are related to any other event; what home remedies, if any, have been tried; any other medications he or she is taking; and whether any acquaintance or relative has recently had similar symptoms.

8. Before leaving a health-care professional's office, a patient should ask questions about anything that is not clear and should understand the diagnosis, the nature of the treatment, and what side effects may occur.

9. Medical professionals agree that periodic checkups of healthy people should vary according to age, sex, and previous medical history. But they do not agree on how often healthy people should have regular checkups. Tests that should be conducted regularly include blood pressure exams, skin tests for tuberculosis, Pap tests for cervical cancer, mammography for breast cancer, and glaucoma tests every two years after age thirty-five.

10. To learn whether a physician is qualified, find out whether he or she is board-certified. To find a new doctor or dentist, ask your present or former doctor or dentist for a referral, ask someone you know, check with the county medical or dental society, or consult your library's reference material.

11. Medical care is expensive for several reasons: It is a limited commodity, physicians and hospitals typically pay high overhead, and the costs of equipment, tests, and even malpractice insurance are passed on to patients.

12. To evaluate a hospital, find out whether it is accredited, is a teaching hospital, provides a wide range of services, and assesses the quality of its own care.

13. For patients, difficulties associated with hospital care include the dehumanization of treatment and the incidence of doctor- or hospital-caused illnesses. The high cost of hospitalization is a serious problem, aggravated by hospitals' reluctance to share expensive equipment and by the high incidence of unnecessary admissions and unnecessary surgery.

14. Because medical care is so expensive, most Americans need health insurance. Most private insurance is provided by nonprofit corporations such as Blue Cross–Blue Shield or by insurance companies. Private insurance is written for individuals and for groups. Basic health insurance pays for hospitalization, medical, and surgical expenses. Major medical insurance covers large

medical bills and usually supplements basic insurance. Disability insurance pays benefits to those who cannot work because of accident or illness.

15. Medicare and Medicaid are public health plans. Medicare covers people sixty-five and older and has two parts. Part A is a compulsory hospitalization plan. Part B is a voluntary program, paid for monthly. Even so, together Parts A and B provide only limited coverage. Medicaid covers part or all of the hospital and medical expenses of those who cannot afford medical care.

16. Health maintenance organizations (HMOs) are prepaid group practices that provide members with all of their health care for a monthly fee. HMOs are structured to promote preventive medicine, and they tend to keep costs low. HMOs offer certain advantages to patients, including less frequent and shorter hospital stays, less surgery, and lower costs.

GLOSSARY

basic health insurance   Insurance that pays benefits for hospitalization and for medical and surgical expenses.

disability insurance   Insurance that pays benefits to a person unable to work because of accident or illness.

glaucoma   A condition in which the pressure inside the eyeball increases.

health maintenance organization (HMO)   A type of prepaid group-practice plan in which consumers pay a set fee every month and in return receive whatever medical services they need at little or no additional cost.

iatrogenic   Referring to illness or injury caused by a doctor's carelessness, error, or poor judgment.

major medical insurance   Insurance designed to provide protection against the high medical expenses that accumulate when a person is seriously injured or ill for a long time.

mamography   An X-ray of the breast to detect abnormalities, especially cancer.

Medicaid   A federal-state health insurance program for people of any age who cannot pay for medical care.

Medicare   A federal health insurance program for people aged sixty-five or older.

nosocomial   Referring to illness or injury caused by contact with a hospital or other health institution, ranging from a fall from bed to an infection to a fatal surgical error.

sign   An objective, observable indication of disease. Compare symptom.

symptom   A subjective indication of disease, experienced by the individual but not necessarily apparent to an observer. Compare sign.

NOTES

1. Lowell Levin, *Self-Care: Lay Initiatives in Health,* 2nd ed. (New York: Protist, 1979), p. 2.

2. John Knowles, *Doing Better and Feeling Worse: Health in the United States* (New York: Norton, 1977), pp. 79–80.

3. Donald Vickery and James Fries, *Take Care of Yourself: A Consumer's Guide to Medical Care,* rev. ed. (Menlo Park, Calif.: Addison-Wesley, 1981) p. 1.

4. Keith Sehnert, *How to Be Your Own Doctor—Sometimes* (New York: Grosset & Dunlap, 1975).

5. Robert J. Benowicz, *Nonprescription Drugs and Their Side Effects* (New York: Grosset & Dunlap, 1977); Joe Graedon, *The People's Pharmacy* (New York: Avon Books, 1976); David R. Zimmerman, *The Essential Guide to Nonprescription Drugs* (New York: Harper & Row, 1983); *Handbook of Nonprescriptions Drugs* (Washington, D.C.: American Pharmaceutical Association, 1977); *Physicians' Desk Reference for Nonprescription Drugs* (Oradell, N.J.: Medical Economics Company, updated annually).

6. Vickery and Fries, *Take Care of Yourself,* see note 3, above, pp. 17–18.

7. Ibid., p. 15.

8. Dodi Schultz, "Prescription Price Survey," *West 77th Street Block Association Newsletter* 2, no. 3. (May–June 1981): 8.

9. *Physicians' Desk Reference* (Oradell, N.J. Medical Economics Company, updated annually); *AMA Drug Evaluations,* 4th ed. (Chicago; American Medical Association, 1980); *The Medical Letter* (The Medical Letter, Inc., 56 Harrison St., New Rochelle, N.Y. 10801); *Physi-*

cians' Drug Alert (M. J. Powers & Co., 38 East 57th St., New York, N.Y. 10022).

10. Vickery and Fries, *Take Care of Yourself,* p. 86.

11. Duane Stroman, *The Medical Establishment and Social Responsibility* (Port Washington, N.Y.: Kennikat Press, 1976), p. 171.

12. Stroman, *Medical Establishment,* p. 52.

13. Ibid., p. 55.

14. "Executive Board Debates Chiropractic," *The Nation's Health,* May 1983, p. 10.

15. "New War on Health Costs," *Newsweek,* May 9, 1983, pp. 24, 29.

16. Duane Stroman, *The Quick Knife: Unnecessary Surgery U.S.A.* (Port Washington, N. Y: Kennikat Press, 1979), p. 6.

17. "Could an HMO Give You Better, Cheaper Health Care?" *Changing Times,* June 1980, pp. 29–32.

18. H. Cornacchia and S. Barrett, *Consumer Health: A Guide to Intelligent Decisions* (St. Louis: Mosby, 1980), p. 251.

19. Cornacchia and Barrett, *Consumer Health: A Guide,* pp. 289–290; Shipley and Plonsky, *Consumer Health,* pp. 152–153.

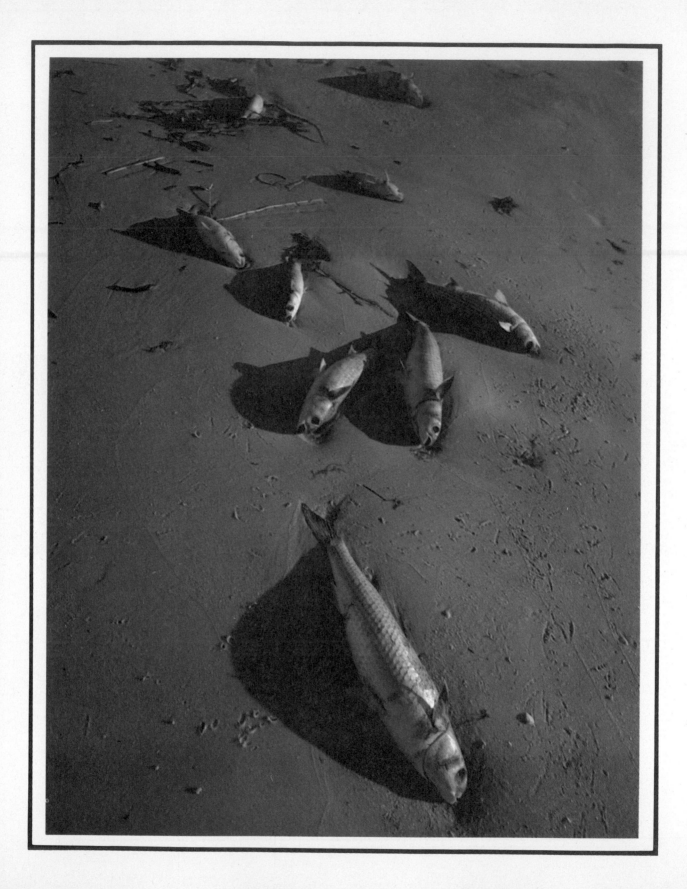

CHAPTER 17

Environmental Health

Pesticides. Drugs. Dyes. Plastics. Fertilizers. Fuels. Synthetic fibers. Building materials. Food additives. Detergents. The list is endless. The spoils of the twentieth-century technological revolution line our cupboards, refrigerators, and medicine cabinets, hang in our closets, cover our lawns, furnish our homes, and occupy our garages. New technology and new chemical compounds—some 1,000 new compounds are developed each year in the United States alone—have been an undeniable boon to humanity. They have increased food production, conquered many infectious diseases, and enabled more people than ever to enjoy "the good life." But it is becoming increasingly clear that all of this progress has a cost. The most glaring consequence is an increase in environmental pollution.

Pollution refers to any substance or energy that contributes to the development of undesirable environmental effects.[1] It includes anything that provides extra energy—in any form—leading to harmful environmental changes. For example, noise is extra energy; sewage adds energy to bodies of water. Radiation adds extra energy that can cause many changes in plants and animals—including human beings.

Our bodies can cope with a certain amount of pollution, via built-in systems for self-cleansing and self-renewal. The body's repair mechanisms are constantly replacing damaged body chemicals, cell parts, and even whole cells. The body also has a system of chemicals known as *enzymes;* they work—particularly in the liver—to break down or metabolize many unwanted or toxic chemicals, both natural and synthetic (see Chapter 3). These protective systems operate constantly. If the damage from toxic substances remains within the normal rate of breakdown and replacement, it will not usually have a harmful effect on the individual. We say that the person's exposure is below the effect's *threshold.*

If the exposure exceeds the threshold, however, the rate at which the individual's body is damaged will exceed the rate at which it can repair itself, and the individual may suffer a loss of body function that may lead to a permanent disability. As Figure 17.1 shows, a given pollutant does not have a single threshold. Rather, as exposure to the pollutant continues, a series of thresholds involving increasingly severe chronic effects, such as weight loss or changed level of enzyme activity, are crossed. Finally, the threshold for the ultimate effect—death—may be reached. (Experts still disagree as to whether this threshold concept applies to cancer-causing chemicals, or whether a single molecule of certain chemicals is sometimes sufficient to cause the disease.)

The threshold concept is the basis for federal and state laws regulating the level of hazardous substances to which people may be exposed in the workplace. Some government regulations also control the substances discharged into the air people breathe. Still others set acceptable levels for contaminants in the water we drink and the food we eat. But the problem is determining what constitutes a "safe" level. Allowances must be made for the lower thresholds of the very young, the very old, the sick, the disabled, and others who are at special risk because of some genetic, developmental, nutritional, physiological, or psychological characteristic.

At this time, government, industry, and private citizens are in the midst of a heated, ongoing debate over all forms of pollution. As you will see in this chapter, we as individuals must make choices as to the types and quantities of pollution

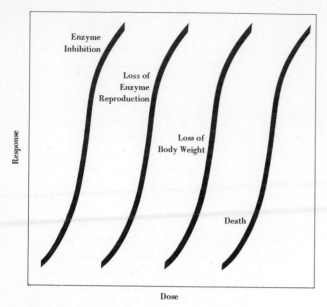

Figure 17.1 There is a relationship between the amount of a chemical substance ingested and the severity of the body's reaction to it. (This is known as the dose-response relationship, discussed in Chapter 5.) The larger the dose, or exposure to a chemical pollutant, the greater the number and severity of adverse responses in the body. Depending on the threshold of exposure and the nature of the pollutant involved, it is believed that these bodily responses may include disrupted enzyme production, weight loss, and death.   Fred Haynes

to which we are exposed; and then we can take action to make our concerns known to those who have some control over pollution.

AIR POLLUTION

Air pollution is the presence in the air of contaminants that do not disperse properly and that interfere with human health.[2] People once believed that Earth had an unlimited supply of breathable air. But now there is widespread doubt: We now know that the air—most vital of our natural resources—must be protected before it is irreversibly fouled.

How Air Pollution Endangers Our Health

Air pollution poses its most immediate threat to the respiratory system, but over time it can also

harm other parts of the body, including the brain and the heart.

CONTAMINATING SUBSTANCES IN AIR

The principal contaminants responsible for air pollution are sulfur oxides, nitrogen oxides, carbon monoxide, hydrocarbons, and particulate matter (see Table 17.1).

SULFUR OXIDES   Sulfur oxides, produced primarily by the burning of fossil fuels such as coal, petroleum, and natural gas, are thought to be a principal cause of excessive deaths during major smog incidents. Sulfur dioxide, in particular, has been implicated in bronchitis, emphysema, and asthma, but all the sulfur oxides cause irritation to the eyes, throat, and upper respiratory system, causing coughing and choking.

NITROGEN OXIDES   Nitrogen oxides come from motor vehicle emissions and the burning of fossil fuels. They are thought to contribute to respiratory difficulties and to reduce the oxygen-carrying capacity of the blood. Further, nitrogen dioxide, upon absorbing energy from sunlight, undergoes a chemical reaction that forms ozone. Ozone causes eye and throat irritation and has been implicated in pulmonary fibrosis, a lung disorder.

CARBON MONOXIDE   Carbon monoxide, a deadly gas that is colorless and odorless, is released from automobile exhausts at the rate of 60,000 tons a year in the United States. It constitutes more than half of all humanmade air emissions. Carbon monoxide levels are especially high in dense traffic, at intersections, and in enclosed areas such as garages and tunnels. The major effect of carbon monoxide is to reduce the oxygen-carrying capacity of our red blood cells. Exposure to significant doses of carbon monoxide causes a deficiency of oxygen in the blood, resulting in impaired respiration and malfunctioning of the brain and the heart. Other effects include impaired hearing, vision, and thought. Excessive exposure to carbon monoxide can lead to unconsciousness and death.

HYDROCARBONS   Hydrocarbons, also produced primarily by automobile emissions, result from incomplete burning of fuel. Hydrocarbons are a significant factor in photochemical smog (discussed in the following section).

TABLE 17.1 ▪ Major Air Pollutants and Their Health Effects

Pollutants	Major Sources	Characteristics and Effects
Carbon Monoxide (CO)	Vehicle exhausts	Colorless, odorless poisonous gas. Replaces oxygen in red blood cells, causing dizziness, unconsciousness, or death.
Hydrocarbons (HC)	Incomplete combustion of gasoline; evaporation of petroleum fuels, solvents and paints	Although some are poisonous, most are not. React with NO_2 to form ozone, or smog.
Lead (Pb)	Anti-knock agents in gasoline	Accumulates in the bone and soft tissues. Affects blood-forming organs, kidneys, and nervous system. Suspected of causing learning disabilities in young children.
Nitrogen Dioxide (NO_2)	Industrial processes, vehicle exhausts	Causes structural and chemical changes in the lungs. Lowers resistance to respiratory infections. Reacts in sunlight with hydrocarbons to produce smog. Contributes to acid rain.
Ozone (O_3)	Formed when HC and NO_2 react	Principal constituent of smog. Irritates mucous membranes, causing coughing, choking, impaired lung function. Aggravates chronic asthma and bronchitis.
Total Suspended Particulates (TSP)	Industrial plants, heating boilers, auto engines, dust	Larger visible types (soot, smoke, or dust) can clog the lung sacs. Smaller invisible particles can pass into the bloodstream. Often carry carcinogens and toxic metals; impair visibility.
Sulfur Dioxide (SO_2)	Burning coal and oil, industrial processes	Corrosive, poisonous gas. Associated with coughs, colds, asthma, and bronchitis. Contributes to acid rain.

Source: Environmental Protection Agency.

PARTICULATE MATTER Particulate matter includes dust, ash, and other fine particles that are by-products of fuel combustion, other types of burning, and abrasion milling. These particles, which are observable components of smog, irritate the eyes, throat, and lungs; some may be carcinogenic.

WHO IS AT GREATEST RISK FROM AIR POLLUTION?

Individuals vary considerably in their susceptibility to unclean air. Those with heart disease and those with respiratory ailments such as asthma, bronchitis, and emphysema are likely to feel the effects of air pollution. But even those who do not have heart disease or respiratory illnesses may be affected by air pollution to some degree: Although there is no proof that air pollution *causes* disease, people in heavily polluted areas suffer more short-term respiratory ailments and chest infections than do those in clean-air zones. Cigarette smokers, in particular, run a higher risk of contracting pollution-related ailments, because the effects of cigarette smoke and air pollution seem to reinforce each other.

THE DANGERS OF SMOG

Sometimes urban authorities issue warnings about the form of air pollution known as **smog** (a made-up word that combines *smoke* and *fog*). Though acute smog episodes are rare, they can be deadly. Twenty people died and thousands fell ill during a smog alert in Donora, Pennsylvania, in 1948; and more than 4,000 people succumbed to London's "killer smog" of 1952.

There are actually two types of smog: the London type and the Los Angeles type. The London variety, blamed for thousands of deaths in Europe

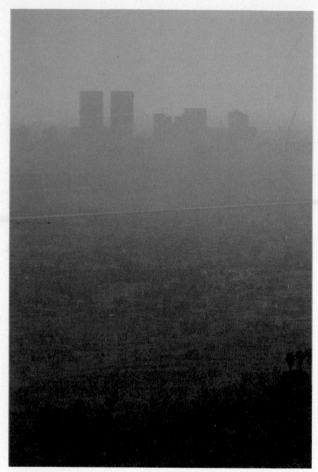

Photochemical smog hovers over Los Angeles. (© Mike Yamashita, 1981/Woodfin Camp & Assoc.)

and the eastern United States, is more correctly termed *sulfur-dioxide smog.* It is caused by the burning of fossil fuels (primarily coal with high sulfur content); high levels of sulfur dioxide and ozone result, combined with particulate matter and foggy air. Sulfur-dioxide smog poses a special threat: It inhibits the sweeping action of the cilia that line our respiratory passages, allowing smog particles to remain and irritate sensitive tissues. These particles and chemicals impair breathing so markedly that people with chronic respiratory problems may die. Impaired breathing can also aggravate heart problems. Reduction of the use of high-sulfur fuels has significantly decreased the occurrence of London-type smog.

Los Angeles-type smog, more properly called *photochemical smog,* results from the interaction of sunlight with temperature inversions and ex-

haust emissions from automobiles. This type of smog occurs in areas with poor air circulation (valleys, for example), especially those where there is sunny weather and low humidity. In Los Angeles, a layer of cool ocean air may slip in under the normally warm, stable air above the city. This cool air becomes trapped by the warmer air, a phenomenon called a **temperature inversion.** Motor vehicle emissions rise through the cool air but cannot penetrate the warm layer, which acts like a lid on the Los Angeles basin. Thus the pollutants are trapped and subjected to the action of sunlight, which produces additional pollutants (such as ozone). The pollutants do not disperse until the weather changes and the inversion lifts.

PROBLEMS WITH FLUOROCARBONS

Although **fluorocarbons**—chemical compounds used as propellants in aerosol spray cans—are not known to have a direct effect on human beings, they are nevertheless considered a threat to health by a growing number of scientists. Evidence has accumulated to suggest that because these compounds are inert and do not react with the other contents of the spray cans, they float up unchanged to the stratosphere, where they set off chemical reactions that may gradually destroy the layer of ozone that lies ten to forty miles above the earth. This ozone layer is important to living things on earth because it absorbs wavelengths of ultraviolet sunlight. Among the possible consequences of ozone depletion, scientists fear an increase in the incidence of skin cancer and a negative effect on human immune responses.

Improving Air Quality: What Is Being Done?

The federal Clean Air Act, passed in 1970 and amended in 1977, signified a major change in our consciousness of the importance of air quality. It established strict air-quality standards based primarily on health rather than economic considerations. The Clean Air Act empowered the Environmental Protection Agency (EPA) to set limits on several major air pollutants, including sulfur oxides and nitrogen oxides, and it mandated reductions of automobile and factory emissions.[3] By the time it came up for renewal by Congress in December 1981, the act had caused dramatic improvement in air quality throughout the United States. But in a time of economic recession, many manufacturers were pressuring the government to relax the costly regulations. Battle lines were drawn: Industrialists claimed that the price of complying with the Clean Air Act (especially the strict limits on automobile emissions) was too high, and environmentalists contended that increased costs were balanced by a reduction in pollution-related illnesses and deaths.[4] At the time of this writing, some 86 percent of the public favor a strong pollution control law; efforts to weaken the measure have so far been defeated.[5]

CHEMICAL POLLUTION

Toxic Wastes

Each year, American industry produces about 126 billion pounds of toxic wastes—enough to fill the New Orleans Superdome from top to bottom every day![6] And, according to the EPA, only about 10 percent of these chemicals are regularly disposed of safely. The remainder are illegally dumped in municipal landfills, open pits, or lagoons (see Figure 17.2).

Toxic wastes can enter the body through the mouth, nose, or skin. Some are stored in the fat of human beings and animals, accumulating in body tissue and causing damage to vital organs, debilita-

tion, and death.[7] Some toxic waste substances, such as asbestos, benzene, vinyl chloride, and arsenic, are carcinogenic. Others are teratogenic (causing birth defects) or mutagenic (triggering mutations in genes). The possible effects of some common hazardous wastes are summarized in Table 17.2.

Among the toxic-waste substances whose health dangers have been documented are polychlorinated biphenyls (PCBs)—poisons whose chemical structure is similar to that of the persistent pesticide DDT. A component of electrical insulators, adhesives, sealants, printing inks, waxes, and many other products, PCBs are believed to produce cancer in laboratory animals, and they have been linked to reproductive disorders, kidney damage, liver ailments, and eye irritations in humans. In 1968, some 1,000 people in Japan became ill after consuming rice oil contaminated with PCBs. Ten years later, in the United States, an EPA survey revealed that nearly one-third of nursing mothers had measurable amounts of PCBs in their milk. In an effort to regulate disposal of PCBs, EPA regulations stipulate that all PCB contaminated material must be specially labeled and disposed of only at EPA-approved waste-disposal sites.[8]

THE LOVE CANAL INCIDENT

One of the most highly publicized toxic-waste disasters took place at Love Canal, a once-pleasant

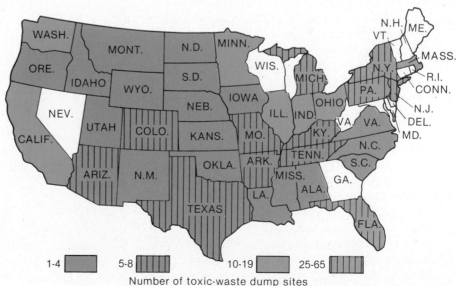

Figure 17.2 In December 1982 the Environmental Protection Agency released a list of the 418 abandoned toxic-waste dump sites—many of them illegal—that posed the greatest threat to people, water, and air and were therefore first in line for federal Superfund cleanup money. This map shows the state-by-state distribution of these dump sites. New Jersey led the list, with 65 sites. The EPA's list did not include the thousands of toxic-waste dump sites that are still in active use or on federal property.
Source: U.S. Environmental Protection Agency.

1-4   5-8   10-19   25-65
Number of toxic-waste dump sites

TABLE 17.2 · Common Hazardous Wastes

Chemical	Use	Hazard
C-56	Bug and insect killer	Acutely toxic, suspected carcinogen
Trichloroethylene (TCE)	Degreaser	Suspected carcinogen
Benzidene	Dye industry	Known human carcinogen
Curene 442	Plastics industry	Suspected carcinogen
Polychlorinated biphenyls (PCBs)	Insulators, paints, and electrical circuitry	Acutely toxic, suspected carcinogen
Benzene	Solvent	Suspected carcinogen
Tris	Fire retardant	Suspected carcinogen
DDT	Bug and insect killer	Acutely toxic
Vinyl chloride	Plastics industry	Known human carcinogen
Mercury	Multiple uses	Acutely toxic
Lead	Multiple uses	Acutely toxic, suspected carcinogen
Carbon tetrachloride	Solvent	Acutely toxic, suspected carcinogen
Polybrominated biphenyls (PBBs)	Fire retardant	Effects unknown

Source: Council on Environmental Quality.

neighborhood near the industrial town of Niagara Falls, New York. The area took its name from William T. Love, an enterpreneur who, as part of a scheme to industrialize Niagara Falls, started building a canal on the site in the late nineteenth century. Love ultimately declared bankruptcy, and soon after World War II the area was acquired by the Hooker Chemical and Plastics Corporation, which dumped approximately 21,800 tons of pesticides, cleaning solutions, and other toxic wastes into the canal between 1947 and 1952. In 1953 Hooker covered the site with dirt and sold it to the Niagara Falls Board of Education for $1.00. The board—which had signed papers stipulating that it would not hold Hooker responsible for any injuries or deaths that might occur at the site—then built a school on the landfill and sold adjoining lots for real estate development. Families settled in the area.[9]

In 1978 heavy rains and snowfalls caused the canal's contents to overflow. Chemicals such as benzene, PCBs, and C-56 (a by-product of the manufacture of pesticides that can cause damage to virtually every organ in the body) were carried by creeks into the neighborhood. Reports told of noxious odors permeating homes, of slime oozing into basements, of children coming home with painful rashes and watering eyes after swimming in a pond on the canal site—and, most alarming of all, of unusually high rates of miscarriages, birth defects, liver ailments, nervous disorders, epilepsy-like seizures, genetic damage, and cancer.

Finally the landfill's topsoil began to wash

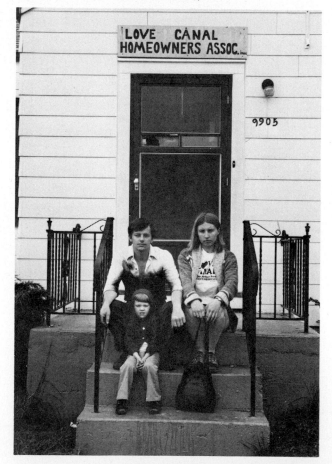

This family lived in the Love Canal area until toxic waste pollution forced them and their neighbors to evacuate. The woman shown here was told by officials that she had suffered chromosomal damage. (©Andy Levin, 1980/Black Star)

away, revealing Hooker's by-then corroded and leaking metal casks and alerting EPA officials to the disaster. Analysis revealed that the dump contained more than eighty chemicals, ten of which were potential carcinogens. There were also solvents that attack the heart and liver, and pesticides so dangerous that their commercial sale has for for years been restricted by the government.[10] In addition to the physical ailments residents have suffered, there has been considerable psychological damage. One study has shown that children who lived near the canal suffer from obsession with fears of premature death. Some adolescent girls have expressed fear of having deformed babies.[11]

President Jimmy Carter declared a state of emergency in the area, and 237 families were evacuated with the help of federal funds in August 1978. Many of those who were left behind, convinced that they, too, were in danger, joined together to take action, forming the Love Canal Homeowners' Association. Angry, frustrated—but persistent—they took their case to whoever would listen: the press, local government, the state, Washington. Finally, in May 1980, President Carter responded to their pleas. He empowered the state and the EPA to relocate 710 families temporarily, while the chemical quagmire was drained and the area made safe for habitation. Untold damage had been done by the time the government took action; nevertheless, the Love Canal homeowners, who were powerless individuals when they started out, demonstrated that a well-organized, persevering group *can* prod a slow-moving government into taking action on their behalf.

DIOXIN: THE TIMES BEACH INCIDENT

In 1971 oil was sprayed on the dirt roads of Times Beach, Missouri, a suburb of St. Louis. The oil was sprayed to keep down dust. This was a routine practice and was quickly forgotten. Eleven years later, however, that oil caused the EPA to buy the entire town of Times Beach and evacuate its residents—at a cost of $36.3 million in government funds.

As it turned out, the oil had been mixed with sludge from a chemical plant—sludge that contained dioxin, which, according to some scientists, is the most dangerous chemical known. Dioxin is really a name for a large number of chemicals that share a basic structure; this group of chemicals is notorious for producing dramatic health problems in incredibly small doses. In animal experiments, doses as small as five parts per 1,000 billion have caused cancer. Thus far, no human deaths have been directly attributed to dioxin, but dioxin has been *associated* with a host of diseases in humans, including cancer and kidney and liver diseases.

The Centers for Disease Control soon determined the source of the dioxin that contaminated Times Beach: It came from a chemical plant in Verona, Missouri, which had since gone out of business. But a crucial problem remains: to find out what has happened to the rest of the dioxin produced at all the chemical plants in America. And though the Times Beach incident is over, we will surely face other large-scale toxic waste problems in the future.

Pesticides and Herbicides

Pesticides such as DDT, aldrin, and dieldrin have become a pervasive part of the world environment: These chemicals have played a major role in increasing food production and in controlling diseases such as malaria and yellow fever throughout the world. Yet pesticides have become a threat, too: They are easily spread, they persist in the environment, and, like PCBs, they tend to accumulate in living tissues, especially in the fatty tissues of animals and humans.

An ongoing debate in this area concerns Agent Orange, a mixture of two potent herbicides— 2,4-D and 2,4,5-T—used to defoliate jungles and destroy crops. Between 1965 and 1970, the Defense Department sprayed 10.7 million gallons of Agent Orange on Vietnam. By 1977 Vietnam veterans had begun to contact the Veterans Administration (VA) about Agent Orange-related health problems, including cancer, liver damage, depression, sleeplessness, miscarriages and stillbirths in their wives, and birth defects in their children.[12] The issue made national headlines in 1978 when a twenty-eight-year-old Chicagoan named Paul Reutershan stunned a TV talk-show audience with the remark, "I died in Vietnam and didn't know it." At that time he was suffering from stomach cancer; two months later, he died. And at that point the organization he had founded, Agent Or-

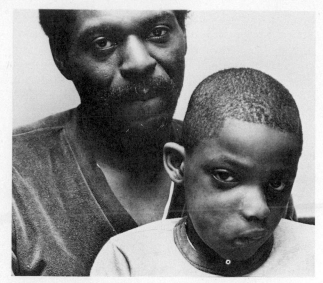

This man was exposed to Agent Orange during his military service in Vietnam in the mid-1960s. He has since been troubled by rashes, nausea, headaches, and numbness in his hands. His son was born with a facial tumor and is "always sick," the father says. (Wendy Watriss, 1981/Woodfin Camp & Assoc.)

ange Victims International, took their case to the public.

A year later, the EPA suspended domestic use of 2,4,5-T, one of the ingredients in Agent Orange, after women in Alsea, Oregon, complained of high rates of miscarriage following use of the herbicide near their homes. Then a study commissioned by the federal Veterans Administration demonstrated a relationship between Agent Orange and the buildup of dioxin in human tissues. But it was not until June 1981 that the efforts of individuals and veterans' groups began to pay off. The House of Representatives passed four veterans' bills, including a measure that ordered the VA to begin free treatment of veterans with conditions attributable to Agent Orange.

At this writing, there is still no ironclad link between Agent Orange and specific disabilities. Nevertheless, the veterans have made believers of many members of Congress, and when the Agent Orange bills were passed, congressional committee members specified, "When a doubt exists, the doubt should be resolved in favor of the veteran."[13]

Other Hazardous Chemicals

ASBESTOS

Asbestos is a naturally occurring mineral that can be processed to form practically indestructible fibers. People who work with asbestos are exposed to a significant hazard, since inhaling or ingesting even very small amounts of asbestos is associated with an increased risk of cancer of the lungs and the intestinal tract in susceptible people. But there is also evidence that relatively small amounts of asbestos fiber pose a threat to the health of the general public. City dwellers breathe in the fibers with the air, and asbestos has also been found in wines filtered with asbestos mesh, in baby powder, and in water supplies. Most of our homes and cars contain some asbestos in insulation, water pipes, brake linings, and the like.

LEAD

Lead, like asbestos, is a naturally occurring element, usually distributed in low concentrations. Since the introduction of the automobile, however, the lead content of the atmosphere has greatly increased, for it has long been an additive in leaded gasoline. Furthermore, until recently lead was used in many paints, automobile batteries, ceramics, glassware, pipes, and other manufactured goods. The basic danger from lead lies in lead poisoning, which causes weakness, loss of appetite, anemia, and damage to the nervous system.

Federal law now requires companies whose products contain lead to use minimal amounts of lead, thus reducing the risks of atmospheric lead poisoning. Of even greater danger is lead poisoning that may occur when children eat lead-based paint and putty, usually off walls and woodwork in older buildings. Hundreds of children have died from this type of poisoning over the years, and thousands of others have suffered chronic symptoms related to it. Studies have found that children whose blood contains elevated levels of lead tend to score lower on intelligence tests than children with normal blood.[14]

MERCURY

Mercury is a naturally occurring element that is widely distributed in the earth's crust. In its elemental form, mercury is a very stable metal, and mercury salts are considered quite insoluble. However, certain microorganisms can convert elemental mercury and other forms of mercury into an organic form, methyl mercury, which, when consumed in large enough quantities, produces devastating symptoms.

Unfortunately, this fact was not discovered until several years after a tragic incident. From the early 1930s until 1971, certain Japanese factories released industrial wastes containing substantial quantities of mercury into the Pacific Ocean. Marine microorganisms metabolized the mercury to its organic form, which became progressively more concentrated as it passed along the food chain to higher organisms. The highest organisms in the chain were human beings—residents of a fishing village on Minamata Bay, whose diet consisted almost solely of fish. The high level of mercury in the fish they ate resulted in fifty-two deaths; more than a hundred other people experienced serious symptoms, including inability to speak, mental retardation, numbness of arms and legs followed by deterioration of muscle tissue, gradual loss of vision and hearing, disruption of equilibrium, loss of coordination, and emotional disturbance. Many of these victims are now permanently disabled, and children born to mothers who consumed the contaminated seafood are severely deformed.

As a result of the Minamata episode and other mercury-related disasters, most industrialized nations have instituted strict regulations prohibiting mercury pollution, and acute mercury poisoning from contaminated food is now far less likely than it was a decade ago.

WATER POLLUTION

Unlike many of the earth's inhabitants, who must haul bacteria-laden water from nearby lakes, creeks, and wells, we enjoy the convenience of having seemingly clean water at our immediate disposal. We expect it to be there—for drinking, cooking, bathing, swimming, fishing. But in recent years, we have become increasingly concerned about chemical pollution of our water. For example, on June 12, 1973, the federal government warned parents in Duluth, Minnesota, not to allow their children to drink the municipal water, which

was found to be laced with asbestos fibers.[15] According to a report published by the Water Resources Research Institute in 1975, half of the water supplies that serve fewer than 500 people did not meet minimum health standards, and nearly 25 percent exceeded federal standards for contamination.[16] In May 1978, four wells in Bedford, Massachusetts, which provide 80 percent of the town's drinking water, were found to be contaminated with toxic chemicals. And as of November 1982, 54 public wells on Long Island had been closed because of organic chemical contamination that exceeded state guidelines.[17]

Sources of Domestic Water

To understand the problems associated with water pollution, we need to look at the water that comes from each source: water from wells, or ground water, and water from lakes, reservoirs, and rivers, or surface water.

Most water pollution in the United States is caused by industrial processing and its resulting wastes, which are often dumped directly into the public water supply. (©George Hall/Woodfin Camp & Assoc.)

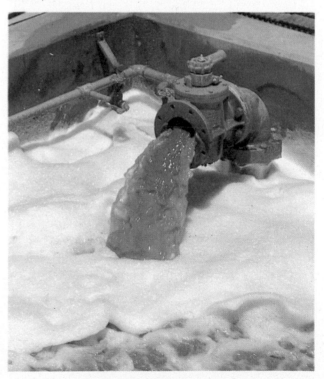

GROUND WATER

Buried from a few feet to a half-mile or more beneath the earth's surface are strata known as *aquifers* (water-bearing layers of porous rock, sand, and gravel). The "ground water" in these aquifers was once believed to be beyond the reach of pollutants. But increasing quantities of synthetic chemicals and other harmful substances—such as cleaning agents, salts used to melt ice and snow from highways, leaks from underground oil and gas tanks, agricultural chemicals, and surface water—are contaminating our subterranean water supplies. These materials filter down from the land surface into the aquifers or directly contaminate unprotected wells.

SURFACE WATER

About half of the U.S. population gets its drinking supply from surface water—that is, from rivers, creeks, lakes, streams, or reservoirs. Pollution of surface water can come from many sources. Air pollutants may enter surface water through rain. Chemicals and other pollutants may be washed into surface water by rain or the action of humans. Finally, we may pollute surface water intentionally by dumping home or industrial wastes.

The Problem of Acid Rain

In many of our lakes and streams, plant and animal life has been choked off by **acid rain**—rain containing nitrogen and sulfur oxides discharged from motor vehicles and coal-burning power plants and factories. Rising upward into the atmosphere, these pollutants circulate, react with moisture, and turn into nitric and sulfuric acids, which eventually fall back to earth—in rain or snow that is as acidic as lemon juice or vinegar. Unfortunately, many of the towering industrial smokestacks that were designed to minimize local pollution have apparently acted to *increase* acid rain: They inject the pollutants higher into the atmosphere, which makes it easier for acidic compounds to form. The effect of acid rain on humans is still unclear, but acid sulfate particles—bits of "acid dust" that float down independent of rain, snow, and sleet—are believed to contribute to a number of respiratory ailments.[18]

NOISE POLLUTION

When we refer to loud noises as "deafening," we are not just using a figure of speech. Noise is now recognized as a form of pollution that can be hazardous to human health. Our ears were simply not made to withstand constant assaults from jet planes, amplified rock music, power lawnmowers, construction sites, and household appliances.

Health Dangers of Noise Pollution

Besides developing hearing problems, persons exposed to noise pollution may experience fatigue, insomnia, irritability, more accidents, and learning difficulties. Excessive noise produces bodily changes, including increased heart rate, digestive spasms, blood vessel constriction, and pupil dilation. In animal studies, continual noise has damaged the heart, brain, liver, reproductive system, and immunological system. Noise may also be a factor in stress-related disorders, including high blood pressure, peptic ulcers, weight loss, and emotional disturbances.

Recent research has also found a connection between noise and socially undesirable behavior. In one experiment, subjects behaved more aggressively after being exposed to noise that they could not escape or control.[19]

Rock music fans should beware of dangerously loud music. If you can't hear what the person next to you is saying over the sound of the music, you are risking hearing impairment.

Controlling Noise Pollution

Control of noise pollution is difficult. European countries have instituted a number of antinoise laws that appear to be successful at curbing harmful noise, and the Japanese carefully monitor the noise levels at busy intersections in urban areas. But in the United States, where average noise levels have increased greatly in the last twenty years, few communities have dealt with the problem

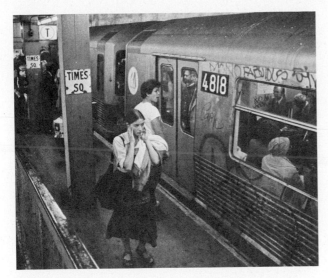

Noise pollution causes physical and psychological stress and can cause hearing loss. (©Jim Anderson/ Woodfin Camp & Assoc.)

successfully. Industries have done better in protecting employees: Workers in high-noise occupations are outfitted with special headgear, and soundproofing and wise architectural planning help to separate office workers from noisy machinery. Nevertheless, the problem is a long way from being completely solved, and insurance companies continue to pay out millions of dollars to workers who have gone deaf from exposure to excessive noise on the job.

RADIATION

Radiation has always been part of our natural environment. It comes to us as a result of radioactive mineral deposits, cosmic radiation, and similar natural phenomena. Today, however, our environment also contains humanmade radiation. It comes from medical X-rays and radiation therapy, microwave ovens, color television sets, industrial isotopes and X-rays, radioactive wastes from nuclear power plants, and nuclear fallout from weapons testing. Natural radiation is responsible for about 58 percent of an average person's exposure to radiation in the environment. Humanmade radiation accounts for 41 percent, and the remaining 1 percent comes from fallout.[20] (Concerns about nuclear fallout led to the 1963 treaty be-

tween the United States and the Soviet Union banning atmospheric testing of atomic weapons.)

Health Effects of Radiation

Radiation may enter the body directly through the skin, but it is usually inhaled or ingested as radioactive particles or substances. The effect of radiation exposure depends on the dose, the length of exposure, the type of radiation, and the individual's degree of sensitivity. Prolonged or excessive exposure produces **radiation sickness** in most people. The symptoms of this disease come in stages: first, diarrhea, nausea, vomiting; second, loss of hair, hemorrhaging beneath the skin surface, ulcers in the mouth and digestive system; third, eye cataracts, high susceptibility to infections, and possible leukemia. In general, women tend to be more vulnerable to the effects of radiation than are men.

VULNERABLE PARTS OF THE BODY

Radiation has its most serious effect on those tissues in which cells normally reproduce rapidly—the lining of the digestive tract, the blood-forming tissues, and so on. Especially vulnerable are sperm and egg cells and developing fetuses. Radiation is thus a major factor in genetic mutations, and significant doses are known to cause infertility, miscarriage, and birth defects. And certain radioactive elements can remain in the body indefinitely, emitting harmful radiation over a long period of time. Strontium-90 accumulates in bones; plutonium collects in the liver, bones, and sex organs.

RADIATION AND CANCER

The tissues of the body vary widely in their sensitivity to radiation. Some tissues are very sensitive to radiation and will become damaged with minimal doses; others are remarkably resistant. Diagnostic radiation—use of radiation as an aid in diagnosing disease—usually presents such a small risk of disease that the benefits are thought to outweigh any risk.

   In doses *below* those that cause radiation sickness but above normal (such as those experienced by people who work with radioactive materials), radiation is thought to be carcinogenic. Because radioactive particles act primarily to alter or destroy individual cells, long-term exposure at normally "nondangerous" levels may promote cancerous growth. Recent studies indicate that there may be *no* safe level of radiation exposure, *no* dose of radiation so low that the risk of cancer is zero.

Some researchers believe that humans are exposed to unnecessary doses of radiation through routine dental and diagnostic X-rays. Reflecting this concern, in November 1982 the American College of Radiologists joined a growing list of clinicians in recommending that chest X-rays be used more sparingly.[21] Other medical professionals have expressed hope that the development of revolutionary techniques for viewing body tissues without X-rays will replace the use of radiation-dependent equipment in clinical diagnosis.[22]

Nuclear Power Plants

Some people see nuclear power as the answer to our energy crisis. Others see it as a growing menace that threatens the entire planet. This debate became more intense following the breakdown of a nuclear reactor on Three Mile Island, located about ten miles from Harrisburg, Pennsylvania—a chain of human and mechanical failures that raised questions about the future of the nuclear power industry in the United States.

DIFFICULT DECISIONS

This chapter has presented an overview of some of the most important issues in environmental health. As we pointed out, this chapter cannot deal effectively with all the issues; you need to do additional reading and studying to understand fully the issues raised. There is, however, one basic point that applies to all the issues that we have discussed here.

In this country we have become used to relying on the fruits of an increasingly technological society. New technologies can greatly improve our quality of life—but always at some cost. The decision that we must make is whether the cost is worth the benefit.

Take, for example, a trash compactor, an appliance that compresses household refuse into smaller, more convenient packages. Although this may be useful to the homeowner, when the compacted trash gets to the sanitary landfill, it presents a problem: Natural breakdown processes such as **biodegradation** (breakdown and assimilation of organic material by microorganisms) are hampered because the refuse is so compacted. What decision is to be made here? Do we accept the reduced effectiveness of the sanitary landfill so that we can have compacted trash that's easy to handle, or do we value the ultimate degradation of the refuse over the convenience?

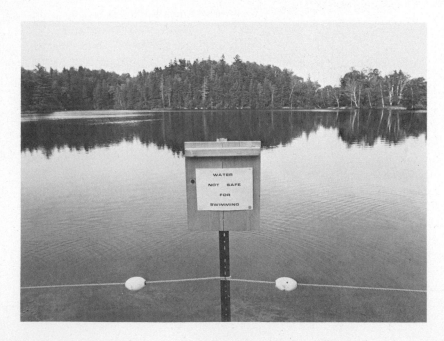

Vermont is not heavily industrialized, yet this lake in that state has become dangerously polluted. Pollution does not recognize any boundaries, so the future of our environment—and the quality of our lives—is up to *all* of us. (© Antonio Mendoza/The Picture Cube)

Nearly all of our environmental issues involve such trade-offs. For agricultural fertilizers, pesticides, and herbicides, we must often choose between higher crop yields and damage to the harmless insects and animals that inhabit farmland. Which choice is better? Obviously there is no clear answer to this question. On the one hand, our society values individual freedom—we believe that we should be free to manage our own affairs as long as we infringe only minimally on the rights of others. On the other hand, we must consider the benefits of keeping our environment intact—benefits the whole community will enjoy in the future.

In such debates we would do well to remember Barry Commoner's four laws of the environment:

1. Everything is connected to everything else.
2. Everything must go somewhere.
3. Nature knows best.
4. There is no such thing as a free lunch.[23]

Generally, individual actions yield inadequate solutions to environmental problems. Thus we have developed the habit of relying on government to solve our environmental problems. The government has helped control many environmentally dangerous situations, but always at the price of a loss of personal—and corporate—freedom. It is likely, and perhaps healthy, that we will continue to debate the values and costs of increasing environmental controls.

MAKING HEALTH DECISIONS

Assessing Your Environment

The term *environment* includes a broad spectrum of forces that affect our daily lives. In our society we constantly interact with environmental forces that have potential for causing us great harm or good. Consider each of the following items carefully. Through your answers, you may come to a clearer understanding of how your environment affects you now—and, more important, what environmental decisions you may face in the future.

I. WHERE YOU LIVE

How would you rate your community on each of the following factors? If poorer than average, put −1 in the blank; if about average, 0; if better than average, +1.

_____ 1. Condition of roads

_____ 2. Availability of playgrounds

_____ 3. Public gardens and parks

_____ 4. Attractive housing

_____ 5. Bicycle trails

_____ 6. Air quality

_____ 7. Amount of sunshine

_____ 8. Adequacy of rain

_____ 9. Severity of winters

_____ 10. Summer heat

_____ 11. Noise

_____ 12. Litter

_____ 13. Water quality

_____ 14. Water availability

_____ 15. Availability of industrial employment

_____ *Total score*

II. WHERE YOU WORK

(If you aren't employed, answer as if you were working in a job you want to have someday.)

What is the major product of your employer?

_____

Would you characterize the work as mainly physical, mainly mental, or both equally?

_____

To what extent are you exposed to the following stresses and hazards in your occupation? Score 0 for not at all; 1 for somewhat; 2 for definitely; 3 for severely; and NA for not applicable.

1. *Stresses*

_____ Noise

_____ Performance pressure

_____ Office politics

_____ Other _____

2. *Hazards*

_____ Accidental injury

_____ Dusts, gases, fumes

_____ Extremes of temperature and humidity

_____ Noise

_____ Infections

_____ Poisons, chemical wastes

_____Total score

III. EXPOSURE TO RADIATION

You can get a rough estimate of your annual exposure to radiation (expressed in units called millirems, or mrems) by filling in each blank as directed and adding up your scores.*

	YOUR ANNUAL DOSE (Mrems)
1. Your community's elevation (26 mrems at sea level + 1 mrem for each 100 feet of elevation)	_____
2. House construction: stone, concrete, or masonry building, add 7	_____
3. Ground (U.S. average)	26
4. Radiation in food, water, and air (U.S. average)	24
5. Weapons tests fallout	4
6. X-ray diagnosis ▪number of chest X-rays_____ × 10	_____

*Adapted from American Nuclear Society, *Nuclear Power and the Environment, Book 1, Radiation: Questions and Answers,* 1982.

	YOUR ANNUAL DOSE (Mrems)
▪number of lower gastrointestinal tract X-rays _____ × 500	
▪other X-rays _____ × 300	_____
7. Jet plane travel: 1 mrem for each 2,500 miles	_____
8. TV viewing: number of hours per day _____ × 0.15	_____
9. Nearness to nuclear power plant ▪at site boundary: average number of hours per day _____ × 0.2= _____ × 365 days	_____
▪1 mile away: average hours per day _____ × 0.02 = 2 _____ × 365 days	_____
▪5 miles away: average hours per day _____ × 0.002=	_____
▪over 5 miles away: 0	_____
Total score	_____

SCORING AND INTERPRETATION

I. Where You Live

What is your net score on items 1–15? Which are the positive aspects of where you live, as revealed by your ratings? Which are the negative aspects?

II. Where You Work

What was your net score on the items dealing with stresses and hazards at work? If you smoke cigarettes, add 6 to your score.

Total score _____.

Which item(s) contributed most to your total score?

III. Exposure to Radiation

The average radiation exposure in the United States is about 180 mrems. How does your estimated total compare with this average? _____

_____

Summary

The information that you have provided in the previous sections indicates the extent to which your environment may be influencing your life and health.

1. Does any of the information you have collected on your environment point to a need for change? Specifically, cite any changes that may be necessary in:

   a. Where you live _____

   _____

   _____

   b. Where you work _____

   _____

   _____

   c. Your exposure to radiation _____

   _____

   _____

   d. Your own behaviors _____

   _____

   _____

   e. Other _____

   _____

   _____

2. If your answers to points *a–e* above suggest that you *should* make certain changes, what would be the costs to you (personal, financial, other) to make these changes? What would be the benefits? Summarize them below:

COSTS	BENEFITS
_____	_____
_____	_____
_____	_____
_____	_____
_____	_____
_____	_____
_____	_____
_____	_____

SUMMARY

1. One consequence of our society's rapid advances in technology has been an increase in environmental pollution. A person's level of exposure to a pollutant can cross a series of effect thresholds, involving increasingly severe damage to the body.

2. Air pollution is the presence in the air of con-taminants that do not disperse properly and that interfere with human health. Major air contaminants are: sulfur oxides, nitrogen oxides, carbon monoxide, hydrocarbons, and particulate matter.

3. Smog is a form of air pollution that can occur in two types. Sulfur-dioxide (London-type) smog is caused by the burning of fossil fuels, which creates high levels of sulfur dioxide and ozone, combined with particulate matter and foggy air. Photo-

chemical (Los Angeles–type) smog is caused by the interaction of sunlight with temperature inversions and auto exhaust emissions.

4. Fluorocarbons used as propellants in aerosol spray cans are believed to be contributing to the destruction of the stratospheric ozone layer that shields the earth from the sun's ultraviolet rays.

5. The Clean Air Act, enforced by the Environmental Protection Agency, has been a major weapon in the battle against air pollution.

6. Chemical pollution involves the production of billions of pounds of toxic wastes each year, most of which are disposed of in an unsafe manner—as the incidents at Love Canal in New York and Times Beach in Missouri made dramatically clear.

7. Among the chemicals known or believed to pose a threat to human health are: PCBs, dioxin, pesticides such as DDT, herbicides such as Agent Orange, asbestos, lead, and mercury.

8. Water pollution is another area of increasing concern. Both ground water and surface water are vulnerable to pollution. Acid rain is a threat to aquatic life in certain parts of the country.

9. Besides damaging hearing, noise pollution can contribute to a variety of physical and psychological problems.

10. Some radiation occurs naturally in the environment, but levels of humanmade radiation—from medical X-rays, microwave ovens, color TVs, and other sources—are increasing at a rate that has caused concern.

11. There is no minimum dose of radiation that can be considered safe in all cases. Radiation sickness develops after prolonged or excessive exposure to radiation. Exposure to radiation may lead to other diseases, including cancer, and can in itself be fatal.

12. Most environmental issues require us to choose between the benefits of a technological innovation and its costs in terms of potential damage to the environment.

GLOSSARY

acid rain Rain containing nitric and sulfuric acid, formed when nitrogen and sulfur oxides from motor vehicles and coal-burning power plants and factories react with moisture in the atmosphere.

air pollution The presence in the air of contaminants that do not disperse properly and that interfere with human health.

biodegradation The breakdown and assimilation of organic material by microorganisms.

fluorocarbons Inert chemical compounds used as propellants in aerosol spray cans and believed to be damaging the ozone layer of the stratosphere that protects the earth from the sun's ultraviolet rays.

pollution Any substance or energy that contributes to the development of undesirable environmental effects.

radiation sickness Disease produced by prolonged or excessive exposure to radiation.

smog A form of air pollution that may occur as either sulfur-dioxide smog (high levels of sulfur dioxide and ozone combined with particulate matter and foggy air) or photochemical smog (the result of the interaction of sunlight, temperature inversion, and exhaust emissions from automobiles).

temperature inversion A phenomenon in which a layer of cool air is trapped under a layer of warm air; pollutants such as motor vehicle emissions also become trapped and are subjected to the action of sunlight, which produces additional pollutants such as ozone.

NOTES

1. Environmental Protection Agency, *Common Environmental Terms* (A-107), November 1977, p. 12.

2. Ibid., p. 2.

3. W. A. — , "The 1977 Clean Air Act Amendments: Their Potential Impact on Economic Growth," *Population and Environment* Spring 1980, p. 21–25.

4. P. De — , "The Clean Air Act: A Realistic Assessment of — Effectiveness," *Harvard Educational Law Review* 1 — : 164–203.

5. *Rolling Stone*, August 6, 1981, p. 24.

6. *Environment and Health* (Washington, D.C.: Congressional Quarterly, Inc., 1981), p. 17.

7. *Environmental Chemicals, Enzyme Function, and Human Disease*, CIBA Foundation Symposium 76 (New Series) (New York: Excerpta Media, 1980).

8. K. Higuchi, ed., *PCB Poisoning and Pollution* (New York: Academic Press, 1976), pp. 3–4; *Environment and Health*, pp. 31, 35.

9. *Environment and Health*, p. 35; M. Brown, "Love Canal and the Poisoning of America," *Atlantic* 224 (December 1979): 35.

10. *Environment and Health*, pp. 35–36.

11. Tracy Freedman, "Love Canal Children: Leftover Lives to Live," *The Nation* 232 (May 23, 1981): 624.

12. *Environment and Health*, p. 32.

13. Ibid., pp. 32–33.

14. J. E. Fielding and P. K. Russo, "Exposure to Lead: Sources and Effects," *New England Journal of Medicine* 297, no. 17 (1977): 943–945.

15. *Environment and Health*, p. 41.

16. Ibid., p. 45.

17. M. McIntyre, "Long Island's Endangered Resource," *Newsday*, November 21, 1982.

18. *Environment and Health*, pp. 21–22.

19. Jane E. Brody, "Noise Poses a Growing Threat, Affecting Hearing and Behavior," *New York Times*, November 16, 1982, pp. C1, C6.

20. A. Turk et al., *Environmental Science* (Philadelphia: Saunders, 1974), pp. 297, 324.

21. Jeanne Kassler, "Radiologists Urge Fewer Chest X-Rays," *New York Times*, November 23, 1982.

22. Jane E. Brody, "Magnetic Device Lifts Hopes for Diagnosis Without X-Ray," *New York Times*, November 28, 1982, p. 1.

23. Barry Commoner, *The Closing Circle: Nature, Man, and Technology* (New York: Knopf, 1971), pp. 33–48.

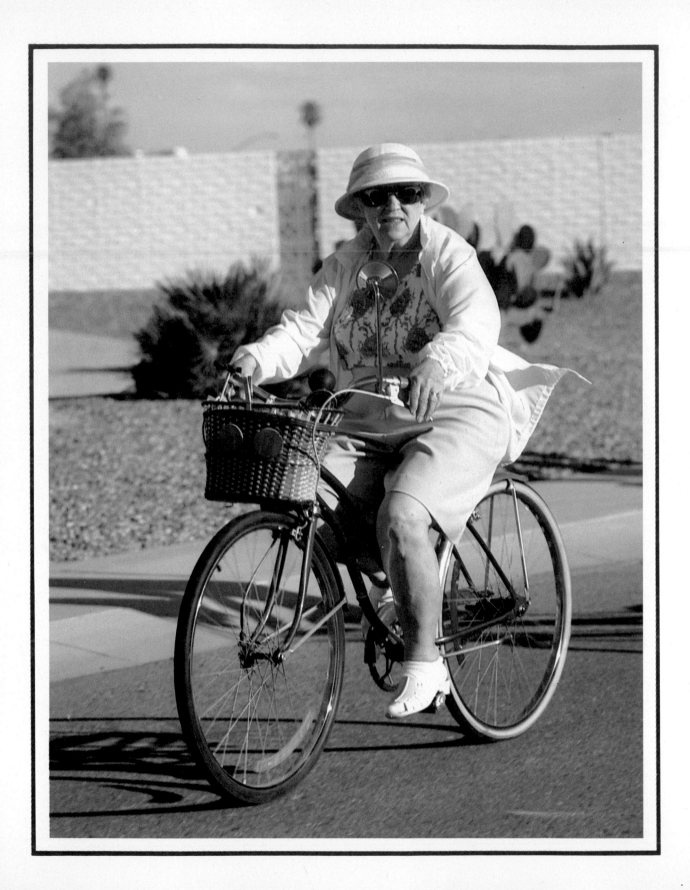

CHAPTER 18

Aging and Death

Advanced age is something all of us will probably experience. Life expectancy has soared since the turn of the century: The average American born in 1900 could not reasonably count on living as many as fifty years, yet a baby born today is likely to live at least seventy-three years, and a person born in the year 2000 will probably be able to look forward, on the average, to eighty-five years of life.[1]

If we are healthy, old age can be rewarding. If, however, old age is marked by pain, disability, loneliness, and fear, it can be unbearable. But while we plan our schooling, our personal lives, and our careers through our forties and fifties, few of us think seriously about how we will spend our late sixties, seventies, and eighties.

Even fewer of us think of our eventual death. Until recently, in fact, few but poets, philosophers, and theologians chose to dwell on the subject. Within the past decade, however, death has become an acceptable topic of discussion—in part because of recent medical advances, which have challenged many of our traditional ideas about death.

This chapter will describe the aging process and some of the problems elderly people face in our society. It will also explore the ways in which people face death—their own and their loved ones'.

THE PROBLEM OF AGEISM

Our society associates the idea of aging and the elderly with many negative qualities. When older persons are depicted on our film and television screens, they are often presented not as individuals but as stereotypes: enfeebled physically, failing mentally, unable to cope with daily routine, bewildered by modern technology, and a burden to a younger, more savvy generation. Even worse than these unflattering and inaccurate depictions in the media is the outright discrimination against elderly people in our society. Companies are often reluctant to consider older persons as candidates for jobs, and landlords sometimes consider them poor prospects as tenants. Even physicians sometimes take a patronizing attitude toward older patients, assuming that they are frail (when they may very well not be) and treating them almost like children.[2]

Many observers feel that the pattern of stereotyping older people and discriminating against them is much the same as the practice of lumping together all persons of a particular race or sex as members of an inferior group—patterns known as *racism* and *sexism*. These observers refer to this looking down on people over a certain age as *ageism*. As they point out, ageism in our society includes the common use of words and phrases that are "put-downs."[3] Sometimes, when people are talking about an older person, they use words that are normally applied to objects that have outlived their usefulness: *rickety, decrepit, outmoded*. Sometimes unpleasant words are used to picture older people of one sex or the other: *biddy* or *hag* for women, *codger* or *geezer* for men.

It is widely—and mistakenly—believed that all persons grow increasingly feeble at a steady, uniform rate. In fact, however, a Duke University study of people over sixty-five established that more than half of these subjects had *no* detectable deterioration in physical condition![4] Further, aging is highly individual: Some elderly people are far healthier and function far better both physically and mentally than their juniors, or even than they themselves did at an earlier age.

Also, age is often mistakenly associated with *senility*, a word that suggests mental disintegration and childlike behavior. In fact, only 5 to 8 percent of elderly Americans actually become senile in the sense that their memory and other mental functions begin to fail.

Why have these prejudices and stereotypes arisen? Why are they shared by so many people? Ageism, like racism and sexism, comes partly from the grim fact that there is competition for scarce resources in our society. When there are not enough jobs, money, and pleasant places to live, one group will unconsciously tend to put another group down, in order to rationalize—without even knowing it—the fact that it is trying to take the larger share of the economic pie. Ageism also comes partly from our fear of the unknown. As one study has pointed out, the premium our society places "on productivity and control makes aging and death a personal affront to the individual." We Americans are very threatened by the gradual loss of vigor and productivity we all must face as we get older, and it's hard for us to accept these losses as part of our normal human experience.[6]

WHAT IS AGING?

To risk stating the obvious, none of us is getting any younger. Nor are we staying the same age from year to year, or even from minute to minute. We are **aging**. Aging is a gradual developmental process of biological, psychological, sociological, and behavioral change that begins, in a sense, the moment we are born. In another sense—the one we'll use here—aging can be said to start at the time that we reach maturity. It is the change that occurs between the time we attain maturity and the end of our life.

Individuals change at different rates and at different points in their life cycle. It is true that as we look at higher and higher age brackets, we can see that a greater percentage of people are infirm or disabled. Among people under forty-five, only 6.8 percent are forced to live with some physical limitation. Among those from forty-five to sixty-four, 23.9 percent (almost a quarter) are disabled; and among those sixty-five and over, 45.2 percent are disabled.[7] If we could break down these data year

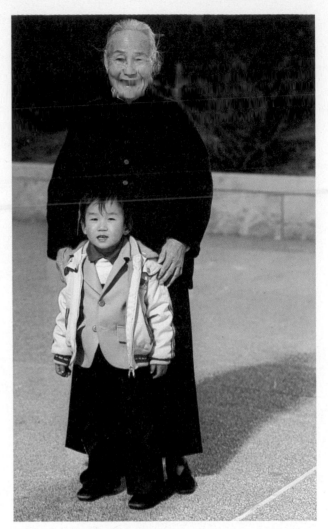

Contrary to widespread belief, a majority of elderly people enjoy good health and suffer from no disabilities. (©Joan Liftin/Archive)

by year, we would see the gradual rise in the percentages. But note that according to these figures, more than half of all people aged sixty-five and over are still able to go about their daily activities with no limitation whatever! Thus, it is difficult to pick a chronological age to serve as a reference point for denoting "old age." The most commonly used age is sixty-five years; but this point, originally established when the social security system was instituted, is rather arbitrary.

Gerontologists use several categories: "young-old," generally between the ages of sixty-five and seventy-four; "middle-old," between seventy-five and eighty-four; and "old-old," eighty-five years and beyond. Alternatively, moving away from the strictly chronological approach, "young-old" can be used to refer to aged persons whose lives are active, creative, vigorous, and productive; at the other extreme are the "old-old" or "frail elderly," who are unable to care for themselves. Clearly, the number of years a person has lived is not the best index of human developmental processes; environmental factors can enhance or erode a person's functional capacity, and the physical, mental, and social components of aging are closely interrelated.

What Causes Aging?

There are many theories about the aging process, but none of them, as yet, fully explains the underlying mechanism or mystery of how and why we age. **Gerontology**—the study of aging—attempts to shed light on this process. (It's important not to confuse that word with **geriatrics**—the area within gerontology that deals with promoting and maintaining the health of elderly people and with preventing and treating their diseases.)

One theory, the "wear-and-tear" theory, maintains that the human body simply wears out with use, as any complex piece of machinery would. Another, the "waste-product" theory, proposes that damaging waste products build up within our body cells and interfere with their functioning. A third theory, the "autoimmune theory," holds that the body's immune system, which is normally directed against foreign substances, begins to attack the body's own cells; the body ages because it can no longer distinguish between its own cells and foreign invaders. According to yet another view, the "free radical" theory, highly reactive fragments of chemical substances in our bodies—called "free radicals"—may cause aging by destroying other essential body chemicals.

Or it may just be that our bodies' genetic reproduction program, which is spelled out at conception in the DNA within the fertilized egg, eventually runs out, so that our body functions simply end. Another possibility is that as body cells divide and redivide, copying their DNA each time, they introduce errors into this genetic material. These errors may build up—much as nicks build up on an often-played phonograph record—

until the cells can no longer function normally. Or, finally, the body may have specific pacemakers, probably in the brain, that control the aging process.[8]

Although these theories are different, they are not necessarily incompatible. It may be that several of them are essentially correct descriptions of different aspects of the aging process.

Physical Aging on the Invisible Level

Many physical changes relating to aging are not visible to the naked eye; they occur within the tissues and the very cells of the body.[9] These changes are largely related to three phenomena. First, the total number of cells in the person's body decreases; second, there is a decrease in the efficiency of the process by which the cells burn fuel to get energy; and third, the cells *use* that energy less efficiently. Not all tissues in the body appear to be equally subject to these changes: The liver and the kidneys, for example, are not usually affected as early as the brain and certain types of muscle tissue, including voluntary muscles and heart muscle. But there is a decrease in the body's capabilities, which is often especially evident in situations where the individual has to respond to physical stress.

Another important change at the cellular level is that active nucleic acids, especially DNA, are present in the cells in lower concentrations. DNA is not merely the material that determines how our bodies will develop from conception on; it also plays a lifelong role in the renewal and repair of tissues, guiding the processes by which our cells create new protoplasm. Because the cells of an older person's body contain less DNA, their protein metabolism changes. This decreases their production of a variety of chemical substances, chiefly those substances that help the body adapt to internal and external conditions to maintain a balanced state (medically called *homeostasis*).

Physical Aging on the Visible Level

Many of the physical changes produced by aging are visible to the observer, though they proceed at very individual rates."[10] They are caused by the deterioration described above. The skin becomes less smooth and more lined; the hair loses color (the gradual admixture of white hairs produces the hue we call gray); the muscles may become flabby; the joints, especially in the hands, often become more prominent; the individual's posture may grow somewhat stooped; the digestion may become "delicate" and the intestines sluggish; all the senses—including hearing, vision, taste, and smell —become less acute.

Some of these changes can create further complications. If the individual's senses of taste and smell are diminished and his or her physical activity decreases at the same time, he or she may fail to eat an adequate diet; the result can be malnutrition, which can, of course, lead to additional problems. Partial loss of hearing or eyesight may make the individual more prone to accidents. Increased bone fragility can in turn make these accidents far more dangerous than they might have been earlier in life.

Aging and Disease

It is often hard to draw the line between those conditions that are caused by the natural aging process and those that are actually disease-related. Experts hotly debate several questions in this area. For example, it is known that blood pressure tends to rise gradually over the years. Some experts believe that this is a natural part of the aging process and that therefore the physician should not rush to treat it. Others feel that higher-than-average blood pressure is an illness, and that it should be treated whether it occurs at age eighteen or eighty. Another example is cataracts (clouding of the lenses of the eyes): It is known that they will afflict many people sooner or later, but why one person not until the age of ninety and another in his late forties? Or take another example—osteoarthritis: Once considered a "wear-and-tear" condition, this disease is now believed by a number of researchers to be preceded by acute problems that might be successfully treated or prevented.[11]

INFECTIOUS DISEASES

As we've said, the body's ability to repair and renew itself lessens with age. Further, our im-

mune system becomes less efficient as well, so that we have less resistance to attack by pathogens— which is why physicians routinely recommend that older people get preventive inoculations against certain infections, particularly pneumococcal pneumonia and influenza, even though most younger people do not need these immunizations.[12]

CHRONIC DISEASES

The highest toll taken among the aged, in terms of both death and disability, is by chronic conditions —disorders that worsen gradually, or perhaps progress as the body's resist-and-repair capabilities decrease.[13]

DISORDERS OF THE CARDIOVASCULAR SYSTEM Cardiovascular disorders, including heart disease, cerebrovascular accident (stroke), hypertension, and atherosclerosis, rank first among chronic diseases of the aged, accounting for more than 60 percent of deaths in those over age sixty-five. Among them, the primary disorder is atherosclerosis, a slowly progressive process that is now considered to be a definite disease rather than a consequence of aging. Atherosclerosis primarily affects the aorta, the arteries branching from it (including those supplying the heart), and the arteries of the brain (see Chapter 12); atherosclerosis is always present to some degree in the elderly. It may, in turn, result in angina, myocardial infarction, strokes, and kidney problems.

CANCER Second-ranking among causes of death in this age group are malignant neoplasms—cancers. While the word *cancer* is often used in the singular, cancers are actually many different diseases, varying widely in seriousness and treatability. Approximately half of *all* cancers are found in those over sixty-five, probably for a number of reasons. One is that certain cancers can be traced to long exposure to triggering factors (for example, sunlight). A second reason for the high incidence of cancers among the aged *may* be that the older person's immune system is less efficient.

OTHER CHRONIC DISEASES Among the other ranking causes of death in the aged, but representing far smaller proportions of fatalities, are influenza and pneumonia (3.6 percent) and diabetes mellitus (2.2 percent).[14] Diabetes is more prevalent among the aged than among younger people, probably because most cases of diabetes are of the maturity-onset type. Diabetes poses a special threat because it contributes to disabilities such as blindness, neurological problems, kidney problems, and heightened susceptibility to infection.

While they do not figure prominently in mortality statistics, two other categories of chronic physical illness associated with aging should be noted. They are among the most important reasons why older people are more likely to be disabled than younger people. One is the group of ills associated with gradual deterioration of the body's various systems, such as digestive malfunction and deterioration of the "control systems" (nerves and hormonal systems). The other is the group of conditions known as *autoimmune* diseases—including rheumatoid arthritis, chronic thyroiditis, and others. These diseases, while by no means limited to the elderly, do increase strikingly with age. In autoimmune disorders, the immune system seems to go out of control and attack the body's own tissues. One reason these disorders are more common in advanced age is probably that the self-recognition mechanisms of the immune system fail more often than in the younger person.

DRUG PROBLEMS OF THE ELDERLY

The elderly often require medication to cope with their increased susceptibility to disease. Although they represent only about 12 percent of the American population, they use 25 percent of the drugs prescribed in this country. Drug problems of the elderly are often not recognized in our society, because they involve the misuse of physician-prescribed medications and over-the-counter drugs, rather than illicit substances such as those associated with drug abuse by younger adults. Moreover, because older people are more likely to have chronic diseases, they tend to take drugs over longer periods of time.[15]

Aging and the Mind

Intelligence does *not* invariably decline with age. There may be *mild* impairment of memory (usually short-term memory), ability to concentrate, and in some cases reaction time.[16] But beyond that, aging in itself does not give rise to intellectual impairment (see Figure 18.1). In fact, in some

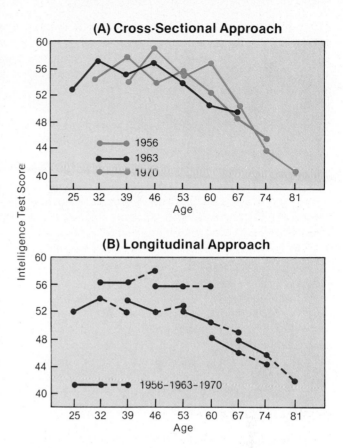

Figure 18.1   The answer to the question of whether intellectual ability declines with age depends largely on the method used to study the matter. Cross-sectional studies suggest more decline than longitudinal studies do. (A) The cross-sectional approach studies groups of people who were born at different times. When this method is used, younger people look smarter than older people. But this method obscures sociocultural differences among generations. The point is not that a twenty-four-year-old is smarter than a sixty-year-old, but that a person born in, say, 1965 instead of 1905 has probably had a better education. (B) The longitudinal method studies the same people at a number of points during their lives. As the bottom graph shows, decline over time from initial test score by sixty- and sixty-seven-year-olds is minimal, although because of generational differences their initial scores were lower than those of younger people.

Source: Adapted from K. Warner Schaie and Gisela Labouvie-Vief, "Generational Versus Ontogenetic Components of Change in Adult Cognitive Behavior: A Fourteen-Year Cross-Sequential Study," *Developmental Psychology* 10 (1974): 305–320.

areas of intellectual functioning, people tend to improve well into their later years. A person's verbal skills (word use and comprehension) are better at sixty-five than at forty or twenty-five. Visual skills (such as finding a simple figure within a complex one) also keep on improving with age, and older people are about as flexible at shifting from one way of thinking to another as the middle-aged.[17] The capacity for creative thought and creative work also persists into the later years. Tolstoy, Voltaire, Chagall, Picasso, and Casals all continued to produce literature, art, and music of high quality into their seventies and eighties. Creativity and productivity are likely to be the result of accumulated knowledge and experience.

"SENILITY" AND ALZHEIMER'S DISEASE

As we noted earlier, there is a myth that most of the elderly are likely to be afflicted by age-related dementia. In fact, there *is* a condition that involves progressive deterioration of memory and other mental functions, associated with advanced age. It was formerly located in the larger category known medically as "senile dementia," and is now properly termed Alzheimer's disease. In this condition, the brain's medium-sized and small blood vessels degenerate. Its cause is unknown, and there is no known prevention, although a correlation has been found between Alzheimer's disease and brain concussions sustained earlier in life. It produces a dementia that gradually increases in severity with advanced age. Alzheimer's disease is now believed, however, to have a gradual onset well *before* the individual grows old. Some experts think it may be related to the individual's genetically determined background, and that it may be associated with a specific biochemical defect (thus, it is potentially treatable).[18]

As we've said, the proportion of those afflicted with what is correctly termed Alzheimer's disease is quite small (only 6 to 8 percent). This point has been increasingly emphasized in the medical literature. Physicians should avoid assuming that an elderly patient is "senile": the patient may have a completely *different* condition that can give rise to some similar symptoms. Emotional problems such as depression, caused by loss of family ties, anxiety over money, and loss of independence, can lead to symptoms that are like those of Alzheimer's disease. So can physical disorders—including malnutrition, glandular dysfunctions such as thyroid problems, drug toxicity (to which the elderly are especially susceptible), and infection. Many cases of "senile dementia" have actually been reversed when physicians realized that the patient had one of these treatable conditions and applied the proper remedies.[19]

PROBLEMS OF THE AGED

Aside from difficulties stemming from illness or physiological change, the elderly in today's society may face a number of other hardships. Some of these problems are related to age itself, others to the societal attitudes we discussed earlier.

Emotional Problems

By and large, age itself does not bring radical emotional change. We continue throughout our lives to adjust to changing circumstances—more or less well, depending on our own abilities. Nor will age in itself change our essential personalities or our attitudes toward life, other people, and ourselves. Nevertheless, new kinds of stresses may occur as the individual grows older—and these stresses may strain the emotional resources of even the most resilient person.

WORK-ROLE LOSS

One stress many older people undergo is the loss of their formal work roles; in the past this loss chiefly affected men, but in the future it is bound to affect women equally. Productivity is basic to the American ethic: Working, especially for pay, is equated with worth in our society. A person deprived of that role—particularly someone who has no other active or productive pursuit that can continue—may feel a profound sense of loss.

LOSS OF LOVED ONES

Another stress factor that may increase in advanced age is bereavement. Most of us have suffered the loss of an older relative or family friend. Some of us have, perhaps once or twice by the time we reach our twenties, found ourselves

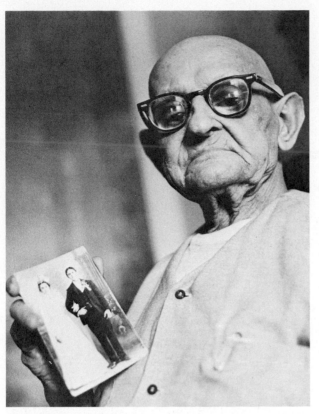

The death of a husband or wife deprives the surviving spouse of a central social role as well as of companionship. (©Michael Malyszko, 1979/Stock, Boston)

mourning a friend our own age, taken from us by an accident or illness. Such losses are far more frequent for those of advanced years, and many old people have to grieve for multiple losses at the same time.

The most devastating is the loss of a spouse, often the companion and confidant of many decades. Losing one's spouse means losing a role as well—one is no longer a husband or wife. Widowhood often brings a loss of social status; worse, the bereaved individual may be cut off from friends and relatives who were used to the couple as a couple and may feel uncomfortable or awkward with the remaining individual.

Profound depression may follow the first reaction of shock and grief, and emotional and even physical illness may ensue. At least one study has found a significantly higher death rate among the widowed in the months following a spouse's death.[20]

OTHER EMOTIONAL PROBLEMS

Other stresses that may occur with advancing years include diminished income, change of residence, and increased fear for one's personal safety (muggers view the elderly as easy targets)—all coupled with loneliness and the consciousness of ebbing strength and vigor, perhaps with the extra burden of physical illness.

In certain respects, advancing age in our society is more of a problem for women than for men. In men, graying hair and lined faces are often viewed as signs of maturity, character, and ruggedness; but in women, they are viewed as signs of loss of beauty and desirability. Men over sixty are said to look distinguished and dignified, while women over sixty are more likely to be viewed as "old." These negative images for women contribute to feelings of decreased worth.

Practical Problems

Poverty and old age are clearly linked. A minority of retirees have company pensions or Individual Retirement Accounts (IRAs), and social security—the sole support of many of America's elderly—is painfully inadequate. Government programs do not fully cover costs relating to disease and disability, particularly costs for home health care and chronic disorders—where most elderly people's greatest needs lie. Much of the poverty of the elderly, furthermore, is due to age discrimination in employment, coupled with the pattern of forced retirement: Though many hope to go on working, they are often required to retire earlier than they had foreseen, and they may not have made adequate financial plans.

For many people, old age brings problems relating to care. According to a Duke University study, the chances are about one in four that an older person will spend time in a home for the aged, a nursing home, or some other institution.[21]

PLANNING FOR SUCCESSFUL AGING

As we have noted, we are *all* aging. We can increase our chances of a tranquil, productive, happy old age if we form good health habits, starting in our teens and twenties.

Forming Good Habits for Lifelong Physical Health

Throughout this book, we've suggested ways you can control disease risk factors: Control your weight, drink only moderately if at all, and do not smoke. Get checkups so that conditions such as diabetes and hypertension can be detected and treated early. Statistics also show that people who are happily married, have stable family relationships, and are able to relax and avoid chronic tension tend to live longer. So do those who stay away from high-risk occupations and recreational activities and who limit their exposure to environmental hazards and toxic substances.

Does exercise help increase one's chances for long life? Animal studies, and a few studies of humans, suggest that regular exercise throughout life *may* help to diminish some of the effects of aging, such as elevated blood pressure and increased prevalence of heart disease. If you start an exercise program now and stick with it, you *may* help increase your longevity.[22] Exercise also helps keep muscles strong and joints supple, and it helps prevent the loss of bone (osteoporosis) often seen in older people.

Another area where you can change your habit patterns now is nutrition. As we noted in Chapter 13, experts believe it's wise to cut down on dietary cholesterol and those foods that encourage our bodies to produce cholesterol.

Thinking Ahead for Your Later Years

Retirement, diminished income, and loss of friends and associates come to many people as surprises for which they are completely unprepared. Retirement alone can cause a serious crisis. Thus, it is wise for everyone to investigate the financial and other options well before retirement age. Books, courses, and individual and group counseling for preretirement people are widely available. Studies show that the most well-adjusted retirees are those whose previous lives have not revolved solely around their jobs. Therefore, it's a good idea to get involved in some nonwork activities now that can be continued with pleasure into retirement.[23]

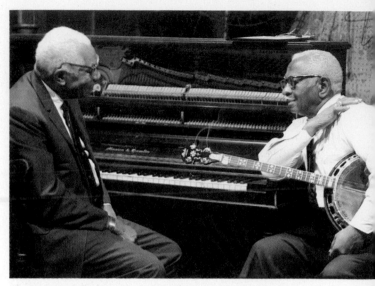

Some elderly people are able to carry their career activities over into retirement. Others never retire at all, but continue to pursue their professions throughout their lives. (©Ethan Hoffman/Archive)

Toward Your Well-Being as a Whole Person

As we've seen, working throughout life to optimize our health is likely to improve the quality of our life in later years. But we are not merely physical mechanisms; we are also sexual, social, intellectual, and emotional beings. Taking an early look at these other areas can enhance our well-being when we're older.

OLDER PEOPLE AND SEXUALITY

Sex, in the later years as in youth, is the subject of an astounding body of myth—notably, that it somehow ceases to exist at all for those over a certain age. This attitude is sometimes accepted by the elderly themselves—with the result that some people, as they grow older, feel that their interest in sex *should* be curtailed. In fact, older people, like younger people, may vary considerably from one to another in their interest and engagement in sexual activity. A person who previously has had little interest in sex will probably continue to feel the same way. But a person who has found sexual activity pleasurable will probably continue to find it so. Physical changes do occur—among them a longer excitement phase (pre-erec-

ACTIVITY: EXPLORING HEALTH

Planning to Deal with Old Age

How do you plan to deal with your parents' old age—and with your own? Try answering these questions and see.

1. If your parents are unable to take care of themselves when they grow old, would you
   a. place them in a home for the aged?
   b. place them in a nursing home?
   c. invite them to move in with you and your family?
   d. hire a live-in caregiver at their residence?
   e. ignore them?

2. When you grow old, would you rather
   a. remain in your own home?
   b. live with your adult children's family?
   c. be placed in a long-term care facility?
   d. live in a retirement village?
   e. live in an adult group home?

3. When you are older, would you like to
   a. retire voluntarily as soon as possible?
   b. retire when you are forced to by established procedures?
   c. retire at age sixty-five?
   d. retire when your retirement income is adequate to support your preretirement lifestyle?
   e. never retire?

4. What age-related health problem do you think would be most difficult for you to adjust to?
   a. loss of mobility
   b. chronic illness
   c. reduced vision or hearing
   d. loss of teeth
   e. reduced mental ability and memory

5. Which of the following styles of grandparenting do you think you will be most likely to follow?
   a. Maintain a constant interest in grandchildren, but be careful not to interfere or offer advice in childrearing.
   b. Emphasize playfulness, having a good time, and sharing enjoyable activities with grandchildren.
   c. Coach your adult children in the care of your grandchildren, and take responsibility for ensuring that your grandchildren have educational opportunities.
   d. Take responsibility for the actual care of your grandchildren, or for whichever grandchild needs care the most.
   e. Appear mainly on special occasions (such as holidays), and have only fleeting and infrequent interaction with grandchildren.

INTERPRETATION

Look again at each of your responses, and list the logical consequences of your particular choice.

_____

_____

_____

_____

_____

Discuss what advantages or disadvantages each choice has over the alternatives. _____

_____

_____

_____

_____

_____

Source: Adapted from D. A. Read, *Looking In: Exploring One's Personal Health Values* (Englewood Cliffs, N.J.: Prentice-Hall, 1977), p. 100.

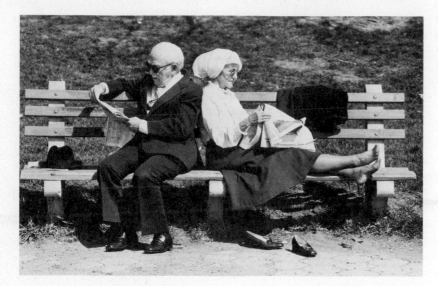

There is no age limit on the pleasure a couple can take in each other's company, including a continued interest in sex. (©Ira Berger/Woodfin Camp & Assoc.)

tion in the male, prelubrication in the female). But they simply mean that sexual activity between a couple may gradually assume somewhat different patterns over the years, not that it will become undesirable or impossible.

OLDER PEOPLE'S SOCIAL NEEDS

Social contacts continue to be important as we grow older, particularly when we are threatened by role loss (loss of work, loss of spouse). Many studies on widowhood, and some on retirement, have demonstrated that older people are more satisfied with life, following such role loss, if they continue to participate in community and other organized groups, and if they continue to associate with friends, especially of the same sex.[24]

Having close friends to talk with becomes even more important when one must face death—either one's own or that of a loved one. Friends can help us come to terms with death's reality.

DEFINITIONS OF DEATH

In the past, a person was considered dead when he or she stopped breathing and the heart ceased to beat. Today, however, medical technology is able to maintain the heartbeat and respiration in people who would otherwise be dead. These developments have raised new questions about whether people have the right to control how they die, and even about when death itself may actually be said to occur. Furthermore, now that today's advanced

surgical procedures make it possible to transplant body parts such as kidneys, it is important to know at what point death really happens and organs can legitimately be removed for transplantation. In 1968 a committee of the Harvard Medical School offered a definition of death based on the concept of **brain death**. A person would be considered dead if he or she was unreceptive and unresponsive; was in an irreversible coma; did not move or did not breathe when off a mechanical respirator; had no reflexes; and had a flat electroencephalogram (EEG), indicating no brain waves. That definition is now widely accepted medically, and a number of states have written it into law.

WHAT DOES DEATH MEAN TO US?

Not all cultures have viewed death with fear. Though some have seen it as a state of eternal misery—and have reflected this view in art and literature, depicting dead people as grisly skeletons—other cultures have viewed death in a neutral or even positive light, seeing it as a state of peace, a sleeplike trance.

What Death Means to Individual People

Just as the meaning of death varies from culture to culture, so it varies from individual to individual.

For some people, the thought of death may even be joyful if they believe it will bring a reunion with a husband, wife, parent, or child who has already died. For others, death means a painful separation, the absence of someone central to their everyday lives.

Since few of us talk to each other about death, we often aren't aware of what others think and feel about death. Too often we assume that others feel the way we do. For example, we may assume that a very sick person is longing for death to bring relief after prolonged suffering, whereas the sick person may dread death because it will cut short a life he or she still finds precious. In making such assumptions, we may offend or hurt someone who is trying to recover from the loss of a loved person.

What Death Means to People of Different Ages

Our reactions to death do vary with our age, but sometimes not in the ways we would expect them to.

CAN CHILDREN COPE WITH THE IDEA OF DEATH?

Adults often assume that children cannot cope with or understand death, and they try to shelter the young from even hearing about a death. Yet there is plentiful evidence that even preschoolers are quite aware of death; these days, children certainly see death on television. They will not necessarily be traumatized by references to death; indeed, research shows that they are *more* likely to be disturbed by death if it is treated like a dark, terrible secret than as a natural part of living.[25]

HOW CAN ADULTS HELP CHILDREN DEAL WITH DEATH?

Talks about death and what it means are best integrated into everyday conversations prompted by the death of a pet animal or a shoot-out on a television show. Having just one dramatic discussion can be unnatural and scary for a child. And it's better to discuss death when both adult and child are relaxed than to wait for the death of a close relative or family member.

When a death does occur, children may react in ways that adults do not always easily comprehend at first. Some experts believe that a reason children may not show grief is that their personalities are not fully developed; instead of mourning, they may become anxious or use defense mech-

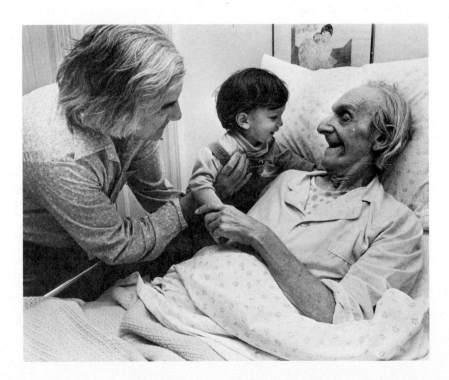

Encouraging the view that death is a natural part of human experience can help children—and adults— cope with it better. (©Abigail Heyman/Archive)

anisms, such as rationalization (see Chapter 1).[26] Very young children can't verbalize their feelings, so they may act them out—for example, by ree-nacting familiar activities of the deceased. Young-sters may also have trouble sleeping or become moody when a family member dies.

A relaxed and patient adult can help the child explore his or her feelings and return to a more normal schedule and moods. The most important thing for parents to remember is that children facing a death need patience and plenty of atten-tion.[27]

HOW ADULTS HANDLE DEATH

Reaching adulthood does not necessarily guaran-tee us a mature attitude toward death. Some peo-ple may ignore serious medical symptoms, such as a persistent weight loss or cough, afraid to admit that they are vulnerable. Such individuals may ac-cept the general idea that other people die, but may not be able to face the fact that they them-selves must die eventually. This denial can keep them from seeking the medical care they need.

OLDER PEOPLE AND DEATH

It's often assumed that the elderly gradually disen-gage themselves from life by reducing their re-sponsibilities and emotional involvements. They are retired, living a less active life. They reevalu-ate their activities to decide what to do in the limited time remaining; an older person may sud-denly take a long trip or develop a new hobby. Friends and relatives may assume that these ac-tivities signal a slow withdrawal from life, even a preparation for death. But many older people cling to life, cherishing it no less than a younger person. So younger people should not act as if the elderly automatically accept a serious or terminal illness as timely and appropriate.

THE PROCESS OF DYING

How do we define the point in time when a person begins to die? It's not easy to say. The exact mo-ment that a disease becomes terminal can rarely be pinpointed, for illness is a process of gradual deterioration.

Psychological Issues: Accepting the News

The first inkling that death is near usually comes via the doctor's office or hospital. It's not unusual for people to take a while to accept the news. Some are not psychologically ready to hear that they are dying, so they misinterpret the central facts. At times, too, doctors have trouble giving us unpleasant news, so they garble the message in clinical terms we don't readily understand. Quite often, then, it takes some time for an individual to understand a terminal diagnosis and to accept it.

How Others Treat the Dying Person

The way both the medical professionals and the family treat the dying person depends very much on the circumstances. Sometimes the quality of the care they give the person depends on how certain death is, and how far off it is thought to be. A cancer patient who lingers for days, weeks, or months in bed is sometimes left isolated, with medical professionals and family allowing him or her to "fade away." The patient typically loses control over his or her care and becomes a low priority to medical personnel.[28] By contrast, the medical system rallies all its resources to rescue the patient when there is a sudden emergency such as a heart attack, a premature birth, or a car accident. The dying person is often surrounded by people intent on ensuring his or her comfort. It is important for us all to become more aware of such differences in treatment, so that more of a balance can be struck and more sensitive care can be given to all dying patients.

Preparing for Death

In recent years, particularly through the well-pub-licized work of Elisabeth Kübler-Ross, there has been a new focus on the "stages" through which some dying people may pass. Following interviews with hundreds of patients, Kübler-Ross concluded

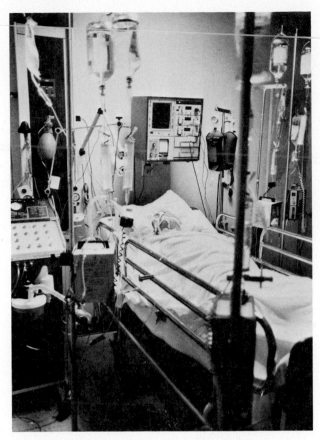

Terminally ill patients may be left isolated, surrounded by machines instead of people. (©Ken Karp)

and forth among various stages, or may exhibit more than one stage of reacting at the same time. Her research has been helpful in its compassionate exploration of what dying people experience.

Still, not every dying person goes through the stages described by Kübler-Ross. Moreover, no one facing death should feel that he or she necessarily *should* go through five stages—or *any* series of stages—to adapt to the situation. Indeed, researchers are finding that most often an individual's distinctive attitude and conduct during dying simply reflect his or her attitudes and conduct throughout life.[30] What researchers *do* find to be a nearly universal fact is that the emotional needs of a dying person are not much different from anyone else's: Like everyone else, dying people want the love and esteem of others.

In some cases the prospect of death does prompt new insights and emotional growth. Some people do use the time to examine their lives and long-held beliefs. Such people may even come close to the stereotypes of dying people glorified in the media and novels, who achieve more love for other people, an intense religious devotion, or a more satisfying integration of their past values with new ones. Driven by a clearer sense of time limits, they try to resolve past conflicts and smooth over estrangements with family and friends.[31] But such an attitude is not universal and should not necessarily be anticipated as an integral part of the process of dying.

The primary psychological state of most dying patients can best be described as ambivalence—a constant wavering between opposites, in which the individual sometimes needs other people and sometimes abhors their presence; is sometimes angry, sometimes serene; sometimes openly confronts the fact of dying and sometimes denies it.

THE ROLE OF THE WILL TO LIVE

There does appear to be a phenomenon that doctors and family members describe as a "will to live," which can be a crucial variable in deciding whether a person will recover from an illness. But those who know they are dying and lose their drive to prolong their lives at any cost are not necessarily depressed or eager to die. One radiologist, for example, noted that several older people begged him to stop medical treatment. Their skin was so fragile that even lying on an X-ray table

that many dying people go through five specific stages.[29] First, there may be a denial of the diagnosis: Frequently, people simply assert that the news cannot be true, saying, "No, not me, I can't be dying." Second, patients often grow angry, asking "Why me?" and raging at their fate. Next the person may try to bargain with fate, asking to be "allowed" to live just long enough for an important event, such as a daughter's graduation or a son's wedding. In the fourth stage, the person may grow depressed, drained by stress and physical suffering, and may withdraw from friends and family. Finally, the dying patient may accept his or her fate. This final stage is not always a happy or blissful one; rather, as the depression lifts, the individual grows more peaceful, resigned to a foreseeable death.

Kübler-Ross found that some people may not get to every stage; some stop along the way, never accepting their death. Some people may go back tore it and made them bleed. It was not that they wanted to die immediately; they were simply reacting to the pain of the treatment.[32]

THE PROBLEM OF PAIN

Anxiety, depression, and fatigue can add to a dying person's pain, making him or her suffer unreasonably in the final days or weeks. Researchers have found that pain is actually a dual phenomenon: The patient is suffering not only because of the physical sensation but also because of a psychological reaction to it. A person who is angry, depressed, or feeling isolated may feel much more pain than one who is given sympathy and understanding. Indeed, studies show that simple emotional support, sleep, and diversions can help alleviate pain that might otherwise become intractable and intolerable over time.[33] (See Figure 18.2.)

SPECIAL PROBLEMS OF THE AMBULATORY DYING

The ambulatory dying—such as some cancer patients whose death may be certain but is being deferred by radiotherapy or chemotherapy—have the same needs as people dying in hospitals or other institutions, but they also have other concerns. Their daily lives may seem on the surface to be the same as they have always been; thus, for them death and dying may have a special unreal-

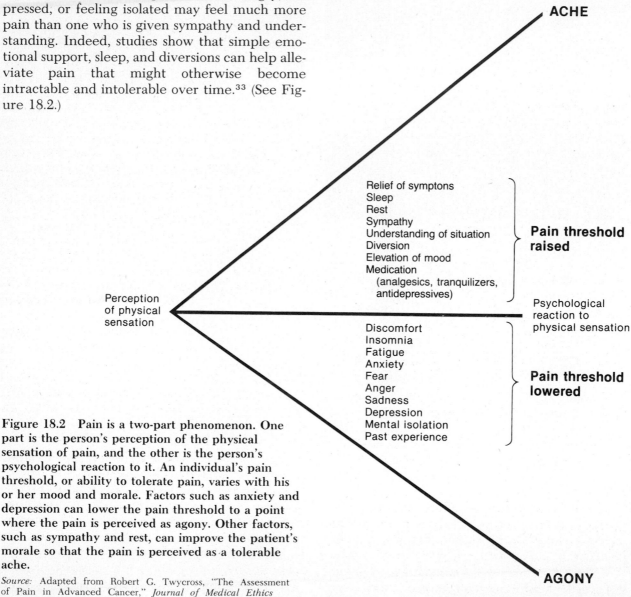

Figure 18.2 Pain is a two-part phenomenon. One part is the person's perception of the physical sensation of pain, and the other is the person's psychological reaction to it. An individual's pain threshold, or ability to tolerate pain, varies with his or her mood and morale. Factors such as anxiety and depression can lower the pain threshold to a point where the pain is perceived as agony. Other factors, such as sympathy and rest, can improve the patient's morale so that the pain is perceived as a tolerable ache.

Source: Adapted from Robert G. Twycross, "The Assessment of Pain in Advanced Cancer," *Journal of Medical Ethics* 4 (1978): 114.

ity. They may hesitate to talk about their condition, for fear of losing their friends or jobs. As death approaches, these people may be sentenced to an island of isolation, created partly by their own fears and partly by the uneasiness that many acquaintances cannot help displaying in their presence.

WHAT DOES IT ACTUALLY FEEL LIKE TO DIE?

As actual death approaches, people are likely to feel increasingly drowsy and may be quite unaware of what is going on around them. Drugs, the disease, and the psychological distancing done by the patient tend to contribute to drowsiness. Only about 6 percent of dying patients are conscious shortly before death, and the moment of death is rarely distressful. There is even some evidence that as death approaches, the brain releases a chemical that makes the moment of death pleasant instead of painful. For most people, death comes as they would wish it—quickly, painlessly, and peacefully.

CARE OF THE DYING: SOME MAJOR ISSUES

In facing death, the patient and family must not only adjust to new emotions, they must also deal with a number of practical issues. Should the dying person be kept at home or in a hospital or nursing home? In some states with "right-to-die" laws, the dying patient may also have some wishes about what equipment should be used to prolong life. These decisions are critical to the final experiences of the dying patient.

Alternatives to Dying in a Hospital

HOSPICES

The term *hospice* refers to a philosophy of care for the dying: It tries to give the dying more control over the care they receive and aims at helping them and their families adapt with dignity to their fatal diagnoses. There are now more than 800 hospice groups in the United States, each different in the setting, staffing, and services it provides. Some

offer day care, some offer home health care, and others have inpatient care.[34]

The primary goals of the hospice movement are to relieve the pain of the dying, to offer emotional support to the family and patient, and to create an environment where those goals can be met. In line with those goals, the movement has set forth some basic guidelines for care of the dying:

- The fatal diagnosis should not be used as a reason to neglect the patient; all efforts should be made to relieve distressful symptoms.
- The dying person should be able to have a sense that he or she is protected and adequately cared for.
- Staff members should be given time to form personal relationships with the patient.
- Visitors should be allowed as often as the patient and family members would like. Furthermore, the patient and family should be given privacy for their visiting and not be interrupted at the convenience of the institution or health-care professionals. Such policies would permit a child to spend time with a dying parent—a practice not allowed at some hospitals with strict limits on the age of visitors.[35]
- The founder of the hospice movement, Dr. Cicely Saunders, has shown that pain—and the attendant anxiety—can be controlled more effectively when painkilling medications are given on a regular schedule than when medications are given after the need for them has developed.

CARE AT HOME

Home care for the dying is seen as a particularly good option if the family is able and willing to provide the care. Studies show that this approach can prove beneficial not only to the dying person but to the family as well: Patients experience more dignity and comfort than in the hospital, and families adjust with less difficulty. Home care costs the family a fraction of what a hospital stay would cost, and programs encouraging such care also benefit the community as a whole by freeing hospital beds for acute care. Recently, there has been a movement to urge third parties such as insurance companies to reimburse families as fully as possible for the various costs involved in home care.[36]

Organ Donation, Euthanasia, and the Right to Die

Today, it is fairly widely accepted that an individual has a right to dictate what is to be done with his or her remains after death. With advances in medical technology, it has become increasingly possible to transplant organs from a dead person to another individual. Many people choose to donate certain body parts to others after death. Others decide to have their bodies sent to medical schools or research institutions.

But there is less general acceptance of the idea that physicians should be allowed to do anything other than fight on for the patient's life, no matter what the circumstances. For example, if a dying individual is suffering great pain or discomfort—and, indeed, would welcome death—should physicians be permitted to speed the death in some painless and humanitarian way, such as by administering a lethal drug or terminating life-sustaining treatment? Such a killing, called **euthanasia**, might be merciful to the dying person but would also place a difficult burden on the family, physicians, judges, and other people who might become involved in the decision. At this time, euthanasia is illegal, but a report published in 1983 by the President's Commission for the Study of Ethical Problems in Medicine and Biomedical and Behavioral Research said that nothing prevents a doctor from giving pain-relieving drugs that will probably hasten death, as long as the sole reason for giving the drug is not to end the patient's life, but to relieve unbearable pain.[37]

A related question is: Can a patient, or a patient's family or physician, refuse medical treatment that might reasonably be expected to save the patient's life—without this action's being legally considered suicide on the part of the patient or homicide on the part of the family or physician? This question became a public issue in the mid-1970s, when the Quinlan family of New Jersey agonized over whether their daughter Karen Ann should be taken off a respirator that was believed to be keeping her alive. Karen Ann Quinlan was bedridden in a deep coma; her parents petitioned the courts to have the respirator shut off, arguing that she no longer had a life worth living. The Quinlan case prompted a public debate, which is still raging, over just what right people have to decide the circumstances of their own dying days, and what rights others may have. In view of the presidential commission, mentally competent patients should be given all the necessary information and then be allowed to decide whether to halt medical treatment that keeps them alive but offers no hope of curing or improving their condition; in the case of mentally incompetent patients (such as the newborn, the retarded, or the comatose), family members should be allowed to make similar decisions.

At the time of this writing, twelve states have "natural death" laws, allowing patients to refuse treatment in terminal illnesses; forty-two states allow patients to appoint surrogates, who can act on their behalf if they are unable to make the decision themselves. A simultaneous movement to develop "living wills" has also emerged, designed to give Americans the right to control the way they die. In a living will a person specifies that he or she does not want to be kept alive by artificial means under certain circumstances. Most often the living will is written as a legal document, witnessed by at least two people, and notarized to ensure that the person who draws it up is of sound mind. More than 750,000 people have drawn up such documents.[38] But most legal authorities doubt that the living wills have the force of law without a law passed specifically to back them up. To date, only California has passed such a law. Living wills also leave the question of recovery up to physicians, and doctors do not always agree on a patient's prognosis—nor are they always correct even when they do. In the case of Karen Ann Quinlan, doctors predicted that she would die shortly after the respirator was withdrawn. But she lived on for years after the courts ordered it removed.

Even beyond these questions of judgment, there are other concerns about the right-to-die laws. Many people question whether anyone can anticipate how he or she will feel about dying when the actual moment approaches. Would a car-accident victim, paralyzed and unable to speak yet fully conscious, want to be taken off a respirator? What if alternative treatments arose that the person had not anticipated when he or she made the decision? Finally, many people worry that right-to-die laws could become smoke screens for inadequate care for the dying. It is difficult enough for a dying person to secure a caring and attentive environment without such laws; they might be used to justify further inattention and neglect, these people fear, as part of a person's "right to die."[39]

BEREAVEMENT

Treatment and care of the dying place their own stress on a family, but the actual death causes a new kind of stress that can have a profound effect on the survivors. There is the stress that comes from **bereavement**—the loss of someone we have loved or valued—and from the change in our own status, as from spouse to widowed person, that results from the death. Then there is the stress of **grief,** our subjective response to bereavement. When we grieve, we may experience symptoms of distress in both our minds and our bodies: Grief affects many, if not all, aspects of our lives, and can in some cases become so intense that it can be considered a disease process. The biochemical and physiological reactions can be so severe that they can precipitate physical illness and even death.[40]

Patterns of Bereavement in Spouses

The way we react to a death depends in part on the way our loved one died. When death comes as a surprise, a spouse may feel as if there are no limits to the grief, and that it may never ease. But studies of widows and widowers have found that a lingering illness before death has given the spouse a chance to anticipate the death and begin to come to terms with it.[41] Researchers have even noted a phenomenon called "anticipatory grief," where a spouse begins to feel the loss and to grieve before the actual death; after the death, a wife or husband may even express some relief that the spouse's suffering is over. Yet even for those who anticipate it, the sense of loss and desolation are still strong when the death actually occurs.[42]

Researchers have found certain patterns among the bereaved; these patterns may not emerge in every case, but they do arise often enough to warrant attention. Soon after the death, a husband or wife often tends to idealize the deceased. Over time, more realistic memories emerge, often followed by surges of anger, which can be quite unexpected and intense. For example, a wife may be angry that her husband has "left" her alone. This reaction can be confusing to the surviving spouse. She may feel guilty at the anger, especially when she had just been idealizing her dead husband. Generally, however, the anger passes; it is only one step toward coming to a more realistic view of life without the deceased. Survivors may also experience loneliness long after the funeral. While there is usually an initial burst of concern and caring from friends and family, these other people often return rather quickly to their daily lives, and the widower or widow is left to face days and months of readjustment.

A sudden death—in a mining accident, for example, as here—is a great shock to surviving family and friends, allowing them no time to prepare themselves psychologically. (©Earl Dotter/Archive)

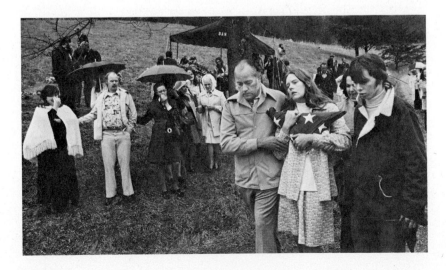

Bereaved Children

The impact of a death on children can be intense and long-lasting. Not only do children feel the loss of the parent or sibling who has died, but they may also suffer from lack of attention from family members during bereavement. Some bereaved parents find it difficult to cope with both their own sorrow and their surviving children's needs. Loss of an important person in childhood can have lingering effects, too: Studies show that people who lose someone dear to them as a child are more likely to suffer physical or mental illness as adults.[43]

What the Bereaved Person Can Do to Cope

No one can predict exactly how long we will grieve for the loss of someone dear to us. Researchers have found, however, that there are ways of coping with the grief that can lessen the stress and help people come through it intact. Perhaps most important of all, studies show that it is crucial to "allow" ourselves to grieve and to verbalize the feelings that accompany the grief. The simple act of talking about how we feel about ourselves, the death, and the person who died can help us survive the most desolate moments.

Coping with the Death of a Child

The death of a child is one of the most wrenching types of deaths to endure. Often, it is seen as hideously unnatural, and many parents refuse to accept the death until they are actually confronted with the body. Accepting the death is often only the beginning of a grieving period filled with intense longings for the youngster and tremendous guilt. Parents ask what they could have done to prevent the death, and even the slightest reminder of the child—a toy in a neighbor's yard—may set off waves of yearning for the child. These feelings can upset the family's normal relationships: A surviving child may feel neglected or afraid, or try to act (or be pushed into acting) as a replacement for the deceased. The strains on the family can become all the more intense because there are few social supports available for them,

especially if a child is stillborn or dies shortly after birth. Authorities are only beginning to recognize the special needs of families who experience such losses and to provide counseling for them.[45]

FUNERALS AND MOURNING

After death comes **mourning**—all those culturally reinforced patterns of thought, feelings, and behaviors that bereaved individuals experience in our society. Part of mourning is the larger society's support for bereaved people and the rituals and expectations with which society responds to bereavement.

Funeral Customs

When death finally arrives, it brings a need for a parting ceremony, a rite of passage, that can help friends and relatives absorb and comprehend their loss. This ritual occurs, in one form or another, in every human society, and like other rituals, satisfies deep-seated human needs.

Funeral customs vary widely, depending on the family's religion, geographic region, preferences, and finances. In some places neighbors bring food to the home of the deceased and visit with the family. In other cases friends and relatives may hold a wake and stay up all night in the room with the body. The ceremony may be religious or secular in nature. Most recently, the trend in the United States is toward participation of the survivors in the ritual. Family members may help plan the actual burial or may write parts of the service.

The decision for cremation or burial of the body also varies widely with local customs and religion. Catholics are now allowed to cremate the deceased, following an authorization from the church in the 1960s. The three modern branches of Judaism differ on what should be allowed. Most Protestants are left to individual preference.

The Psychological Value of the Funeral

There is evidence that funerals are of psychological value to survivors. The funeral provides an important emotional release in the first few days after death, giving the survivors something concrete to do. It also helps to confirm the reality of the death and simultaneously provides a network of people who may be called on later for support. Funerals also seem to fulfill several important functions for the society at large. They bring families together and affirm the importance of family networks within the society.

The Cost of Dying

The traditional funeral often means a sizable expense. As a ceremonial expenditure it ranks second only to the amount Americans spend each year on weddings.

Extravagant and elaborate practices have brought the funeral industry under strong attack for inducing people to spend exorbitant amounts of money in their most vulnerable moments. Jes-

sica Mitford's book *The American Way of Death* attacked many practices by funeral directors as deceptive and unscrupulous.[46] More recently, the Federal Trade Commission has called certain practices into question and has drawn up proposals regulating the funeral industry with the aim of protecting consumers from exploitation. One questionable practice targeted by the FTC is the automatic embalming of the body without the family's prior permission. Contrary to popular belief, embalming is not required by law; the underlying motive for the embalming appears to be to make more money from the funeral, since a funeral with a body maximizes the funeral director's services and usually means that the family will buy a more expensive casket to put on display. The FTC has also suggested that changes be made in the way caskets are marketed, that no casket be required for cremation, and that all funeral homes offer low-cost containers for cremation.[47]

MAKING HEALTH DECISIONS

How Ready Are You for Death?

How prepared are you to face your own death or that of others? Answering the following questions may help you assess your readiness.

YES   NO

_____ _____ 1. Have you ever attended a funeral?

_____ _____ 2. Have you ever viewed a dead person?

_____ _____ 3. Have you ever read a book on death and dying?

_____ _____ 4. Have you written a "living will"?

_____ _____ 5. Have you ever helped a mourning person deal with his or her grief over the loss of a loved one?

_____ _____ 6. Have you ever visited a nursing home for the terminally ill?

YES   NO

_____ _____ 7. Have you ever visited a hospice?

_____ _____ 8. Have you ever visited a terminally ill relative or friend?

_____ _____ 9. Have you considered whether you would want to be hooked up to a life-support system if you were unable to make a satisfactory recovery from an accident or illness?

_____ _____ 10. Have you provided for this decision (question 9) in your will? (For example, have you set up instructions for doctors attending you in your final moments?)

_____ _____ 11. Have you examined your lifestyle recently in terms of possible modifications in your

YES   NO   YES   NO

_____ _____ goals and your means of   _____ _____ 18. Have you ever visited a
              achieving them?   cemetery to mourn the loss
_____ _____ 12. Have you executed a plan to   of a loved one?
              modify or alter your lifestyle, _____ _____ 19. Have you made
              on the basis of question 11?   arrangements for the disposal
_____ _____ 13. Have you ever thought of   of your own body in case of
              death as something other   death (for example, bought a
              than the end of life (for   cemetery plot, arranged for
              example, a new beginning, a   cremation)?
              different state of being)?   _____ _____ 20. Have you considered
_____ _____ 14. Have you ever experienced a   donating any body parts to
              near-fatal episode, or some   a medical school or an
              other event in your life that   organ bank, for purposes of
              made you feel lucky you're   scientific research or
              alive?   transplantation?
_____ _____ 15. Have you acknowledged the
              inevitability of death?   *Interpretation:* Some people might feel that
_____ _____ 16. Have you ever witnessed the the more *yes* responses you have, the better pre-
              death of a pet, or grieved for pared you probably are to face death. What do you
              the loss of one?   think?
_____ _____ 17. Have you ever talked with a *Discussion:* Check over your *no* responses.
              dying person about his or   Would you like to modify your behavior in some
              her philosophy of life and   way regarding any or all of these?
              readiness for death?

Source: Adapted from Walter D. Sorochan, *Promoting Your Health* (New York: Wiley, 1981), p. 447.

SUMMARY

1. Our society associates aging with many negative qualities. The elderly are stereotyped and discriminated against in a pattern that has been labeled "ageism." The myths about aging include the false notions that people grow increasingly feeble at a steady and uniform rate and that all people grow senile as they age. In fact, many older people are not enfeebled at all, and relatively few lose their memory or other cognitive functions.

2. Aging is a gradual developmental process of psychological, sociological, and behavioral change that begins at maturity and continues until death. Individuals change at different rates, and it is therefore very difficult to pinpoint the beginning of old age.

3. Gerontologists, who study the aging process,

have offered several theories of how and why people age, but none fully explains it. One theory holds that the body simply wears out; another, that harmful waste products build up and interfere with cell function; a third, that the body's immune system begins to attack the body's own cells; a fourth, that chemical fragments called "free radicals" destroy other, essential body chemicals. It is also possible that we are genetically programmed to age, or that dividing cells introduce errors into genetic material, or that the body has pacemakers that control aging.

4. Aging is not the same as disease, although the line between them is sometimes blurred. Older people can be more susceptible to infectious diseases than younger people. Chronic conditions cause the greatest amount of disability and death among older people, especially disorders of the cardiovascular system, cancer, influenza and

pneumonia, diabetes, deterioration of the body's various systems, and autoimmune diseases.

5. Aging does not necessarily impair mental functioning. "Senility," the loss of memory and other mental functions, affects only 6 to 8 percent of older people. Properly called Alzheimer's disease, the condition may eventually be treatable. But physicians must make sure that apparent confusion or disorientation in older people are not due to depression, malnutrition, or other conditions.

6. The aged may face emotional problems, including loss of formal work roles, loss of loved ones, and the stresses that accompany changes in income or residence, loneliness, illness, or fear for their safety.

7. Practical problems that many aging people encounter include financial difficulties and the need for special care. About one in twenty people over age sixty-five actually need care in a home for the aged, nursing home, or other facility.

8. A tranquil and productive old age can depend on habits acquired early in life. Thus younger people should begin the lifelong habits of controlling their weight, exercising regularly, not smoking, drinking moderately or not at all, and avoiding situations of chronic tension or high risk. People who plan ahead financially and who enjoy activities besides their jobs do best after retirement.

9. Although sexual patterns may change with age, healthy people can be sexually active well into old age. Social needs also persist in old age; the elderly benefit from friendships and participation in self-help groups.

10. Cultures vary in their views of death, some portraying it as a state of misery and others regarding it as peaceful or trancelike. People of different ages also view death differently: Children may not be able to verbalize their grief; adults may deny their own vulnerability; and older people do not necessarily accept death more readily than anyone else.

11. Some people prepare for death in a series of stages: denial, anger, bargaining with fate, depression, and acceptance. But most people's reactions to the prospect of death grow naturally out of each person's characteristic attitudes and behavior patterns. Doctors recognize a phenomenon called "the will to live" that may crucially affect a person's chances of recovery from an illness. Anxiety, depression, and fatigue can increase the perception of pain. Emotional support, sleep, and diversions can help dying people to cope with pain that might otherwise grow intolerable.

12. When it comes to caring for the dying, patients and their families must make certain practical decisions. Is the dying person to be cared for in a hospital, nursing home, hospice, or at home? Are his or her organs to be donated for transplants after death? More generally, can a patient or a patient's family refuse treatment for terminal illness?

13. Bereavement is the loss of a loved or valued person. Grief is the subjective response to bereavement. Grief can be so intense as to be considered a disease process.

14. The sudden death of a spouse or other loved person may be more of a blow than a death that allows survivors time for "anticipatory grief." Bereaved spouses tend to idealize the dead person at first, and then begin to produce more realistic memories and even anger toward the dead person for "leaving" them. Children may suffer not only from grief at the death of a loved one but also from neglect by other grieving family members.

15. Bereaved people can be helped to cope by being allowed simply to talk about their grief. It is important that they allow themselves to grieve and to put their feelings into words. The death of a child is especially difficult to endure, and families who lose children, especially those whose children are stillborn or die soon after birth, have special needs for social support.

16. After death comes a period of mourning, beginning with the ritual of the funeral. Funeral customs vary with the family's geographic region, religion, preferences, and finances. Funerals may help people to give up the dead person, provide emotional release and a social network of supporters, confirm the reality of death, affirm religious and ethnic values, and reinforce the social order.

GLOSSARY

aging A gradual developmental process of biological, psychological, sociological, and behavioral changes that occurs between the time we reach maturity and the end of our life.

bereavement The loss, through death, of a person one has loved or valued.

brain death The concept that a person may be considered dead when the brain is no longer functioning, as determined by a number of objective indicators.

euthanasia The deliberate killing of a sick person with the intention of ending his or her suffering.

geriatrics The area within gerontology that deals with promoting and maintaining the health of the elderly and with preventing and treating their diseases.

gerontology The study of aging.

grief The subjective response to bereavement.

mourning The culturally reinforced patterns of thought, feelings, and behaviors that bereaved individuals experience.

NOTES

1. Joan Arehart-Treichel, "Life Expectancy: The Great Twentieth-Century Leap," *Science News* 121, no. 11 (March 13, 1982): 186–188.

2. James J. Strain, "Ageism in the Medical Profession," *Geriatrics* 36, no. 4 (April 1981): 158–165.

3. The discussion that follows is based on Frank H. Nuessel, Jr., "The Language of Ageism," *The Gerontologist* 22, no. 3 (1982): 273–275.

4. George Maddox and Ewald M. Busse, "The Duke University Longitudinal Studies: An Integrated Investigation of Aging and the Aged, Ancillary Studies and Research Support Services, 1950–1980" (in preparation), cited in R. H. Neuhaus and R. H. Neuhaus, *Successful Aging* (New York: Wiley, 1982), p. 17.

5. Gina Kolata, "Alzheimer's Research Poses Dilemma," *Science* 215, no. 4528 (January 1, 1982): 47.

6. Nancy L. Jose and Glenn E. Richardson, "Ageism: Need We Discriminate?" *Journal of School Health*, September 1980, p. 419.

7. Metropolitan Life Foundation, *Statistical Bulletin* 63, no. 1 (January–March 1982): 2.

8. Summarized in Neuhaus and Neuhaus, *Successful Aging.*

9. The discussion that follows is based on Howard C. Hopps, "Pathologic versus Nonpathologic Aspects of Senescence," in National Research Council, *Panel on Aging and the Geochemical Environment* (Washington, D.C.: National Academy Press, 1981), pp. 25–41.

10. The discussion that follows is based on ibid.

11. Ibid.

12. Martin S. Finkelstein, "Unusual Features of Infections in the Aging," *Geriatrics* 37, no. 4 (April 1982): 65–78.

13. The discussion that follows is based on Hopps, "Pathologic and Nonpathologic Aspects."

14. Neuhaus and Neuhaus, *Successful Aging.*

15. M. R. Levy and K. Glanz, "Drug Misuse Among the Elderly: An Educational Challenge for Health Professionals," *Journal of Drug Education* 11, no. 1 (1981): 61–75.

16. Strain, "Ageism in the Medical Profession."

17. Neuhaus and Neuhaus, *Successful Aging*, pp. 67–69.

18. John M. Last, ed., *Maxcy-Rosenau's Public Health and Preventive Medicine*, 11th ed. (New York: Appleton-Century-Crofts, 1980), p. 1338.

19. T. D. Sabin, A. J. Vitug, and V. H. Mark, "Are Nursing Home Diagnosis and Treatment Adequate?" *Journal of the American Medical Association* 248, no. 3 (July 16, 1982): 321–322.

20. M. C. Parkes, B. Benjamin, and R. G. Fitzgerald, "Broken Heart: A Statistical Study of Increased Mortality Among Widowers," *British Medical Journal* 1 (1969): 740–743.

21. Maddox and Busse, "Duke University Longitudinal Studies."

22. Saul Kent, "Exercise and Aging," *Geriatrics* 37, no. 6 (June 1982): 132–135.

23. Raymond Bossé and David J. Ekerdt, "Change in Self-Perception of Leisure Activities with Retirement," *The Gerontologist* 21, no. 6 (1981): 650–654.

24. Cited in F. Elwell and Alice D. Maltbie-Crannell, "The Impact of Role Loss Upon Coping Resources and Life Satisfaction of the Elderly," *Journal of Gerontology* 16, no. 2 (1961): 223–232.

25. Maria H. Nagy, "The Child's Theories Concerning Death," *Journal of Genetic Psychology* 73 (1948): 3–27.

26. R. J. Kastenbaum, *Death, Society, and the Human Experience,* 2nd ed. (St. Louis: Mosby, 1981), pp. 10–17, 19–20, 25–26, 32, 45.

27. Ibid., pp. 131–132.

28. Barrie R. Cassileth and James L. Stinnett, "Psy-

chosocial Problems," in Barrie R. Cassileth and Peter A. Cassileth, eds., *Clinical Care of the Terminal Cancer Patient.* (Philadelphia: Lea & Febiger, 1982), pp. 108–118.

29. Elisabeth Kübler-Ross, *On Death and Dying* (New York: Macmillan, 1969).

30. Kastenbaum, *Death, Society,* p. 191.

31. Russell A. Meares, "On Saying Good-bye Before Death," *Journal of the American Medical Association* 246, No. 11 (September 11, 1981): 1227–1229.

32. Richard A. Kalish, "Non-Medical Interventions in Life and Death," *Social Science and Medicine* 4 (1970): 655–665.

33. Robert G. Twycross, "The Assessment of Pain in Advanced Cancer," *Journal of Medical Ethics* 4 (1978): 112–116.

34. Marian Osterweis and Daphne S. Champagne, "The U.S. Hospice Movement: Issues in Development," *American Journal of Public Health* 69, no. 5 (May 1979): 492–496.

35. Kastenbaum, *Death, Society,* pp. 199–201.

36. Barbara J. Ward, "Hospice Home Care Program," *Nursing Outlook,* October 1978, pp. 646–649; S. Malkin, "Care of the Terminally Ill at Home," *Canadian Medical Journal* 115 (July 1976): 129–130; Anthony Amado, Beatrice A. Cronk, and Rich Mileo, "Cost of Terminal Care," *Nursing Outlook,* August 1979, pp. 522–526; R. G. Benton, *Death and Dying: Principles and Practice in Patient Care* (New York: Van Nostrand-Reinhold, 1978), pp. 64–66.

37. Harold M. Schmeck, Jr., "U.S. Panel Calls for Patients' Right to End Life," *New York Times,* March 22, 1983, pp. A1, C7.

38. Marguerite Mancini, "Death with Dignity: Are Living Wills the Answer?" *American Journal of Nursing,* December 1978, pp. 2133–2144.

39. Marc Lappé, "Dying While Living," *Journal of Medical Ethics* 4 (1978): 195–199; Joan Gibson et al., "Right to Die: A Medical, Moral, or Legal Decision?" *Journal of Family Practice* 7, no. 5 (1978): 1047–1051.

40. G. L. Engel, "A Unified Concept of Health and Disease," in D. Ingle, ed., *Life and Disease* (New York: Basic Books, 1963); J. F. Frederick, "Grief as a Disease Process," *Omega* 7 (1976): 297–306; W. D. Rees and S. G. Lutkins, "The Mortality of Bereavement," *British Medical Journal* 4 (1967): 13–16.

41. C. M. Parkes, *Bereavement* (New York: International Universities Press, 1972).

42. I. O. Glick, R. S. Weiss, and C. M. Parkes, *The First Year of Bereavement* (New York: Wiley-Interscience, 1974).

43. E. F. Furman, *A Child's Parent Dies* (New Haven, Conn.: Yale University Press, 1974); Robert Bendiksen and Robert Fulton, "Death and the Child," *Omega* 6 (1975): 45–60.

44. Charles E. Hollingsworth and Robert O. Pasnau, *The Family in Mourning: A Guide for Health Professionals* (New York: Grune & Stratton, 1977), pp. 145–147; Benton, *Death and Dying,* pp. 88–91.

45. Hollingsworth and Pasnau, *Family in Mourning,* pp. 63–67, 152–153; Stanley E. Weinstein, "Sudden Infant Death Syndrome," *American Journal of Psychiatry* 135, no. 7 (July 1978): 831–834; Thomas A. Helmrath and Elaine M. Steinitz, "Death of an Infant," *Journal of Family Practice* 6, no. 4 (1978): 785–790.

46. Jessica Mitford, *The American Way of Death* (New York: Fawcett, 1979).

47. Rebecca A. Cohen, "The FTC Assault on the Cost of Dying," *Business and Society Review* 27 (Fall 1978): 48–53.

GLOSSARY

A

abortion The termination of a pregnancy by removal of the uterine contents before the embryo or fetus is developed enough to survive on its own.

abscess A pus-filled cavity formed in the body as a result of destruction of local tissue in the inflammatory response.

acid rain Rain containing nitric and sulfuric acid, formed when nitrogen and sulfur oxides from motor vehicles and coal-burning power plants and factories react with moisture in the atmosphere.

ACTH (adrenocorticotrophic hormone) A pituitary hormone that stimulates the cortex of the adrenal glands to produce hormones called corticosteroids.

active immunity Long-lasting resistance to an infectious disease acquired through the body's production of antibodies as a result of either having the disease or being vaccinated against it. Compare **passive immunity**.

addiction A compulsive pattern of drug use, marked both by tolerance and by psychic and physical dependence. Compare **dependence, habituation.**

adenocarcinomas Cancers arising from glandular epithelial cells, such as the cells lining the milk duct in the breast.

adjustment disorder A nonpsychotic disorder in which the individual's response to a painful event is more extreme than would ordinarily be expected or considered normal.

adrenal glands Two glands located just above the kidneys; the inner portion (medulla) secretes the hormones epinephrine and norepinephrine in response to stress; the outer portion (cortex) secretes corticosteroids.

aerobic exercise Sustained exercise during which the body is able to meet its oxygen needs continually. Compare **anaerobic exercise.**

affective disorders Devastatingly painful psychotic disorders of mood or feeling, such as major depression and bipolar disorder.

aging A gradual developmental process of biological, psychological, sociological, and behavioral change that occurs between the time we reach maturity and the end of our life.

air pollution The presence in the air of contaminants that do not disperse properly and that interfere with human health.

alcoholic A person whose drinking is associated with serious disruptions in his or her personal and social life and with loss of behavioral control *and* who has developed a preoccupation with alcohol and a physical and psychological dependence on it. Compare **problem drinker.**

alcoholic hepatitis An alcohol-related disease in which the liver becomes inflamed and swollen.

allergy (hypersensitivity) An acquired overreaction to a specific substance by the body's immune system.

amniocentesis Procedure in which a doctor withdraws some amniotic fluid from a pregnant woman's uterus to test for certain genetic disorders in the fetus.

amnion (amniotic sac) Fluid-filled sac within the uterus that encloses and protects the developing baby.

amphetamines A group of synthetic stimulant drugs ("uppers," "pep pills").

amyl nitrite A prescription drug used in the treatment of angina; used recreationally as a euphoriant and presumed sexual stimulant.

anaerobic exercise Exercise in which the body's demand for oxygen exceeds its supply, producing "oxygen debt." Compare **aerobic exercise.**

analgesic A substance that eliminates or reduces the sense of pain.

anaphylactic shock A life-threatening allergic reaction in which blood pressure can drop so low that the person dies.

anaplastic Referring to cancers whose cellular structure is so abnormal that they no longer resemble the cells from which they originated, and no identification is possible.

angina pectoris A tightness, pressure, and intense pain in the chest caused by insufficient blood flow through partially blocked coronary arteries.

animal parasite An organism that lives in or on the body of another animal (the **host**), obtaining food from it and in the process weakening it and causing disease.

anorexia nervosa An eating disorder in which people severely limit the amount of food they eat, virtually starving themselves.

anthropometric measurements Measurements taken, using calipers, of various parts of the body to calculate the proportion of fat in the body.

antibiotics A group of drugs that destroy or inhibit the growth of disease-causing bacteria.

antibodies Chemical substances produced in response to an invading microorganism (the **antigen**) that can inactivate the microorganism.

antigen An invading microorganism that stimulates the body to produce chemical substances (**antibodies**) that can inactivate the microorganism.

anxiety disorder A nonpsychotic disorder, involving a severe and persistent fear or worry that interferes with the individual's everyday functioning and that may have physical effects as well.

anxiolytics (relaxants) Hypnosedative drugs used as anxiety reducers; some also used as muscle relaxants and to control specific types of convulsive seizures; formerly known as "minor tranquilizers."

aorta The main vessel of the circulatory system, carrying blood from the heart to the arteries.

arrhythmia An abnormal rhythm in the heartbeat.

arterioles The smallest arteries.

arteriosclerosis A condition in which the arteries become thick and hard and lose their elasticity; caused by calcium deposits.

artery A blood vessel that carries blood from the heart to the various parts of the body.

atherosclerosis A disease process in which fatty deposits circulating in the blood accumulate on the intima (the lining of the artery walls), forming plaque which causes the walls to become rough and thickened.

autonomic nervous system A part of the nervous system that works with the central nervous system to produce emotions.

B

bacteria (singular: **bacterium**) Single-celled, plantlike microorganisms.

barbiturates Hypnosedatives used primarily to treat insomnia and less often for daytime sedation; some also have anticonvulsive properties.

basic health insurance Insurance that pays benefits for hospitalization and for medical and surgical expenses.

benign tumor A tumor that grows relatively slowly and remains localized.

benzopyrene A chemical found in tobacco smoke; one of the deadliest carcinogens known.

bereavement The loss, through death, of a person one has loved or valued.

biodegradation The breakdown and assimilation of organic material by microorganisms.

biofeedback A technique for developing conscious control over involuntary body processes such as blood pressure and heartbeat.

biotransformation (metabolism) The process by which reactions inside the body change chemical substances, such as drugs, into different compounds.

bipolar disorder An affective disorder in which the individual exhibits mania, with or without depressive symptoms, alternating—sometimes rapidly—with anger or depression.

blood alcohol level (BAL) The concentration of alcohol in the blood at a given time.

blood pressure The force exerted by the blood on the walls of the arteries. See **diastolic, systolic.**

brain death The concept that a person may be considered dead when the brain is no longer

functioning, as determined by a number of objective indicators.

bulimia A type of anorexia nervosa characterized by eating binges followed by purges.

butyl nitrite An analog of amyl nitrite used recreationally as a euphoriant and presumed sexual stimulant.

C

Caesarean section Delivery of a baby through surgical incisions made in the mother's abdomen and uterus.

caffeine A stimulant drug found in coffee, cola drinks, chocolate, tea, and other beverages as well as some OTC drugs.

cancer A condition of abnormal cell growth.

capillaries Very small blood vessels that serve as links between arterioles and venules.

carbohydrates One of the four basic components of food, found in the form of sugars and starches in bread, potatoes, most fruits and vegetables, and other foods. Carbohydrates are the body's source of ready energy.

carbon monoxide One of the most hazardous gases in tobacco smoke. It impairs the blood's capacity to carry oxygen and concentrates in the blood of the fetus of a woman who smokes.

carcinogenic Cancer-producing.

carcinomas Cancers that arise from epithelium.

cardiac arrest Any stoppage of the heartbeat.

cardiorespiratory endurance The ability of the heart, lungs, and blood vessels to mobilize the body's energy and sustain movement over a period of time.

cerebrovascular accident (stroke, cerebrovascular occlusion) A sudden loss of brain function resulting from interference with the blood supply to one part of the brain.

cervix The narrow lower end of the uterus, at the upper end of the vagina.

chemotherapy A course of treatment using chemicals that destroy cancerous cells.

cholesterol A fatlike substance that is found in all foods from animal sources and is also manufactured by the human body.

circumcision Surgical removal of the foreskin.

cirrhosis of the liver A chronic inflammatory disease that causes scarring of the liver and impairs liver function; frequently associated with alcoholism.

classical conditioning A type of learning in which an individual comes to associate an originally neutral stimulus with a meaningful one, then responds to the neutral one as if it were the meaningful one.

clitoris Extremely sensitive external female sexual organ located under a hood formed by the upper joining of the labia minora.

cocaine A stimulant drug extracted from the leaves of the coca bush of South America.

cognitive dissonance An uncomfortable conflict between two realities that don't match; often leads to use of the defense mechanism of rationalization.

cognitively mediated stress Perceived stress that occurs when we label something negatively in our minds.

cohabitation An arrangement in which an unrelated man and woman live together without marrying.

collateral circulation A system of smaller blood vessels, which develop to provide alternative routes for blood when a main artery is blocked.

complete protein Protein that includes all eight of the essential amino acids.

conditioned anxiety Perceived stress that comes from having learned to fear specific situations.

condom A thin rubber or natural skin sheath that is placed over the erect penis just before intercourse to prevent conception.

congeners Substances other than alcohol that are natural products of the fermentation and preparation of some alcoholic beverages.

congenital heart disease Defects of the heart that are present at birth.

congestive heart failure A condition in which the heart cannot pump enough blood, resulting in a congestion of blood in the lungs.

coronal ridge The rim of tissue between the glans and the shaft of the penis.

coronary atherosclerosis A disease process characterized by fatty thickening of the intima (the lining) of the coronary arteries.

coronary embolism A blockage of a coronary artery that occurs when a piece of clotted material breaks away from the artery wall and dams up a narrowed coronary artery.

coronary thrombosis A blood clot in a coronary artery.

corticosteroids Hormones produced by the cortex of the adrenal glands.

Cowper's glands Two pea-sized organs that sometimes produce a few drops of fluid at the end of the penis during sexual arousal.

cross-sensitivity A situation in which allergy to one drug warns of possible similar reactions to other, chemically related ones.

D

defense mechanism One of a number of mental strategies for protecting oneself from experiencing the anxiety associated with painful emotions.

denial A defense mechanism in which an individual refuses to recognize truths about the outer world, ignoring those which threaten his or her self-esteem or create anxiety.

densimetric method Technique for assessing the proportion of lean and fat tissue in the body by weighing the person first in air, then again when submerged in water, to determine overall body density in relation to water.

dependence A situation in which an individual becomes so accustomed to a drug that he or she cannot function without it; may be physical, psychic, or both. Compare **addiction**, **habituation**.

depersonalization A defense mechanism in which an individual is unable to recognize that other people are fully human, with human feelings and emotions.

detoxification The process of weaning a person from physical dependence on alcohol and repairing the toxic effects of alcohol in the body.

diabetes mellitus A chronic illness characterized by abnormal processing of carbohydrates as a result of the body's inability to produce enough insulin (**juvenile-onset diabetes**) or to use insulin properly (**adult-onset diabetes**).

diaphragm A shallow rubber cup that is inserted into the vagina, where it completely covers the cervix, forming a mechanical barrier that prevents sperm from entering the woman's uterus.

diastolic Referring to blood pressure inside the arteries when the left ventricle of the heart is relaxed and filling with blood between beats. Compare **systolic**.

disability insurance Insurance that pays benefits to a person unable to work because of accident or illness.

disulfiram (Antabuse) A drug that disrupts the body's ability to metabolize alcohol; causes a person to feel ill if he or she drinks alcohol while taking it.

drug A nonfood substance that is deliberately introduced into the body in order to produce some specific physiological or psychological effect.

dual-career marriage A marriage in which both partners seriously pursue professional careers.

E

ectomorphy Degree of "linearity" or "long-bonedness" of a person's body build.

ectopic pregnancy Condition in which a fertilized egg implants and begins to develop in the Fallopian tube rather than the uterus.

edema Swelling caused by fluid collecting in the tissues.

ejaculation Contractions of the urethra, penis, and prostate gland that usually accompany orgasm in the male, forcing semen out of the tip of the penis.

ejaculatory ducts Two structures formed by the ends of the seminal vesicles and of the vas deferens that, in turn, join the urethra.

embryo A developing baby in the uterus during the first two months following conception.

emotional health A state in which we are not troubled by ongoing conflicts among our emotions, so that our emotions do not interfere with our everyday existence.

endemic Describing a disease that usually occurs in just one geographical area.

endocrine glands Body cells and tissues that produce hormones.

endocrine system The body's mechanism for producing and secreting (releasing) hormones.

endogenous microorganisms Microscopic organisms that normally live within the human body, usually causing it no harm and often contributing to its welfare, but sometimes causing disease.

endometrium The inner lining of the uterus.

endomorphy Degree of fatness of a person's body build.

endorphins Natural brain chemicals that are similar to morphine.

endurance The number of times the muscles can contract against a moderate force.

enkephalins Natural opiatelike chemicals manufactured by the body.

enrichment The restoring to food of specific nutrients that were lost in processing or the addition of nutrients that were not originally present in a food.

epidemic An outbreak of disease that affects more people in a certain geographical area than would be expected on the basis of previous experience.

epidemiology The systematic study of the distribution and dynamics of disease as it affects large groups of people.

epididymis Highly coiled network of tubing in the back of each testicle through which sperm cells travel as they mature.

epinephrine (adrenaline) One of the hormones secreted by the medulla of the adrenal glands in response to stress.

episiotomy A surgical incision made between a mother's vaginal opening and anus to prevent undue tearing of the tissues during delivery of a baby.

epithelium The cells forming the skin, the glands, and the membranes that line the respiratory, urinary, and gastrointestinal tracts.

erogenous Exciting sexual desire or producing sexual arousal.

essential fat Fat that is necessary for the body's normal physiological functioning in the storage and usage of nutrients. Compare **storage fat.**

estrogen An ovarian hormone that helps to regulate the menstrual cycle.

ethyl alcohol The active ingredient in alcoholic beverages (distilled spirits, wine, beer) prepared from natural plant products such as fruits and grains.

euthanasia The deliberate killing of a sick person with the intention of ending his or her suffering.

exogenous microorganisms Microscopic organisms that are not normally residents of the human body, many of which can cause disease if they enter the body.

F

Fallopian tube (oviduct) One of two tiny, muscular tunnels that transport ova from the ovary to the uterus.

fats (lipids) One of the four basic components of food, found in oils, meats, and other foods. Fats are essential as a source of energy, for insulation and protection of the body, and for many body processes (such as hormone synthesis and blood clotting).

fat-soluble vitamins One of the two major types of vitamins, consisting of vitamins A, D, E, and K. Excess consumption of these vitamins is dangerous because surplus amounts cannot be excreted, but rather are stored in fatty tissue, where they may build to toxic levels. Compare **water-soluble vitamins.**

fertilized ovum (fertilized egg) A cell formed by the union of a sperm cell and an ovum, from which a new human being eventually develops.

fetal alcohol syndrome Characteristic adverse effects (including mental retardation, slow growth before and after birth, and a wide range of physical defects) exhibited by children born to women who drink heavily.

fetus A developing baby in the uterus from the beginning of the third·month of pregnancy until birth.

fibrillation An arrhythmia in which the ventricles of the heart beat irregularly at an extremely fast rate.

flashbacks Brief, sudden unexpected perceptual distortions and bizarre thoughts—similar to those experienced while on an LSD trip—that occur long after the immediate effects of the drug have worn off.

flexibility The freedom with which the body's muscles, bones, tendons, and ligaments are able to move.

fluorocarbons Inert chemical compounds used as propellants in aerosol spray cans and believed to be damaging the ozone layer of the stratosphere that protects the earth from the sun's ultraviolet rays.

foreskin The flap of tissue at the head of the penis.

frenulum The triangular region on the underside of the penis.

fungi (singular: **fungus**) Many-celled, plantlike organisms that lack chlorophyll and must therefore obtain food from organic material—in some cases, from humans.

G

gamma globulin Certain blood proteins that contain antibodies.

general adaptation syndrome (GAS) Hans Selye's term for the series of stages that occur in the body's efforts to adapt to stress; it consists of the alarm stage, the resistance stage, and the stage of exhaustion.

geriatrics The area within gerontology that deals with promoting and maintaining the health of the elderly and with preventing and treating their diseases.

gerontology The study of aging.

glans The head of the penis.

glaucoma A condition in which the pressure inside the eyeball increases.

glucose A type of sugar.

glycogen The form in which glucose is stored in the liver and muscles; it is released into the bloodstream when blood sugar levels fall too low.

grief The subjective response to bereavement.

H

habituation A pattern of compulsive drug use that arises from psychic dependence but does not usually involve tolerance. Compare **addiction, dependence**.

hashish A concentrated and potent resin of *Cannabis sativa* (the hemp plant).

health maintenance organization (HMO) A type of prepaid group-practice plan in which consumers pay a set fee every month and in return receive whatever medical services they need at little or no additional cost.

heart A four-chambered, muscular organ that continuously pumps blood throughout the circulatory system.

heart attack The death of a portion of the heart muscle due to lack of oxygen.

heart block A sudden slowing or stopping of the heartbeat, caused by a failure of the electrical connection between the atria and ventricles of the heart.

hemorrhage Profuse bleeding.

heroin A narcotic analgesic derived from morphine and more than twice as powerful.

heterosexuality Sexual or emotional preference for persons of the opposite sex.

homeostasis A state in which bodily functions are in normal balance.

homosexuality A sexual or emotional preference for persons of one's own sex.

hormones Chemical substances that are produced by glands and that act as messengers within the body and help regulate the body's functioning.

host The human or animal in or on which an animal parasite lives.

hydrogenation The process of changing a liquid fat to a solid by bubbling hydrogen gas through it.

hymen Circular membrane that narrows the opening of the vagina in some females who have never had sexual intercourse.

hypertension (high blood pressure) An elevation of blood pressure above the normal range, which increases the risk of cardiovascular disease.

hyperthermia Cancer treatment in which body tissues are superheated to make cancerous cells more sensitive to radiation therapy.

hypnosedatives A group of drugs that have both sedative (calming) and hypnotic (sleep-inducing) effects ("downers").

hypoarousal A state in which the body is less aroused than normal.

hypoglycemia Low blood sugar. Temporary low blood sugar is a normal condition; the disease hypoglycemia is a rare condition caused by malfunctioning of the pancreas.

hypothalamus A structure in the brain that produces certain hormones that, in turn, stimulate the pituitary gland to secrete hormones.

I

iatrogenic Referring to illness or injury caused by a doctor's carelessness, error, or poor judgment.

immunity A group of mechanisms that help protect the body against specific diseases.

immunotherapy Cancer treatment that involves strengthening the body's own immune system.

impotence Sexual dysfunction in which a man is unable to achieve or maintain an erection long enough to reach orgasm with a partner. See **primary impotence, secondary impotence.**

incomplete protein Protein that lacks one or more of the eight essential amino acids.

incubation period The time between first exposure to a virus or other disease-causing organism and the appearance of symptoms.

infection The invasion of the body by disease-causing organisms and the reaction of the body to their presence.

inflammatory response (inflammation) A general defense mechanism in the blood and tissues aimed at warding off any irritant or foreign body.

inhalants A group of substances containing volatile chemicals that have psychoactive (and other) effects when inhaled.

inhalation A route of administration that involves breathing a drug into the lungs.

insulin A substance produced by the body that enables it to take sugar (in the form of glucose) from the bloodstream and use it for energy.

interferon A substance produced by the body to help protect it against viruses.

internal locus of control A person's belief that he or she, not outside forces or other people, is largely responsible for what happens to him or her in life.

intima The lining of the arteries.

intrauterine device (IUD) A soft, flexible plastic device that is inserted into the uterus by a physician to prevent pregnancy.

intravenous injection Injection of a substance into a vein. Compare **subcutaneous injection.**

isokinetic Referring to the strength training of muscles through the use of specialized apparatus that, throughout a complete range of motion, provides resistance that is exactly equal to the force the user applies.

isometric Referring to the strength training of muscles by pushing or pulling against a fixed resistance or an immovable object through a relatively narrow range of motion.

isotonic Referring to the strength training of muscles through exercises that involve muscle contractions throughout a complete range of motion.

L

labia Two soft, sensitive folds of skin at either side of the opening of the vagina. The outer broad folds are called the *labia majora;* the inner, hairless lips are called the *labia minora.*

laparoscopy Surgical sterilization technique for women, in which a small electrode is used to sever the Fallopian tubes.

leukemias Cancers arising from blood-forming cells.

lipoproteins Substances containing both fat and protein that transport fat molecules through the body. **Low-density lipoprotein (LDL)** contains little protein and is the major medium of cholesterol transport. **High-density lipoprotein (HDL)** is heavier and higher concentrations of it in the body seem to offer some protection from heart disease.

LSD (lysergic acid diethylamide) A synthetic psychedelic/illusionogen drug used recreationally ("acid").

lymphocytes White blood cells that fight infection.

lymphomas Cancers arising from lymphatic cells.

M

major depression An affective disorder in which the individual experiences a dysphoric mood, loses interest in all aspects of life, and may suffer other incapacitating symptoms.

major medical insurance Insurance designed to provide protection against the high medical expenses that accumulate when a person is seriously injured or ill for a long time.

malignant tumor A tumor whose cells grow in abnormal ways and may break away and spread to other parts of the body.

mammography An X-ray of the breast to detect abnormalities, especially cancer.

mania A mood of extreme excitement; an aspect of bipolar disorder.

marijuana Material from *Cannabis sativa* (the hemp plant) dried and prepared for smoking; has a variety of mind-altering and physiological effects that may resemble those of a mild sedative or a mild stimulant, depending on the individual and the setting ("pot," "grass").

Medicaid A federal-state health insurance program for people of any age who cannot pay for medical care.

Medicare A federal health insurance program for people aged sixty-five or older.

meditation A technique by which a person can induce in himself or herself a state of deep physiological and mental repose.

melanomas Cancers of pigment-carrying cells of the skin.

menopause Gradual, permanent cessation of a woman's menstruation and therefore of the reproductive phase of her life; also known as the *climacteric.*

menstrual cycle The monthly cycle in which the lining of the uterus thickens and prepares to receive a fertilized ovum then is discharged in menstruation if a pregnancy does not occur.

menstruation The sloughing off of

the thickened lining of the uterus that occurs about once a month if the woman is not pregnant.

mescaline A psychedelic/illusionogen drug derived from the peyote cactus of the U.S. Southwest.

mesomorphy Degree of muscularity of a person's body build.

metabolites The products of biotransformation.

metastases Secondary tumors that form when cancerous cells break away from the original malignant tumor and transfer to a new location in the body.

metastatic growth The process by which cancerous cells break away from the original malignant tumor and transfer to a new location in the body.

methadone An opioid used in treatment of heroin addiction.

minerals With vitamins, one of the four basic components of food, consisting of inorganic elements that humans need in trace amounts daily to help form tissues and various chemical substances in the body.

mitosis The orderly division of a cell into two new cells.

molecule The smallest unit of a chemical substance such as a drug.

mons veneris A sensitive cushion of fatty tissue covered with skin and hair, located in the female vulva over the pubic bone.

morphine A narcotic analgesic that is the active ingredient in opium.

mourning The culturally reinforced patterns of thought, feelings, and behaviors that bereaved individuals experience.

myocardial infarction Death of a section of the heart muscle caused by reduction in the supply of blood to the area.

myotonia Generalized sexual response in which muscles throughout the body increase tension.

N

narcotic analgesics A group of drugs—including the opiates and the opioids—that act on the central nervous system to eliminate or relieve pain without causing loss of consciousness.

natural family planning A method of contraception in which a couple avoids intercourse during the time when the woman may be ovulating.

neoplasm A group of cells growing in an uncontrolled fashion to form a tumor.

nicotine A toxic drug found in tobacco that acts as a stimulant and is responsible for many of the harmful effects of smoking.

nitrous oxide An anesthetic gas sometimes used recreationally as an inhalant.

nonemissive erection Sexual dysfunction in which a man is able to achieve an erection but not to ejaculate.

nonpsychotic disorders Mental disorders in which the individual's functioning is seriously inhibited but in which thought processes are not as grossly distorted as in some of the psychotic disorders and the individual recognizes and is disturbed by the symptoms.

norepinephrine (noradrenaline) One of the hormones secreted by the medulla of the adrenal glands in response to stress.

nosocomial Referring to illness or injury caused by contact with a hospital or other health institution, ranging from a fall from bed to an infection to a fatal surgical error.

nutrition The science of food, its use within the body, and its relationship to good health.

O

obese Weighing 20 percent or more above the recommendation

in insurance-company tables. Compare **overweight**.

oncogenes Individual tumor cells.

opiates A group of narcotic analgesics, including opium, morphine, and heroin.

opioids A group of synthetic narcotic analgesics, including methadone and meperidine, that are chemically similar to the opiates.

opium A narcotic analgesic that is the parent substance of the opiates; derived from the juice of the opium poppy.

oral administration The introduction of a drug into the body through the mouth.

oral contraceptives ("the Pill") Synthetic equivalents of natural sex hormones that are medically prescribed to prevent ovulation and thus prevent conception.

organic mental disorders Psychotic disorders caused by actual physical disorders of the brain.

orgasm The climactic stage of sexual response.

ovaries Two small internal female sexual organs that produce ova (egg cells).

overload Subjecting muscles to a greater-than-normal load to increase their size and strength.

overweight Weighing 15 percent or more above the recommendation in insurance-company tables. Compare **obese**.

ovulation The process by which ova periodically ripen and leave the ovaries.

ovum Female reproductive cell.

P

pancreatitis Inflammation of the pancreas associated with heavy alcohol intake.

pandemic An epidemic that affects people in a huge area, such as an entire country or continent.

paranoid disorder A psychotic disorder involving delusions of persecution.

parasitic worms Many-celled animals such as pinworms, tapeworms, and flukes that live in human hosts, causing illness.

parenteral administration The introduction of a drug into the body in such a way as to bypass the digestive system, usually by injection.

passive immunity Short-term resistance to infectious disease acquired through the administration of antibodies formed by another person or an animal. Compare **active immunity.**

passive smoking Breathing in air polluted by the tobacco smoke of other people. Especially dangerous to children whose parents smoke.

pathogen An organism, such as a bacterium or virus, that can be an agent of infectious disease.

PCP (phencyclidine) An animal anesthetic used recreationally as a psychedelic/illusionogen drug ("angel dust").

penis The external male organ of sexual intercourse and urination.

perineum Hairless area of skin at the lower end of the labia, near the anus.

personality disorders Deeply ingrained maladaptive reactions that impair an individual's social or occupational functioning.

phagocytes White blood cells that protect the body from infection by engulfing and digesting invading microorganisms, toxins, and other foreign substances.

pharmacokinetics The study of what happens to drugs once they are in the body.

pituitary gland The tiny "master gland," located at the base of the brain, that is stimulated by the hypothalamus to secrete hormones that, in turn, stimulate other glands to secrete other hormones.

placenta A mass of tissue attached to the uterine lining that, during pregnancy, absorbs nutrients from the mother's bloodstream and transfers them to the bloodstream of the developing baby, and carries away fetal wastes.

plaque Fatty deposits, made up largely of cholesterol, that can build up on the walls of blood vessels, narrowing them and eventually perhaps closing them completely.

pollution Any substance or energy that contributes to the development of undesirable environmental effects.

premature ejaculation The expulsion of semen before or immediately after insertion of the penis into the vagina.

premenstrual syndrome (PMS) A pattern of physiological symptoms, irritability, lethargy, and depression that precedes menstruation in some women.

prenatal Before birth.

primary impotence Sexual dysfunction in which a man has never been able to achieve an erection.

primary orgasmic dysfunction Sexual dysfunction in which a woman has never experienced an orgasm by any method.

problem drinker A person whose drinking is associated with serious disruptions in his or her personal and social life and with loss of behavioral control. Compare **alcoholic.**

progesterone An ovarian hormone that helps to regulate the menstrual cycle, stimulating the uterus each month to prepare to receive a fertilized ovum if one is present.

proof A number indicating the concentration of ethyl alcohol in a beverage; can be converted to percent by dividing by two (thus, 80-proof whiskey is 40 percent alcohol).

projection A defense mechanism in which an individual attributes his or her own undesirable motives and feelings to other people or even inanimate objects.

prostate gland Male organ located just below the urethra that produces about 30 percent of the seminal fluid.

protein One of the four basic components of food, consisting of amino acids and found in meat, eggs, dairy products, and some other foods. Protein is necessary for growth and repair of the body.

protozoa (singular: **protozoon**) Single-celled parasitic animals, some of which produce illness in human and animal hosts.

psilocybin A psychedelic/illusionogen drug derived from a Mexican mushroom.

psychedelic/illusionogen A group of drugs that create illusions, distorting the user's mind by creating moods, thoughts, and perceptions that would otherwise take place only in a dream state (also known as *hallucinogens, deliriants, psychotogens, psychotomimetics*).

psychic contactlessness A defense mechanism in which an individual is unable to communicate with or become intimate with others.

psychoactive drugs Drugs that alter a person's moods, consciousness, and behaviors.

psychotic disorders Mental disorders in which the individual has significantly lost contact with reality.

pus A sticky, yellow-white substance that fills an abscess as a result of the inflammatory response; it consists of fluid in which active and dead white blood cells are suspended.

R

radiation sickness Disease produced by prolonged or excessive exposure to radiation.

radiation therapy The use of very high, concentrated doses of radiation to destroy cancer cells.

rationalization A defense mechanism in which an individual asserts acceptable motives for questionable behavior; often used in situations of cognitive dissonance.

receptor sites Specific spots within cells where the molecules of a specific drug "fit."

refractory period A temporary state following orgasm during which most males cannot respond to renewed sexual stimulation.

reinforcers Responses from the environment that strengthen a particular behavior, making an individual more likely to repeat it.

relaxation response A method of stress management similar to meditation, developed by Herbert Benson of Harvard University.

renin A disease-related enzyme, produced by the kidneys, that helps the body retain sodium instead of excreting it.

repression A defense mechanism in which an individual rejects all awareness of threatening thoughts, feelings, memories, or wishes.

rheumatic fever Inflammatory disease of connective tissue throughout the body; can cause scarring of heart muscle and valves.

Rh factor A substance in the red blood cells which, if lacking in the mother and inherited by the first baby from the father, can cause the mother's blood to produce antibodies that result in a blood disorder called erythroblastosis fetalis in second and later children.

rickettsiae Infectious organisms that grow in the intestinal tracts of insects and insectlike creatures and may be transmitted to humans through insect bites.

route of administration The method by which a drug is introduced into the body. See **inhalation, oral administration,** and **parenteral administration.**

S

sarcomas Cancers that arise from supporting or connective tissues, such as bones, cartilage, and the membranes covering muscles and fat.

saturated fat A fat that has all the hydrogen atoms it is capable of holding; usually solid at room temperature. Compare **unsaturated fat.**

schizophrenia A psychotic disorder in which the individual seems totally removed from reality.

scrotum The loose pouch of skin that hangs behind and under the penis and contains the testicles.

secondary impotence Sexual dysfunction in which a man who has previously been able to achieve an erection is now unable to do so in some or all sexual encounters.

secondary (situational) orgasmic dysfunction Sexual dysfunction in which a woman frequently has difficulty achieving an orgasm.

semen (seminal fluid) Sperm-carrying liquid expelled from the penis during ejaculation.

seminal vesicles Two small structures located at the base of the bladder that produce about 70 percent of the seminal fluid.

setpoint The weight range that is natural to an individual's body which, according to the "setpoint theory," the body strives to maintain by adjusting its metabolic rate.

sex (1) gender (maleness or femaleness); (2) physical expression of affectionate or erotic feelings. Compare **sexuality.**

sexual dysfunction Any problem that prevents a person from engaging in sexual relations or from reaching orgasm.

sexuality Masculinity or femininity; the way in which one's gender is integrated into one's personality. Compare **sex.**

sexually transmitted diseases (STDs) Infectious diseases that are almost always transmitted during sexual intercourse, homosexual relations, or other sexual activity.

side effects Effects of a drug that are unwanted and are not related to the essential purpose of the drug.

sidestream smoke Smoke from the burning end of a cigarette.

sign An objective, observable indication of disease. Compare **symptom.**

simple sugars Chemicals that are an intermediate step between carbohydrates and glucose.

skill-related stress Perceived stress that occurs when we are uncertain whether we have the skills to do a task.

smog A form of air pollution that may occur as either sulfur-dioxide smog (high levels of sulfur dioxide and ozone combined with particulate matter and foggy air) or photochemical smog (the result of the interaction of sunlight, temperature inversion, and exhaust emissions from automobiles).

socialization The process by which people learn the ways of a given society or social group so that they can function within it.

social learning (modeling) Behavior learned by observing the experience of others.

sperm Male reproductive cell.

spermatic cords Muscular structures from which the testicles are suspended within the scrotum.

spermatogenesis The process of continual sperm production.

sphygmomanometer Instrument used to measure blood pressure.

spontaneous abortion   Expulsion of an improperly implanted or defective embryo or fetus from the uterus; commonly called a *miscarriage.*

starches   A group of chemicals that are one of the two major types of carbohydrates. See **sugars.**

stimulants   Drugs that activate the sympathetic division of the autonomic nervous system.

stimulus   Any marked change in an organism's environment.

storage fat   Fat deposited under the skin and around the internal organs to protect them; although it is sometimes called *excess fat,* some storage fat is necessary to the body's well-being. Compare **essential fat.**

strength   The amount of force the muscles can generate.

stress   Certain physical reactions that human beings (and other animals) exhibit in response to any stimulus.

stroke   See **cerebrovascular accident.**

subcutaneous injection   Injection of a substance under the skin. Compare **intravenous injection.**

sublimation   A defense mechanism in which an individual substitutes socially acceptable behavior for unacceptable impulses, such as hostility or aggression.

sugars   A group of chemicals that are one of the two major types of carbohydrates. See **starches.**

symptom   A subjective indication of disease, experienced by the individual but not necessarily apparent to an observer. Compare **sign.**

synergism   A type of drug interaction in which two drugs, when taken at the same time or in rapid sequence, have more powerful effects than the two drugs would have if taken alone.

synesthesia   The blending of two senses so that, for example, a person using LSD "hears" colors and "sees" sounds.

systolic   Referring to blood pressure inside the arteries when the left ventricle of the heart is contracting at each beat. Compare **diastolic.**

T

tar   A sticky residue from burning tobacco, consisting of more than 200 chemicals, many of which are hazardous.

temperature inversion   A phenomenon in which a layer of cool air is trapped under a layer of warm air; pollutants such as motor vehicle emissions also become trapped and are subjected to the action of sunlight, which produces additional pollutants such as ozone.

teratogenic drugs   Drugs that, if taken by a pregnant woman, can interfere with crucial stages of a baby's prenatal development and are thus associated with birth defects.

testicles (testes)   Male organs that produce sperm.

THC (tetrahydrocannabinol)   The chief psychoactive ingredient in marijuana and hashish.

therapeutic index   The safety margin between the effective dose of a drug and the lethal dose.

tissue   A collection of cells in the body that are specialized to perform certain functions.

tolerance   A situation in which the body becomes adapted to a drug, so that increasingly larger doses are needed to produce the original desired effect.

toxins   Poisonous substances, such as those produced by disease-causing organisms.

toxoids   Modified toxins, which are no longer poisonous, used to induce the production of antibodies that will inactivate specific microbial disease-producing toxins.

transient ischemic attack (TIA)   A very mild stroke, causing temporary dizziness or slight weakness or numbness.

triglycerides   One of a number of fatty acids into which excess glucose is converted and stored in the body's fat tissue.

tubal ligation   Surgical sterilization technique for women, in which the Fallopian tubes are severed or tied off.

tumor   A swelling or mass formed by a group of cells within a tissue that grow to an abnormal size and shape and begin to multiply in an uncontrolled fashion.

U

umbilical cord   A ropelike tissue that connects the developing baby to the placenta.

unsaturated fat   A fat that is capable of holding more hydrogen atoms than it does; usually liquid at room temperature. Compare **saturated fat.**

urethra   The tube from the urinary bladder through which urine is passed out of the body; in males, the urethra is also the canal through which semen is discharged.

uterus   The womb; a hollow, muscular internal female sex organ that contributes to sexual response and that shelters and nourishes the fetus during pregnancy.

V

vaccine   Killed or weakened viruses that are taken orally or by injection to stimulate the body to produce antibodies that give immunity to the specific disease caused by the virus.

vagina   The canal-like structure of the female body that extends from the bottom of the uterus to the vulva; it receives the penis during sexual intercourse and acts as a passageway for a baby during birth.

vaginal spermicides Nonprescription foams, creams, or jellies that a woman inserts in her vagina, against the cervix, to prevent conception by killing sperm.

vaginismus Sexual dysfunction involving involuntary muscle spasms that cause the vagina to shut so tightly that penetration by a penis is impossible or painful.

vas deferens Long tubes that carry sperm from the epididymis to the seminal vesicles.

vasectomy Surgical sterilization technique for men, in which the vas deferens are cut and tied off.

vasocongestion Increased blood flow, as to genital organs during sexual arousal.

vector A carrier of an infectious agent; insects, ticks, and rats are vectors of some human infectious diseases.

vein Blood vessel that carries blood from the body back to the heart.

venules The small veins.

virus A microorganism that can reproduce only in living cells of a person or animal.

vitamins With minerals, one of the four major components of food, needed in very small amounts but essential for triggering vital bodily functions.

vulva The external genital region surrounding the opening of the vagina.

W

water-soluble vitamins One of the two major types of vitamins, consisting of vitamin C and the B-complex vitamins. Because these vitamins are soluble in water, any excess amount can be excreted. Compare **fat-soluble vitamins.**

withdrawal A method of contraception in which the man withdraws his penis from the woman's vagina before he ejaculates; also known as *coitus interruptus.*

withdrawal syndrome An unpleasant and possibly painful condition that an individual who is physically dependent on a drug experiences when deprived of the drug.

INDEX

A

abdominal circumference test, taking, 341 (how-to)
abdominal pain, 189, 191, 241, 243, 246, 255, 389
  care of, 390 (how-to)
abortion, 108, 149, 197, 198, 208–209, 416, 417
accidents, 49, 99, 222, 389
  See also automobile accidents; injuries
acid indigestion, care of, 390 (how-to)
acid rain, 420
acquired immune deficiency syndrome (AIDS), 251
acquired immunity, 3, 246, 251–253
  guarding one's, 252–253 (how-to)
acupuncture, 401
acyclovir (Zovirax), 259
adaptation, 20, 55–56
addiction, 85
  See also drug dependence, tolerance, and habituation
adenocarcinoma, 270
administration of drugs, 75 (how-to), 76 (how-to)
adolescents, *see* young adults
adrenal hormones, 20, 52, 54, 55, 63, 143
adrenaline, 20, 54, 55, 143
adrenocorticotropic hormone (ACTH), 54
adults:
  coping with death by, 440
  See also young adults
aerobic exercise, 369
affective disorders, 33–34
  See also depression
ageism, 429–430
  See also old age
Agent Orange, 417–418
agoraphobia, 35

AIDS (acquired immune deficiency syndrome), 251
airplane glue, 76, 108
air pollution, 3, 412–415
alarm stage of adaptation to stress (Selye), 55
alcohol, 5, 71, 75, 78, 84–87, 93, 98–100, 112, 117–130, 143
  avoiding drug interaction with, 81 (how-to)
  cancer and, 271, 273–274
  drug interactions with, 80, 81, 99, 110, 123–124, 208
  facts and fallacies about, 120 (activity)
  long- and short-term effects of, 121–130
  marijuana compared with, 109, 110
  mechanism of action of, 118–121
  nutrition and, 129, 330, 331
  in pregnancy, 110, 124–125, 197
  safe and sensible consumption of, 118 (how-to), 122 (how-to), 123 (how-to), 126 (how-to), 133–135 (activity)
alcoholism, 3, 129–133
  cancer and, 271, 273–274
  causes of, 132
  defining, 130–132
  and determining if one has a drinking problem, 129 (activity)
  spotting, 131–132 (how-to)
  stress and, 7, 8, 47, 56
  treatment of, 39, 132–133
allergies, 59, 72, 74, 149, 155, 251
alveoli of lungs, 291
Alzheimer's disease, 32, 434
amantadine, 246
ambulatory-care clinics, 402
ambulatory dying patients, 442–443
amenorrhea, coping with, 191 (how-to)
amino acids, 315

amniocentesis, 196–197
amobarbital (Amytal), 98
amoebic dysentery, 247
amphetamines, 78, 80, 102–103, 105
amyl nitrite, 108–109
anaerobic exercise, 369
anal stage of development (Freud), 25
anaphylactic shock, 74
anaplastic cancer, 270
anemia, 108, 321, 346, 418
  sickle-cell, 3, 194
anesthesia, in childbirth, 199
aneurysms, 145
angel dust (phencyclidine, PCP), 106, 107
anger, 34
  coping with, 28, 29 (how-to)
  See also violence
angina pectoris, 108, 296, 432
animal parasites, 247
anorexia nervosa, 351, 354
antacids, 74
anthropometric measurements, 341
antianxiety drugs, 37, 84, 98–99
antibiotics, 72, 74, 80, 83, 243–245, 255, 299, 385
antibodies, 250–252, 315
anticipatory grief, 445
antidepressants, 35, 37–38, 93
antigens, 59
antihistamines, 72, 124
anti-inflammatory drugs, 72
antipsychotic drugs (major tranquilizers), 35, 39, 92
anxiety, 34–35, 37, 51, 106, 113, 180
  coping with, 27, 28 (how-to)
  See also stress
anxiolytic drugs, 37, 84, 98–99
aorta, 291
aortic aneurysms, 145
Appetrol, 103
arrhythmia, *see* heart rate and heartbeat

CREDITS AND ACKNOWLEDGMENTS

Except where noted below or in the figure captions, all line illustrations are by Vantage Art, Inc., Massapequa, New York.

Chapter-Opening Photos: Introduction, P. 2 © Stacy Pick 1982/Stock, Boston; **Ch. 1,** p. 18 © David Pollack; **2,** p. 46 © Dan McCoy/Rainbow; **3,** p. 70 Paul Kotz 1982/West Stock; **4,** p. 92 © Erich Lessing/Magnum; **5,** p. 116 © Burt Glinn/Magnum; **6,** p. 140 Birgit Pohl; **7,** p. 162 © Leonard Speier; **8,** p. 186 © George Malave/Stock, Boston; **9,** p. 214 © Frank J. Staub/The Picture Cube; **10,** p. 238 © James J. Broderick 1983/Int'l Stock Photo; **11,** p. 266 © Martin M. Rotker/Taurus Photos; **12,** p. 288 © Bill Pierce/Rainbow; **13,** p. 312 © Leonard Speier 1983; **14,** p. 339 © Mark Bolster 1982/Int'l Stock Photo; **15,** p. 362 © Chris Brown/Stock, Boston; **16,** p. 384 © Gabe Palmer/1983 Palmer-Kane Inc.; **17,** p. 410 © Frank Siteman/The Picture Cube; **18,** p. 428 © Alan Reininger/Contact Press Images

Introduction   The Concept of Health
P. 7—© Lenono Music, Inc.; 8—From *The Wellness Workbook* by Regina Sara Ryan and John W. Travis, M.D., copyright 1981, used with permission, available from Ten Speed Press, Box 7123, Berkeley, CA 94707 ($9.95 paper, $15.95 cloth, plus $1.00 for postage and handling); 12–15—Adapted from the publication "Your Lifestyle Profile," produced by the Department of Health and Welfare, Government of Canada.

Chapter 3   Patterns of Drug Use
P. 81—Reproduced by kind permission of *Nursing Times.*

Chapter 4   Psychoactive Drugs
P. 104—Adapted by permission of Joel Fort, M.D., author, *The Addicted Society* (New York: Grove Press, 1981) and *To Dream the Perfect Organization* (Oakland, Calif.: Third Party Pub., 1981), professor, Golden Gate University and University of California Extension, consultant, and sociatrist.

Chapter 5   Alcohol
Pp. 123, 124, 126—Adapted with permission of Macmillan Publishing Company from *Responsible Drug and Alcohol Use* by Ruth C. Engs, copyright © 1979 by Ruth C. Engs; 126—Reprinted by permission of Lippincott/Harper & Row.

Chapter 6   Smoking
P. 148—Courtesy American Cancer Society, Inc.; 155—Reprinted by permission of *The New England Journal of Medicine.*

Chapter 7   Human Sexuality
P. 170—Doug Armstrong, after William H. Masters and Virginia E. Johnson, *Human Sexual Response,* Little, Brown and Company, 1966; 180–182—Adapted from Robert F. Valois, "Sexual Attitude Questionnaire," in Cox, Doyle, Kammerman, and Valois, *Wellness R.S.V.P.,* 1st ed., copyright © 1981 by the Benjamin/Cummings Co., Inc., Menlo Park, Calif., reprinted by permission of the author and the publisher.

Chapter 10   Infectious Diseases
P. 250—Tom Lewis.

Chapter 11   Cancer
Pp. 268, 278, 280—Courtesy American Cancer Society, Inc.; 272—© 1982 by The New York Times Company, reprinted by permission.

Chapter 12   Cardiovascular Diseases
Pp. 290, 294, 301, 306–307—By permission of the American Heart Association, Inc.; 295—Adapted with permission of Macmillan Publishing Company from *Introduction to Public Health,* 7th ed., by Daniel M. Wilner, Rosabelle Price, and Edward O'Neill, copyright © 1978 by Macmillan Publishing Company.

Chapter 13   Diet and Nutrition
Pp. 326–327—Adapted from the *Guide to Good Eating* by permission of the National Dairy Council.

Chapter 14   Weight Management
P. 342—Courtesy Metropolitan Life Insurance Company; 356–357—Adapted by permission from Jack D. Osman, *Thin from Within* (Washington, D.C.: Review & Herald, 1981), Fat Control, Inc., P.O. Box 10117, Towson, MD 21204, $8.00 postage paid.

Chapter 15   Exercise and Physical Fitness
P. 364—Adapted by permission of Yorke Medical Books, Technical Publishing, a division of Dun-Donnelley Publishing Corporation, a Company of Dun & Bradstreet Corporation.

Chapter 16   Health Care and the Consumer
P. 389—Reprinted by permission of Addison-Wesley Publishing Co., Inc.; 406—© 1982 by The New York Times Company, reprinted by permission.

Chapter 17   Environmental Health
P. 424—Reprinted by permission of the American Nuclear Society.

Chapter 18   Aging and Death
P. 433—Copyright 1974 by the American Psychological Association, adapted by permission of the authors; 442—Reprinted by permission of the author, R. G. Twycross, and the Society for the Study of Medical Ethics; 447–448—Reprinted by permission of Walter Sorochan.

ABOUT THE AUTHORS

Marvin R. Levy is a professor in the Department of Health Education and holds a secondary appointment as Professor of Family Practice and Community Health in the School of Medicine of Temple University. He served as chairman of the Department of Health Education from its inception until 1981 and is currently Director of the Health Education Research Center at the university. He received an M.A. (1956) and an Ed.D. (1968) in health education from Columbia University and an M.P.H. from The Johns Hopkins University in 1983. He was director of Health and Safety for the New Jersey State Department of Education and served as Director of the National Drug Abuse Education Project in Washington, D.C. Professor Levy's research has focused on dependency behavior prevention, human sexuality and family living, lifestyle analysis, and health problems of aging. His publications include more than two dozen articles, several book chapters, and four monographs. He has served on the editorial boards of several professional journals. He has been director and principal investigator for eleven government-funded grants and contracts. He serves on several advisory boards and as consultant to numerous public and private organizations. Professor Levy has received the Lindback Award for Distinguished University Teaching and has been named an honorary member of the Institute of the History of Medicine and Medical Research, New Delhi.

Mark Dignan is Associate Professor of Public Health Education at the University of North Carolina at Greensboro. He received a bachelor's degree from the University of New Mexico in 1971, an M.S. from the University of Utah in 1974, a Ph.D. from the University of Tennessee in 1977, and an M.P.H. in biostatistics from the University of North Carolina at Chapel Hill in 1982. Professor Dignan's research has focused on understanding the mechanisms through which individuals make decisions about their health. He has published articles in many professional journals and is the co-author of *Introduction to Program Planning: A Basic Text for Community Health Education* (Lea & Febiger, 1982). In January 1984 he became affiliated with the Bowman Gray School of Medicine, Wake Forest University.

Janet H. Shirreffs is Associate Professor of Health Science at Arizona State University at Tempe. She was graduated *cum laude* from Ithaca College in 1967 and received a Ph.D. from Texas Woman's University in 1973. She was a member of the Health Science faculty at Ball State University for four years prior to joining the Arizona State faculty in 1976. Professor Shirreffs' writing and research interests are in the behavioral aspects of health and in the philosophy of health education. Her published works include more than twenty articles in major professional journals, several book chapters, and three books, including *Community Health: Contemporary Perspectives* (Prentice-Hall, 1982). On the basis of her service as a member of the Board of Directors, she has received a Certificate of Appreciation Award from the Association for the Advancement of Health Education.